# Chronic Obstructive Pulmonary Disease Exacerbations

# LUNG BIOLOGY IN HEALTH AND DISEASE

*Executive Editor*

**Claude Lenfant**

*Former Director, National Heart, Lung, and Blood Institute*
*National Institutes of Health*
*Bethesda, Maryland*

*The opinions expressed in these volumes do not necessarily represent the views of the National Institutes of Health.*

# Chronic Obstructive Pulmonary Disease Exacerbations

edited by

**Jadwiga A. Wedzicha**
*University College London*
*London, UK*

**Fernando J. Martinez**
*University of Michigan Health System*
*Ann Arbor, Michigan, USA*

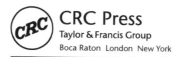

CRC Press
Taylor & Francis Group
Boca Raton London New York

CRC Press is an imprint of the
Taylor & Francis Group, an **informa** business

CRC Press
Taylor & Francis Group
6000 Broken Sound Parkway NW, Suite 300
Boca Raton, FL 33487-2742

First issued in paperback 2019

ISBN-13: 978-1-4200-7086-6 (hbk)
ISBN-13: 978-1-138-37245-0 (pbk)

---

### Library of Congress Cataloging-in-Publication Data

Chronic obstructive pulmonary disease exacerbations / edited by Jadwiga A. Wedzicha, Fernando J. Martinez.
     p. ; cm. — (Lung biology in health and disease; 228)
    Includes bibliographical references and index.
    ISBN-13: 978-1-4200-7086-6 (hardcover : alk. paper)
    ISBN-10: 1-4200-7086-X (hardcover : alk. paper) 1. Lungs—Diseases, Obstructive—Complications. I. Wedzicha, Jadwiga Anna. II. Martinez, Fernando J. III. Series: Lung biology in health and disease ; v. 228.
    [DNLM: 1. Pulmonary Disease, Chronic Obstructive. 2. Recurrence. W1 LU62 v.228 2008 / WF 600 C5524 2008]
    RC776.O3C477 2008
    616.2′4—dc22

                               2008021270

---

**Visit the Taylor & Francis Web site at**
**http://www.taylorandfrancis.com**

**and the CRC Press Web site at**
**http://www.crcpress.com**

# Introduction

The first, or certainly one of the first, definition of chronic obstructive pulmonary disease (or chronic obstructive lung disease as it is also called) was proposed in the 1959 Ciba Foundation Symposium on "the definition and classification of chronic obstructive pulmonary emphysema and related conditions." Since, the journey of COPD (or COLD) has been remarkable; but the 1980s marked the beginning of a multinational research effort that has been most productive. Quite broad and diversified, this effort has focused on the pathology and possible treatments of this disease. Although it was recognized that the disease is irreversible and relentlessly progressive, delaying this progression and maintaining the best possible quality of life of the patients has been among the major goals.

As the editors of this volume point out in their Preface, it was reported "in the late 1990s that COPD exacerbations are an important determinant of health-related quality of life in COPD (patients)" and also of the speed and severity of the disease progression. Exacerbations are defined by a sudden worsening of the symptoms, and they may be life threatening in many instances. Yet, if appropriately managed, the patients may return to the same symptom and physiological levels as before the exacerbation. Much research at the fundamental as well as clinical levels has been conducted with the aim of understanding what triggers these exacerbations, how to prevent them, and how best to treat them. Indeed, much has been learned that can assist the practicing physicians and benefit the patients.

This volume titled *Chronic Obstructive Pulmonary Disease Exacerbations* and edited by Drs. Jadwiga A. Wedzicha and Fernando J. Martinez presents the most up-to-date knowledge about the mechanism and treatment of COPD exacerbations to the readership of this new volume. Contributors from North America, Europe, Asia, and the South Pacific report their experience on the basis of years of successful research and clinical care. All of the contributors to this volume are known and respected pioneers in their respective fields.

In their Preface, the editors predict that this volume will stimulate more investigations to better understand and manage COPD exacerbations. Of particular interest is the interdependency of COPD exacerbations and comorbid conditions. But, in addition, and most important, this book can help general practitioners make use of research outcomes, which can benefit their patients.

The series of monographs Lung Biology in Health and Disease has presented many volumes on COPD over the years, with the first monograph on this topic published in 1978. Directly, or indirectly, the knowledge they have reported has contributed to better care of COPD patients. This volume, however, has very special messages that specifically address how to manage the worsening of the disease and, hopefully, maintain a better quality of life. As the Executive Editor of this series, I am grateful to the editors and the contributors for the opportunity to introduce this volume to our readership.

Claude Lenfant, M.D.
*Vancouver, Washington, U.S.A.*

# Preface

It is now recognized that exacerbations are a major cause of the global morbidity and mortality associated with chronic obstructive pulmonary disease (COPD). They are also a cause of hospital admission and readmission and thus lead to considerable health care costs. Following the observation in the late 1990s that exacerbations are an important determinant of health-related quality of life in COPD, there has been considerable interest in the study of exacerbations. Over the last few years, studies have shown that exacerbations contribute to disease progression and mortality and that they are an important outcome for new therapies in COPD.

For this book, we have assembled international experts, both clinicians and scientists with an interest in COPD exacerbations, to review critically the current literature and provide up-to-date reviews on the various issues as well as highlight the many controversies and bottlenecks in the study of exacerbations.

COPD exacerbations are episodes of worsening of symptoms, accompanied by inflammatory and physiological changes. In this book, we have firstly covered issues of definition, diagnosis, and epidemiology and then presented a number of chapters on the many diverse mechanisms, including the role of bacterial and viral infection to the development of respiratory failure, associated with COPD exacerbations, which are heterogeneous events. It is now recognized that systemic inflammation and comorbidity play a prominent role in COPD and affect exacerbation outcome. Environmental issues, including air pollution, are difficult to study, but there is considerable recent information on their relation to COPD exacerbation in this book.

Both management of the acute exacerbation and exacerbation prevention have been addressed in separate sections. We now have a wide variety of pharmacological and nonpharmacological interventions to treat and prevent exacerbations, yet many clinicians are confused about how to use these therapies and for which patients. The section on exacerbation management will also cover new models of care for COPD exacerbations, integration of home and hospital care for these patients, and, importantly, end-of-life issues. Studies investigating new therapies for either reducing severity or frequency of COPD exacerbations have proved problematic to design and often conduct, with specific statistical considerations, and we have addressed these issues in the last section of the book.

We know that you will very much enjoy reading this book and that it will stimulate many of you to further study this fascinating and important topic. In view of their significance, COPD exacerbations will be the subject of much future research and clinical trial activity. The book will be useful as a reference to all clinicians involved in the care of patients with COPD.

Finally, we would like to thank all the authors for agreeing to write the chapters and contributing to this high quality book. We also express our gratitude to Sandra Beberman and her team for allowing us to proceed with this project and supporting us throughout the commissioning and production.

*Jadwiga A. Wedzicha*
*Fernando J. Martinez*

# Contributors

**Antonio Anzueto**   Division of Pulmonary and Critical Care Medicine at the South Texas Veterans Health Care System, Audie L Murphy Division and the University of Texas Health Science Center at San Antonio, San Antonio, Texas, U.S.A.

**Shawn D. Aaron**   The Ottawa Health Research Institute, University of Ottawa, Ottawa, Ontario, Canada

**Simonetta Baraldo**   Department of Cardiac, Thoracic, and Vascular Sciences, University of Padova, Padova, Italy

**Peter J. Barnes**   National Heart and Lung Institute, Imperial College, London, U.K.

**Bianca Beghé**   Section of Respiratory Diseases, Department of Oncology, Haematology and Respiratory Diseases, University Hospital of Modena, University of Modena and Reggio Emilia, Modena, Italy

**Erik W. M. A. Bischoff**   Department of Primary Care, Centre of Evidence Based Medicine, Radboud University Nijmegen Medical Centre, Nijmegen, The Netherlands

**Jean Bourbeau**   Respiratory Epidemiology and Clinical Research Unit, Montreal Chest Institute, McGill University Health Center, Montréal, Québec, Canada

**Peter M. A. Calverley**   Division of Infection and Immunity, Clinical Sciences Centre, University Hospital Aintree, Liverpool, U.K.

**Gaetano Caramori**   Department of Clinical and Experimental Medicine, Research Center on Asthma and COPD, University of Ferrara, Ferrara, Italy

**Paul J. Christensen**   Pulmonary and Critical Care Medicine Section, Medical Service, Department of Veterans Affairs Health System and the Division of Pulmonary and Critical Care Medicine, Department of Internal Medicine, University of Michigan Health System, Ann Arbor, Michigan, U.S.A.

**Marco Contoli** Department of Clinical and Experimental Medicine, Research Center on Asthma and COPD, University of Ferrara, Ferrara, Italy

**Borja G. Cosio** Department of Respiratory Medicine, Hospital Universitario Son Dureta, Palma de Mallorca, Spain

**Gerard J. Criner** Division of Pulmonary and Critical Care Medicine, Temple University School of Medicine, Philadelphia, Pennsylvania, U.S.A.

**Jeffrey L. Curtis** Pulmonary and Critical Care Medicine Section, Medical Service, Department of Veterans Affairs Health System and the Division of Pulmonary and Critical Care Medicine, Department of Internal Medicine and the Graduate Program in Immunology, University of Michigan Health System, Veterans Administration Medical Center, Ann Arbor, Michigan, U.S.A.

**A. G. Davison** Southend University Hospital, Prittlewell Chase, Westcliff-on-Sea, Essex, U.K.

**Marc Decramer** Department of Respiratory Medicine, University of Leuven, Leuven, Belgium

**Himanshu Desai** Division of Pulmonary, Critical Care, and Sleep Medicine, Department of Medicine and University of Buffalo, State University of New York, Buffalo, New York, U.S.A.

**Gavin C. Donaldson** Academic Department of Respiratory Medicine, Royal Free and University College Medical School, London, U.K.

**Mark W. Elliott** Department of Respiratory Medicine, St. James's University Hospital, Leeds, U.K.

**Andrés Esteban** Intensive Care Unit, Hospital Universitario de Getafe, Madrid, Spain

**Leonardo M. Fabbri** Section of Respiratory Diseases, Department of Oncology, Haematology and Respiratory Diseases, University Hospital of Modena, University of Modena and Reggio Emilia, Modena, Italy

**W. Bradley Fields** Division of Pulmonary and Critical Care Medicine, Department of Internal Medicine, University of Michigan Health System, Ann Arbor, Michigan, U.S.A.

**Joseph Footitt**   Department of Respiratory Medicine, National Heart and Lung Institute, Imperial College, London, U.K.

**Christine M. Freeman**   Division of Pulmonary and Critical Care Medicine, Department of Internal Medicine, University of Michigan Health System, Ann Arbor, Michigan, U.S.A.

**Fernando Frutos-Vivar**   Intensive Care Unit, Hospital Universitario de Getafe, Madrid, Spain

**Judith Garcia-Aymerich**   Centre for Research in Environmental Epidemiology (CREAL), Institut Municipal d'Investigació Mèdica (IMIM), Barcelona, Spain

**Rachel Garrod**   Faculty of Health and Social Care Sciences, St. George's, University of London and Kingston University, Tooting, U.K.

**James J. P. Goldring**   Academic Department of Respiratory Medicine, Royal Free and University College Medical School, London, U.K.

**Karin Groenewegen**   Department of Respiratory Medicine, University Hospital Maastricht, Maastricht, The Netherlands

**Meilan Han**   Division of Pulmonary and Critical Care Medicine, Department of Internal Medicine, University of Michigan Health System, Ann Arbor, Michigan, U.S.A.

**Luke Howard**   Hammersmith Hospital, Imperial College Healthcare NHS Trust and National Heart and Lung Institute, Imperial College London, London, U.K.

**David SC Hui**   Department of Medicine and Therapeutics, The Chinese University of Hong Kong, Prince of Wales Hospital, Hong Kong

**John R. Hurst**   Academic Unit of Respiratory Medicine, University College London, London, U.K.

**Wim Janssens**   Department of Respiratory Medicine, University of Leuven, Leuven, Belgium

**Andrea K. Johnston**   Department of Pulmonary, Critical Care, and Sleep Medicine, University of Kentucky Medical Center, Lexington, Kentucky, U.S.A.

**Sebastian L. Johnston**    Department of Respiratory Medicine, National Heart and Lung Institute, Imperial College, London, U.K.

**Fanny WS Ko**    Department of Medicine and Therapeutics, The Chinese University of Hong Kong, Prince of Wales Hospital, Hong Kong

**Nancy Kline Leidy**    United BioSource Corporation, Bethesda, Maryland, U.S.A.

**Kim Lokar-Oliani**    Department of Cardiac, Thoracic, and Vascular Sciences, University of Padova, Padova, Italy

**Fabrizio Luppi**    Section of Respiratory Diseases, Department of Oncology, Haematology and Respiratory Diseases, University Hospital of Modena, University of Modena and Reggio Emilia, Modena, Italy

**John Maclay**    ELEGI/Colt Research Laboratories, MRC/University of Edinburgh Centre for Inflammation Research, Queens Medical Research Institute, Edinburgh, U.K.

**William Macnee**    ELEGI/Colt Research Laboratories, MRC/University of Edinburgh Centre for Inflammation Research, Queens Medical Research Institute, Edinburgh, U.K.

**Patrick Mallia**    Department of Respiratory Medicine, National Heart and Lung Institute, Imperial College, London, U.K.

**William D-C. Man**    Respiratory Muscle Laboratory, Royal Brompton Hospital, London, U.K.

**David M. Mannino**    Department of Preventive Medicine and Environmental Health, University of Kentucky College of Public Health, Lexington, Kentucky, U.S.A.

**Nathaniel Marchetti**    Division of Pulmonary and Critical Care Medicine, Temple University School of Medicine, Philadelphia, Pennsylvania, U.S.A.

**Brunilda Marku**    Department of Clinical and Experimental Medicine, Research Center on Asthma and COPD, University of Ferrara, Ferrara, Italy

**Fernando J. Martinez**    Division of Pulmonary and Critical Care Medicine, Department of Internal Medicine, University of Michigan Health System, Ann Arbor, Michigan, U.S.A.

**David McAllister**   ELEGI/Colt Research Laboratories, MRC/University of Edinburgh Centre for Inflammation Research, Queens Medical Research Institute, Edinburgh, U.K.

**Christine Mikelsons**   Physiotherapy Department, Royal Free Hospital, London, U.K.

**Stanley D. W. Miller**   Department of Respiratory Medicine, St. James's University Hospital, Leeds, U.K.

**Marc Miravitlles**   Department of Pneumology, Clinical Institute of Thorax (IDIBAPS), Hospital Clínic, Barcelona, Spain

**Dennis E. Niewoehner**   Pulmonary Section, Minneapolis Veterans Affairs Medical Center, Department of Medicine, University of Minnesota, Minneapolis, Minnesota, U.S.A.

**Mitzi Nisbet**   Royal Brompton Hospital, London, U.K.

**Denis E. O'Donnell**   Department of Medicine, Queen's University, Kingston, Ontario, Canada

**Ronan O'Driscoll**   Respiratory Medicine, Salford Royal University Hospital, Salford, Great Manchester, U.K.

**Anita Pandit**   Royal Glamorgan Hospital, Llantrisant, U.K.

**Alberto Papi**   Department of Clinical and Experimental Medicine, Research Center on Asthma and COPD, University of Ferrara, Ferrara, Italy

**Chris M. Parker**   Department of Medicine, Queen's University, Kingston, Ontario, Canada

**Martyn R. Partridge**   Department of Respiratory Medicine, NHLI Division, Imperial College London and Honorary Consultant Respiratory Physician, Imperial College Healthcare NHS Trust, London, U.K.

**Michael I. Polkey**   Respiratory Muscle Laboratory, Royal Brompton Hospital, London, U.K.

**Phillippa J. Poole**   Department of Medicine, Faculty of Medical and Health Sciences, University of Auckland, Auckland, New Zealand

**J. K. Quint**   Academic Unit of Respiratory Medicine, University College London, London, U.K.

**Roberto Rabinovich**   ELEGI/Colt Research Laboratories, MRC/University of Edinburgh Centre for Inflammation Research, Queens Medical Research Institute, Edinburgh, U.K.

**Stephen I. Rennard**   Pulmonary and Critical Care Medicine, University of Nebraska Medical Center, Omaha, Nebraska, U.S.A.

**Kathryn Rice**   Pulmonary Section, Minneapolis Veterans Affairs Medical Center, Department of Medicine, University of Minnesota, Minneapolis, Minnesota, U.S.A.

**Roberto Rodríguez-Roisin**   Department of Pneumology, Hospital Clínic, University of Barcelona, Barcelona, Spain

**Marina Saetta**   Department of Cardiac, Thoracic, and Vascular Sciences, University of Padova, Padova, Italy

**Maria Sedeno**   Respiratory Epidemiology and Clinical Research Unit, Department of Medicine, McGill University, Montréal, Québec, Canada

**Terence A. R. Seemungal**   Department of Clinical Medical Sciences, University of the West Indies, St Augustine Campus, Trinidad and Tobago

**Sanjay Sethi**   Division of Pulmonary, Critical Care, and Sleep Medicine, Department of Medicine, Veterans Affairs Western New York Health Care System, and University of Buffalo, State University of New York, Buffalo, New York, U.S.A.

**Anita K. Simonds**   Academic Department of Sleep & Breathing, Royal Brompton Hospital, London, U.K.

**R. A. Stockley**   Queen Elizabeth Hospital, Edgbaston, Birmingham, U.K.

**Annemarie Sykes**   Department of Respiratory Medicine, National Heart and Lung Institute, Imperial College, London, U.K.

**Graziella Turato**   Department of Cardiac, Thoracic, and Vascular Sciences, University of Padova, Padova, Italy

**Scott S. Wagers**  Department of Respiratory Medicine, University Hospital Maastricht, Maastricht, The Netherlands

**Jadwiga A. Wedzicha**  Academic Unit of Respiratory Medicine, University College London, London, U.K.

**Robert Wilson**  Royal Brompton Hospital, London, U.K.

**Emiel F. Wouters**  Department of Respiratory Medicine, University Hospital Maastricht, Maastricht, The Netherlands

**Renzo Zuin**  Department of Cardiac, Thoracic, and Vascular Sciences, University of Padova, Padova, Italy

# Contents

# 1

## Definitions and Severity of Exacerbations

**STEPHEN I. RENNARD**
Pulmonary and Critical Care Medicine, University of Nebraska Medical Center, Omaha, Nebraska, U.S.A.

**NANCY KLINE LEIDY**
United BioSource Corporation, Bethesda, Maryland, U.S.A.

## I. Introduction

Acute exacerbations of chronic obstructive pulmonary disease (COPD) are relatively frequent events that have a major impact on patient well-being, both at the time of the event and in the long term. Recent observations have clearly shown that therapeutic interventions can, to some extent, prevent exacerbations as well as modify their course. This has created both the opportunity and the imperative to develop more effective interventions to mitigate the burden of acute exacerbations, which, in turn, has created a need for precise and operationally tractable definitions. Crucially, a definition of exacerbations is needed that permits the events to be adequately quantified, both in terms of frequency and severity. This has proven difficult for a variety of reasons. First, exacerbations are heterogeneous. In addition, they are primarily a patient-reported event. Objective confirmatory tests based on bio-markers have yet to be satisfactorily developed. The problem of definition is exacerbated by the distinction between definition and diagnosis. As pointed out by Prof. Gordon Snider:

> It is important to realize the difference between the definition of a disease and its diagnostic criteria (1). The defining characteristics of a disease are the common properties specifying the group of abnormal persons on whom the description of the disease is based. The definition of a disease is important in communication.
>
> Diagnostic criteria are features of the disease chosen from its description that are found by empirical research to best distinguish the disease from others which resemble it. The diagnostic criteria may or may not include features of the defining characteristics and frequently include features that do not appear in the definition (1).

Current efforts to establish a consensus definition of acute exacerbation of COPD have been primarily developed for one of three purposes: (*i*) understanding the etiology and mechanisms of exacerbations, (*ii*) determining the impact of exacerbations on the course of COPD, and (*iii*) determining if interventions alter the incidence or the clinical course of exacerbations. These studies are most often conducted in preselected populations that have a high incidence of events. Defining exacerbations in this population is a different problem than that of diagnosis in a more general problem. Distinguishing between an acute exacerbation of COPD and events that may resemble it to varying degrees and in varying ways is a major clinical problem that has received very little attention (see chap. 3 for a more detailed discussion).

The current chapter will review the history of definitions of acute exacerbations of COPD, discuss the various types of definitions, and review current attempts to develop definitions that will facilitate the understanding of these events and expedite the development of therapies to mitigate them.

## II. Definitions

Definitions can take various forms, reflecting their underlying purpose. Conceptual definitions are based in theory; while they may inform empirical and clinical practice, they often reflect a limited evidence-based understanding. Empirical definitions, in contrast, are operational. They permit development of quantitative instruments to describe events and are useful for hypothesis testing. In the case of exacerbations of COPD, which are patient-reported events, instruments to detect exacerbations should be based on the conceptual definition and patient descriptions and experiences of these events and show evidence of reliability, validity, and responsiveness. Practical applications in clinical settings require definitions that are empirically grounded and validated and applicable to individuals, in contrast to populations.

There are four dimensions of exacerbations to consider when defining exacerbations. Definitions that summarize the essential features of exacerbations inform the development of empirical methods for capturing the presence or *frequency* of these events. Descriptions of variability in magnitude inform operational definitions of *severity* and *duration*. Duration, in turn, involves two important components of exacerbation that are of clinical and empirical interest: *recovery* and *resolution*. Finally, the *impact* of an exacerbation includes its effect on health status, morbidity, mortality, and trajectory of disease.

### A. Conceptual Definitions of Exacerbation

A number of groups and professional organizations have developed conceptual or working definitions of exacerbations on the basis of consensus in an effort to clarify the concept and guide research efforts to understand exacerbations and treatment effects and to inform clinical practice (Table 1). The definition proposed by the 1999 Aspen Lung Conference that refers to a *sustained* worsening of the patient's condition, implying an event that lasts at least 24 hours (2) while worsening *beyond normal day-to-day* variations, seeks to differentiate the severity of exacerbations from "bad days" or acute, short-term episodes of cough, breathlessness, or other manifestations within a given day. This group also proposed that mild exacerbations are characterized by an increased need for medication (which patients manage themselves), moderate are those for which the patients seek medical assistance, and severe are those in which the patient or caregiver recognizes clear and/or rapid deterioration and requires hospitalization.

The American Thoracic Society and the European Respiratory Society proposed definition was similar, specifying dyspnea, cough, and sputum as characteristic features (3). The first GOLD (Global Initiative for Chronic Obstructive Lung Diseases) report of 2001 did not define exacerbation, but described the signs and symptoms associated with the event (4). Breathlessness was identified as the main symptom, with wheezing, chest tightness,

**Table 1**  Consensus Definitions of Exacerbation

| Source | Definition |
|---|---|
| British Thoracic Society, 1997 | A *worsening* of the previous stable situation. Important symptoms include increased *sputum purulence, sputum volume, dyspnea or wheeze, chest tightness, and fluid retention.* |
| Aspen Lung Conference, 1999 | A sustained *worsening* of the patient's condition, from the stable state and beyond normal day-to-day variations, that is acute in onset and necessitates a change in regular medication in a patient with underlying COPD. |
| GOLD, 2001[a] | *Increased breathlessness*, the main symptom of an exacerbation, is often accompanied by *wheezing and chest tightness, increased cough and sputum, change of the color and/or tenacity of sputum, and fever.* Exacerbations may also be accompanied by a number of nonspecific complaints, such as *malaise, insomnia, sleepiness, fatigue, depression, and confusion.* A *decrease in exercise tolerance, fever,* and/or new radiological anomalies suggestive of pulmonary disease may herald a COPD exacerbation. An *increase in sputum volume and purulence* points to a bacterial cause, as does a prior history of chronic sputum production |
| ATS/ERS, June 2004 | An event in the natural course of the disease characterized by a *change* in the patient's baseline *dyspnea, cough, and/or sputum beyond day-to-day variability* sufficient to warrant a change in management. |
| NICE, Feb 2004 | A sustained *worsening* of the patient's symptoms from their usual stable state, which is beyond normal day-to-day variations and is acute in onset. Commonly reported symptoms are *worsening breathlessness, cough, increased sputum production, and change in sputum color.* The change in these symptoms often necessitates a change in medication. |
| GOLD, 2006 (Rabe et al. 2007) | An event in the natural course of the disease characterized by a *change* in the patient's baseline *dyspnea, cough, and/or sputum* that is beyond normal day-to-day variations, is acute in onset, and may warrant a change in regular medication in a patient with underlying disease. |

[a]Description rather than definition.
Italicized text highlights characteristic features.
*Abbreviation*: COPD, chronic obstructive pulmonary disease.

sputum tenacity, and fever as frequent accompanying features, with or without other nonspecific complaints. The description also pointed to reduction in exercise tolerance, fever, or radiologic anomalies as potential indicators of exacerbation onset. The most recent GOLD definition is similar to the 1999 Aspen Conference definition and again specifies changes in dyspnea, cough, and/or sputum as the characteristic or cardinal features of the event (5,6). It also specifies that the change *may* be sufficient to warrant a change in treatment, recognizing unreported events and permitting clinic contact for evaluation with an option to maintain current therapy.

On the basis of this work, there is consensus that an exacerbation of COPD is a state characterized by a worsening of the patient's underlying condition, including, but not limited to, an increase in respiratory symptoms. The requirement of a change in treatment varies across definitions and may actually reflect severity rather than define the event. With this definition in mind, how have exacerbations been measured in clinical research?

## B.  Empirical Definitions of Exacerbations

### Event-Based

In epidemiologic studies and some prevention-targeted clinical trials, frequency of exacerbation has been defined in terms of health care utilization. This approach, often referred to as an event-based definition, operationalizes exacerbation in terms of the number of clinic visits, emergency room or urgent care visits, or hospitalizations for an exacerbation. These events are not only patient-initiated, but require action as determined by the physician. Time to first visit or hospitalization has also been used as an outcome in clinical trials testing interventions designed to prevent or reduce the frequency of exacerbations. The use of a change in treatment, generally oral steroids or antibiotics, as an additional criterion for the presence of an exacerbation has been varied.

Health care events have also been used as a proxy for exacerbation severity. It has been suggested, for example, that exacerbations requiring an unscheduled clinic or emergency room visit are "moderate," and those requiring hospitalization are "severe" (2,7). The addition of systemic corticosteroids and/or antibiotics to maintenance therapies has been used to signify the presence of an exacerbation or to rate an exacerbation as "moderate" (7).

There are a number of relatively serious limitations associated with an event-based definition of exacerbation. First, the initial clinic contact and visit is initiated by the patient on the basis of his or her assessment of the episode. With as many as 50% of exacerbations unreported (8,9), event-based definitions seriously underestimate exacerbation frequency. Admission to hospital is directly related both to the underlying health of the patient and to health policy or coverage within a given country or region. Patients undergoing treatment in regions with relatively liberal admission policies will have more frequent and more "serious" exacerbations, while those in regions with conservative admission policies will have less frequent and/or fewer "serious" episodes. This bias has serious implications for prevalence estimates in epidemiologic studies, effect estimates in studies examining the link between exacerbations and disease trajectory, and site selection and treatment outcomes in clinical trials. Finally, this definition does not take into consideration, standardize, or control for, the patient or physician assessment of exacerbation, including its elements or magnitude using the features outlined in the consensus definition. Symptom-based methods attempt to address these limitations.

### Symptom-Based

Attempts at characterizing exacerbations for empirical purposes are often traced back to definitions used by Anthonisen et al., who used an empirical definition to identify and classify exacerbations in a clinical trial designed to test the benefits of antibiotic therapy (10). In this study, exacerbations were defined in terms of symptoms and classified into three types: Type 1—presence of dyspnea, sputum volume, and sputum purulence; Type 2—presence of two of these three symptoms; and Type 3—presence of one of these three symptoms, with at least one of the following findings: upper respiratory infection (sore throat, nasal discharge) in the previous five days, fever without other cause, increased wheezing, increased cough, or increase in respiratory rate or heart rate by 20% over baseline. Patients who experienced an increase in symptoms were to notify the center and were examined by a nurse-practitioner who determined whether the symptoms fulfilled these criteria, indicating that the patient was eligible for intervention as outlined in the study protocol.

Seemungal et al. extended this definition for the East London (U.K.) prospective cohort study, designed to understand causes and mechanisms of exacerbations of COPD (9). These investigators defined exacerbation as two new symptoms of COPD present for two days, as recorded on a diary card, one of which must be dyspnea, sputum volume, and/or sputum purulence. Other symptoms could also be present and included cough, wheeze, sore throat, nasal discharge, or fever (9).

Diary Cards.   The definition put forth by Seemungal requires the use of a daily reporting system, generally in the form of diary cards, to establish baseline levels for the patient's health status and to detect change indicative of an exacerbation. Diary cards have been used in a significant number of prospective clinical studies and trials to document symptom severity and to identify unreported exacerbations. Unfortunately, there is substantial variability in the content and structure of these diaries. Although most cards include dyspnea, cough, and sputum, the actual items used to capture these symptoms vary greatly. For example, some measures of dyspnea ask patients to rate their breathlessness with one or more activities while others ask them to rate their shortness of breath on a scale of "none" to "maximum," with no reference to activity. Similarly, cough has been assessed as frequent or severe, or the extent to which it interferes with activity or sleep, while sputum evaluations may include one or more items referencing color, consistency, volume, or difficulty, or a single item asking patients to rate their sputum "production" from none to severe. This measurement variability makes comparison of information across studies virtually impossible and may account for some of the inconsistency in findings across otherwise similar investigations.

Although cross-study comparisons are difficult, examining the general content of diary cards across studies contributes to the consensus-building process. Dyspnea, cough, and sputum production have been included in virtually all diary cards. Additional symptoms include chest tightness or discomfort, sleep disturbance or nighttime awakenings, fatigue (using terms such as weariness, tiredness, or faintness), and activity, including activities of daily living (ADLs) and work. Key questions include the following: What is the core set of clinical indicators of an exacerbation that are experienced by the patient and that should be assessed in order to determine the presence, severity, and recovery pattern of an exacerbation? What combination of these indicators constitutes or is consistent with an exacerbation, particularly those that are unreported? And finally, are exacerbations heterogeneous, and are there "phenotypes" of exacerbations that reflect different sets of features?

Identifying an exacerbation through diary cards requires an algorithm based on the definition of exacerbation and its clinical indicators, and an accumulation of data to create confidence in the sensitivity of the algorithm. In the absence of a standard, Seemungal et al. as described above, defined exacerbation *a priori* as the presence for at least two consecutive days of increase in any two "major" symptoms (dyspnea, cough, sputum) or increase in one "major" and one "minor" symptom (8). The first of the days was taken as the day of onset. Symptoms were binary coded and summed to give a daily symptom score.

## C.  The Patient's Perspective

Results from qualitative studies and patient surveys can provide important insight into patient perspectives of exacerbation and further inform definitions and measurement. Qualitative research is a hypothesis generating empirical method involving focus groups or 1:1 interviews in which the words and phrases of the study participants, recorded and transcribed, serve as the data (11,12). Systematic analytical methods are applied to identify and cluster information, formulate themes, and summarize the findings. In the case of exacerbations, qualitative research can provide a rich source of information about patient descriptions of their experiences, the terminology they use as they refer to these events, the manifestations or attributes that define them, and the actions they may or may not take when they occur. A limited number of studies using this methodology to understand and define exacerbations from the patient's perspective has been reported to date (13–15).

In a multinational cross-sectional interview-based qualitative study by Kessler et al. of 125 patients with moderate to severe COPD, the most common terms patients used when referring to a worsening of their condition were "chest infection" (16%; $n = 20$), "crisis" (16%; $n = 20$), or an "attack" (6.4%; $n = 8$) (13). Only two patients understood what the term "exacerbation" meant. Despite the varied terminology, patients clearly understood the concept and were able to identify and describe their exacerbation experiences.

The seriousness with which patients view an exacerbation is evident in their terminology (crisis, attack), the description of dread and fear related to their occurrence, and the anxiety and concern that accompany them (14). Patients participating in individual interviews in a qualitative study by Adams et al. (13) ($n = 23$) described a "frightening change" that led to consultation with a physician (13). Patients in focus groups of experiences with acute exacerbations of chronic bronchitis (AECB) associated panic and dread with the onset of the "attack" (15). The sudden and alarming nature of these events led Celli to suggest that the medical community adopt the term "lung attack" (Celli B, personal communication, 2005)(16).

Patients have described warning signs of an onset of exacerbation, including breathlessness, fatigue or tiredness, cough, or—in a relatively small number of patients (10%)—pain (14). When these warning signs occurred, they initiate various forms of self-care, including taking additional medication or resting, with relatively few patients (18%) in the Kessler et al. study indicating they would contact their physician (14).

Manifestations of exacerbation described by patients include respiratory symptoms (breathing difficulty, changes in phlegm, increased cough, difficulty coughing up phlegm, coughing up blood, runny nose, sneezing, and wheeziness), changes in daily activity (slower, difficulty performing), systemic signs and symptoms (anorexia, exhaustion, feeling weak, generally unwell, dizziness, sweating, cramping pain, and "other" ("grey" color, headaches, unable to speak) (13). A significant reduction in activity is also a characteristic feature of exacerbations. Nearly all of the patients (90%; $n = 107$) in the Kessler et al. study reported an adverse impact on ADLs, with half of these patients indicating that they required additional help with tasks during exacerbations (14). Forty-seven percent of the patients ($n = 59$) reported that all activities were stopped, and a third (38%; $n = 47$) could do nothing at all. Over a third (39%; $n = 49$) reported being bedridden.

There is also qualitative evidence to suggest that there may be within-patient consistency in how exacerbations are manifested. Most patients (85%, $n = 106$) in the Kessler et al. study reported consistency in symptoms from exacerbation to exacerbation. In contrast, it is unknown if those who report varying manifestations are experiencing different types of events. Quantitative assessment of these qualitative findings could assist phenotyping and further clarify definitions and testing targeted treatment.

Patient surveys can also provide insight into patient perception of exacerbations and why they may go unreported. Miravitilles et al. for example, conducted a telephone survey of 1100 subjects reporting symptoms consistent with COPD and/or taking medication for a respiratory problem other than asthma (17). Symptoms of exacerbation with the greatest impact on well-being were increased coughing (42%), increased shortness of breath (37%), increased fatigue (37%), increased sputum production (35%), increased frequency of chest pains (20%), and fever (13%). Serious activity limitations were also reported, with nearly half (45%) reporting having to stay in bed or on the couch all day.

## D. A Consensus Definition

Across all of the work outlined above, there is general agreement that exacerbations of COPD are events or episodes in which patients experience a remarkable, sustained worsening of the primary respiratory manifestations of the disease (dyspnea, cough, and/or sputum) beyond normal daily variability. There is also general consensus that a patient may experience a worsening of one or any combination of these symptoms, and that this respiratory symptom or symptom complex may be accompanied by other nonrespiratory symptoms or signs of exacerbation. Specifying these additional signs and symptoms is likely to contribute to a better understanding of the full range of attributes associated with exacerbations, the variability in presentation across patients, possible consistency within patients, and the role-specific etiologic or mechanistic processes may play in this variability. Standardizing the evaluation and scaling of exacerbations through a common tool and metric will help further characterize and perhaps classify exacerbations, including the prodromal, acute, and recovery phases.

## III. Standardizing Measurement of Exacerbations

The consensus regarding definitions can inform the development and selection of measurement tools for various types of studies including large, population-based epidemiologic and economic studies estimating the frequency and burden of exacerbations in a population, as well as clinical studies examining frequency, quality, and impact of exacerbations and the effect of interventions to treat or prevent these events.

In the absence of a standardized metric or biomarker for exacerbations, the determination of whether or not an exacerbation is present in any individual patient is made by both the patient and the clinician. The patient's decision is first, as the individual experiencing the change in his/her condition must make a judgment that the change is sufficiently different or serious to warrant either a change in self-care practice or contact with a health care provider. The clinician's determination is based on the patient's report of his/her condition in the context of the consensus definitions outlined above, and any additional data gathered through physical examination or laboratory testing that may suggest alternative explanations for the patient's change in health state. Determining the severity and duration (resolution) of exacerbations are also left to the judgment and discretion of the clinician and patient, who may have different opinions. Clearly, there is a need for a common definition and standardized tool for evaluating exacerbations of COPD.

### A. Patient-Reported Outcome Tools

Because exacerbations are defined in terms of signs and symptoms experienced by the patient, and the event itself is initially recognized and treated by the patient, either independently or with the assistance of a health care provider, they come under the rubric of a patient-reported outcome, or PRO. In the United States, this means that any tool used in a drug registration trial to evaluate the effect of treatment on frequency, severity, and/or duration of exacerbations must meet the criteria set forth in the Food and Drug Administration (FDA) draft guidance on patient-reported outcomes. This includes making certain the instrument is grounded in the patient's experience, using data gathered through focus groups and/or 1:1 interviews, and assuring that patients understand the tool and interpret it correctly using cognitive interviewing methodology. The latter includes an in-depth 1:1 interview with patients to evaluate their understanding of the directions, recall period, item stems, and response options to make certain the respondents are interpreting the tool as it was intended and in a manner consistent with the underlying concept being measured. Empirical evidence of reliability, including internal consistency and reproducibility, validity, and responsiveness to change, is also required.

The EXACT-PRO (Exacerbations of Chronic Pulmonary Disease Test—Patient-Reported Outcome) initiative was developed to address the need for a standardized, validated instrument to evaluate the frequency, severity, and duration of exacerbations. This project brought together international experts in COPD, clinical trial design, and measurement and representatives from the FDA to discuss the key elements of a tool to operationalize exacerbations for use in pharmaceutical trials and regulatory submissions with the potential for more widespread use by the clinical research community. The initiative was launched in 2006, with unrestricted sponsorship from multiple pharmaceutical companies. It began with a large qualitative study involving over 70 patients with COPD in focus groups and 1:1 interviews to determine the essential attributes of an exacerbation from the perspective of the patients themselves and formulate the structure and content of the EXACT measure (18).

Figure 1 shows a heuristic for understanding the evolution of an exacerbation from the patient's perspective based on the qualitative work. This heuristic is consistent with the consensus definition in that it shows a sustained worsening of the patient's underlying condition with rising levels of breathlessness, cough, and sputum production together with other signs and symptoms that improve over time. According to the qualitative data analysis, exacerbations of COPD can be defined as follows:

> An event characterized by a rapid, persistent (at least two or three days), and disconcerting increase in the frequency and severity of symptoms, including respiratory symptoms (difficulty breathing, cough with sputum, chest discomfort), feelings of being weak or tired, and sleep disturbance, with a dramatic reduction in activity. Improvement or recovery is gradual and resolution is often indicated by the resumption of normal daily activities.

The qualitative data gathered during Phase I of the EXACT-PRO initiative were used to develop a pool of 23 items to evaluate exacerbations of COPD. These items were

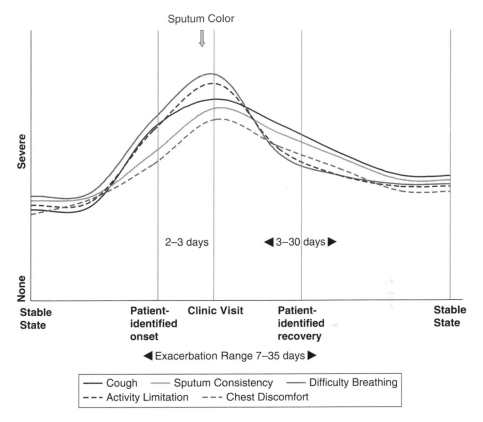

**Figure 1** Qualitatively-based heuristic for depicting exacerbations of COPD.

subjected to an empirically-based item reduction process with reliability and validity testing in a prospective study. The study involved over 400 patients, 200 of whom experienced an exacerbation and 200 of whom were stable and had no clinic visit or hospitalization for an exacerbation during the previous 60 days. Patients completed the draft (23-item) tool daily using a personal data assistant (PDA). On the basis of this, nine items were eliminated. The final 14-item EXACT offers a comprehensive assessment during an exacerbation, evaluating breathlessness, cough and sputum, chest symptoms, difficulty with sputum, feeling tired or weak, sleep disturbance, and feeling scared or worried, and requires less than five minutes for patients to complete. A shorter tool made up of a subset of items from the EXACT is under development to ease patient burden during long-term prospective studies. This item subset is designed to signal the worsening of a patient's condition suggestive of an exacerbation and requiring a more comprehensive evaluation through the 14-item assessment. The entire process would be handled through PDA programming that would detect the signal and automatically display the additional items comprising the tool. Patients would complete the 14-item EXACT daily, until the score returned to the defined tolerance level, at which time the diary would convert back to the shorter subset of items. The PDA could also be programmed to randomly administer the 14-item set to gather additional data throughout the study period.

The EXACT, therefore, is an instrument that is well designed to capture a patient-reported outcome dataset that can determine the incidence, severity, and duration of COPD exacerbations. The availability of a validated instrument with satisfactory measurement properties will greatly facilitate the evaluation of COPD exacerbations.

## B.  Laboratory Tests

While exacerbations are critically patient-reported events, the availability of laboratory tests for exacerbation would be a tremendous advance. There are several, nonexclusive uses for "tests" in the assessment of acute exacerbations of COPD. These include tests that could serve as defining features, as pathognomonic diagnostic points, and as gauges to quantify exacerbation severity. While no test currently available can be used for these purposes, much has been learned recently regarding the cellular and molecular mechanisms that underlie exacerbations and their physiologic consequences. These advances are reviewed in detail in other chapters (see chaps. 6 on inflammatory markers, 7 on physiologic changes, and 8 on systemic consequences). While all these represent potential objective tests for exacerbations, all share certain problems with regard to their use, which are highlighted here.

It is clear that acute exacerbations of COPD are, in most cases, inflammatory events. Increased inflammation can be gauged by increased neutrophils, cytokines, and inflammatory mediators in the sputum during exacerbations (19,20). Systemic inflammation is also supported by observation made in peripheral blood. Neutrophils show signs of activation and increased cytokines are readily observed (20–24). Importantly, the increase in cytokines is related to clinical features of the exacerbated patient (25). Moreover, the purulence of the sputum, which reflects local inflammation, is thought to be related to both clinical outcome and response to treatment (10,25). All these observations suggest that measures of inflammation have the potential to be useful biomarkers for COPD exacerbations. Unfortunately, many of these markers are also increased in stable COPD, with further increases during the acute event. As with symptoms, an acute event may be characterized by an increase from the "usual baseline." For these measures to be used to define events, it will be necessary to determine the magnitude of change that is meaningful. Similarly, it is likely that these measures are not specific to COPD exacerbations, as increased inflammation in the lung can result from other causes (e.g., pneumonia and systemic inflammation). This will complicate the diagnostic utility of inflammatory biomarkers. However, as current technology to assess inflammation provides readily quantifiable data, inflammatory measures are appealing as gauges of severity, if an event can be properly defined and diagnosed. Standardized PRO measures will facilitate the latter.

Increased respiratory rate in COPD patients can lead to dynamic hyperinflation (26). This may develop during an exacerbation due to an increased drive to breathe because of increased demand, anxiety, or other causes and may be independent of acute decrements in airflow, which would synergize to worsen the problem. Decrements in inspiratory capacity are likely to occur during acute exacerbations as improvement is observed with resolution (27,28). Thus, inspiratory capacity measurement is also an appealing "test" that could be used to assess exacerbations. As with measures of inflammation, however, dynamic hyperinflation is not specific to acute exacerbation; therefore, reductions in inspiratory capacity are likely to be more easily used as gauges of severity than as definitive diagnostic features.

Radiologic assessment has not usually been used to gauge COPD exacerbations. The major purpose of a chest radiograph in this clinical setting is to exclude another problem, such as pneumonia, which would preclude the diagnosis of an acute exacerbation (29). Advances in imaging of the lungs, however, have the potential to alter this approach. Aggressive diagnostic assessment has, in some studies, revealed the presence of pulmonary emboli in otherwise "unexplained" acute exacerbations (30). In addition, CT scanning can reveal evidence of pneumonitis when chest radiographs are normal, further confounding the distinction between an acute exacerbation and pneumonia (31). The ability of CT scanning to distinguish airway from alveolar disease (32) and to quantify dynamic changes on inspiratory and expiratory studies (33) suggests that this technology may have application to the assessment of acute exacerbations.

The application of "tests" to the assessment of COPD exacerbations is also complicated by the heterogeneity of exacerbations. For example, while most exacerbations are associated with inflammation, it is not clear that increased inflammation is present in *all* exacerbations. Of course, whether such "an-inflammatory" exacerbations are similar to or distinct from inflammatory exacerbations is also unknown. With the well-recognized etiologic and clinical heterogeneity of exacerbations, it seems plausible that biomarkers, physiologic, and radiographic assessments will be able to delineate among various types of exacerbations.

## IV. Heterogeneity and Phenotypes of Exacerbations

Exacerbations of COPD are heterogeneous at several levels. The etiology may relate to viral or bacterial infection or to other causes (see chaps. 10 and 11). More importantly, individual patients may respond to an exacerbation differently. It seems likely that there will be underlying genetic differences that could contribute to clinical response, but few studies on this topic have been conducted. Patients also may respond differently because of their underlying pathophysiology. Individuals with greater heterogeneity in time constants (i.e., greater heterogeneity of obstruction across the various airways of the lung) should be more likely to develop dynamic hyperinflation and, therefore, should be more likely to experience dyspnea with increasing respiratory rate (34). Similarly, individuals with concurrent bronchiectasis may be expected to produce more sputum and be more likely to have chronic bacterial colonization, although this remains to be tested rigorously (20,35).

Patients with COPD are also heterogeneous with respect to their systems of social support. Those with able caregivers may have generally better care, particularly as their health status worsens. This may allow them to avoid some encounters with the health care system. Alternatively, better support may also allow patients to survive with otherwise more severe disease. Such individuals may necessitate greater intensity of intervention when an exacerbation occurs.

The heterogeneity of underlying disease can affect the assessment of exacerbations in several ways. First, patients with comorbidities may have conditions (e.g., congestive heart failure) that confound the diagnosis of COPD exacerbation. Second, many comorbid conditions may also confound the management of exacerbations. Diabetes, for example, may worsen in those in whom systemic glucocorticoids are required. The presence of these comorbidities may dramatically influence the impact of an exacerbation and may also affect the way in which therapy for exacerbation should be implemented. Unfortunately, many clinical trials systematically exclude individuals with serious comorbidities, and thus clinical information on concurrent management of comorbid conditions is often limited.

The underlying severity of the lung disease has a dramatic effect on the nature of clinical intervention required for an exacerbation. An individual who has seriously compromised lung function and who requires high-flow nasal oxygen at baseline may need intubation with a minimal decrement in lung function. In contrast, an individual with excellent lung function may be able to tolerate considerable compromise and still be able to work. This heterogeneity in response confounds the use of health care utilization as a gauge of exacerbation severity.

The clinical response to an exacerbation may also be heterogeneous. Specifically, it is unclear to what degree individuals experience a prodrome or temporal consistency or variations within or across symptoms. Similarly, little is known if specific exacerbations due to specific etiologies are associated with specific symptom sets, although viral infections have been associated with "cold" symptoms and with more severe symptoms (36). It is also unknown to what degree the clinical features of exacerbation are stable within a given individual, or if they change as the disease progresses. These questions could be addressed through a standardized tool for assessing exacerbations.

The duration of an exacerbation is also problematic. Just as there is no consensus definition for onset, there is none for resolution, and it is difficult to determine duration. Nevertheless, duration is likely a measure of severity in some sense. An important issue, which also remains unresolved, is the distinction between resolution and recovery. In this context, the precipitating events that lead to an exacerbation may lead to a number of impacts. The initial precipitating event may resolve and the patient may recover from the impacts at very different rates. At present, no standardized definition or measurement tool has been applied to these clinical problems.

## V.  Summary

This chapter has reviewed a number of issues relating to COPD exacerbations. Both conceptual and empiric definitions have been applied to COPD exacerbations, and a consensus has emerged on what should be included as an exacerbation. The development of rigorous measurement instruments will help advance understanding of COPD exacerbations and can refine understanding of these events. A number of important questions will need to be addressed with a few examples shown in Table 2. Advances are being made toward addressing many of these, which are the subject of many of the chapters that follow.

**Table 2**  Sample Empirical Questions

- Is there within-patient consistency in exacerbation expression?
- Is there an identifiable symptom-based phenotype? Breathlessness-dominant, cough-dominant, with or without systemic manifestations?
- Can patients recognize exacerbations early? Or, which patients can recognize exacerbations early and why? What signals do they use?
- When patients choose to manage an exacerbation themselves, what do they do? When do they decide to seek care? Who decides to seek care and when?
- Are there biomakers that can identify exacerbations? Can they measure severity?
- How should resolution of exacerbation be defined?
- Can biomarkers distinguish phenotypes of exacerbations?
- Is there genetic or physiologic heterogeneity that contributes to predisposition to exacerbation?

## Acknowledgment

The authors gratefully acknowledge the assistance of Jill Duncan with the formatting and editorial review of this chapter.

## References

1. Snider GL. Nosology for our day: its application to chronic obstructive pulmonary disease. Am J Respir Crit Care Med 2003; 167(5):678–683.
2. Rodriguez-Roisin R. Toward a consensus definition for COPD exacerbations. Chest 2000; 117 (5 suppl 2):S398–S401.
3. Celli BR, MacNee W. Standards for the diagnosis and treatment of patients with COPD: a summary of the ATS/ERS position paper. Eur Respir J 2004; 23(6):932–946.
4. Global Initiative for Chronic Obstructive Lung Disease (GOLD). Executive summary: Global strategy for the diagnosis, management and prevention of chronic obstructive pulmonary disease. NHLBI/WHO Workshop Reprint 2001. Available at: http://www.goldcopd.com/exec-summary-2001. Accessed December, 2007.
5. Global Initiative for Chronic Obstructive Lung Disease (GOLD). Global strategy for diagnosis, management and prevention of COPD, 2006. Available at: http://www.goldcopd.org. Accessed December, 2007.
6. Rabe KF, Hurd S, Anzueto A, et al. Global strategy for the diagnosis, management, and prevention of chronic obstructive pulmonary disease: GOLD executive summary. Am J Respir Crit Care Med 2007; 176(6):532–555 [Epub May 16, 2007].
7. Calverley P, Pauwels Dagger R, Lofdahl CG, et al. Relationship between respiratory symptoms and medical treatment in exacerbations of COPD. Eur Respir J 2005; 26(3):406–413.
8. Seemungal TA, Donaldson GC, Bhowmik A, et al. Time course and recovery of exacerbations in patients with chronic obstructive pulmonary disease. Am J Respir Crit Care Med 2000; 161 (5):1608–1613.
9. Seemungal TA, Donaldson GC, Paul EA, et al. Effect of exacerbation on quality of life in patients with chronic obstructive pulmonary disease. Am J Respir Crit Care Med 1998; 157(5 pt 1): 1418–1422.
10. Anthonisen NR, Manfreda J, Warren CPW, et al. Antibiotic therapy in exacerbations of chronic obstructive pulmonary disease. Ann Int Med 1987; 106:196–204.
11. Creswell JW. Qualitative Inquiry and Research Design: Choosing Among Five Methods. Thousand Oaks, CA: Sage Publications, 1998.
12. Marshall C, Rossman GB. Designing Qualitative Research. 2nd ed. Thousand Oaks, CA: Sage Publications, 1995.
13. Adams R, Chavannes N, Jones K, et al. Exacerbations of chronic obstructive pulmonary disease: a patients' perspective. Prim Care Respir J 2006; 15(2):102–109.
14. Kessler R, Stahl E, Vogelmeier C, et al. Patient understanding, detection, and experience of COPD exacerbations: an observational, interview-based study. Chest 2006; 130(1):133–142.
15. Nicolson P, Anderson P. The patient's burden: physical and psychological effects of acute exacerbations of chronic bronchitis. J Antimicrob Chemother 2000; 45:25–32.
16. Celli BR, Barnes PJ. Exacerbations of chronic obstructive pulmonary disease. Eur Respir J 2007; 29(6):1224–1238.
17. Miravitlles M, Anzueto A, Legnani D, et al. Patient's perception of exacerbations of COPD—the PERCEIVE study. Respir Med 2007; 101:453–460.
18. Leidy NK, Howard K, Petrillo J, et al. The EXAcerbation of Chronic Pulmonary Disease Tool (EXACT): a patient-reported outcome, phase I. Presented at: the American Thoracic Society International Conference; May18–23, 2007; San Francisco, CA.

19. Aaron SD, Angel JB, Lunau M, et al. Granulocyte inflammatory markers and airway infection during acute exacerbation of chronic obstructive pulmonary disease. Am J Respir Crit Care Med 2001; 163(2):349–355.

20. Gompertz S, O'Brien C, Bayley DL, et al. Changes in bronchial inflammation during acute exacerbations of chronic bronchitis. Eur Respir J 2001; 17(6):1112–1119.

21. Koenderman L, Kanters D, Maesen B, et al. Monitoring of neutrophil priming in whole blood by antibodies isolated from a synthetic phage antibody library. J Leukoc Biol 2000; 68(1):58–64.

22. Pinto-Plata V, Toso J, Lee K, et al. Profiling serum biomarkers in patients with COPD: associations with clinical parameters. Thorax 2007; 62(7):595–601.

23. Pinto-Plata VM, Livnat G, Girish M, et al. Systemic cytokines, clinical and physiological changes in patients hospitalized for exacerbation of COPD. Chest 2007; 131(1):37–43.

24. Selby C, Drost E, Lannan S, et al. Neutrophil retention in the lungs of patients with chronic obstructive pulmonary disease. Am Rev Respir Dis 1991; 143:1259–1264.

25. White AJ, O'Brien C, Hill SL, et al. Exacerbations of COPD diagnosed in primary care: changes in spirometry and relationship to symptoms. COPD 2005; 2(4):419–425.

26. O'Donnell DE. Hyperinflation, dyspnea, and exercise intolerance in chronic obstructive pulmonary disease. Proc Am Thorac Soc 2006; 3(2):180–184.

27. Parker CM, Voduc N, Aaron SD, et al. Physiological changes during symptom recovery from moderate exacerbations of COPD. Eur Respir J 2005; 26(3):420–428.

28. Stevenson NJ, Walker PP, Costello RW, et al. Lung mechanics and dyspnea during exacerbations of chronic obstructive pulmonary disease. Am J Respir Crit Care Med 2005; 172(12): 1510–1516.

29. Sherman S, Skoney JA, Ravikrishnan KP. Routine chest radiographs in exacerbations of chronic obstructive pulmonary disease. Diagnostic value. Arch Intern Med 1989; 149(11):2493–2496.

30. Tillie-Leblond I, Marquette CH, Perez T, et al. Pulmonary embolism in patients with unexplained exacerbation of chronic obstructive pulmonary disease: prevalence and risk factors. Ann Intern Med 2006; 144(6):390–396.

31. van Strijen MJ, Bloem JL, de Monye W, et al. Helical computed tomography and alternative diagnosis in patients with excluded pulmonary embolism. J Thromb Haemost 2005; 3(11):2449–2456.

32. Fujimoto K, Kitaguchi Y, Kubo K, et al. Clinical analysis of chronic obstructive pulmonary disease phenotypes classified using high-resolution computed tomography. Respirology 2006; 11 (6):731–740.

33. Jensen SP, Lynch DA, Brown KK, et al. High-resolution CT features of severe asthma and bronchiolitis obliterans. Clin Radiol 2002; 57(12):1078–1085.

34. Niewoehner D. Structure-function relationships: the pathophysiology of airflow obstruction. In: Stockley R, Rennard SRK, Celli B, eds. Chronic Obstructive Pulmonary Disease. Malden, MA: Blackwell, 2007:3–19.

35. Patel IS, Vlahos I, Wilkinson TM, et al. Bronchiectasis, exacerbation indices, and inflammation in chronic obstructive pulmonary disease. Am J Respir Crit Care Med 2004; 170(4):400–407.

36. Seemungal T, Harper-Owen R, Bhowmik A, et al. Respiratory viruses, symptoms, and inflammatory markers in acute exacerbations and stable chronic obstructive pulmonary disease. Am J Respir Crit Care Med 2001; 164(9):1618–1623.

# 2
# Epidemiology of COPD Exacerbations

**ANDREA K. JOHNSTON**
Department of Pulmonary, Critical Care, and Sleep Medicine, University of Kentucky Medical Center, Lexington, Kentucky, U.S.A.

**DAVID M. MANNINO**
Department of Preventive Medicine and Environmental Health, University of Kentucky College of Public Health, Lexington, Kentucky, U.S.A.

## I. Introduction

Chronic obstructive pulmonary disease (COPD) is expected to be the third cause of death worldwide by the year 2020, behind only cardiovascular disease and cerebrovascular disease (1), and the fifth leading cause of disability-adjusted life years lost (2). In the United States, COPD accounted for 8 million outpatient visits, 1.5 millions emergency department (ED) visits, 726,000 hospitalizations, and 119,000 deaths in 2000, with the number of women dying from COPD surpassing the number of men for the first time (3). In the United Kingdom, COPD exacerbations are now the most common cause of hospital admission (4). Acute exacerbations of COPD (AECOPD) account for a large proportion of the economic, medical, and psychosocial impact of this chronic disease and are often associated with physician visits, hospitalizations, medication prescriptions, functional decline, and mortality.

The term exacerbation may be used inconsistently in clinical practice, leading to difficulty assessing the true rate and outcomes of exacerbations. Definitions of exacerbations in epidemiologic or clinical studies have ranged from self-recorded patient diary cards of symptoms to physician-charted documentation and from outpatient treatment or medication prescribed to hospital and ICU admissions. One of the most commonly used definitions of an AECOPD was developed by Anthonisen et al. in 1986 and consists of a triad of respiratory symptoms: increased dyspnea, sputum volume, and sputum purulence (5). This definition continues to be used today, often with a modification of time symptoms have persisted (i.e., 2 or 3 days).

The current ATS/ERS (American Thoracic Society/European Respiratory Society) consensus statement is based on these criteria and states "an exacerbation of COPD is an event in the natural course of disease characterized by a change in the patient's baseline dyspnea, cough and/or sputum beyond day-to-day variability sufficient to warrant a change in management (6)." Exacerbations can be classified by levels, with level 1 requiring outpatient treatment, level 2 requiring hospitalization, and level 3 requiring ICU care.

Another obstacle encountered when examining the frequency of exacerbations is identifying when one exacerbation ends and another begins. One outpatient study of 101 COPD patients showed that at 35 days of follow-up after an AECOPD, 25% still had peak flow lower than baseline and 14% had symptoms worse than baseline. In some (7.1%), the symptoms never returned to baseline level (7). Another study of 73 COPD patients found that 22% of subjects with moderate to severe COPD had a recurrent exacerbation event within 50 days of the initial event (8). In these patients who have a recurrent exacerbation before completely returning to normal from the initial exacerbation or whose respiratory symptoms never return to baseline, it raises the possibility of a "chronic exacerbation" state that may be associated with an accelerated lung function decline and worse outcomes.

Our goal in this chapter is to provide an overview of the epidemiology of AECOPD with particular attention to the overall estimated rates of exacerbations, proportion requiring hospitalizations, comorbid factors, and mortality. Subsequent chapters will focus more on the pathophysiology, etiologies, burden, and prevention of exacerbations.

## II.  Methods

In order to examine the overall rates of COPD exacerbations, we performed a PubMed search using the terms COPD, exacerbation, and epidemiology. We limited the search to articles with human subjects published in English. We selected articles that quantified the number of AECOPD in a population over time or mortality related to AECOPD. We limited the number of pharmaceutical-funded studies that were primarily looking at medication efficacy to a few larger, more recent, and commonly cited studies (9–11). Ultimately, we selected 30 articles for further review. In cases where the annual rate of AECOPD was not stated in the study, we estimated this by dividing the study population by the total number of AECOPD and adjusted for time to estimate the number of exacerbations per person per year. For mortality, we divided the total number of subjects studied by the total number of deaths and adjusted this for time to get an annual estimated mortality percentage.

## III.  Exacerbation Frequency

The wide variation in the definition of AECOPD is evident in Table 1: In the 30 selected studies, 16 different definitions were used. The annual rate of AECOPD ranged from 0.99 to 3.83 per person-year. As expected, the reported incidence of AECOPD varied depending on the definition used and the population studied (outpatient vs. ED vs. hospitalized) (Fig. 1).

Donaldson et al. has found that using diary cards yielded a higher exacerbation frequency than other methods, presumably because patients often self-manage exacerbations without presenting to medical attention. In the East London study, about 50% of exacerbations diagnosed by diary cards were unreported to the research team though the symptoms experienced between reported and unreported events were similar (12). This lack of reporting may explain the higher rate of exacerbations (2.92–3.36 per person-year) observed in studies using diary cards for diagnosis compared with other less sensitive methods (13,14). Hospitalized or ED patients also appear to, subsequently, have higher exacerbation rates (2.2–2.8 per person-year) possibly because of a more impaired population at baseline or lack of access to a primary care provider (15,16) (Fig. 2).

**Table 1** Definitions of AECOPD Used in Selected Studies

| Study (Ref.) | Medical chart coding or ICD codes (491, 492, 496) | Symptoms[a] | Time | Treatment | Physician or ED visit | Hospitalization | Radiographic infiltrate | Notes |
|---|---|---|---|---|---|---|---|---|
| A (5) | | D, V, P, T, N, F, W, RR, HR | 3 days | + moderate | + moderate | + | + | |
| B (22,27) | | B, D, V | | | | + severe | | |
| C (36) | | D, +/- VFW | | | | | | |
| D (16,21,23,26,28, 30,37,38) | + | | | | | | | |
| E (24) | + | D, RF, MS, H | | | | + | | |
| F (29) | | D, V, P, F, B | | | | | – | |
| G (18,33,39) | | D,V, P | | | | | | |
| H (9,10) | | + | | + | | | | |
| I (13,14) | | D, V, P, N, B, F, T | ≥2 days | | | | | Diary cards |
| J (25,34,40) | | D, V, P | | | | + | | |
| K (41) | | | | + | | + | | |
| L (35) | | D, V, P | ≥2 days | | | | | |
| M (31) | | | | | | | | |
| N (42) | | + | ≥2 days | + | | +/- | | |
| O (19) | | + | | + | + | – | | SGRQ |
| P (15) | | + | | | + | | | |

aSymptoms are indicated as follows:

D = dyspnea.

V = sputum volume.

P = sputum purulence.

F = fever.

B = bronchospasm.

N = nasal discharge.

T = sore throat.

W = weight change.

RR = Inc respiratory rate by 20% of baseline.

HR = Inc heart rate by 20% of baseline.

M = malaise.

H = hypercapnia.

RF = respiratory failure.

MS = decreased mental status.

*Abbreviations*: AECOPD, acute exacerbations in chronic obstructive pulmonary disease; ICD, International Classification of Diseases; ED, emergency department; SGRQ, St. George's Respiratory Questionnaire.

Exacerbations per person per year

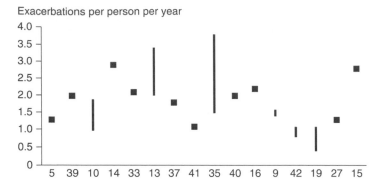

**Figure 1** Estimated annual exacerbation rates of COPD based on selected studies (number under-neath estimate corresponds to reference number) and ordered by year of publication. Estimates are presented as either a point estimate (*square*) or range of estimates (*bar*) from each study.

Hospitalizations per person per year

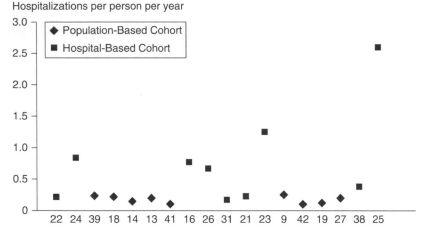

**Figure 2** Estimates of annual hospitalization rates for acute exacerbation COPD in selected studies (number underneath estimate corresponds to reference number) and ordered by year of publication. Cohorts originally derived from outpatient populations are indicated with diamonds, and those derived from ED or hospitalized populations are indicated with squares. *Abbreviation*: ED, emergency department

## IV.  Frequent Vs. Infrequent Exacerbators

Acknowledging the variability in the rates of AECOPD related to definitions, there are also risk factors leading to more frequent exacerbations. Donaldson et al. has classified patients as infrequent ($\leq$2 in the previous year) or frequent exacerbators (3–8 in the previous year) to identify the differences between these two groups (14). Quality of life scores were lower, while daily cough and sputum productions were higher in frequent exacerbators (14). Respiratory symptoms such as chronic dyspnea and wheeze (17) and chronic mucous hypersecretion (18) are also increased among "frequent exacerbators" in other cohorts studied. This observation suggests a possible etiologic or epidemiologic link between chronic respiratory symptoms and COPD exacerbations.

The proportion of patients with COPD who are "frequent exacerbators" depends upon the definition used: In one cohort, 55% were considered frequent exacerbators with more than two AECOPD in the past year (18), whereas 63% of another cohort were classified as frequent exacerbators with more than one AECOPD in the past year (19). In the latter, frequent exacerbators had a lower forced expiratory volume in one second ($FEV_1$) (1.14L, 37.6%, vs. 1.36L, 42.6%), were more steroid (16% vs. 13%) and oxygen (38% vs. 21%) dependent, and had worse gas exchange. Exacerbations were significantly correlated with prior COPD hospitalization, $FEV_1$ percent predicted, BODE index (body mass index, airflow obstruction, dyspnea, and exercise capacity), and GOLD (Global Initiative for Chronic Obstructive Lung Diseases) stage (19).

Lung function decline in frequent (>2.92/yr) versus infrequent (<2.92/yr) exacerbators with similar baseline lung function has also been examined. Frequent exacerbators experienced a median exacerbation rate of 4.2/yr and had a faster decline in $FEV_1$ of 40.1 mL/yr (4.22% per year) over four years of follow-up, whereas infrequent exacerbators had a median rate of 1.9/yr and a decline in $FEV_1$ of 32.1 mL/yr (3.59% per year) (17).

In summary, more frequent AECOPD, despite the definition used, is associated with more chronic respiratory symptoms, more severe COPD at baseline, and an accelerated decline in lung function over time.

## V.  Lung Function Impairment

A lower $FEV_1$ is associated with an increased risk of exacerbations (18) (Table 2). As noted above, more frequent exacerbations are associated with a greater decline in $FEV_1$ (17), and smokers may experience a more significant decline in lung function as compared with nonsmokers (20). Recurrent AECOPD may be an integral part of the decline in lung function over time observed in COPD patients.

## VI.  Emergency Care

AECOPD accounted for over 1 million ED visits in 2000 in the United States (3), which significantly contributes to the economic and medical impact of this disease. The factors associated with ED visits are crucial to identify, since ED visits are associated with a higher one-year mortality (21). Of those seen in the emergency department with a presumed diagnosis of AECOPD, approximately 45% will be admitted. However, as many as 17% who are treated and discharged home may relapse within 48 hours and require admission upon re-presentation (22). Identifying factors that predict the need for hospital admission is needed to help decrease the number of relapses. One study looking at the predictive value of spirometry in ED patients concluded that a posttreatment $FEV_1$ of less than 40% predicted was an indicator for admission with a sensitivity of 0.96, specificity of 0.58 and overall accuracy of 0.78 (22). A recent prospective multicenter cohort study involving 15 states and 3 Canadian provinces looked at factors associated with frequent ED visits for COPD in 379 patients. Those who were nonwhite, uninsured, on Medicaid, had less than a high school

**Table 2** Studies Looking at the Epidemiology of COPD Exacerbations, by Publication Year

| Author et al. (Ref.), publication yr | Country | Study type | N | Definition no. | Lung function (mean FEV$_1$) | Estimated exacerbation rate (no./person/yr) | Estimated hospitalization for AE-COPD (no./person/yr) | All-cause mortality in study population/yr |
|---|---|---|---|---|---|---|---|---|
| Anthonisen (5), 1987 | Canada | Randomized double blind crossover | 173 | A | 33.9% | 1.3 | – | 5.2% |
| Emerman (22), 1991 | United States | Prospective observational | 83[b] | B | 40.7% discharged 23% admitted | – | 0.22 | – |
| Fuso (36), 1995 | Italy | Retrospective chart review | 590[a] | C | – | – | – | 14.4% in-hospital |
| Seneff (28), 1995 | United States | Prospective cohort | 362[a] | D | – | – | – | ICU mortality 9.4%; hospital mortality 24%; 59% overall mortality at 1 yr |
| Connors (24), 1996 | United States | Prospective observational; randomized controlled (phase 2) | 1016[a] | E | 0.80L (% not available) | – | 0.84 | 11% in-hospital; 43% 1 yr |
| Vittaca (29), 1996 | Italy | Prospective observational | 39[a] | F | 26% MV 41% no MV | – | – | 43% in-hospital |
| Miravitlles (39), 1999 | Spain | Cross-sectional observational | 1001 | G | 47% | 2 median | 0.24 | – |
| Burge(10), 2000 | United Kingdom | Randomized double blind placebo controlled | 751 | H | 44–47% | 0.99–1.32 median | – | 3.1%; 0.67% from COPD |
| Miravitlles (18), 2000 | Spain | Cross sectional observational | 896 | G | 49.7–53.3% | 1.43–1.90 mean | 0.22 | – |

| Study | Country | Study type | N | | % | Rate | Value | Outcome |
|---|---|---|---|---|---|---|---|---|
| Donaldson (14), 2002 | United Kingdom | Prospective observational | 109 | I | 38.2% | 2.92 median | 0.15 | — |
| Lieberman (34), 2002 | Israel | Prospective observational | 219[a] | J | 40.7–41.6% | — | — | 2.1% in-hospital |
| Sethi (33), 2002 | United States | Prospective observational | 81 | G | 47.3% | 2.1 | — | — |
| Donaldson (13), 2003 | United Kingdom | Prospective observational | 132 | I | 38.4% | 3.36 calculated 2.52 median GOLD 2–2.68 GOLD 3–3.43 | 0.20 | — |
| Patil (30), 2003; Tata (37), 2003 | United States United Kingdom | Cross-sectional Self-controlled case series | 71,130[a] 5918 | D D | — — | — 1.8 | — — | 2.5% in-hospital — |
| De Melo (41), 2004 | Canada | Prospective cohort | 5645 | K | — | 1.12 | 0.102 | — |
| Hurst (35), 2005 | United Kingdom | Cohort | 105 | L | 39.6% | 1.77 overall (1.55—infrequent; 3.83—frequent) | — | — |
| Stevenson (40), 2005 | United Kingdom | Prospective observational | 22[a] | J | 36% | 1.97 | — | — |
| Wang (16), 2005 | Canada | Retrospective chart review | 282[a] | D | 35.9% | 2.2 | 0.77 | 9.9% in-hospital; 18% overall 1-yr mortality; 14% overall due to COPD |
| Cao (26), 2006 | Singapore | Cross sectional | 186[a] | D | — | — | 0.67 | — |
| Gudmundsson (31), 2006 | Scandinavia | Prospective observational | 416[a] | M | 40.6% alive 33.5% dead | — | 0.18 | 14.7% |
| Kim (21), 2006 | United States | Retrospective cohort | 482[b] | D | — | — | 0.23 ED visit or hospitalization | 15% |
| Price (23), 2006 | United Kingdom | Prospective | 7529[a] | D | — | — | 1.25 | In-hospital mortality 7.4%; 15.3% 90 days |

*(Continued)*

**Table 2** Studies Looking at the Epidemiology of COPD Exacerbations, by Publication Year (*Continued*)

| Author et al. (Ref.), publication yr | Country | Study type | N | Definition no. | Lung function (mean FEV$_1$) | Estimated exacerbation rate (no./person/yr) | Estimated hospitalization for AE-COPD (no./person/yr) | All-cause mortality in study population/yr |
|---|---|---|---|---|---|---|---|---|
| Aaron (9), 2007 | Canada | Randomized double blind placebo controlled | 449 | H | 38.0% | 1.37–1.61 | 0.25 | 3.5% |
| Calverley (42), 2007 | International | Randomized double blind | 6112 | N | 43.6–43.1% post bronchodilator | 0.85–1.13 | 0.09 | 4.7% 1.9% from COPD |
| Cote (19), 2007 | United States | Prospective observational | 205 | O | 39.5% | 1 median | 0.12 | 4.9% |
| | | | | | | GOLD 1 and 2–0.41 GOLD 3–1.05 GOLD 4–1.08 | | 2.9% from COPD |
| Fitzgerald (27), 2007 | Canada | Prospective observational | 524 | B | 43.9% | 1.31 | 0.2 | – |
| Kinnunen (38), 2007 | Finland | Retrospective database review | 12,597[a] | D | – | – | 0.39 | 6.87% |
| Ng (25), 2007 | Singapore | Prospective cohort | 376[a] | J | 47.3–48.2% | – | 2.6 | 15% |
| Tsai (15), 2007 | United States and Canada | Observational | 388[b] | P | – | 2.8 | – | – |

Definition numbers classified in Table 1.

[a]Hospitalized population.

[b]Emergency department population.

*Abbreviations*: AECOPD, acute exacerbations in chronic obstructive pulmonary disease; MV, mechanical ventilation; GOLD, Global Initiative for Chronic Obstrusive Lung Diseases.

education, and lacked a primary care provider were more likely to have frequent ED visits. In this study, having a primary care provider lowered the frequency of ED visits (15).

## VII. Hospitalizations

Hospitalization rates for AECOPD, in the majority of studies, range between 0.15 and 0.25/patient/yr (Table 2, Fig. 2), and the average length of stay is 8.7 days (23). Studies with higher rates included populations drawn from hospitalized patients that would, probably, include patients with more severe disease or comorbidities (16,23–25) (Fig. 2). For example, the study by Connors, which had a 0.84 rate of hospitalization/person/yr was performed in seriously ill, hospitalized patients with a median APACHE III (Acute Physiology and Chronic Health Evaluation) score of 39 and a 43% one-year mortality (24).

Of admitted patients, 53% of one cohort spent at least one day in an ICU and 35% required mechanical ventilation (24). The burden of exacerbations is not limited to the hospital length of stay. Approximately 5% to 10% of patients will need long-term care facilities upon discharge (16,24) and some patients may benefit from pulmonary rehabilitation before returning home.

## VIII. Comorbidities

Respiratory symptoms and decreased $FEV_1$ are associated with exacerbation frequency, but comorbidities also affect exacerbation severity and prognosis (18). The presence of comorbid conditions (cardiac insufficiency, ischemic heart disease, or diabetes mellitus) was the most important factor predicting hospital admission for AECOPD with an odds ratio of 1.97 in a cross-sectional observation study of 896 patients in Spain. Of admitted patients, 35.7% had at least one comorbid condition in contrast to 22.8% of nonadmitted patients (18). This relationship has been consistently observed. Seventy-four percent of those with frequent hospital readmissions for COPD have at least one comorbid condition (26), 34% to 39% have two or more comorbid diseases (24,26), and 42% have three or more (24).

Aside from physical illness, AECOPD is also associated with depression (27). Depressed patients and those taking psychotropic medications are more likely to be frequently admitted for AECOPD (26). In one study, the prevalence of depression was 44.4% at admission for AECOPD, and depression was significantly associated with mortality and hospital stay (25). Conversely, exacerbations themselves lead to depression and decreased quality of life. At six months after discharge, only 26% one cohort was alive and able to report a good, very good, or excellent quality of life (24).

## IX. Mortality

Hospital admissions for AECOPD are associated with a 2.5% to 24% mortality, with up to 43% mortality noted in those requiring mechanical ventilation (Table 2). On average, a 14% to 18% one-year mortality is seen in those hospitalized with AECOPD (Table 2). The highest mortality rates noted in Table 2 (15% 90-day and 43% in-hospital mortality) are in ICU patients (28,29). As previously noted, visiting an emergency department for AECOPD may be associated with an increased one-year mortality rate. One study looked at mortality, following an ED visit for AECOPD and found a 30-day, 90-day, and one-year mortality of 5%, 11% and 23%, respectively (21).

In one study of 282 patients hospitalized for AECOPD, 9.9% died during hospitalization, 85.5% were discharged home and 4.6% needed long-term care facilities (16). These rates are consistent with the SUPPORT (Study to Understand Prognoses and Preferences for Outcomes and Risks of Treatments) trial by Connors et al., which showed an 11% in-hospital mortality rate with 81% of survivors being discharged home, 10% to a nursing home, and 2% to a rehabilitation hospital (24). Mortality is higher with older age (21,28,30,31), male sex (30), decreased lung function (31), and comorbid illness (21,28,31). Compared with hospitalized patients without COPD, a diagnosis of COPD is also associated with a higher age-adjusted in-hospital mortality for pneumonia, hypertension, heart failure, ventilatory failure, and thoracic malignancies (32). The relationship between AECOPD and mortality due to other causes needs additional research.

## X. Conclusions

COPD is an increasingly common chronic illness associated with a significant burden, largely because of exacerbations. Our recognition of AECOPD is influenced by how we define an exacerbation event and the type of population studied. According to our literature review, most people with COPD will have between one and three acute exacerbations per year and approximately 0.2 hospitalizations per year due to AECOPD, with a significant related mortality. Characteristics associated with more frequent exacerbations and health care utilization patterns have been identified. Although an exacerbation event may be "acute," the resulting effects, such as an accelerated decline in lung function, psychosocial impairments, and functional decline, are "chronic." Future research is needed to look at those with "chronic exacerbations," examine the mechanisms of AECOPD in lung function decline, and identify the various socioeconomic factors influencing treatment and outcomes in AECOPD.

### References

1. Gulsvik A. The global burden and impact of chronic obstructive pulmonary disease worldwide. Monaldi Arch Chest Dis 2001; 56(3):261–264.
2. Murray CJ, Lopez AD. Alternative projections of mortality and disability by cause 1990-2020: Global Burden of Disease Study. Lancet 1997; 349(9064):1498–1504.
3. Mannino DM, Homa DM, Akinbami LJ, et al. Chronic obstructive pulmonary disease surveillance– United States, 1971–2000. MMWR Surveill Summ 2002; 51(6):1–16.
4. Wedzicha JA, Seemungal TA. COPD exacerbations: defining their cause and prevention. Lancet 2007; 370(9589):786–796.
5. Anthonisen NR, Wright EC, Hodgkin JE. Prognosis in chronic obstructive pulmonary disease. Am Rev Respir Dis 1986; 133(1):14–20.
6. Celli BR, Macnee W. Standards for the diagnosis and treatment of patients with COPD: a summary of the ATS/ERS position paper. Eur Respir J 2004; 23(6):932–946.
7. Seemungal TA, Donaldson GC, Bhowmik A, et al. Time course and recovery of exacerbations in patients with chronic obstructive pulmonary disease. Am J Respir Crit Care Med 2000; 161(5): 1608–1613.

8. Perera WR, Hurst JR, Wilkinson TM, et al. Inflammatory changes, recovery and recurrence at COPD exacerbation. Eur Respir J 2007; 29(3):527–534.
9. Aaron SD, Vandemheen KL, Fergusson D, et al. Tiotropium in combination with placebo, salmeterol, or fluticasone-salmeterol for treatment of chronic obstructive pulmonary disease: a randomized trial. Ann Intern Med 2007; 146(8):545–555.
10. Burge PS, Calverley PM, Jones PW, et al. Randomised, double blind, placebo controlled study of fluticasone propionate in patients with moderate to severe chronic obstructive pulmonary disease: the ISOLDE trial. BMJ 2000; 320(7245):1297–1303.
11. Calverley P, Pauwels R, Vestbo J, et al. Combined salmeterol and fluticasone in the treatment of chronic obstructive pulmonary disease: a randomised controlled trial. Lancet 2003; 361(9356): 449–456.
12. Seemungal TA, Donaldson GC, Paul EA, et al. Effect of exacerbation on quality of life in patients with chronic obstructive pulmonary disease. Am J Respir Crit Care Med 1998; 157(5 pt 1): 1418–1422.
13. Donaldson GC, Seemungal TA, Patel IS, et al. Longitudinal changes in the nature, severity and frequency of COPD exacerbations. Eur Respir J 2003; 22(6):931–936.
14. Donaldson GC, Wilkinson TM, Hurst JR, et al. Exacerbations and time spent outdoors in chronic obstructive pulmonary disease. Am J Respir Crit Care Med 2005; 171(5):446–452.
15. Tsai CL, Griswold SK, Clark S, et al. Factors associated with frequency of emergency department visits for chronic obstructive pulmonary disease exacerbation. J Gen Intern Med 2007; 22 (6):799–804.
16. Wang Q, Bourbeau J. Outcomes and health-related quality of life following hospitalization for an acute exacerbation of COPD. Respirology 2005; 10(3):334–340.
17. Donaldson GC, Seemungal TA, Bhowmik A, et al. Relationship between exacerbation frequency and lung function decline in chronic obstructive pulmonary disease. Thorax 2002; 57(10): 847–852.
18. Miravitlles M, Guerrero T, Mayordomo C, et al. Factors associated with increased risk of exacerbation and hospital admission in a cohort of ambulatory COPD patients: a multiple logistic regression analysis. The EOLO Study Group. Respiration 2000; 67(5):495–501.
19. Cote CG, Dordelly LJ, Celli BR. Impact of COPD exacerbations on patient-centered outcomes. Chest 2007; 131(3):696–704.
20. Kanner RE, Anthonisen NR, Connett JE. Lower respiratory illnesses promote FEV(1) decline in current smokers but not ex-smokers with mild chronic obstructive pulmonary disease: results from the lung health study. Am J Respir Crit Care Med 2001; 164(3):358–364.
21. Kim S, Clark S, Camargo CA Jr. Mortality after an emergency department visit for exacerbation of chronic obstructive pulmonary disease. COPD 2006; 3(2):75–81.
22. Emerman CL, Effron D, Lukens TW. Spirometric criteria for hospital admission of patients with acute exacerbation of COPD. Chest 1991; 99(3):595–599.
23. Price LC, Lowe D, Hosker HS, et al. UK National COPD Audit 2003: Impact of hospital resources and organisation of care on patient outcome following admission for acute COPD exacerbation. Thorax 2006; 61(10):837–842.
24. Connors AF Jr., Dawson NV, Thomas C, et al. Outcomes following acute exacerbation of severe chronic obstructive lung disease. The SUPPORT investigators (Study to Understand Prognoses and Preferences for Outcomes and Risks of Treatments). Am J Respir Crit Care Med 1996; 154(4 pt 1): 959–967.
25. Ng TP, Niti M, Tan WC, et al. Depressive symptoms and chronic obstructive pulmonary disease: effect on mortality, hospital readmission, symptom burden, functional status, and quality of life. Arch Intern Med 2007; 167(1):60–67.
26. Cao Z, Ong KC, Eng P, et al. Frequent hospital readmissions for acute exacerbation of COPD and their associated factors. Respirology 2006; 11(2):188–195.

27. FitzGerald JM, Haddon JM, Bradly-Kennedy C, et al. Resource use study in COPD (RUSIC): a prospective study to quantify the effects of COPD exacerbations on health care resource use among COPD patients. Can Respir J 2007; 14(3):145–152.
28. Seneff MG, Wagner DP, Wagner RP, et al. Hospital and 1-year survival of patients admitted to intensive care units with acute exacerbation of chronic obstructive pulmonary disease. JAMA 1995; 274(23):1852–1857.
29. Vitacca M, Clini E, Porta R, et al. Acute exacerbations in patients with COPD: predictors of need for mechanical ventilation. Eur Respir J 1996; 9(7):1487–1493.
30. Patil SP, Krishnan JA, Lechtzin N, et al. In-hospital mortality following acute exacerbations of chronic obstructive pulmonary disease. Arch Intern Med 2003; 163(10):1180–1186.
31. Gudmundsson G, Gislason T, Lindberg E, et al. Mortality in COPD patients discharged from hospital: the role of treatment and co-morbidity. Respir Res 2006; 7:109.
32. Holguin F, Folch E, Redd SC, et al. Comorbidity and mortality in COPD-related hospitalizations in the United States, 1979 to 2001. Chest 2005; 128(4):2005–2011.
33. Sethi S, Evans N, Grant BJ, et al. New strains of bacteria and exacerbations of chronic obstructive pulmonary disease. N Engl J Med 2002; 347(7):465–471.
34. Lieberman D, Lieberman D, Gelfer Y, et al. Pneumonic vs nonpneumonic acute exacerbations of COPD. Chest 2002; 122(4):1264–1270.
35. Hurst JR, Donaldson GC, Wilkinson TM, et al. Epidemiological relationships between the common cold and exacerbation frequency in COPD. Eur Respir J 2005; 26(5):846–852.
36. Fuso L, Incalzi RA, Pistelli R, et al. Predicting mortality of patients hospitalized for acutely exacerbated chronic obstructive pulmonary disease. Am J Med 1995; 98(3):272–277.
37. Tata LJ, West J, Harrison T, et al. Does influenza vaccination increase consultations, cortico-steroid prescriptions, or exacerbations in subjects with asthma or chronic obstructive pulmonary disease? Thorax 2003; 58(10):835–839.
38. Kinnunen T, Saynajakangas O, Keistinen T. The COPD-induced hospitalization burden from first admission to death. Respir Med 2007; 101(2):294–299.
39. Miravitlles M, Mayordomo C, Artes M, et al. Treatment of chronic obstructive pulmonary disease and its exacerbations in general practice. EOLO Group. Estudio Observacional de la Limitacion Obstructiva al Flujo aEreo. Respir Med 1999; 93(3):173–179.
40. Stevenson NJ, Walker PP, Costello RW, et al. Lung mechanics and dyspnea during exacer-bations of chronic obstructive pulmonary disease. Am J Respir Crit Care Med 2005; 172(12): 1510–1516.
41. de Melo MN, Ernst P, Suissa S. Rates and patterns of chronic obstructive pulmonary disease exacerbations. Can Respir J 2004; 11(8):559–564.
42. Calverley PM, Walker P. Chronic obstructive pulmonary disease. Lancet 2003; 362(9389): 1053–1061.

# 3

# Differential Diagnosis of COPD Exacerbations

**PETER M. A. CALVERLEY**
Division of Infection and Immunity, Clinical Sciences Centre, University Hospital Aintree, Liverpool, U.K.

## I. Introduction

As this volume demonstrates, exacerbations of chronic obstructive pulmonary disease (COPD) are important events that contribute to progressive ill health and mortality in these patients (1,2). A variety of increasingly robust definitions have been developed to allow us to capture information about when these events occur and how they relate to other aspects of the COPD patient's life (1,3–5). Such definitions have considerable utility when collecting data in clinical trials but have not yet translated themselves into routine clinical practice where treatment for COPD, presently dictated by some identifiable symptomatic change, does not always match up with discreet step changes in predefined symptoms, physical findings, or laboratory measurements. The potential for diagnostic overlap is considerable, even in clinical trial populations. Thus, in the large multicenter TORCH study (TOwards a Revolution in COPD Health), which looked, among other things, at the occurrence of health care–defined exacerbations, all episodes treated with antibiotics and/or oral corticosteroids were classed as exacerbations (6). Hence, those episodes that the physician thought were due to, or were associated with, pneumonia were also counted as exacerbations, despite their presumably rather different clinical course and management. This highlights our neglect of issues related to the differential diagnosis of these episodes, and while it may be inevitable that operational definitions applied to clinical trial data produce this sort of confusion, it cannot be considered acceptable in clinical practice.

This chapter will look at what disorders can be most readily confused in an exacerbation of COPD and how they can be distinguished. There is a paucity of data directly relevant to this question, especially for exacerbations managed in the community. This may reflect the perception that diagnosing exacerbations is either a relatively straightforward or an important task. However, this review will highlight that this is not the case.

## II. Clinical Features of COPD Exacerbations

Many of the key features that identify COPD exacerbation have been considered in the chapter discussing the definition of these episodes. Exacerbations usually involve patient-reported symptoms such as increased cough, the production of sputum when this is not normally present, or an increase in its volume or change in its color, the development of green sputum being a good marker of increased numbers of neutrophils (7). Commonly there is a perception of worsening breathlessness, although this is not always seen (8), and the presence of symptoms suggested of an associated upper respiratory tract infection or fever. Two factors make it hard to be extremely restrictive when diagnosing exacerbation. First, there is no set pattern to the way in which symptoms are reported. Some patients focus on increased cough and sputum, others on increased cough and breathlessness, and yet others on increased breathlessness and cold symptoms. The range of potential combinations is large, although the approach adopted by those defining exacerbations from diary cards has proven to be robust, with an increase in two symptoms, one of which must be a major one being required before an episode can be confidently diagnosed (9). The second factor is the need for an increase in symptoms itself, which always involves some subjective judgement about the patient and/or the doctor as to whether the difference is really different from the normal day-to-day variation, which many patients experience as COPD progresses.

These considerations become relevant when the differential diagnosis of an exacerbation is considered. The variable onset of symptoms accompanied by differences in the time before the patient acts upon them makes it hard to distinguish exacerbations in their early stages from other conditions that may share a similar etiology. The wide range of possible symptom combinations makes an absolute distinction on the basis of the timing and contribution of the patient's complaints very difficult. Finally, the relative lack of physical signs specific to an exacerbation, the nonspecific nature of the ones that do occur (e.g., tachypnea, accessory muscle use, wheeze), and the ability of the overinflated chest to mask new physical signs arising from other causes (e.g., new crackles) add to the diagnostic challenge.

Despite these drawbacks, it is possible in many cases to identify alternative explanations for what might otherwise be called a COPD exacerbation and to institute more appropriate treatment. Often the patients themselves will say that this is not their normal "attack," and this insight is always worth reporting. Fortunately, the number of alternative conditions that can mimic a COPD exacerbation is modest. Identifying these may completely change the management approach in mild to moderate severe disease. In severe or very severe COPD, it is more common to add in additional management options to deal with these alternative diagnoses that can be much harder to identify.

## III.  Principal Alternative Diagnoses

Table 1 provides a brief list of the main conditions that can mimic exacerbations of COPD and some of the symptoms with which they commonly present. Each of these conditions will be considered in more detail below.

### A.  Cardiac Failure

The occurrence of pulmonary congestion due to impaired left ventricular function with or without fluid overload from other causes is an extremely common clinical problem and results from many of the same predisposing factors as those leading to COPD. The impairment of left ventricular emptying secondary to ischemic heart disease or hypertension is more common in older smokers and is often unaccompanied by more specific

**Table 1**  A Symptomatic Approach to the Differential Diagnosis of COPD Exacerbations

| Alternative diagnosis | Principal symptoms |
| --- | --- |
| Cardiac failure | Dyspnea especially when lying flat, cough, wheezing |
| Pulmonary embolism | Dyspnea especially of sudden onset, cough, chest pain (pleuritic sometimes), hemoptysis (sometimes) |
| Pneumonia | Dyspnea, fever, cough with purulent sputum, chest pain (often pleuritic) |
| Bronchiectasis | Sputum volume increased and worse purulence, chest pain (usually pleuritic), fever, dyspnea |
| Pneumothorax | Dyspnea of sudden onset, cough |
| Metabolic acidosis | Dyspnea plus atypical clinical symptoms |

pointers to ischemic heart disease such as exertional chest pain. A strong link between COPD and the risk of cardiovascular disease has now emerged from population studies, and the risk of the two pathologies coexisting is greater than will be predicted by chance alone (10). Additionally, pulmonary infection whether viral or bacterial, remains a major trigger to COPD exacerbations and also worsens cardiac function, either by direct effect on the myocardium but secondary to increased inspiratory efforts, which in the case of COPD can decrease cardiac failing by shifting blood to the periphery (11). Additionally worsening gas exchange and especially arterial hypoxemia increase the pulmonary artery pressure and when accompanied by $CO_2$ retention promotes fluid retention, which is evident as an increased jugular venous pressure and peripheral edema (12). These changes reflect an impact on right heart function, which can itself result from COPD (13). It does create diagnostic confusion about what processes are driving the deteriorating symptom, and it is often impossible without specific cardiac functional studies to know exactly how much of a given exacerbation is a result of cardiac decompensation and how much a consequence of worsening pulmonary mechanics.

Studies in primary care where the majority of COPD cases identified are of mild to moderate severity managed by family physicians suggest that left ventricular impairment is frequently overlooked (14,15). In patients admitted to the intensive care unit with a COPD exacerbation, almost half have evidence of cardiac failure, and this can be identified by increased levels of the peptide NT-proBNP (amino terminal pro-brain natriuretic peptide) (16).

Confirming the diagnosis of coexisting heart failure can be a challenge, as echocardiography is often technically difficult in hyper inflated COPD patients, while gated radionuclide scanning is more accurate but not widely available for clinical purposes. Thus, the frequency with which impaired cardiac function contributes to the symptomatology of exacerbations remains an unclear area and one that merits further study.

### B.  Pulmonary Embolism

Like heart failure, the assessment of pulmonary embolisms in COPD is likely to be underdiagnosed. COPD is itself a risk factor for thromboembolic disease, although this is most likely to cause diagnostic confusion in severe COPD. Traditionally secondary polycythemia is thought of as the main risk factor for pulmonary embolism, but this complication is seen less frequently than previously, although red cell mass can be increased in heavy smokers with COPD (17). A potentially more common factor is immobility, which predisposes to peripheral venous thrombosis and is more common in COPD than in age-matched control subjects (18). Leg movement appears to be particularly reduced in these patients. Reduced levels of self-recorded activity identify patients at risk of COPD exacerbations (19) so that a connection between exacerbations and thromboembolism risk is plausible.

Direct evidence of thromboembolism is rather contentious. The use of the D-dimer blood test is confounded by the potential increase associated with infection and acute stress, which often accompanies exacerbations, and this has not been systematically investigated in well-defined COPD populations. Autopsy studies have shown that antemortem thrombus occurs in the pulmonary arteries of patients with advanced COPD (20), and this is seldom recognized clinically. Data from CT-PA studies have produced apparently contradictory information, with one French study identifying up to 25% of patients who have unsuspected pulmonary embolism when they presented with exacerbations with atypical clinical features or otherwise had a risk factor such as previous malignancy (21). However, data from Switzerland are rather more reassuring. Routine CT-PA measurement in 123 patients consecutive exacerbations and found only 1% of cases where a previously unsuspected pulmonary embolism was present (22). These contradictory results reflect the patient selection in each study. The French patients all exhibited atypical features of a COPD exacerbation while the patients in Switzerland were more typical of patients presenting to the emergency room. This suggests that CT-PA is a valuable tool when presentation is not as the clinician expects. It is certainly to be preferred to ventilation perfusion scanning, which is uninterpretable in patients with even moderate COPD and can lead to over-diagnosis of disease if other imaging methods are not used to support it.

### C.  Pneumonia

Pneumonia is not uncommon in COPD and has a worse prognosis than other forms of community (23). The symptoms of pneumonia in the COPD patient are very similar to those used to define an exacerbation with increased breathlessness, cough, and the onset of purulence sputum being common to both. Complaints of shivering, rigors, or feverishness, especially if confirmed by a raised temperature, are useful clinical pointers to an underlying pneumonia. However, strict criteria to separate the two conditions have not been established and whether the sensitivity and specificity have potentially useful clinical signs such as fever or basal crackles remains to be tested. A patient who developed new alveolar shadowing on a chest X ray must be assumed to have pneumonia, but how often such changes occur in otherwise "uncomplicated exacerbations" is entirely unknown. To further confuse the issue, the treatment of episodes where cough and increased sputum, volume, or purulence occur is with broad-spectrum antibiotics that are likely to be the same ones used as first-line treatment for community-acquired pneumonia.

Clinically, pneumonia is a significant event and often leads to hospitalisation in patients with more severe disease, although the diagnosis of pneumonia may itself be made for the first time when the patient presents with exacerbation symptoms to the hospital. Recent studies have defined an increased risk of hospitalization due to pneumonia in patients using inhaled corticosteroids for COPD (24), although it is difficult to avoid confounding issues due to disease severity in reports using administrative database information. More robust evidence comes from the TORCH study (6). This was a three-year multicenter randomized controlled trial comparing inhaled corticosteroids, long-acting β-agonists by inhalation, a combination of the two, and a placebo, although the main aim of the study was to test the effects of treatment on all course mortality. Exacerbation data were collected at three-month intervals throughout. Physician reported that pneumonia was found to be significantly less frequent than COPD exacerbation, occurring in approximately 5% of exacerbations in placebo-treated patients. By contrast, exacerbations classed as pneumonia were significantly common in patients randomized to receive inhaled corticosteroids, either alone or with the long-acting bronchodilator, with a 60% greater chance of having an event reported during the three years of the study if this treatment was given. From this study, all episodes treated with antibiotic were classed as being exacerbation and that almost all of the pneumonias were double counted. Physicians did not need to perform a chest X ray to confirm the diagnosis of pneumonia, although a radiograph had been performed in approximately two-thirds of the cases. There was no regional difference to suggest different diagnostic approaches between the 42 different countries contributing patients. The surprising observation was that use of inhaled corticosteroids reduced the overall exacerbation frequency in improved health status, while its combination with the long-acting β-agonist was associated with fewer hospitalizations and a lower overall mortality.

The association of pneumonia and inhaled corticosteroids has been confirmed in a further large randomized control trial, the INSPIRE study where the combination of β-agonist and inhaled steroids were compared with the long-acting bronchodilator tiotropium (25). Again, pneumonia was significantly commoner in corticosteroid-treated patients, while the use of corticosteroids to treat exacerbations was significantly less frequent in those receiving tiotropium. Daily diary cards were available in this study and the initial analysis of these data suggests differences in the symptoms that precede many of the pneumonic events. In both the bronchodilator and the corticosteroid groups, there were similar numbers of pneumonias that began abruptly without extended prodromal symptoms. However, there were far more episodes in patients taking inhaled corticosteroids where a prior exacerbation did not appear to resolve, and then a diagnosis of pneumonia was made than was true for those treated with tiotropium. Whether this represents a difference in diagnostic classification or a modification of the presentation of an exacerbation in patients using inhaled corticosteroids remains to be established. Alternative immunological mechanisms exist that might also account for the increase in the clinically diagnosed pneumonia and further work will be needed to resolve this issue.

### D. Bronchiectasis

Patients with clinically evident bronchiectasis are usually readily distinguished from those suffering from full COPD by the large volume of persistently purulent sputum they produce. Exacerbations in these patients are usually associated with fever, lethargy, and malaise as well as a change in sputum volume and an increase in the number of coarse crackles that can be heard on auscultation. However, there is overlap between bronchiectasis and COPD. Studies of infective COPD exacerbations have identified in a community population by primary care physicians suggest that episodes of sputum purulence in those with COPD confirmed by spirometry are more frequent in individuals with CT evidence of bronchiectasis (26). The changes on the CT in these patients were due to a combination of tubular and saccular airway enlargement. Other studies have suggested that tubular bronchiectasis is more often seen in COPD patients attending hospital, and the significance of airway dilatation in this setting is less clear (27). The relationship of structural changes in the airways to persistent lower respiratory tract colonization is still to be clarified, but it is reasonable to believe that a number of patients who have persistent purulent sputum production will have colonized lower airways (28), and these individuals are more likely to have typical symptoms of exacerbation (29).

Clinically, patients with persistent sputum production and a pattern of recurrent pneumonic episodes, especially if it occurs in the same region on the plain chest X ray, require further investigation with high-resolution CT to exclude localized bronchiectasis as a cause. This may change the treatment approach favoring the use of antibiotics earlier in the exacerbations of these patients and potentially by the parenteral route. However, the incidental finding of CT-defined bronchiectasis on a scan performed for some other purpose is not at present an indication to adjust a routine management to the exacerbation.

### E.  Pneumothorax

Patients with COPD, especially those with significant emphysema, are prone to develop a pneumothorax. This may occur when a relatively peripheral emphysematous area is partially occluded during an infected episode. In these circumstances, reabsorption of the distal gas does not occur and the area is exposed to significant local alveolar wall stress because of its inability to fully empty during expiration. Further acute increases in intrathoracic pressure because of coughing may be sufficient to trigger local wall rupture, with a consequent general loss of elastic recoil, as the visceral and parietal pleural surfaces are uncoupled. The consequent loss of lung recoil favors airway closure, which may trigger a coughing attack, but most commonly, breathlessness predominates, and this can be quite sudden in onset and severe. A pneumothorax can also occur if there is local chest trauma, especially when there is an accompanying rib fracture where the associated pleuritic chest pain further complicates the management and increases the risk of distal pneumonic infection.

The physical signs of pneumothorax are often difficult to interpret in COPD because of the background of pulmonary hyperinflation. Detecting tracheal deviation in a patient with a short trachea who is using their accessory muscles can be particularly hard. Similarly, the identification of reduced inspiratory breath sounds can be almost impossible when breath sounds are generally decreased because of severe emphysema. In this setting, the suddenness of the clinical presentation is often the trigger to obtain a chest radiograph. How often smaller self-limiting air leaks occur and are treated as "exacerbations" is not known. Some patients do have local pleural adhesions, which limit the degree to which pulmonary collapse occurs. In this setting the differential diagnosis of a localized pneumothorax from an emphysematous bulla can be almost impossible without more detailed imaging such as CT.

### F.  Chronic Asthma

Although the existence of an "overlap" between COPD and bronchial asthma appears likely, the data that clearly demonstrate that this occurs is scarce. The patients with chronic asthma clinically strongly resemble those with COPD, although they do tend to show somewhat greater but still-incomplete degrees of bronchodilator reversibility and more sputum eosinophilia, which favor a diagnosis of chronic asthma (30). As yet we do not have good clinical studies that show that these patients pursue a different clinical course and in practice the therapy for both chronic asthma and acute COPD is very similar. The presence of wheezing during inspiration and expiration may suggest involvement of the muscular airways, but this can occur in COPD when expiratory flow limitation is present and flow-limiting choke points are relatively proximal. Serial monitoring of spirometry or at least peak expiratory flow during treatment is often the best clue to the presence of responsive bronchial asthma and is worth doing in any patient who presents with their first exacerbation or those with atypical features or a history suggestive of prior asthma.

### G. Metabolic Acidosis

Most COPD exacerbations occur as a result of viral and/or bacterial infection, although there is increasing evidence that exposure to environmental oxidant stress or temperature change also contributes in a significant number of cases (31,32). In a few individuals, usually patients with severe or very severe disease, the symptoms of an exacerbation can result from other illness that is not immediately apparent but that is typically associated with an increased respiratory drive to breath, normally the result of metabolic acidosis. This can arise for many reasons, including occult renal disease, decompensated diabetes, or any form of severe sepsis. Although the clinical presentation suggests that the patient has had further COPD exacerbation, the arterial blood gas analysis shows a low or lower than usual for that patient, $CO_2$, a low pH, and a reduced bicarbonate or calculated base excess. A careful clinical history and search for alternative explanations for this problem is needed whenever abnormalities of this type are identified.

## IV. Clinical Approach to Differential Diagnosis

The relatively nonspecific nature of the symptoms that lead the patients to start new therapy or seek medical help have been a considerable challenge to investigators who have tried to understand and quantify them. Diary cards have been the most effective way to do this and scoring rules have been developed to identify when an event has occurred or simply result that patient's normal symptom fluctuation. In a clinical setting, such a precise information is usually lacking and instead the doctors make an overall assessment of whether the patient's "chest" is now worse than usual and, if so, why.

Several factors influence this decision. If the patient has had previous episodes where the event proved to be an exacerbation (a conclusion usually influenced by the course and resolution of the episode), then it is likely that the present episode will also be an exacerbation. Detailed reports of the between-episode consistency of specific symptoms are presently lacking, but in general, individuals with exacerbations are more likely to have had an episode earlier; however, that has been defined (33). The patients who seldom exacerbate but now present with a new episode require a more searching review to ensure that this is indeed due to the COPD. As noted above, the patient's perception of whether this episode corresponds to their "normal attack" is also important and it is useful to document in what way it differs, if it does. Finally, the severity of the underlying disease and the time since the last exacerbation are important. In general, patients with less severe spirometric impairment where symptoms have been settled for weeks and months are less likely to present with a new exacerbation. In contrast, those with severe or very severe disease frequently relapse because of their COPD, especially if they have required hospitalization in the preceding six weeks (34). This may reflect the use with which such patients become unstable following relatively minor environmental or bacterial strain change (35) or from failure of the original episode to resolve. As patients like this have usually been assessed in some detail previously, it is often the case that the new episode is a further exacerbation rather than the onset of an additional new problem.

There are several useful clinical pointers to alternative explanations for new symptoms, and these are also influenced by disease severity. Pulmonary edema of rapid onset can lead to acute breathlessness at any stage of COPD and is a real possibility when the severity of the symptoms is disproportionate to the known degree of airflow obstruction. Breathlessness when lying flat, the need to sleep with more pillows than usual, new onset, nocturnal breathlessness, all suggest pulmonary edema. Cardiovascular instability, especially tachycardia or a new arrhythmia such as atrial fibrillation (which often occurs in infective episodes and can be quite refractory to treatment), or a reduction in blood pressure suggests significant coexisting heart disease. An increased jugular venous pressure and peripheral edema point to fluid overload but the former can be a difficult sign to elicit when the respiratory rate and accessory muscle use are increased at rest. As noted already, these changes can reflect worsening hypoxic corpulmonalae.

A chest X ray can usually resolve any diagnostic confusion, and the presence of cardiomegaly, upper lobe blood diversion, and especially an increase in the pulmonary lymphatics or alveolar filling can be conclusive. The ECG provided supplementary information and is especially useful in identifying unsuspected ventricular hypertrophy and signs of acute cardiac ischemia. The specificity of other markers of cardiac function like BNP or troponin in the absence of chest pain remains to be resolved for the COPD patients. If pulmonary edema is present, hypoxemia may be disproportionately severe, and in some COPD patients, pulmonary edema can cause $CO_2$ retention and impair respiratory muscle performance. Although echocardiography is often performed, it is seldom useful in the acute evaluation of these patients.

Both pulmonary embolism and pneumothorax can be accompanied by rapid onset worsening of breathlessness. This is also seen in patients with rapidly developing consolidation due to pneumonia. Conversely, breathlessness may occur less dramatically and still be the result of any of these processes. Involvement of the parietal pleura whether by consolidation due to pneumonia or a pulmonary infarction gives rise to typical pleuritic chest pain, although this is only seen in a minority of cases in COPD patients. Dry cough is often reported in patients with pneumothorax and in some patients with pulmonary emboli, while hemostasis always requires further investigation and can result in pulmonary infarction or pneumonia. The most useful physical signs are hemodynamic instability for pulmonary embolism, new onset of crackles, fever and, very occasionally, bronchial breathing with pneumonia, and a unilateral difference in breath sound, which has not been noted previously where pneumothorax develops. Differences in the percussion node may be present with pneumonia or a pleural infusion secondary to pulmonary infarction, but this too can be a difficult sign to elicit.

Once again the chest X ray will resolve most problems related to pneumonia and pneumothorax. Pulmonary embolism is more challenging and, as noted already, atypical features and disproportionate hypoxemia point to the need for CTPA study, and an increase in the size of the P waves on the ECG can occur with a large pulmonary embolism but are also seen in patients with poor pulmonary embolism.

By contrast, asthma is usually part of the differential diagnosis of only the first exacerbation, as it does not usually develop once COPD is well established. Wheezing and coughing, which are prominent at night or specifically first thing in the morning, especially accompanied by chest tightness, are useful pointers here. When patients do complain of new onset wheezing on a background of established COPD, this is all too often the result of an occult neoplasm compromising a large airway and unilateral chest sounds, especially a fixed wheeze, is a strong indication for further imaging and perhaps bronchoscopy. Symptoms that occur gradually over week or are recurrent can be due to a pleural infusion that may result from an empyema or again may be malignant in nature. The rarer but serious complication are often accompanied by more systemic ill health and weight loss, which is always a marker of the need for further investigation.

Illnesses that mimic exacerbations by promoting metabolic acidosis can be very varied and should be considered when there is no known renal disease or diabetes or when the exacerbation is accompanied by symptom of acute illness affecting systems beyond the lungs. Arterial blood gas analysis is the main diagnostic aid here and will require the patient to be seen in an environment where this can be conducted.

## V.  Conclusion

In all of the above settings, alternative diagnoses are identified because of the atypical nature of the symptoms, signs, or investigations when the exacerbation is assessed. Unusually severe or sudden onset symptomatology, especially when breathlessness is the symptom concerned, should always prompt a consideration of other explanations, although in many cases no alternative explanation will be found apart from severe exacerbation of COPD. Alternative diagnoses need to be borne in mind in more severe disease, but in this setting they can often be hard to identify, hence the low index of diagnostic suspicion is likely to be the most effective way in which important alternative or comorbid condition can be picked up. Developing a systematic and readily applied diagnostic algorithm will be a major step forward in the routine care of COPD patients as would data about how frequently alternative diagnosis explains some or all the apparent episode of exacerbation. Until this is available, our best approach is to be aware of the possibility that other common conditions can mimic COPD exacerbations and to consider these when the patient presents acutely.

## References

1.  Wedzicha JA, Seemungal TA. COPD exacerbations: defining their cause and prevention. Lancet 2007; 370(9589):786–796.
2.  Soler-Cataluna JJ, Martinez-Garcia MA, Roman SP, et al. Severe acute exacerbations and mortality in patients with chronic obstructive pulmonary disease. Thorax 2005; 60(11):925–931.
3.  Rabe KF, Hurd S, Anzueto A, et al. Global strategy for the diagnosis, management, and prevention of chronic obstructive pulmonary disease: GOLD executive summary. Am J Respir Crit Care Med 2007; 176(6):532–555.
4.  Pauwels R, Calverley P, Buist AS, et al. COPD exacerbations: the importance of a standard definition. Respir Med 2004; 98(2):99–107.
5.  Calverley P, Pauwels DR, Lofdahl CG, et al. Relationship between respiratory symptoms and medical treatment in exacerbations of COPD. Eur Respir J 2005; 26(3):406–413.
6.  Calverley PM, Anderson JA, Celli B, et al. Salmeterol and fluticasone propionate and survival in chronic obstructive pulmonary disease. N Engl J Med 2007; 356(8):775–789.
7.  Stockley RA, O'Brien C, Pye A, et al. Relationship of sputum color to nature and outpatient management of acute exacerbations of COPD. Chest 2000; 117(6):1638–1645.

8. Seemungal TA, Donaldson GC, Bhowmik A, et al. Time course and recovery of exacerbations in patients with chronic obstructive pulmonary disease. Am J Respir Crit Care Med 2000; 161(5): 1608–1613.

9. Burge S, Wedzicha JA. COPD exacerbations: definitions and classifications. Eur Respir J Suppl 2003; 41:46s–53s.

10. Hole DJ, Watt GC, Davey-Smith G, et al. Impaired lung function and mortality risk in men and women: findings from the Renfrew and Paisley prospective population study. BMJ 1996; 313 (7059):711–715 (comments).

11. Aliverti A, Kayser B, Macklem PT. A human model of the pathophysiology of chronic obstructive pulmonary disease. Respirology 2007; 12(4):478–485.

12. Calverley PMA. Chronic respiratory failure. In: Warrell DA, Cox TM, Firth JD, eds. Oxford Textbook of Medicine. Oxford: OUP, 2003:1397–1403.

13. MacNee W, Xue QF, Hannan WJ, et al. Assessment by radionuclide angiography of right and left ventricular function in chronic bronchitis and emphysema. Thorax 1983; 38(7):494–500.

14. Rutten FH, Cramer MJ, Lammers JW, et al. Heart failure and chronic obstructive pulmonary disease: An ignored combination? Eur J Heart Fail 2006; 8(7):706–711.

15. Rutten FH, Moons KG, Cramer MJ, et al. Recognising heart failure in elderly patients with stable chronic obstructive pulmonary disease in primary care: cross sectional diagnostic study. BMJ 2005; 331(7529):1379.

16. Abroug F, Ouanes-Besbes L, Nciri N, et al. Association of left-heart dysfunction with severe exacerbation of chronic obstructive pulmonary disease: diagnostic performance of cardiac biomarkers. Am J Respir Crit Care Med 2006; 174(9):990–996.

17. Calverley PM, Leggett RJ, McElderry L, et al. Cigarette smoking and secondary polycythemia in hypoxic cor pulmonale. Am Rev Respir Dis 1982; 125(5):507–510.

18. Pitta F, Troosters T, Spruit MA, et al. Characteristics of physical activities in daily life in chronic obstructive pulmonary disease. Am J Respir Crit Care Med 2005; 171(9):972–977.

19. Garcia-Aymerich J, Monso E, Marrades RM, et al. Risk factors for hospitalization for a chronic obstructive pulmonary disease exacerbation. EFRAM study. Am J Respir Crit Care Med JID - 9421642 2001; 164(6):1002–1007.

20. Calverley PM, Howatson R, Flenley DC, et al. Clinicopathological correlations in cor pulmonale. Thorax 1992; 47(7):494–498.

21. Tillie-Leblond I, Marquette CH, Perez T, et al. Pulmonary embolism in patients with unexplained exacerbation of chronic obstructive pulmonary disease: prevalence and risk factors. Ann Intern Med 2006; 144(6):390–396.

22. Rutschmann OT, Cornuz J, Poletti PA, et al. Should pulmonary embolism be suspected in exacerbation of chronic obstructive pulmonary disease? Thorax 2007; 62(2):121–125.

23. Restrepo MI, Mortensen EM, Pugh JA, et al. COPD is associated with increased mortality in patients with community-acquired pneumonia. Eur Respir J 2006; 28(2):346–351.

24. Ernst P, Gonzalez AV, Brassard P, et al. Inhaled corticosteroid use in chronic obstructive pulmonary disease and the risk of hospitalization for pneumonia. Am J Respir Crit Care Med 2007; 176(2):162–166.

25. Wedzicha JA, Calverley PM, Seemungal TA, et al. The prevention of COPD exacerbations by salmeterol/fluticasone propionate or tiotropium bromide. Am J Respir Crit Care Med 2008; 177:19–26.

26. O'Brien C, Guest PJ, Hill SL, et al. Physiological and radiological characterisation of patients diagnosed with chronic obstructive pulmonary disease in primary care. Thorax 2000;55(8):635–642.

27. Patel IS, Vlahos I, Wilkinson TM, et al. Bronchiectasis, exacerbation indices, and inflammation in chronic obstructive pulmonary disease. Am J Respir Crit Care Med 2004; 170(4):400–407.

28. Soler N, Agusti C, Angrill J, et al. Bronchoscopic validation of the significance of sputum purulence in severe exacerbations of chronic obstructive pulmonary disease. Thorax 2007; 62(1):29–35.

29. Wedzicha JA. Exacerbations: etiology and pathophysiologic mechanisms. Chest 2002; 121(5 suppl): 136S–141S.

30. Fabbri LM, Romagnoli M, Corbetta L, et al. Differences in airway inflammation in patients with fixed airflow obstruction due to asthma or chronic obstructive pulmonary disease. Am J Respir Crit Care Med 2003; 167(3):418–424.

31. Delfino RJ, Murphy-Moulton AM, Burnett RT, et al. Effects of air pollution on emergency room visits for respiratory illnesses in Montreal, Quebec. Am J Respir Crit Care Med 1997; 155(2): 568–576.

32. Ko FW, Tam W, Wong TW, et al. Temporal relationship between air pollutants and hospital admissions for chronic obstructive pulmonary disease in Hong Kong. Thorax 2007; 62(9): 780–785.

33. Donaldson GC, Seemungal TA, Patel IS, et al. Longitudinal changes in the nature, severity and frequency of COPD exacerbations. Eur Respir J 2003; 22(6):931–936.

34. Davies L, Wilkinson M, Bonner S, et al. "Hospital at home" versus hospital care in patients with exacerbations of chronic obstructive pulmonary disease: prospective randomised controlled trial. BMJ 2000; 321(7271):1265–1268.

35. Sethi S, Evans N, Grant BJ, et al. New strains of bacteria and exacerbations of chronic obstructive pulmonary disease. N Engl J Med 2002; 347(7):465–471.

# 4
## Symptom Changes at COPD Exacerbation

**TERENCE A. R. SEEMUNGAL**
Department of Clinical Medical Sciences, University of the West Indies, St Augustine Campus, Trinidad and Tobago

## I. Introduction

Chronic obstructive pulmonary disease (COPD) is defined in terms of spirometry (1). Obstruction is thought to be of importance by the patient when there are associated symptoms, and in fact this is when the patient frequently comes to the attention of the physician and the diagnosis is made. Patients older than 40 years usually present with COPD (1). The cardinal symptoms of COPD are dyspnea of effort, cough, and sputum production (1). Other symptoms though present are not thought to be as important, and these include wheeze and chest discomfort. Pedal edema portends right ventricular dysfunction and is an indicator of severity (1).

How a COPD exacerbation is identified has historically been dependent on the type of study being undertaken and at least 18 definitions have been used in the various studies mentioned in this chapter. Thus in the early etiological studies of the 1960s many researchers did not use what we would now call a precise definition, relying on the doctor to make the diagnosis on nonexplicit criteria (2,3). Fletcher, for instance, referred to an undefined term called "chest cold" (4).

Many researchers in the 1970s and 1980s considered cough and sputum to be the most important features of COPD exacerbations, though many of these studies were attempting to determine the contribution of viruses to exacerbations of COPD (5–7). One of the first studies to use explicit symptom criteria was that of McHardy et al. who thought that the most important symptoms were cough, sputum, and wheeze (8). However from Anthonisen onward dyspnea has been considered a prominent symptom of COPD exacerbations. The London COPD study has considered the most important exacerbation symptoms to be increased dyspnea, increased sputum volume, and increased sputum purulence and has conducted a series of studies of patients with COPD yielding some very useful information on several of these symptoms of COPD exacerbation.

## II.  Common Symptoms at Exacerbation

Table 1 shows the symptoms present at exacerbation for four long-term studies. The Anthonisen study was a randomized study of antibiotic use in COPD (9). The Ball and Papi studies (10,11) were cross-sectional studies, with the Ball study being a General Practitioner Database study of exacerbations of chronic bronchitis, which included COPD, but the Seemungal study (12) like the Anthonisen study was a cohort study. The differences in symptoms between the four studies have more to do with study design than actual incidence. The Seemungal study shows symptoms at onset of exacerbation and the Ball study at presentation to the general physician. However the Anthonisen study gives the peak incidence during the exacerbation. All of these studies suggest that increased dyspnea is very common in COPD exacerbation. Sputum changes are also important occurring in most exacerbations (9,10,12,13). Other symptoms such as chest tightness and chest pain have not been much studied, though they are mentioned in the GOLD document (1). By including a cold as an exacerbation symptom (though not by itself) both the Anthonisen and Seemungal studies attempted to relate exacerbations to colds, a point on which we shall expand later.

**Table 1**  Frequency of Different Symptoms at COPD Exacerbation in Four Large-Scale Studies

|  |  | Anthonisen 1987 | Ball 1995 | Seemungal 2000 | Papi 2006 |
|---|---|---|---|---|---|
| Disease and severity |  | COPD | Chronic bronchitis | COPD | COPD |
| Mean $FEV_1$ % |  | 34 | N/A | 42 | 50 |
| Setting |  | Cohort community study | General practitioner database | Cohort community study | Cross-sectional hospital |
| Number of patients |  | 173 | 471 | 101 | 64 |
| Number of exacerbations |  | 448 | 471 | 504 | 64 |
| Major |  |  |  |  |  |
|  | Increased SOB (%) | 90 | 45 | 64 | 95 |
|  | Increased sputum volume (%) | 70 | 76 | 26 | 75 |
|  | Increased sputum purulence (%) | 60 | 66 | 42 | 52 |
| Minor |  |  |  |  |  |
|  | Colds (%) | 52 | N/A | 35 | N/A |
|  | Increased wheeze (%) | 73 | N/A | 35 | N/A |
|  | Increased cough (%) | 82 | N/A | 20 | 75 |

*Abbreviation*: N/A, not available.

## III. Time Course of Symptom Changes

If symptoms change at exacerbation, then it should be possible to plot a time course of these changes. The first study to examine such a time course was the London COPD group (12,14). Daily symptoms were monitored by patient-recorded diary cards, which allowed the patient to score symptom changes in binary code as worsened or not (12,14). A typical diary card is illustrated in Figure 1 (15).

From this study it is possible to define a periexacerbation period of 50 days from 14 days before exacerbation onset to 35 days after onset (Fig. 2). A detailed explanation of the pattern shown in this figure is given below for one exacerbation. In the study of Seemungal et al. (12), the day of onset of exacerbation was defined in terms of the simultaneous occurrence of at least two major symptoms or one major and one minor symptom (Table 1). Figure 2 shows that the frequency of symptoms was maximal at the day of onset and gradually decreased thereafter. Over the prodromal period (the 7 days prior to onset of exacerbation), dyspnea, symptoms of a common cold, sore throat, and cough increased significantly (12). The median time taken for return of symptoms to baseline called the symptom recovery time was seven days.

---

**LONDON COPD STUDY DIARY CARD**
**STUDY NO:**

**NAME:**
**INSTRUCTIONS**

1. On waking, please record your bedroom temperature on your daily record sheet. Please remember to record this from the same locality each morning.

2. At approximately 10 am please record your peak flow reading. Please record only the best of three readings.

3. Please also note to the nearest half hour the amount of time you spend outside of your house daily (to include travelling time).

4. Should you experience any changes in your health as noted below, please contact The Doctor on:

   **0181 528 9001 pager No: 856928.**

Please record any of the following changes in your health in the space provided in this card using the correlating codes A to E2 on the appropriate day.

**A** = Increased shortness of breath
**B1** = Increased sputum colour
**B2** = Increased sputum amount
**C** = Colds
**D** = Increased wheeze and/or chest feels tighter
**E1** = Sore throat
**E2** = Increased cough

**NAME** .................          **DATE NEXT VISIT**.............

---

(A)

**Figure 1** (A) The front page of the diary given to patients in the study. Each patient was given a new diary every month. (**B** continued on page 42) Page 2 of the London COPD study diary card. *Source*: Modified from Ref. 15.

| MONTH_____ | | | | | | | | | | | |
|---|---|---|---|---|---|---|---|---|---|---|---|
| **DATE** | **1** | **2** | **3** | **4** | **5** | **6** | **7** | **8** | **9** | **10** | **11** |
| FEV$_1$<br>FVC<br>**PEAK FLOW (BEST OF 3 READINGS)** | | | | | | | | | | | |
| A.M Bedroom Temperature | | | | | | | | | | | |
| **CHANGE IN SYMPTOMS (A to E2)** | | | | | | | | | | | |
| **NO OF HOURS OUTSIDE OF HOME** | | | | | | | | | | | |
| **DATE** | **12** | **13** | **14** | **15** | **16** | **17** | **18** | **19** | **20** | **21** | **22** |
| FEV$_1$<br>FVC<br>**PEAK FLOW (BEST OF 3 READINGS)** | | | | | | | | | | | |
| A.M Bedroom Temperature | | | | | | | | | | | |
| **CHANGE IN SYMPTOMS (A to E2)** | | | | | | | | | | | |
| **NO OF HOURS OUTSIDE OF HOME** | | | | | | | | | | | |
| **DATE** | **23** | **24** | **25** | **26** | **27** | **28** | **29** | **30** | **31** | | |
| FEV$_1$<br>FVC<br>**PEAK FLOW (BEST OF 3 READINGS)** | | | | | | | | | | | |
| A.M TEMPERATURE | | | | | | | | | | | |
| **CHANGE IN SYMPTOMS (A to E2)** | | | | | | | | | | | |
| **NO OF HOURS OUTSIDE OF HOME** | | | | | | | | | | | |

**(B)**

**Figure 1** (*Continued*)

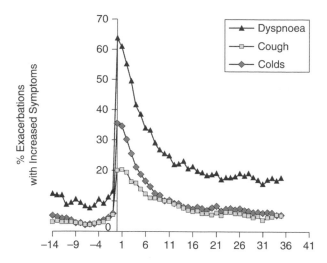

**Figure 2** Time course of symptom changes from 14 days to 35 days after onset of COPD exacerbation. *Source*: Modified from Ref. 12.

## IV. Physiological Basis of Dyspnea and Symptom Recovery

### A. Dyspnea

During exacerbations of COPD, there is reduced elastic recoil of the lung and increased airways resistance leading to sputum retention, mucosal edema, and bronchospasm, and these in turn lead to worsening of baseline expiratory flow limitation (16). Time course studies of physiological variables during and after COPD exacerbations all show that forced expiratory volume ($FEV_1$), forced vital capacity (FVC), inspiratory capacity, and total lung capacity all increase following an exacerbation, while there is a decrease in functional residual capacity and residual volume (12,17). During COPD exacerbations the primary mechanical anomalies are (*i*) worsening expiratory airflow limitation, which gives rise to (*ii*) dynamic hyperinflation, and both of these lead to inspiratory muscle dysfunction. Airflow limitation leads to hypoxia and hypercarbia, but the ensuing increased ventilatory drive is ineffective because of factors (*i*) and (*ii*). Neuromechanical uncoupling then occurs leading to the sensation of dyspnea (16).

### B. Lung Function

It has been suggested that change in resting inspiratory capacity postbronchodilator is the strongest predictor of subsequent improvement in exercise capacity (18). Also, Stevenson et al. (19) found that patients reporting less breathlessness at the time of discharge from hospital for a COPD exacerbation were those in whom inspiratory capacity improved most during recovery. However this result is not consistent between all studies of inspiratory capacity (20). Studies using expiratory flow measures such as peak expiratory flow (PEF) or FEV$_1$ appear to have more reproducible results. Significantly greater fall in PEF at onset of exacerbation have been related to increased dyspnea, increased wheeze, and presence of a cold (12).

## V.  The Concept of Recovery of Symptoms and Lung Function

Figure 3 shows two daily plots for London COPD study patient during one exacerbation. Figure 3A shows the daily PEF on the vertical axis and time before and after exacerbation onset on the horizontal axis. Analysis of daily PEF in COPD patients during an exacerbation revealed early on a wide day-to-day variability in this parameter (12). Thus the London COPD study used a three-day moving average PEF to avoid false early recoveries when PEF improved for just a single day (as occurred on day 14 for this patient) but then

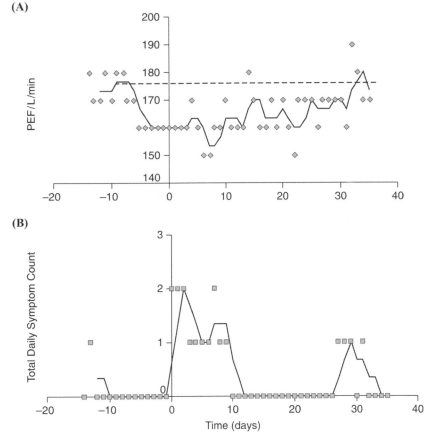

**Figure 3**  Time course of peak expiratory flow and daily total symptom count before and after a COPD exacerbation for one patient from the London COPD cohort: the moving average is shown by the continuous line. For explanation please see text.

remained below baseline for a few more days. The three-day moving average PEF was calculated as follows: e.g., for this patient, the three-day moving average PEF for day 5 is the mean of the sum of three parameters, actual PEF on day 4, actual PEF on day 5, and actual PEF on day 6. The three-day moving average PEF is shown as a continuous line in Figure 3A. Finally, the baseline PEF was taken as the mean PEF for the seven days from days 14 to 8 prior to onset of exacerbation, and this is shown by the doted line in Figure 3 A. Using this approach recovery is said to occur on the first day that the three-day moving average PEF reached baseline as occurred at about day 32 in Figure 3A. Thus the PEF recovery time for this exacerbation is 32 days.

PEF was a continuous variable, but a deterioration in symptoms was measured as a discrete variable and scored on an "on or off" basis as 1 or 0, respectively (12). Thus the total number of symptoms present could be scored as the total daily symptom count, and this is shown in Figure 3B. A three-day moving average was calculated as for PEF, and this is shown as a continuous line in Figure 3B. Here we see that the total daily symptom score was 2 at the day of onset of exacerbation (day, 0) and that this had recovered to baseline by day 12 using the three-day moving average approach. By comparing the Figures 3A and 3B, we can see that symptom recovery was complete by day 12 and so for this exacerbation, the symptom recovery time was 12 days for this patient but the PEF recovery time was much longer. This illustrates the lag of PEF recovery behind symptoms referred to earlier.

Figure 3B also illustrates another feature of COPD and this is a deterioration in symptoms around day 30, but this did not constitute an exacerbation and demonstrates the daily variability in COPD symptomatology. Comparison of PEF at two weeks prior to onset of exacerbation with that during an exacerbation also allows us to illustrate a further feature of COPD. Figure 3A shows that though the overall change in PEF between stable state and exacerbation is just about 20 L/min, a relatively small difference, there is a marked difference in lung function variability between stable state at two prior to onset of exacerbation and during the exacerbation.

## A.  Recovery of Lung Function and Symptoms

Using expiratory flow measures, Seemungal et al. related symptom changes at exacerbation to lung function changes, which showed a similar time course as measured by PEF and $FEV_1$ (12). The median PEF recovery time to baseline was seven days. Recovery time for PEF was longer in the presence of dyspnea or symptoms of a common cold at exacerbation onset, though there was no effect of sputum purulence or increased sputum volume. Exacerbations associated with wheeze had a shorter PEF recovery time. Though these relationships were all highly significant, the correlation coefficients were all low (<0.25), thus indicating that the contribution to prolonged recovery time is low. By 90 days 91% of exacerbations had recovered to baseline symptoms but only 75% had recovered to baseline PEF (12). Thus symptom recovery appears to lag behind lung function recovery.

## B.  Failure to Recover

One of the interesting outcomes of the study of time course of an exacerbation was that 14% of exacerbations had not returned to baseline symptoms at 35 days and further that at three months 9.3% or 3.1% of exacerbations had failed to return to baseline PEF or symptoms, respectively. These patients have been referred to as nonrecoverers (21).

## VI.  Changes in Symptoms and Airway and Systemic Inflammation

The symptoms of a common cold (rhinorrhea and/or nasal congestion) are associated with increased exacerbation sputum IL-6 levels: median levels being 177.7 pg/mL with a cold and 70.6 pg/mL without (22). Wedzicha and colleagues also showed that plasma fibrinogen, a marker of systemic inflammation, was higher in exacerbations associated with colds, purulent sputum, and increased cough (23). Thus symptom changes at exacerbations are related both to systemic and sputum inflammatory markers. These studies also support the notion that cold symptoms are important contributors to the symptom complex at COPD exacerbation.

Perera and colleagues studied inflammatory mediators associated with failure to recover to baseline symptoms after an exacerbation (21). They found that 23% of exacerbations had not recovered to baseline symptoms by day 35, with no differences in treatment between the two groups. They then showed that patients who did not recover to baseline symptoms at day 35 had a persistently higher serum C-reactive protein (CRP), sputum IL-6, and sputum IL-8 during the recovery period, thus indicating that in the patients in whom exacerbations do not recover to baseline symptoms at day 35, there is prolonged systemic and airway inflammation. The magnitude of the increase in sputum IL-8 at exacerbation was directly related to the symptom recovery time. This may well indicate a failure to respond to short-course therapy at exacerbation. These studies have now established relationships between the nonrecovery of airway inflammation and symptom changes at exacerbation of COPD (21).

## VII.  Frequency of Symptom Changes and Recurrent Exacerbations

Exacerbations as defined by symptom changes have been shown to be more frequent in COPD patients with poorer quality of life scores (14). Quality of life scores are symptom dependent, and so this may not have been unexpected. However Bhowmik and colleagues successfully showed for the first time in 2000 that these frequent exacerbators have a higher baseline sputum IL-6 (22). Using serum CRP, Perera and colleagues later showed that there was slower resolution of exacerbation inflammatory markers in the frequent exacerbator group (21). Perera also studied the exacerbations, following closely upon an index exacerbation, i.e., within 50 days of onset of the index exacerbation and found that common cold symptoms were significantly associated with both events. This suggests that patients who develop recurrent exacerbations may be more susceptible to viral respiratory infections, as observed in one large-scale epidemiological study (24).

## VIII.  Symptom Changes and New and Colonizing Strains of Bacteria

Patel and colleagues examined the sputum of COPD patients for several species of bacteria and found that COPD patients colonized by *Haemophilus influenzae* in the stable state reported more symptoms and increased sputum purulence at exacerbation than those not colonized (25). There was also a trend in these patients toward more cough symptoms at exacerbation and a longer time to recovery of peak flow than those not colonized, although these findings just failed to reach statistical significance (25). Sethi and colleagues, defining exacerbations similarly but with more sputum producers in their cohort, have found that worsening of symptoms are associated with the acquisition of new strains of bacteria; however, these authors did not attempt to relate specific symptom changes to detection of bacteria (26).

## IX.   Symptom Changes and Viruses

In a study of 168 COPD exacerbations, the occurrence of a cold, sore throat, or cold with increased dyspnea as well as the presence of more symptoms at onset of exacerbation were all related to detection of a virus in nasal aspirates by polymerase chain reaction (PCR). A similar study of viruses using sputum sampling found that virus detection was related to the presence of a cold with increased sputum volume at exacerbation (27). Figure 4 shows that when a virus was detected the proportion of exacerbations recovering to baseline symptoms was much smaller than when a virus was not detected, suggesting that virus detection in these patients was related to severity of exacerbation (28). In the presence of viruses, the median daily total symptom count recovery time was 13 days, which was longer than that of six days for nonviral exacerbations. Further, the rate of recovery was faster in the absence of a virus detected by PCR. Their data suggest that viruses are associated with prolonged COPD exacerbations and thus with greater morbidity. Further, most virus infections are

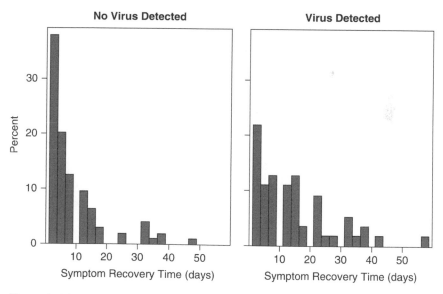

**Figure 4**   Histograms showing the proportions of exacerbations recovering at different times after onset of exacerbation when a virus was detected in nasal aspirates and when a virus was not detected. Within the first 10 days 60% of nonviral exacerbations had recovered as opposed to 44% of viral exacerbations. *Source*: Based on Ref. 2828.

generally more common during the winter, when hospitalization for COPD exacerbation is more frequent.

## X.  Symptom Changes and Environmental Factors

In a one-year study of COPD subjects, Donaldson and colleagues found that nasal congestion and exacerbation were significantly related to low outdoor temperatures and that nasal congestion and increased sputum volume were related low bedroom temperatures (29). Air pollutant changes and symptom changes in COPD have not been prospectively studied, but relationships may be inferred from the work of Anderson et al. in the APHEA project in which they showed that air pollution is associated with daily admissions for chronic obstructive pulmonary disease in European cities with widely varying climates (30). Their results were broadly consistent with those from North America, though the coefficients for particulates were substantially smaller (31–35). These studies show that symptom changes at COPD exacerbation are related to environmental stimuli.

## XI.  Symptoms and Treatment

### A.  Treatment

Several randomized controlled trials of systemic steroids have considered the effects of treatment on exacerbations of COPD but most have used hospitalization as an indication without studying symptom evolution (36–38). However Sayiner and colleagues compared methyl prednisolone 0.3 mg/kg for three days with a 10-day regime of the same treatment and found that the 10-day treatment group had a faster recovery in dyspnea with no difference in relapse rates (39). The London COPD study also reported that exacerbations treated with oral prednisolone were less likely to have symptom relapse (12) and that early treatment was associated with faster symptom resolution (40).

### B.  Untreated Exacerbations

The use of a symptom approach to the detection of exacerbation allows for the diagnosis of exacerbations not treated by a clinician. By their very nature these untreated exacerbations are unlikely ever to have been sampled for biomarkers. No consensus has so far emerged on the importance of these so-called untreated exacerbations but they may contribute to a lower quality of life (40). Thus one can infer from the randomized controlled trials above that an exacerbation associated with treatment should always be treated with systemic steroids, but these data may not be as robust as they initially appear.

### C.  Severity

There is no consensus on exacerbation severity indicators. The relationship of recovery time to inflammation and relation of inflammation to COPD pathogenesis would support a hypothesis that duration of an exacerbation (recovery time) is a severity indicator (12). Further, the level of treatment and occurrence of new signs have both been included in the GOLD document as indicators of severity. However of all indicators studied so far, the only one that has been related to mortality has been level of treatment determined by admission to hospital or not (41).

## XII. Conclusion and Recommendations

COPD exacerbations have been detected by changes in symptoms for at least 30 years. Results of several studies have revealed useful information using this approach. This has lead to the discovery of several different phenotypes of COPD exacerbations: exacerbations characterized mainly by dyspnea without sputum changes, nonrecovered exacerbations, and recurrent exacerbations. Further work has revealed raised levels inflammatory markers in the airways of patients who are slow to recover from their exacerbations. Because of the inherent variability in COPD symptomatology, a plot of symptoms against time may lead to underestimation of the total recovery time. Thus the smoothing of the day-to-day variability allowed for by a moving average approach avoids this underestimation. There have been no studies of what the size of the moving average should be. Intuitively it would seem obvious that if median recovery is about one week, then a three-day moving average would be optimal.

Finally, we consider those patients who do not recover. There are no clear predictive factors for the nonrecoverer nor are there any epidemiological studies of the health burden of nonrecovery. However until the implications of nonrecovery are clarified, it may be advised that patients with COPD exacerbations should be routinely seen at about five weeks after an exacerbation to determine recovery status. Though there is no consensus on how failure to recover should be managed, results of randomized controlled trials of treatment and relapse of exacerbations and the work of Perera et al. would appear to support further treatment with systemic steroids if a nonrecoverer is detected at that stage (21).

## References

1. Global Initiative for Chronic Obstructive Lung Disease, . Global Strategy for the Diagnosis, Management, and Prevention of COPD. Summary of GOLD recommendations, with citations from the scientific literature. Revised 2006. Available at: http://www.goldcopd.com/Guide-lineitem.asp?ll=2&l2=1&intId=996.
2. Stark JE, Heath RB, Curwen MP. Infection with influenza and parainfluenza viruses in chronic bronchitis. Thorax 1965; 20:124–127.
3. Stott EJ, Grist NR, Eadie MB. Rhinovirus infections in chronic bronchitis: isolation of eight possible new rhinovirus serotypes. J Med Microbiol 1968; 1:109–117.
4. Fletcher C, Peto R. The natural history of chronic airflow obstruction. BMJ 1977; 1:1645–1648.
5. Monto AS, Higgins MW, Ross HW. The Tecumseh study of respiratory illness. VIII. Acute infection in chronic respiratory disease and comparison groups. Am Rev Infect Dis 1975; 111:27–36.
6. Smith CB, Golden C, Klauber MR, et al. Interactions between viruses and bacteria in patients with chronic bronchitis. J Infect Dis 1976; 134:552–561.
7. Gump DW, Phillips CA, Forsyth BR. Role of infection in chronic bronchitis. Am Rev Respir Dis 1976; 113:465–473.
8. McHardy VU, Inglis JM, Calder MA, et al. A study of infective and other factors in exacerbations of chronic bronchitis. Br J Dis Chest 1980; 74:228–238.
9. Anthonisen NR, Manfreda J, Warren CP, et al. Antibiotic therapy in exacerbations of chronic obstructive pulmonary disease. Ann Intern Med 1987; 106:196–204.

10. Ball P, Harris JM, Lowson D. Acute infective exacerbations of chronic bronchitis. Q J Med 1995; 88:61–68.
11. Papi A, Bellettato CM, Braccioni F, et al. Infections and airway inflammation in chronic obstructive pulmonary disease severe exacerbations. Am J Respir Crit Care Med 2006; 173:1114–1121.
12. Seemungal TAR, Donaldson GC, Bhowmik A, et al. Time course and recovery of exacerbations in patients with chronic obstructive pulmonary disease. Am J Respir Crit Care Med 2000; 161:1608–1618.
13. Woolhouse IS, Hill SL, Stockley RA. Symptom resolution assessed using a patient directed diary card during treatment of acute exacerbation of chronic bronchitis. Thorax 2001; 56:947–953.
14. Seemungal T, Donaldson GC, Paul EA, et al. Effect of exacerbation on quality of life in patients with chronic obstructive pulmonary disease. Am J Respir Crit Care Med 1998; 157:1418–1422.
15. Seemungal TAR. COPD exacerbations: aetiology and effects on the airways and plasma fibrinogen. A dissertation for the degree of Doctor of Philosophy. University of London. 2002:70–71.
16. O'Donnell DE, Parker CM. COPD exacerbations 3: pathophysiology. Thorax 2006; 61:354–361.
17. Parker CM, Voduc N, Aaron SD, et al. Physiological changes during symptom recovery from moderate exacerbations of COPD. Eur Respir J 2005; 26:420–428.
18. O'Donnell DE, Lam M, Webb KA. Spirometric correlates of improvement in exercise performance after anticholinergic therapy in chronic obstructive pulmonary disease. Am J Respir Crit Care Med 1999; 160:542–549.
19. Stevenson NJ, Walker PP, Costello RW, et al. Lung mechanics and dyspnoea during exacerbations of chronic obstructive pulmonary disease. Am J Respir Crit Care Med 2005; 172:1510–1516.
20. Johnson MK, Birch M, Carter R, et al. Measurement of physiological recovery from exacerbation of chronic obstructive pulmonary disease using within-breath forced oscillometry. Thorax 2007; 62(4):299–306 (epub 2006, Nov 14).
21. Perera WR, Hurst JR, Wilkinson TMA, et al. Inflammatory changes, recovery and recurrence at COPD exacerbation. Eur Respir J 2007; 29(8):527–534.
22. Bhowmik A, Seemungal TAR, Sapsford RJ, et al. Relation of sputum inflammatory markers to symptoms and lung function changes in COPD exacerbations. Thorax 2000; 55:114–120.
23. Wedzicha JA, Seemungal TAR, MacCallum PK, et al. Acute exacerbations of chronic obstructive pulmonary disease are accompanied by elevations of plasma fibrinogen and serum IL-6 levels. Thromb Haemost 2000; 84:210–215.
24. Hurst JR, Donaldson GC, Wilkinson TMA, et al. Epidemiological relationships between the common cold and exacerbation frequency in COPD. Eur Respir J 2005; 26:846–852.
25. Patel SI, Seemungal TAR, Wilks M, et al. Relation of haemophilus influenzae colonisation to exacerbation frequency in COPD. Thorax 2002; 57:759–764.
26. Sethi S, Evans N, Grant BJ, et al. New strains of bacteria and exacerbations of chronic obstructive pulmonary disease. N Engl J Med 2002; 347:465–471.
27. Seemungal TAR, Harper-Owen R, Bhowmik A, et al. Detection of rhinovirus in induced sputum at exacerbation of chronic obstructive pulmonary disease. Eur Respir J 2000; 16:677–683.
28. Seemungal TAR, Harper-Owen R, Bhowmik A, et al. Respiratory viruses and symptoms, inflammatory markers in acute exacerbations of COPD. Am J Respir Crit Care Med 2001; 1618–1623.
29. Donaldson GC, Seemungal T, Jeffries DJ, et al. Effect of temperature on lung function and symptoms in chronic obstructive pulmonary disease. Eur Respir J 1999; 13:844–849.
30. Anderson HR, Spix C, Medina S, et al. Air pollution and daily admissions for chronic obstructive pulmonary disease in 6 European cities: results from the APHEA project. Eur Respir J 1997; 10: 1064–1071.
31. Burnett RT, Dales R, Kewski D, et al. Associations between ambient particulate sulfate and admissions to Ontario hospitals for cardiac and respiratory diseases. Am J Epidemiol 1995; 142: 15–22.
32. Schwartz J. Air pollution and hospital admissions for the elderly in Birmingham, Alabama. Am J Epidemiol 1994; 139:589–598.

33. Schwartz J. Air pollution and hospital admissions for the elderly in Detroit Michigan. Am J Respir Crit Care Med 1994; 150:648–655.
34. Schwartz J. Air pollution and hospital admissions for the elderly in Minneapolis-St. Paul, Minnesota. Arch Environ Health 1994; 49:366–374.
35. Schwartz J. Air pollution and hospital admissions for respiratory disease. Epidemiology 1996; 7:20–28.
36. Aaron SD, Vandemheen KL, Hebert P, et al. Outpatient oral prednisone after emergency treatment of chronic obstructive pulmonary disease. N Engl J Med 2003; 348:2618–2625.
37. Davies L, Angus RM, Calverley PMA. Oral corticosteroids in patients admitted to hospital with exacerbations of chronic obstructive pulmonary disease: a prospective randomised controlled trial. Lancet 1999; 354:456–460.
38. Niewoehner DE, Erbland ML, Deupree RH, et al. Effect of systemic glucocorticoids on exacerbations of chronic obstructive pulmonary disease. Department of Veterans Affairs Cooperative Study Group. N Engl J Med 1999; 340:1941–1947.
39. Sayiner A, Aytemur ZA, Cirit M, et al. Systemic glucocorticoids in severe exacerbations of COPD. Chest 2001; 119:726–730.
40. Wilkinson TMA, Donaldson GC, Hurst JR, et al. Early therapy improves outcomes of exacerbations of chronic obstructive pulmonary disease. Am J Respir Crit Care Med 2004; 169:1298–1303 (epub 2004, Feb 27).
41. Soler-Cataluña JJ, Martínez-García MA, Román Sánchez P, et al. Severe acute exacerbations and mortality in patients with chronic obstructive pulmonary disease. Thorax 2005; 60:925–931.

# 5

# Airway Pathology at Exacerbations

**GRAZIELLA TURATO, SIMONETTA BARALDO, KIM LOKAR-OLIANI, RENZO ZUIN, and MARINA SAETTA**
Department of Cardiac, Thoracic, and Vascular Sciences, University of Padova, Padova, Italy

## I. Introduction

COPD is a chronic disease, which is characterized by not fully reversible airflow limitation and progressive decline of lung function, exercise capacity, and health status. Stable COPD is characterized by a chronic inflammation of the entire bronchial tree with increased numbers of macrophages and $CD8^+$ T lymphocytes in the airway wall and of neutrophils in the airway lumen (1–4). Episodes of symptom exacerbations punctuate the natural course of the disease and are associated with acute worsening of the existing airway inflammation (5). Exacerbations of COPD may be defined by a change in the patient's baseline dyspnea, cough, and/or sputum that is beyond day-to-day variations, is acute in onset and may require a change in regular medication (6,7).

Clinical signs of COPD exacerbations are highly variable and the impending onset of an exacerbation is difficult to predict. Changes in lung function immediately before exacerbation are small and not very useful in predicting the worsening of COPD symptoms. In fact, decreases in peak expiratory flow rate (PEFR) or forced expiratory volume in 1 second ($FEV_1$) are also poorly sensitive in detecting the onset of the exacerbations, even when these parameters are measured daily. This may be due to individual variability, which is larger than the mean change occurring during an exacerbation (5). On the other hand, it should be highlighted that large decreases in PEFR are associated with both degree of dyspnea during the exacerbation and duration of hospitalization (8,9).

The frequency of exacerbations has an impact on a patient's health status and quality of life. Recently, Donaldson and coworkers pointed out that the frequency of exacerbation plays a role in the natural history of the disease. Indeed, they demonstrated for the first time that the frequency of acute exacerbations is an important contributing factor to long-term decline in lung function in COPD (10). Moreover, patients who experience frequent exacerbations in one year are likely to have a higher exacerbation frequency in the following years (11), and those affected by severe COPD are most likely to develop severe exacerbations characterized by acute respiratory failure (12).

The etiology of COPD exacerbations is associated with trigger factors. Recent studies have shown that viral or bacterial infections may trigger these episodes (13,14). Non-infective agents may also play a role. In fact, air pollution may account for approximately

6% to 9% of hospital admissions (15), and reduced temperatures have been associated with a decline in lung function and frequency of exacerbation (16).

## II.  Airway Pathology During Exacerbations

The pathological hallmark of COPD exacerbations is the worsening of the underlying chronic airway inflammation that characterizes the disease. To better understand the nature of this acute-on-chronic inflammation, it is important to briefly highlight the pathological milieu of stable COPD. The presence of a marked inflammatory infiltrate has been observed in the airway and lung tissue of patients in a stable state of the disease. An increase of CD8$^+$ T lymphocytes and macrophages is an important feature of the inflammatory process present in the subepithelium of central airways, which are the main sites of mucus hypersecretion, clinically expressed as chronic bronchitis (1–3). Neutrophils, which are scanty in the subepithelium, are increased in airway lumen (4) and in bronchial glands of COPD subjects (17). This latter location suggests that neutrophils may have a crucial role in mucus hypersecretion, since neutrophil elastase is a remarkably potent secretagogue.

Mucus hypersecretion in patients with stable COPD may have important functional consequences not only in the central but also in the peripheral airways, which are the main sites of increased resistance and, therefore, of airflow obstruction. Indeed, an increased number of mucus-secreting goblet cells associated with an increased number of neutrophils has been reported in the peripheral airway epithelium of COPD patients (18). The resulting excess production of mucus has the potential to alter the surface tension of the airway-lining fluid, rendering the peripheral airways unstable and thereby facilitating their closure. Moreover, the excess of mucus may also cause lumen occlusion by the formation of mucus plugs. Hogg and coworkers have recently shown that, in patients with severe COPD, occlusion of peripheral airways by inflammatory exudates containing mucus is predictive of early death (19). In addition to goblet cell hyperplasia, other pathological lesions are present in peripheral airways of patients with COPD, including airway remodeling (fibrosis and smooth muscle hypertrophy) and airway wall inflammation (1), in particular, CD8$^+$ T-lymphocyte infiltration (20). It should be highlighted that this cell type is also increased in the central airways as well as in lung parenchyma, suggesting that it plays a crucial role in the pathophysiology of COPD (3,21). Indeed, the accumulation of CD8$^+$ T cells in all these compartments is correlated to the degree of airflow limitation (3,20,21).

The inflammatory process in COPD is promoted by the coordinated action of different proinflammatory cytokines, including interleukin 8 (CXCL8), which enhances neutrophil chemotaxis; tumor necrosis factor alpha (TNF-$\alpha$) and interleukin-1$\beta$(IL-1$\beta$), which activate adhesion molecules; leukotriene B4 (LTB4) and growth-related oncogene alpha (GRO-$\alpha$), which are powerful chemoattractants for neutrophils and T lymphocytes.

The inflammatory process is amplified during exacerbations with recruitment of neutrophils and eosinophils, which become the major component of the inflammatory response (22,23). Hence, the worsening of inflammation, not only in the lung but also systemically, is now thought to be the key factor in the pathogenesis of exacerbations of COPD.

### A.  Neutrophils

Only a few pathological studies have examined COPD patients close to or during an exacerbation, because of the difficulty to collect bronchial biopsies from patients in such a compromised clinical condition. Nevertheless, examination of bronchial biopsies, bronchoalveolar lavage, and spontaneous or induced sputum has consistently revealed increased airway inflammation and elevated levels of inflammatory cytokines in these patients (22–27). In particular, exacerbations of COPD are characterized by a notable recruitment of neutrophils (22,23), which appear to be mediated by different molecules. Indeed, the upregulation of the neutrophil chemoattractants CXCL5 (ENA-78) and CXCL8 (IL-8) and of their receptors CXCR1 and CXCR2 has been observed in studies performed on bronchial biopsy and airway secretions in severe and very severe exacerbations of COPD (22,23). Furthermore, an increase in the expression of LTB4, mieloperoxidase, and TNF-$\alpha$ is also associated with exacerbations (28–30). LTB4 is an important mediator of neutrophil recruitment, mieloperoxidase is a marker of neutrophil activation, and TNF-$\alpha$ is an inducer of endothelial cell adhesion molecules, which facilitate the influx of leukocytes into the airway tissue.

Augmented neutrophilic inflammation seems to be a feature of COPD exacerbations, independent of the presence of bacterial and/or viral infection. In a recent study, sputum analysis was performed in patients experiencing severe exacerbations requiring hospitalization (14). The presence of respiratory infection (viral, bacterial, or concomitant viral and bacterial infections) was found in 78% of cases. Interestingly, neutrophilia and neutrophil elastase levels were equally increased in bacterial, viral, and no-detected agent exacerbations. Although sputum purulence was found to be higher in infective than in noninfective exacerbations, it was not different in patients with viral or bacterial infections. Therefore, it appears that, in contrast with previous reports (30,31), sputum purulence may be unable to identify the infective agent involved in COPD exacerbation.

The emerging concept today is that an amplification of airway inflammation is of key importance in the pathogenesis of exacerbations. Neutrophil inflammation causes mucus gland hyperplasia and mucus hypersecretion and a consequent worsening of respiratory symptoms. Moreover, elevated markers of neutrophilic inflammation in sputum are associated with an increased vascular protein leakage, which may lead to edema of the airway wall, thereby contributing to airway narrowing.

The importance of neutrophils in exacerbation of COPD is further supported by the observation that the percentage of neutrophils in the distal airspace is correlated with the severity of airflow obstruction. In fact, the ratio $FEV_1/FVC$ was found to decrease as neutrophilic inflammation increased (5). This suggests that neutrophil recruitment during exacerbations may play a significant role in the progression of COPD and that patients with repeated exacerbations are more likely to experience a faster decline in lung function.

Indeed, activated neutrophils migrate through connective tissue and release enzymes, which can degrade extracellular matrix, leading to a proteinase/antiproteinase imbalance. Therefore, the increased recruitment of neutrophils during COPD exacerbations and the consequent release of enzymes may lead to the tissue damage that is believed to be crucial to disease progression.

## B. Eosinophils

The analysis of bronchial biopsies obtained from patients with mild-to-severe COPD exacerbations showed an increase of eosinophils in the airway bronchial mucosa (26,27) (Fig. 1). This finding was initially debated until further studies demonstrated the importance of eosinophilic inflammation in COPD exacerbation (24,32,33). In particular, a subsequent study found that the expression of RANTES, a known inducer of eosinophil recruitment,

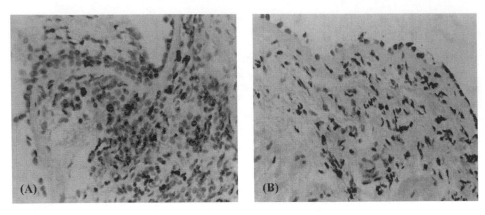

**Figure 1** Bronchial biopsies sections showing eosinophil infiltration in a COPD subject examined during an exacerbation (panel **A**) as compared with a COPD subject in stable conditions (panel **B**). Immunostaining with anti-EG2. *Abbreviation*: COPD, chronic obstructive pulmonary disease.

was increased in airway mucosa at exacerbations of the disease (24). The higher expression of RANTES may be mediated by TNF-$\alpha$, which is upregulated during exacerbations (29), thereby potentially driving the recruitment of eosinophils. Enhanced levels of eotaxin-1, a chemokine involved in eosinophil recruitment and activation, and its receptor CCR3 have also been reported at exacerbation (24). These cytokine pathways could further contribute to eosinophil recruitment in airway wall. Furthermore, several studies have shown that eosinophils are also increased in sputum during exacerbations (32,33), and levels of eosinophil cationic protein in serum and sputum are higher in patients with exacerbations than in those with stable COPD (14,33).

Although the importance of the eosinophilia remains to be clarified, it is known that several eosinophil products (eosinophil peroxidase, major basic protein, eosinophil cationic protein, metalloproteinases, platelet-activating factor, and cysteinyl leukotrienes) may cause inflammatory damage to the airways and worsen bronchial obstruction.

It is also well known that viral infections are able to induce lower airway eosinophilia and production of proinflammatory mediators, which promote eosinophil recruitment (34,35). Interestingly, an increased number of eosinophils in sputum were observed only in exacerbations associated with viral infections, suggesting that sputum eosinophilia may be a marker for a viral trigger of exacerbation (14).

## C. T Lymphocytes

T-cell-mediated immunity performs a crucial task in stable COPD; however, the role it plays in exacerbations is still relatively unknown. Recently, changes in sputum T-lymphocyte subpopulations were examined in severe COPD exacerbations (36), and results showed a decrease of the cell ratio CD4$^+$/CD8$^+$ as compared with stable conditions. This observation suggests an imbalance in T-lymphocyte subpopulations with a further shift toward the CD8$^+$ cell-mediated immune response in severe COPD exacerbations.

Moreover, evidence exists that $CD8^+$ cells may cooperate with RANTES to enhance apoptosis of virally infected cells, and it has been shown that RANTES is increased at exacerbations (24). Thus, as hypothesised by Zhu and coworkers, viral exacerbations and the consequent RANTES overexpression may promote $CD8^+$ cell-mediated tissue damage (24). Therefore, increased frequency of viral exacerbations may destroy airway and alveolar tissue directly, encouraging the development of microscopic emphysema. In this way, repeated exacerbations may accelerate the decline in lung function in smokers. Support for this hypothesis is given by the recent observation that the frequency of exacerbations is an important factor in determining the decline of $FEV_1$ in COPD (10).

### D.  Soluble Mediators in COPD Exacerbations

Several inflammatory markers are increased in the lung during COPD exacerbations.

TNF-$\alpha$ is increased in sputum at exacerbation (29) and could facilitate cell migration by contributing to the upregulation of endothelial adhesion molecules. Moreover, it may be able to increase the expression of RANTES and may indirectly modulate eosinophil recruitment and $CD8^+$ cell-mediated tissue damage (24).

Sputum IL-6 is also increased, especially in exacerbations associated with the common cold (5,34,37,38). Moreover, increased levels of sputum IL-6 are associated with experimental rhinovirus infection in healthy subjects and in patients with asthma (5,37,38). These findings suggest that elevated levels of IL-6 in sputum could be markers of virus-related exacerbation.

Excessive production of elastases and other proteinases, produced by increased numbers of neutrophils and macrophages, may cause epithelial damage, reduce ciliary beat frequency, stimulate mucus secretion by goblet cells, and increase the permeability of the bronchial mucosa, resulting in airway edema and protein exudation into the airways (5). These changes, especially in the small airways, may adversely affect airflow and lead to increased breathlessness as well as to the mucus secretion and purulence that are characteristic of most exacerbations.

Among soluble mediators, endothelin-1 has been proposed as a possible mediator for increased airflow obstruction through the induction of bronchospasm. In addition, endothelin-1 may stimulate mucus secretion, promote airway edema, increase vascular and airway smooth muscle proliferation, and upregulate production of cytokines (5,39). Recently, concentrations of endothelin-1 were shown to be increased in induced sputum at exacerbation, suggesting that it may have a role in the pathophysiology of the worsening of COPD symptoms during acute episodes (39).

Oxidative stress is also increased in the lung during COPD exacerbations, possibly due to a large burden of activated inflammatory cells (5). The newly recruited neutrophils participate in oxidative stress through the activation of oxidant-sensitive transcription factors that lead to increased expression of proinflammatory genes. Critical to the effects of oxidative stress is the protective counterbalance of antioxidant systems. A shift in this oxidant-antioxidant balance could result in an increase in oxidative stress that may cause cellular damage. In this regard, glutathione appears to be an important antioxidant in the lungs and is present in high concentrations in the epithelial-lining fluid (40). During severe COPD exacerbations, glutathione is depleted, indicating increased oxidative stress (28). Several other indirect markers of oxidative stress have been investigated in exhaled breath condensate: notably, both hydrogen peroxide and 8-isoprostane concentrations are increased at exacerbation (41,42), suggesting the involvement of oxidative stress in acute episodes.

The inflammatory changes occurring in the lung during exacerbations may be associated with concomitant systemic events. Plasma biomarkers of inflammation, even though not useful in predicting/determining the clinical severity of exacerbation, have been demonstrated to increase during these acute events (43). In particular, serum C-reactive protein (CRP), in the presence of aggravated symptoms, is a potential marker for the confirmation of COPD exacerbation and, therefore, useful in the choice of therapeutic management. Moreover, patients with frequent exacerbations showed a faster rise in plasma fibrinogen over time (44), and increased levels of CRP and plasma fibrinogen are known to be associated with a higher risk for cardiovascular morbidity. These data support the recently proposed theory that the systemic inflammation present in COPD patients is associated with cardiovascular and systemic effects (45). The increase of this systemic inflammation during exacerbation may aggravate these extrapulmonary diseases, leading to important chronic and acute clinical manifestations.

## III. Summary

Chronic obstructive pulmonary disease (COPD) is a disabling disease that places a social and economic burden on health care systems around the world. It is a major cause of chronic morbidity, mortality, and a decline in health status. The disease is characterized by fixed airflow limitation and progressive reduction in lung function and is punctuated by exacerbations. These episodes of worsening of symptoms are an important cause of hospitalization, and they have a considerable impact on quality of life.

In stable COPD, the airflow limitation is associated with an ongoing inflammatory response involving the entire tracheobronchial tree, characterized by an increase of CD8[+] T lymphocytes, macrophages, and neutrophils. During exacerbation, this inflammatory pattern changes; it is more marked with recruitment of neutrophils and eosinophils, which become the major component of the inflammatory response. Moreover, COPD exacerbations may accelerate the progression of lung function deterioration, which makes prevention of these episodes a priority. Finally, the increased systemic inflammation present in COPD patients during an exacerbation may lead to aggravation of the extrapulmonary complications, adding further to the burden of patients and health care providers.

### References

1. Saetta M, Turato G, Maestrelli P, et al. Cellular and structural bases of chronic obstructive pulmonary disease. Am J Respir Crit Care Med 2001; 163:1304–1309.
2. Saetta M, Di Stefano A, Maestrelli P, et al. Activated T-lymphocytes and macrophages in bronchial mucosa of subjects with chronic bronchitis. Am Rev Respir Dis 1993; 147:301–306.
3. O'Shaughnessy TC, Ansari TW, Barnes NC, et al. Inflammation in bronchial biopsies of subjects with chronic bronchitis: inverse relationship of CD8[+] T lymphocytes with FEV1. Am J Respir Crit Care Med 1997; 155:852–857.
4. Martin TR, Raghu G, Maunder RJ, et al. The effects of chronic bronchitis and chronic air flow obstruction on lung cell populations recovered by bronchoalveolar lavage. Am Rev Respir Dis 1985; 132:254–260.

5.  Papi A, Luppi F, Franco F, et al. Pathophysiology of exacerbations of chronic obstructive pulmonary disease. Proc Am Thorac Soc 2006; 3:245–251.
6.  Rabe KF, Hurd S, Anzueto A, et al. Global strategy for the diagnosis, management, and prevention of chronic obstructive pulmonary disease: GOLD executive summary. Am J Respir Crit Care Med 2007; 176:532–555.
7.  Wedzicha JA, Seemungal TA. COPD exacerbations: defining their cause and prevention. Lancet 2007; 370:786–796.
8.  Garcia-Aymerich J, Monsò E, Marrades RM. Risk factors for hospitalization for a chronic obstructive pulmonary disease exacerbation. Am J Respir Crit Care Med 2001; 164:1002–1007.
9.  Seemungal TA, Donaldson GC, Bhowmik A, et al. Time course and recovery of exacerbations in patients with chronic obstructive pulmonary disease. Am J Respir Crit Care Med 2000; 161:1608–1613.
10. Donaldson GC, Seemungal TA, Bhowmik A, et al. Relationship between exacerbation frequency and lung function decline in chronic obstructive pulmonary disease. Thorax 2002; 57:847–852.
11. Ball P, Harris JM, Lowson D, et al. Acute infective exacerbations of chronic bronchitis. QJM 1995; 88:61–68.
12. Stevenson NJ, Walker PP, Costell RW, et al. Lung mechanics and dyspnea during exacerbations of chronic obstructive pulmonary disease. Am J Respir Crit Care Med 2005; 172:1510–1516.
13. Seemungal TA, Harper-Owen R, Bhowmik A, et al. Detection of rhinovirus in induced sputum at exacerbation of chronic obstructive pulmonary disease. Eur Respir J 2000; 16:677–683.
14. Papi A, Bellettato CM, Braccioni F, et al. Infections and Airway Inflammation in Chronic Obstructive Pulmonary Disease Severe Exacerbations. Am J Respir Crit Care Med 2006; 173:1114–1121.
15. Anderson HR, Spix C, Medina S, et al. Air pollution and daily admissions for chronic obstructive pulmonary disease in 6 European cities: results from the APHEA project. Eur Respir J 1997; 10:1064–1071.
16. Donaldson GC, Seemungal T, Jeffries DJ, et al. Effect of temperature on lung function and symptoms in chronic obstructive pulmonary disease. Eur Respir J 1999; 13:844–849.
17. Saetta M, Turato G, Facchini FM, et al. Inflammatory cells in the bronchial glands of smokers with chronic bronchitis. Am J Respir Crit Care Med 1997; 156:1633–1639.
18. Saetta M, Turato G, Baraldo S, et al. Goblet cell hyperplasia and epithelial inflammation in peripheral airways of smokers with both symptoms of chronic bronchitis and chronic airflow limitation. Am J Respir Crit Care Med 2000; 161:1016–1021.
19. Hogg JC, Chu FSF, Tan WC et al. Survival after lung volume reduction in chronic obstructive pulmonary disease. Am J Respir Crit Care Med 2007; 176:454–459.
20. Saetta M, Di Stefano A, Turato G. CD8$^+$ T-lymphocytes in peripheral airways of smokers with chronic obstructive pulmonary disease. Am J Respir Crit Care Med 1998; 157:822–826.
21. Saetta M, Baraldo S, Corbino L, et al. CD8$^+$ve cells in the lungs of smokers with chronic obstructive pulmonary disease. Am J Respir Crit Care Med 1999; 160:711–717.
22. Saetta M, Baraldo S, Zuin R. Neutrophil chemokines in severe exacerbations of chronic obstructive pulmonary disease: fatal chemo-attraction? Am J Respir Crit Care Med 2003; 168: 911–913.
23. Qiu Y, Zhu J, Bandi V, et al. Biopsy neutrophilia, neutrophil chemokine and receptor gene expression in severe exacerbations of chronic obstructive pulmonary disease. Am J Respir Crit Care Med 2003; 168:968–975.
24. Zhu J, Qiu YS, Majumdar S, et al. Exacerbations of bronchitis: bronchial eosinophilia and gene expression for interleukin-4, interleukin-5, and eosinophil chemoattractants. Am J Respir Crit Care Med 2001; 164:109–116.
25. Stockley RA, Bayley D, Hill SL, et al. Assessment of airway neutrophils by sputum colour: correlation with airways inflammation. Thorax 2001; 56:366–372.

26. Saetta M, Di Stefano A, Maestrelli P, et al. Airway eosinophilia in chronic bronchitis during exacerbations. Am J Respir Crit Care Med 1994; 150:1646–1652.

27. Saetta M, Di Stefano A, Maestrelli P, et al. Airway eosinophilia and expression of interleukin-5 protein in asthma and in exacerbations of chronic bronchitis. Clin Exp Allergy 1996; 26:766–774.

28. Drost EM, Skwarski KM, Sauleda J, et al. Oxidative stress and airway inflammation in severe exacerbations of COPD. Thorax 2005; 60:293–300.

29. Aaron SD, Angel JB, Lunau M, et al. Granulocyte inflammatory markers and airway infection during acute exacerbation of chronic obstructive pulmonary disease. Am J Respir Crit Care Med 2001; 163:349–355.

30. Gompertz S, O'Brien C, Bayley DL, et al. Changes in bronchial inflammation during acute exacerbations of chronic bronchitis. Eur Respir J 2001; 17:1112–1119.

31. Stockley RA, O'Brien C, Pye A, et al. Relationship of sputum color to nature and outpatient management of acute exacerbations of COPD. Chest 2000; 117:1638–1645.

32. Bocchino V, Bertorelli G, Bertrand CP, et al. Eotaxin and CCR3 are up-regulated in exacerbations of chronic bronchitis. Allergy 2002; 57:17–22.

33. Fujimoto K, Yasuo M, Urushibata K, et al. Airway inflammation during stable and acutely exacerbated chronic obstructive pulmonary disease. Eur Respir J 2005; 25:640–646.

34. Fraenkel DJ, Bardin PG, Sanderson G, et al. Lower airways inflammation during rhinovirus colds in normal and in asthmatic subjects. Am J Respir Crit Care Med 1995; 151:879–886.

35. Trigg CJ, Nicholson KG, Wang JH, et al. Bronchial inflammation and the common cold: a comparison of atopic and non-atopic individuals. Clin Exp Allergy 1996; 26:665–676.

36. Tsoumakidou M, Tzanakis N, Chrysofakis G, et al. Changes in sputum T-lymphocyte sub-populations at the onset of severe exacerbations of chronic obstructive pulmonary disease. Respir Med 2005; 99:572–579.

37. Bhowmik A, Seemungal TA, Sapsford RJ, et al. Relation of sputum inflammatory markers to symptoms and lung function changes in COPD exacerbations. Thorax 2000; 55:114–120.

38. Wedzicha JA. Exacerbations: etiology and pathophysiologic mechanisms. Chest 2002; 121:136S–141S.

39. Roland M, Bhowmik A, Sapsford RJ, et al. Sputum and plasma endothelin-1 levels in exacerbations of chronic obstructive pulmonary disease. Thorax 2001; 56:30–35.

40. Cantin AM, North SL, Hubbard RC, et al. Normal alveolar epithelial lining fluid contains high levels of glutathione. J Appl Physiol 1987; 63:152–157.

41. Biernacki WA, Kharitonov SA, Barnes PJ. Increased leukotriene B4 and 8-isoprostane in exhaled breath condensate of patients with exacerbations of COPD. Thorax 2003; 58:294–298.

42. Gerritsen WB, Asin J, Zanen P, et al. Markers of inflammation and oxidative stress in exacerbated chronic obstructive pulmonary disease patients. Respir Med 2005; 99:84–90.

43. Hurst JR, Donaldson GC, Perera WR, et al. Use of Plasma Biomarkers at Exacerbation of Chronic Obstructive Pulmonary Disease. Am J Respir Crit Care Med 2006; 174:867–874.

44. Gan WQ, Man SFP, Senthilselvan A, et al. Association between chronic obstructive pulmonary disease and systemic inflammation: a systematic review and a meta-analysis. Thorax 2004; 59:574–580.

45. Agustí AG. Systemic Effects of Chronic Obstructive Pulmonary Disease. Proc Am Thorac Soc 2005; 2:367–370.

# 6

# Airway and Systemic Inflammatory Markers at Exacerbation

**JOHN R. HURST**
Academic Unit of Respiratory Medicine, University College London, London, U.K.

## I. Introduction

Definitions of chronic obstructive pulmonary disease (COPD) make reference to an abnormal inflammatory response within the lung (1). It is now widely accepted that stable COPD is also associated with heightened systemic inflammation (2). The first part of this chapter examines evidence that exacerbations of COPD are associated with further rises in airway and systemic inflammatory markers. Examining changes in inflammation at exacerbation might be considered an academic pursuit, providing insights into the underlying mechanisms of disease but of little use to the practicing clinician. However, if changes in inflammation also inform on parameters of clinical utility, such as exacerbation etiology or severity, then such a phenomenon, objectively measured and evaluated, would fulfill the definition of a 'biomarker' (3) and be of considerable practical importance. The second part of this chapter therefore considers the utility of measuring airway and systemic biomarkers at exacerbation of COPD.

## II. Changes in Airway and Systemic Inflammatory Markers at Exacerbation of COPD

As research interest in COPD has increased, a large number of studies have reported on changes in airway and systemic inflammatory markers during exacerbations. A major problem has been variation in results across studies. This likely reflects the reality that COPD is a heterogeneous disease and that exacerbations are heterogeneous events ranging from little more than a troublesome increase in symptoms to life-threatening episodes of respiratory failure. However, many studies are poorly designed, and this also undoubtedly contributes to the conflicting results observed. How should a study be best designed to investigate changes in inflammatory markers between the stable and exacerbated state and during recovery of an exacerbation with treatment? The ideal study might include some of the following features:

- Confirmed diagnosis of COPD
- Stable samples obtained when truly in the baseline state
- Stable samples obtained prior to exacerbation samples in the same patients
- Standardized collection and processing of specimens

- Exacerbation confirmed as a clinical diagnosis of exclusion
- Exacerbation samples obtained prior to additional treatment being commenced
- A standardized treatment protocol
- Samples obtained at multiple timepoints during exacerbation recovery
- Adequate statistical power and techniques to avoid type I and type II errors

With these concepts in mind, Table 1A summarizes those studies reporting changes in airway inflammatory markers between the baseline state and exacerbation. Cellular changes are not considered. Only studies in which paired preexacerbation baseline and exacerbation samples were examined are described. Table 1B describes the related studies in which postexacerbation baseline samples were reported, thereby reflecting changes with exacerbation recovery and treatment. A novel alternative approach is to model exacerbations using experimental infection, and the one study that has employed this technique is also included (11). The primary search strategy employed the terms COPD, exacerbation, and inflammation in the PubMed Central database and was conducted during August 2007. Additional manuscripts were located from reference lists and the departmental collection. Abbreviations are listed at the end of this chapter. Tables 2A and 2B describe changes occurring in the systemic compartment at exacerbation onset (Table 2A) and recovery (Table 2B). The cause of systemic inflammation at exacerbation of COPD remains unclear, but most likely represents 'spillover' from that in the airways, and a direct correlation between inflammatory markers in the airway and systemic compartments has now been described (12).

The tables suggest a number of important conclusions. First, exacerbation of COPD is associated with modulation of a variety of inflammatory markers, which generally return toward stable concentrations with treatment and recovery. However, results across studies are discordant, and many studies are small, with low statistical power. Future studies must therefore be adequately powered to examine changes in markers at exacerbation compared to the baseline state. Regarding airway markers, it is interesting to note that the most highly significant and frequently reproduced results were for samples assayed in exhaled breath. This may reflect the complexity and variability of sputum as a substrate (and different methods for obtaining and processing samples), though the reproducibility of exhaled samples remains a concern and analytes are often present in concentrations at the lower limits of detection (37). Results in the systemic compartment are more consistent, and certainly there is now robust evidence that exacerbations of COPD are associated with an acute inflammatory response.

The changes described in Tables 1 and 2 reflect those occurring between two timepoints only: baseline and exacerbation onset or exacerbation onset and subsequent recovery. Some studies have gone further and examined the evolution of inflammatory markers in airway and systemic compartments at multiple timepoints as the exacerbation recovers with treatment (13,15–17,29). The largest of these studies (13) recruited 73 patients and demonstrated increases in sputum IL-6 (but not sputum IL-8) and serum IL-6 and C-reactive protein (CRP) concentration between baseline and exacerbation onset. Seven days later, following therapy with corticosteroids and/or antibiotics, the concentration of serum IL-6 had decreased significantly below the baseline value. Concentrations of the remaining three markers at day 7 were not significantly different from baseline, and the serum IL-6 concentration had returned to baseline by day 14. This is illustrated in Figure 1. Such studies suggest that there is generally a rapid resolution of airway and systemic inflammatory markers following the institution of exacerbation therapy, which may occur more quickly than the recovery in

(*text continues on page 67*)

**Table 1A** Studies Reporting Differences in Airway Inflammatory Markers Between Baseline and Exacerbation. Sputum Unless Otherwise Stated

| First author | | Decreased at exacerbation | | | | Increased at exacerbation | | | | |
|---|---|---|---|---|---|---|---|---|---|---|
| | Ref. | $p < 0.001$ | $p < 0.01$ | $p \leq 0.05$ | No change | $p \leq 0.05$ | $p < 0.01$ | $p < 0.001$ | $n =$ | Remarks |
| Seemungal 2000 | 4 | | | | IL-8 | | IL-6 | | a | [a]43 exacerbations in 33 patients; 22 baselines |
| Roland 2001 | 5 | | | | IL-6, IL-8 | ET-1 | | | 14 | |
| Aaron 2001 | 6 | | | | MPO | IL-8, TNF-$\alpha$ | | | 14 | |
| Fujimoto 2005 | 7 | | | | Eotaxin, tryptase | ECP, IL-8, RANTES | Elastase | | 30 | |
| Bhowmik 2005 | 8 | | | | | | | eNO | 38 | Exhaled breath |
| Mercer 2005 | 9 | | | | TIMP-1 | | MMP-9 | | 12 | |
| Wilkinson 2006 | 10 | | | | IL-6 | IL-8 | | | 39 | |
| Mallia 2006 | 11 | | | | Nasal GM-CSF, IFN-$\gamma$, IL-1, IL-2, IL-4, IL-5, IL-6, IL-10, TNF-$\alpha$ | Nasal IL-8 | | | 4 | Experimental rhinovirus exposure study, nasal lavage |
| Hurst 2006 | 12 | | | | IL-6, nasal IL-6, nasal IL-8, nasal MPO | | | MPO | 21 | Sputum and nasal lavage |
| Perera 2007 | 13 | | | | IL-8 | IL-6 | | | 73 | |

**Table 1B** Studies Reporting Differences in Airway Inflammatory Markers Between Exacerbation and Subsequent Baseline (Recovery). Sputum Unless Otherwise Stated

| First author | Ref. | Increased at recovery | | | | Decreased at recovery | | | $n =$ | Remarks |
|---|---|---|---|---|---|---|---|---|---|---|
| | | $p < 0.001$ | $p < 0.01$ | $p \leq 0.05$ | No change | $p \leq 0.05$ | $p < 0.01$ | $p < 0.001$ | | |
| Agusti 1999 | 14 | | | | | | | eNO | 17 | Exhaled breath |
| Hill 1999 | 15 | SLPI | | | | | Elastase, IL-8, LTB$_4$, MPO, α-1AT | | 11 | α$_1$-antitrypsin deficiency. |
| Crooks 2000 | 16 | | | | | Elastase | IL-8, LTB$_4$, MPO | | 8 | |
| Aaron 2001 | 6 | | | | MPO | IL-8, TNF-α | | | 14 | |
| Gompertz 2001 | 17 | | | | IL-8 | | Elastase, LTB$_4$, MPO | | 31 | Purulent exacerbations |
| Biernacki 2003 | 18 | | | | | | | LTB$_4$, 8-isoprostane | | EBC |
| White 2003 | 19 | | | SLPI[a] | Elastase, IL-8, MPO | | LTB$_4$[a] | | 40 | [a]Only significant if bacterial persistence |
| Gerritsen 2005 | 20 | | | | | | | H$_2$O$_2$ | 14 | EBC |
| Boschetto 2005 | 21 | | | Neurokinin A, substance P | | | | | 8 | |
| Tsoumakidou 2005 | 22 | | | | ECP, GM-CSF | IL-8, MPO | | | 12 | |
| Papi 2006 | 23 | | | | ECP | eNO | | Elastase | 64 | Exhaled breath (eNO) and sputum |
| Oudijk 2006 | 24 | | | | | | | H$_2$O$_2$ | 10 | EBC |

**Table 2A** Studies Reporting Differences in Systemic Inflammatory Markers (serum/plasma) Between Baseline and Exacerbation

| First author | Ref. | Decreased at exacerbation | | | No change | Increased at exacerbation | | | $n =$ | Remarks |
|---|---|---|---|---|---|---|---|---|---|---|
| | | $p < 0.001$ | $p < 0.01$ | $p \leq 0.05$ | | $p \leq 0.05$ | $p < 0.01$ | $p < 0.001$ | | |
| Shindo 1997 | 25 | | | | | $LTE_4$ | | | 8 | |
| Wedzicha 2000 | 26 | | | | | | IL-6 | Fibrinogen | 67 | 120 exacerbations in 67 patients |
| Roland 2001 | 5 | | | | | | ET-1 | | 28 | |
| Hurst 2006 | 12 | | | | | IL-6 | CRP | | 21 | |
| Hurst 2006 | 27 | | | Eotaxin-2 | Amphiregulin, BDNF, βNGF, ENA-78, Erb-B2, Fibronectin, IFN-γ, IL-1β, IL-2Rγ, IL-8, IL-12p40, IL-15, IL-17, IP-10, ITAC, MCP-1, MIP-1β, MMP-9, MPO, Prolactin, RANTES, L-selectin, TGF-α, TIMP-1, TNF-α, TNF-R2, VEGF | IL-1ra, TNF-R1 | aCRP-30, PARC, s-ICAM-1 | CRP, IL-6, MPIF-1 | 90 | |
| Wilkinson 2006 | 10 | | | | IL-6 | | | | 39 | |
| Perera 2007 | 13 | | | | | | CRP, IL-6 | | 73 | |

**Table 2B** Studies Reporting Differences in Systemic Inflammatory Markers Between Exacerbation and Subsequent Baseline (Recovery). Serum/Plasma Unless Otherwise Stated

| Author | Ref. | Increased at recovery | | | | Decreased at recovery | | | $n =$ | Remarks |
|---|---|---|---|---|---|---|---|---|---|---|
| | | $p < 0.001$ | $p < 0.01$ | $p < 0.05$ | No change | $p < 0.05$ | $p < 0.01$ | $p < 0.001$ | | |
| Dev 1998 | 28 | | | | | | | CRP | 50 | |
| Hill 1999 | 15 | | | | | CRP, α-1AT | | | 22 | 11 had $\alpha_1$-antitrypsin deficiency |
| Wedzicha 2000 | 26 | | | | | | | Fibrinogen, IL-6 | 67 | 120 exacerbations in 67 patients |
| Crooks 2000 | 16 | | | | | α-1ACP, α-1PI | CRP | | 8 | |
| Creutzberg 2000 | 29 | | | | IL-6, sTNF-R55, sTNF-R75 | CRP, leptin | glucose | | 17 | |
| Dentener 2001 | 30 | | | s-IL1R-II | | CRP, LBP | | | 13 | 7-day study |
| Gompertz 2001 | 17 | | | | | CRP[a] | CRP[a] | | 69 | [a]Greater fall in purulent than mucoid exacerbations |
| Fiorenza 2002 | 31 | | | | | Desmosine | | | 9 | Urine |
| Malo 2002 | 32 | | | | CRP, IL-6, IL-8 | | | | 10 | |
| Spruit 2003 | 33 | | IGF-1 | | | | | CRP | | |
| Gerritsen 2005 | 20 | | | | E-selectin | | IL-8 | s-ICAM-1 | 14 | |
| Pinto-Plata 2007 | 34 | | | | SLPI, TNF-α | | IL-8, LTB₄ | IL-6 | 20 | |
| Stolz 2007 | 35 | | | | | | | Copeptin, CRP, procalcitonin | 167 | |
| Groenewegen 2007 | 36 | | | BPI | IL-6, s-IL-1RII, sTNF-R55, sTNF-R75 | | | | 21 | 3-mo data reported here |

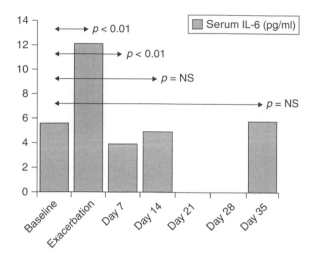

**Figure 1** Time course of median serum IL-6 in 73 exacerbations of COPD. *Source*: From Ref. 13.

symptoms and physiology. In addition, Perera et al. also defined a relationship between nonrecovery of symptoms and persistently elevated systemic inflammatory markers (13).

## III. Utility of Changes in Airway and Systemic Inflammatory Markers at Exacerbation of COPD

Having established that many inflammatory markers may be present at different concentration during exacerbation compared to the baseline state, the important question that arises is whether measuring such markers is useful in clinical practice.

A useful biomarker might inform on one or more of the following aspects of exacerbation:

- To provide objective confirmation of exacerbation, differentiating exacerbation from stable disease or exacerbation from other causes of breathlessness in a patient with underlying COPD, and therefore avoiding the need to consider exacerbation as a clinical diagnosis of exclusion (38)
- To reflect exacerbation etiology and specifically the role of bacteria and viruses, which may therefore inform on the rational use of drugs such as antibiotics
- To predict or quantify the clinical severity of exacerbation, which might usefully guide decisions about the level of treatment required and where this should be delivered
- To predict outcomes later in the evolution of disease, such as the likelihood of reexacerbation or associated cardiovascular risk

A number of studies have reported results suggesting that various biomarkers may indeed have roles in all of the areas described above. However, once again, many of these studies have methodological flaws. In particular, most are observational, which while useful at forming hypotheses do not provide robust evidence of the validity of that biomarker. An ideal biomarker should be sensitive and specific, with well-defined reference limits, and be easily and reliably measured at reasonable cost. Therefore, validation of a biomarker requires assessment in properly designed clinical trials, and there are very few such studies reported at exacerbation of COPD. Given the inherent difficulties of reliably assessing airway inflammatory markers, most studies have chosen to examine biomarkers in the systemic compartment.

## A. Biomarkers That Confirm Exacerbation

There is currently no validated biomarker that can differentiate stable from exacerbated disease or exacerbation from other causes of breathlessness in a patient with underlying COPD. Such an assay would clearly be of utility, both in the clinic and the context of clinical trials.

In the largest study of its kind, Hurst et al. (27) reported the ability of 36 plasma biomarkers in retrospectively differentiating stable from exacerbated disease by comparing paired stable and exacerbation concentrations of markers from 90 patients. No marker was more sensitive or specific than an assessment of symptoms alone, and the best marker was CRP, which while moderately sensitive remains limited by the presence of raised concentrations in stable disease. In addition, CRP assay would not be specific in differentiating exacerbation of COPD from other causes of breathlessness associated with a raised acute-phase response such as pneumonia. Moreover, no combination of markers performed better than CRP alone.

Cardiac causes of increased breathlessness in patients with underlying COPD might be identified using biomarkers of cardiac dysfunction such as troponin and amino terminal pro-brain natriuretic peptide (NT-proBNP) (39). The utility of D-dimer testing at exacerbation of COPD remains controversial, as indeed does the precise prevalence of pulmonary emboli in patients with COPD who present with increased breathlessness (40). Moreover, given that a definitive study of patients with COPD who present with increased breathlessness and are investigated for causes and mimics of exacerbation is yet to be performed, exacerbation of COPD must remain, for the moment, a clinical diagnosis of exclusion (38).

## B. Biomarkers That Inform on Exacerbation Etiology

A biomarker that could differentiate infective from noninfective causes of exacerbation and bacterial from viral disease has the potential to reduce inappropriate use of antibiotics and therefore the health care costs and side effects associated with such therapy.

In one of the few prospective studies of biomarkers at exacerbation of COPD, Stolz et al. examined the role of procalcitonin (PCT), a systemic marker of bacterial infection, in reducing the prescription of antibiotics (41). The trial enrolled 208 patients with exacerbation of COPD requiring hospitalization and randomized them to PCT-guided antibiotic therapy or antibiotics given at the sole discretion of the attending physician. In the intervention group, antibiotics were discouraged when PCT was low (<0.1 µg/L). The primary outcome was antibiotic exposure, and the trial reported a 0.56 (95% CI, 0.43–0.73, $p < 0.0001$) relative risk of exposure to antibiotics at the index exacerbation in the intervention group, which persisted out to six months. Moreover, this was achieved without apparent detriment to clinical outcomes, including exacerbation recovery and the risk of reexacerbation. There are a number of practical issues relating to PCT assay, and intriguingly, the study noted that PCT levels were not different between subjects who did and did not have sputum purulence or the presence of positive sputum bacteriology. Nevertheless, this trial provides robust evidence that biomarker assay is able to reduce antibiotic prescription at exacerbation of COPD.

There is currently no validated biomarker of viral infection, and while such a development might also be important in avoiding inappropriate antibiotic therapy, it should be recalled that exacerbations may be associated with bacterial and viral coinfection (10) such that an approach relevant to both bacteria and viruses may prove to be the most effective. Initial reports using multiple cytokine assays to distinguish bacterial from viral exacerbations require further evaluation (42).

### C. Biomarkers That Inform on Exacerbation Severity

The ability of biomarkers to inform on exacerbation severity is limited by the absence of a widely accepted method of grading exacerbation severity. Severity might be assessed by the magnitude of changes in symptoms or lung function, the duration of such changes, or the need for specific treatments such as systemic corticosteroids or interventions such as hospitalization. One attempt to summarize associations between biomarkers and exacerbation severity (43), including 268 individual studies, found no consistent relationships. More recently, Stolz et al. (35) has reported the utility of copeptin (a vasopressin precursor) in 167 exacerbations and observed relationships between copeptin concentration and the need for intensive care, length of hospital stay (both assessments of exacerbation severity) and longer-term 'clinical failure': a composite endpoint defined as death from any cause or rehospitalization for a subsequent exacerbation. Copeptin is therefore promising as a biomarker of short- and long-term outcomes at exacerbation of COPD, but such results require further prospective confirmation.

### D. Biomarkers That Predict Postexacerbation Events

A number of studies have examined whether airway and systemic markers might predict postexacerbation events. In a prospective study of 1016 patients hospitalized for exacerbation of COPD, serum albumin (among other physiological variables) was independently associated with death over the subsequent six months (44). Serum albumin has also been associated with survival in patients requiring intubation and mechanical ventilation at the time of exacerbation (45). These results, however, reflect patients with the most severe exacerbations and are not generalizable to a wider population.

A recent paper by Perera et al. (13) examined associations between markers of airway and systemic inflammation with exacerbation severity and subsequent outcomes in an ambulatory cohort. Among a number of potentially important observations, the serum CRP concentration measured 14 days after exacerbation onset was directly associated with the risk of recurrent exacerbation, and in a similar analysis, an inverse linear relationship was described between the CRP concentration at 14 days and time to the next exacerbation. The study was observational, and therefore such results require further confirmation in appropriately designed trials. However, these findings do suggest that early follow-up of patients following exacerbation, and assessment of biomarkers such as CRP, may be important in detecting those patients most at risk from reexacerbation.

## IV. Summary

COPD is an inflammatory disease, and there is abundant evidence suggesting that the concentrations of many airway and systemic inflammatory markers are further modulated during exacerbations. Most existing studies are observational, and there is now the need to extend this preliminary knowledge, using well-designed trials to validate clinically useful biomarkers that might confirm exacerbation, reflect exacerbation etiology, or predict the severity or complications of the event. Only in this way can we achieve the goal of translational research and improve patient-focused outcomes by the application of basic science.

## Abbreviations

| | |
|---|---|
| aCRP-30 | adiponectin |
| BDNF | brain-derived neurotrophic factor |
| BPI | bactericidal/permeability-increasing protein |
| BNGF | nerve growth factor-$\beta$ |
| CRP | C-reactive protein |
| EBC | exhaled breath condensate |
| ECP | eosinophil cationic protein |
| ENO | exhaled nitric oxide |
| ENA-78 | epithelial-derived neutrophil-activating protein-78 |
| Erb-B2 | erythroblastic leukaemia viral oncogene homolog 2 |
| ET-1 | endothelin-1 |
| IFN-$\gamma$ | interferon-gamma |
| IGF-1 | insulin-like growth factor-1 |
| IL | interleukin |
| IL-1ra | IL-1 receptor antagonist |
| IL-2R$\gamma$ | IL-2 receptor gamma |
| IP-10 | interferon gamma-induced protein-10 |
| ITAC | interferon gamma-inducible T-cell $\alpha$-chemoattractant |
| GM-CSF | granulocyte-macrophage-colony stimulating factor |
| LBP | lipopolysaccharide-binding protein |
| LTB$_4$ | leukotriene B4 |
| LTE$_4$ | leukotriene E4 |
| MCP-1 | monocyte chemoattractant protein-1 |
| MIP-1$\beta$ | macrophage inflammatory protein 1-$\beta$ |
| MMP | matrix metalloproteinase |
| MPIF-1 | myeloid progenitor inhibitory factor-1 |
| MPO | myeloperoxidase |
| PARC | pulmonary and activation-regulated chemokine |
| RANTES | regulated on activation normal T-cell expressed and secreted |
| s-ICAM-1 | soluble intercellular adhesion molecule-1 |
| s-IL-1RII | soluble interleukin-1 receptor II |
| SLPI | secretory leukoprotease inhibitor |
| sTNF-R | soluble tumor necrosis factor receptor |
| TGF-$\alpha$ | transforming growth factor-$\alpha$ |
| TIMP | tissue inhibitor of metalloproteinase-1 |
| TNF-$\alpha$ | tumor necrosis factor-$\alpha$ |
| TNFR | tumor necrosis factor receptor |
| VEGF | vascular endothelial growth factor |
| $\alpha_1$-ACP | $\alpha_1$-antichymotrypsin |
| $\alpha_1$-AT | $\alpha_1$-antitrypsin |
| $\alpha_1$-PI | $\alpha_1$-proteinase inhibitor |

## References

1. GOLD Executive committee. Global Strategy for Diagnosis, Management, and Prevention of COPD (Revised 2006). Available at: http://www.goldcopd.com. Accessed 23rd August 2007.
2. Gan WQ, Man SF, Senthilselvan A, et al. Association between chronic obstructive pulmonary disease and systemic inflammation: a systematic review and a meta-analysis. Thorax 2004; 59: 574–580.
3. Atkinson AJ, Colburn WA, DeGruttola VG, et al. Biomarkers and surrogate endpoints: preferred definitions and conceptual framework. Clin Pharmacol Ther 2001; 69:89–95.
4. Seemungal TA, Harper-Owen R, Bhowmik A, et al. Detection of rhinovirus in induced sputum at exacerbation of chronic obstructive pulmonary disease. Eur Respir J 2000; 16:677–683.
5. Roland M, Bhowmik A, Sapsford RJ, et al. Sputum and plasma endothelin-1 levels in exacerbations of chronic obstructive pulmonary disease. Thorax 2001; 56:30–35.
6. Aaron SD, Angel JB, Lunau M, et al. Granulocyte inflammatory markers and airway infection during acute exacerbation of chronic obstructive pulmonary disease. Am J Respir Crit Care Med 2001; 163:349–355.
7. Fujimoto K, Yasuo M, Urushibata K, et al. Airway inflammation during stable and acutely exacerbated chronic obstructive pulmonary disease. Eur Respir J 2005; 25:640–646.
8. Bhowmik A, Seemungal TA, Donaldson GC, et al. Effects of exacerbations and seasonality on exhaled nitric oxide in COPD. Eur Respir J 2005; 26:1009–1015.
9. Mercer PF, Shute JK, Bhowmik A, et al. MMP-9, TIMP-1 and inflammatory cells in sputum from COPD patients during exacerbation. Respir Res 2005; 6:151.
10. Wilkinson TM, Hurst JR, Perera WR, et al. Effect of interactions between lower airway bacterial and rhinoviral infection in exacerbations of COPD. Chest 2006; 129:317–324.
11. Mallia P, Message SD, Kebadze T, et al. An experimental model of rhinovirus induced chronic obstructive pulmonary disease exacerbations: a pilot study. Respir Res 2006; 7:116.
12. Hurst JR, Perera WR, Wilkinson TM, et al. Systemic and upper and lower airway inflammation at exacerbation of chronic obstructive pulmonary disease. Am J Respir Crit Care Med 2006; 173:71–78.
13. Perera WR, Hurst JR, Wilkinson TM, et al. Inflammatory changes, recovery and recurrence at COPD exacerbation. Eur Respir J 2007; 29:527–534.
14. Agusti AG, Villaverde JM, Togores B, et al. Serial measurements of exhaled nitric oxide during exacerbations of chronic obstructive pulmonary disease. Eur Respir J 1999; 14:523–528.
15. Hill AT, Campbell EJ, Bayley DL, et al. Evidence for excessive bronchial inflammation during an acute exacerbation of chronic obstructive pulmonary disease in patients with $\alpha_1$-antitrypsin deficiency (PiZ). Am J Respir Crit Care Med 1999; 160:1968–1975.
16. Crooks SW, Bayley DL, Hill SL, et al. Bronchial inflammation in acute bacterial exacerbations of chronic bronchitis: the role of leukotriene B4. Eur Respir J 2000; 15:274–280.
17. Gompertz S, O'Brien C, Bayley DL, et al. Changes in bronchial inflammation during acute exacerbations of chronic bronchitis. Eur Respir J 2001; 17:1112–1119.
18. Biernacki WA, Kharitonov SA, Barnes PJ. Increased leukotriene B4 and 8-isoprostane in exhaled breath condensate of patients with exacerbations of COPD. Thorax 2003; 58:294–298.
19. White AJ, Gompertz S, Bayley DL, et al. Resolution of bronchial inflammation is related to bacterial eradication following treatment of exacerbations of chronic bronchitis. Thorax 2003; 58:680–685.
20. Gerritsen WB, Asin J, Zanen P, et al. Markers of inflammation and oxidative stress in exacerbated chronic obstructive pulmonary disease patients. Respir Med 2005; 99:84–90.
21. Boschetto P, Miotto D, Bononi I, et al. Sputum substance P and neurokinin A are reduced during exacerbations of chronic obstructive pulmonary disease. Pulm Pharmacol Ther 2005; 18:199–205.
22. Tsoumakidou M, Tzanakis N, Chrysofakis G, et al. Nitrosative stress, heme oxygenase-1 expression and airway inflammation during severe exacerbations of COPD. Chest 2005; 127: 1911–1918.

23. Papi A, Bellettato CM, Braccioni F, et al. Infections and airway inflammation in chronic obstructive pulmonary disease severe exacerbations. Am J Respir Crit Care Med 2006; 173:1114–1121.

24. Oudijk EJ, Gerritsen WB, Nijhuis EH, et al. Expression of priming-associated cellular markers on neutrophils during an exacerbation of COPD. Respir Med 2006; 100:1791–1799.

25. Shindo K, Hirai Y, Fukumura M, et al. Plasma levels of leukotriene E4 during clinical course of chronic obstructive pulmonary disease. Prostaglandins Leukot Essent Fatty Acids 1997; 56:213–217.

26. Wedzicha JA, Seemungal TAR, MacCallum PK, et al. Acute exacerbations of chronic obstructive pulmonary disease are accompanied by elevations of plasma fibrinogen and serum IL-6 levels. Thromb Haemost 2000; 84:210–215.

27. Hurst JR, Donaldson GC, Perera WR, et al. Use of plasma biomarkers at exacerbation of chronic obstructive pulmonary disease. Am J Respir Crit Care Med 2006; 174:867–874.

28. Dev D, Wallace E, Sankaran R, et al. Value of C-reactive protein measurements in exacerbations of chronic obstructive pulmonary disease. Respir Med 1998; 92:664–667.

29. Creutzberg EC, Wouters EF, Vanderhoven-Augustin IM, et al. Disturbances in leptin metabolism are related to energy imbalance during acute exacerbations of chronic obstructive pulmonary disease. Am J Respir Crit Care Med 2000; 162:1239–1245.

30. Dentener MA, Creutzberg EC, Schols AM, et al. Systemic anti-inflammatory mediators in COPD: increase in soluble interleukin 1 receptor II during treatment of exacerbations. Thorax 2001; 56:721–726.

31. Fiorenza D, Viglio S, Lupi A, et al. Urinary desmosine excretion in acute exacerbations of COPD: a preliminary report. Respir Med 2002; 96:110–114.

32. Malo O, Sauleda J, Busquets X, et al. Systemic inflammation during exacerbations of chronic obstructive pulmonary disease. Arch Bronconeumol 2002; 38:172–176.

33. Spruit MA, Gosselink R, Troosters T, et al. Muscle force during an acute exacerbation in hospitalised patients with COPD and its relationship with CXCL8 and IGF-I. Thorax 2003; 58:752–756.

34. Pinto-Plata VM, Livnat G, Girish M, et al. Systemic cytokines, clinical and physiological changes in patients hospitalized for exacerbation of COPD. Chest 2007; 131:37–43.

35. Stolz D, Christ-Crain M, Morgenthaler NG, et al. Copeptin, C-reactive protein, and procalcitonin as prognostic biomarkers in acute exacerbation of COPD. Chest 2007; 131:1058–1067.

36. Groenewegen KH, Dentener MA, Wouters EF. Longitudinal follow-up of systemic inflammation after acute exacerbations of COPD. Respir Med 2007; 101(11):2409–2415.

37. Horvath I, Hunt J, Barnes PJ, et al. Exhaled breath condensate: methodological recommendations and unresolved questions. Eur Respir J 2005; 26:523–548.

38. Hurst JR, Wedzicha JA. What is (and what is not) an exacerbation of COPD: thoughts from the new GOLD guidelines. Thorax 2007; 62:198–199.

39. Abroug F, Ouanes-Besbes L, Nciri N, et al. Association of left-heart dysfunction with severe exacerbation of chronic obstructive pulmonary disease. Am J Respir Crit Care Med 2006; 174:990–996.

40. Wedzicha JA, Hurst JR. Chronic obstructive pulmonary disease exacerbation and risk of pulmonary embolism. Thorax 2007; 62:103–104.

41. Stolz D, Christ-Crain M, Bingisser R, et al. Antibiotic treatment of exacerbations of COPD: a randomized, controlled trial comparing procalcitonin-guidance with standard therapy. Chest 2007; 131:9–19.

42. Dal Negro RW, Micheletto C, Tognella S, et al. A two-stage logistic model based on the measurement of pro-inflammatory cytokines in bronchial secretions for assessing bacterial, viral, and non-infectious origin of COPD exacerbations. COPD 2005; 2:7–16.

43. Franciosi LG, Page CP, Celli BR, et al. Markers of exacerbation severity in chronic obstructive pulmonary disease. Respir Res 2006; 7:74.
44. Connors AF, Dawson NV, Thomas C, et al. Outcomes following acute exacerbation of severe chronic obstructive lung disease. Am J Respir Crit Care Med 1996; 154:959–967.
45. Menzies R, Gibbons W, Goldberg P. Determinants of weaning and survival among patients with COPD who require mechanical ventilation for acute respiratory failure. Chest 1989; 95:398–405.

# 7

# Pathophysiology of Acute Exacerbations of COPD

**CHRIS M. PARKER and DENIS E. O'DONNELL**
Department of Medicine, Queen's University, Kingston, Ontario, Canada

## I. Introduction

Acute exacerbations are the most frequent cause of medical visits, hospitalization, and death among patients with chronic obstructive pulmonary disease (COPD) (1). Although it is generally regarded that worsening airway inflammation is the primary inciting event of an exacerbation, the recent evidence suggesting that long-acting bronchodilators and mucolytics reduce the frequency and severity of exacerbations (2,3) indicates that factors other than airway inflammation may be important as well. Our knowledge of the pathophysiologic changes that occur at the time of exacerbation continues to grow. Although detailed studies of patients who have been hospitalized with acute respiratory failure requiring mechanical ventilation have provided clearer insights into the mechanisms that underlie severe exacerbations, considerably less is known about the physiologic derangements that accompany the mild-to-moderate exacerbations, which are more commonly encountered in clinical practice. It is reasonable to assume, however, that exacerbations share common pathophysiologic mechanisms and that these changes may occur along a spectrum of severity that is determined by both host factors (including severity of underlying disease) and environmental influences (such as severity of the inciting illness or insult). This review will summarize our current understanding of the effects of exacerbation on pulmonary function, mechanics [including the central concept of worsening expiratory flow limitation (EFL) and dynamic hyperinflation (DH)], gas exchange, and cardiopulmonary interactions in patients with COPD.

## II. Pulmonary Function

Exacerbations of COPD are associated with acute worsening of lung function indices, including expiratory flows (4). Representative spirometric tracings from a patient at baseline and during an exacerbation are shown in Figure 1. However, the use of pulmonary function tests (PFTs) or spirometry in the diagnosis, management, and prognostication of COPD exacerbations is still uncertain. Unlike asthma, where indices of EFL [such as peak expiratory flow rate (PEFR) or forced expiratory volume in 1 second ($FEV_1$)] can be used to guide patient management, changes in spirometric variables measured at exacerbation in

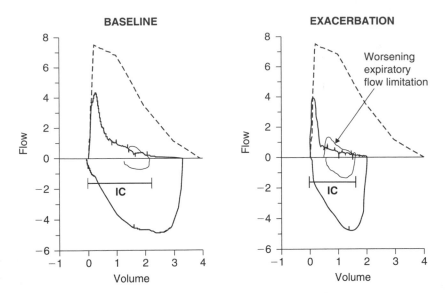

**Figure 1** Representative flow-volume curves obtained during spirometry from a patient with COPD at baseline and during exacerbation. Note the characteristic worsening EFL and the presence of DH during exacerbation as suggested by the reduction in IC. *Abbreviations*: EFL, expiratory flow limitation; DH, dynamic hyperinflation; IC, inspiratory capacity.

patients with COPD are generally small (5–8) and do not necessarily correlate temporally with improvements in symptoms (9); as such, considerable interest has emerged in the use of other spirometric variables [such as the inspiratory capacity (IC)] in the setting of COPD exacerbations (4). Although bedside spirometry is becoming increasingly available, more detailed assessment of pulmonary function (such as measurements of static lung volumes or mechanics) requires the use of cumbersome equipment and a level of patient cooperation that is often not feasible during periods of acute clinical deterioration. For these reasons, it is only recently that data have emerged to characterize these changes in greater detail.

## A. Time Course of PFT Changes During Exacerbation

A prospective cohort study followed 101 patients with moderate to severe COPD (mean $FEV_1$ 41.9% predicted) for a period of 2.5 years (10). Daily diary cards were used to record symptoms and PEFR values; daily spirometry was also performed in a smaller ($n = 34$) subset of this cohort. During the follow-up period, a total of 504 exacerbations were diagnosed on the basis of symptomatic deterioration. At the onset of exacerbation, relatively small changes were noted in PEFR, $FEV_1$, and forced vital capacity (FVC) ($-8.6$ L/min, $-24.0$ mL, and $-76.0$ mL, respectively), and there was only weak correlation between deterioration of PEFR at exacerbation and worsening breathlessness ($r = 0.12$, $p = 0.014$). However, patients with more severe reductions in expiratory flows and volumes at the time of exacerbations took longer to recover ($p < 0.001$), and 35 days after the onset of exacerbation, PEFR had returned to baseline in only 75.2% of patients. Furthermore, at 91 days postexacerbation, 7.1% of patients had not reattained their preexacerbation PEFR baseline, highlighting the potential for significant and sustained physiologic impact after an exacerbation.

A recent study from our laboratory followed 20 patients during symptom recovery from an acute exacerbation (11). All patients were evaluated within 72 hours of the onset of symptomatic deterioration, were classified as having a moderately severe exacerbation using the definition proposed by Rodriguez-Roisin (12), and were evaluated using full pulmonary function testing to evaluate static lung volumes as well as expiratory volumes and flows. Testing was performed at study entry (day 0) and again after 7, 14, 30, and 60 days. At day 0, patients had severe airflow obstruction (mean $FEV_1$ 41% predicted) and evidence of hyperinflation [total lung capacity (TLC) 119% predicted, functional residual capacity (FRC) 164% predicted, and residual volume (RV) 197% predicted]. During recovery, improvements were noted in PEFR (by $0.60 \pm 0.14$ L/sec), $FEV_1$ (by $0.19 \pm 0.05$ L), and FVC (by $0.35 \pm 0.10$ L) as compared with day 0. Furthermore, as symptoms resolved, there was progressive improvement in indices of hyperinflation and gas trapping. Specifically, between day 0 and the final visit, RV and FRC were reduced (by $-0.31 \pm 0.10$ L and $-0.20 \pm 0.06$ L, respectively). These changes were associated with improvements in the IC (by $0.30 \pm 0.05$ L) but no change in TLC, suggesting that IC measurements obtainable with spirometry can reliably track changes in end-expiratory lung volume (EELV) (and hence are reflective of changes in hyperinflation) during recovery. The majority of improvement in PFT parameters was noted during the first 14 days of recovery (Fig. 2). Interestingly, in this study, the $FEV_1$/FVC ratio did not change during the follow-up period, suggesting that the improvement in $FEV_1$ may be predominantly reflective of an improved VC; in other words, volume recruitment as a consequence of reduced air trapping may be responsible for the improved expiratory flows and $FEV_1$. Two additional studies (using spirometry to track physiologic changes during recovery from exacerbation) have found similar findings, noting improvements in $FEV_1$ and PEFR (but no change in $FEV_1$/FVC) and improvements in IC during symptom recovery indicative of a reduction in lung hyperinflation (13,14).

## B. Effects of Exacerbations on Decline of Lung Function

It has been suggested that there is a relationship between the frequency of acute exacerbations of COPD (AECOPD) and the rate of longitudinal decline in $FEV_1$, although this is controversial. Early studies suggested that there was no relationship between pulmonary infections decline in lung function, although many of these studies enrolled both smokers and nonsmokers, and included younger subjects with minimal or no objective evidence of airflow obstruction (15–17). More recently, Kanner et al. found that in a population of patients with mild COPD, there was a greater decline of $FEV_1$ over time in subjects who experienced lower respiratory tract infections, although this effect seemed to be confined to current smokers or nonsustained quitters (18). In a study of 109 COPD patients with moderate to severe COPD (baseline median $FEV_1$ = 38.2%), Donaldson and colleagues demonstrated that subjects who experienced frequent exacerbations (defined as >2.92/yr) had a significantly greater rate of decline in lung function when compared with infrequent exacerbators, although the magnitude of this difference was relatively small (19). Specifically, $FEV_1$ declined by 40.1 mL/yr in frequent exacerbators compared with 32.1 mL/yr in infrequent exacerbators ($p < 0.05$) and PEFR declined by 2.9 L/min/yr versus 0.7 L/min/yr in frequent and infrequent exacerbators, respectively ($p < 0.001$).

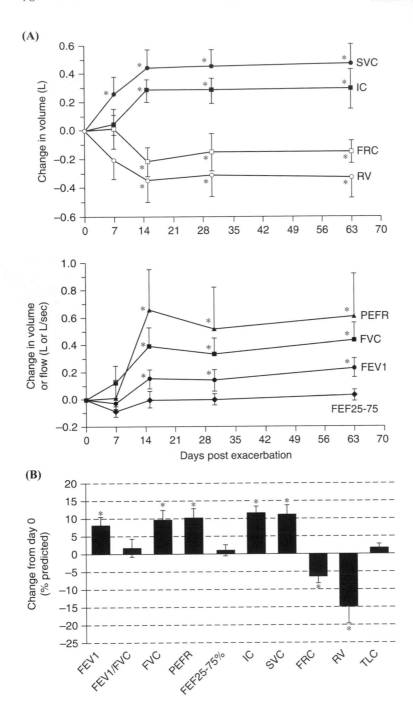

## III. Dynamic Hyperinflation

EFL is characteristic of COPD. In the presence of EFL, expiratory flows rates are independent of expiratory muscle effort. The time constant ($\tau$) for lung emptying during expiration is determined by the product of lung compliance and airway resistance, and hence increases in either lung compliance or airway resistance will contribute to flow limitation. In COPD, EFL arises as a consequence of emphysematous parenchymal destruction of the lung that decreases recoil pressure (and hence increases pulmonary compliance) and an increase in airway resistance due to inflammation, edema, mucus inspissation, chronic remodeling of the airways, and possibly increased cholinergic tone in airway smooth muscle (20). In advanced COPD, expiratory flows may be significantly limited even with spontaneous tidal breathing at rest, and lung emptying is incomplete at the end of expiration. As a result, the EELV (which is synonymous with FRC) is increased. Even in patients with less severe disease, however, increases in ventilatory demand or tachypnea (which may further limit the time available for expiration) may precipitate dynamic increases in EELV after flow limitation exceeds a critical level. As such, in flow-limited patients, any factor that increases minute ventilation (e.g., exercise, voluntary hyperventilation, anxiety, hypoxemia) may contribute to the development of acute lung hyperinflation. This is termed "dynamic hyperinflation" and is defined as a temporary and variable increase in EELV above its baseline resting value. DH has emerged as a central concept in our understanding of the pathophysiology of COPD. During an exacerbation, airway resistance may be abruptly increased (because of worsening bronchoconstriction, edema, and retained secretions), worsening EFL (14). Indeed, it has recently been demonstrated that DH occurs during COPD exacerbations, resulting in increased static lung volumes (including RV and EELV/FRC), which improve with resolution of the exacerbation (11,13,14). Measurement of lung volumes using body plethysmography is difficult and impractical during an exacerbation, and inert gas dilution techniques may underestimate absolute lung volumes in the presence of noncommunicating airways. However, we have recently shown that TLC does not change during exacerbation, suggesting that the IC (which can be obtained more simply using spirometry) is a reliable surrogate for DH in this setting (11). Other authors have also found that the IC improves during symptomatic recovery from an exacerbation, indicative of improvement in lung hyperinflation during convalescence (13,14).

---

**Figure 2** Time course and magnitude of change in lung volumes and flows during recovery from exacerbation. Subjects were studied (day 0) within 72 hours of onset of symptomatic deterioration. (**A**) During recovery from exacerbation, there was progressive improvement in PFT parameters, the majority of which occurred during the first 14 days after the onset of the exacerbation ($n$ =12). Symbols are as marked in the panel. (**B**) Final magnitude of change (% predicted) of lung volumes and flows in 20 patients (mean $FEV_1$ at day 0 = 0.92 ± 0.06 L) recovering from exacerbation, measured 60 ±5 days after onset of exacerbation. Note the lack of change in TLC during recovery, suggesting that the IC is a reliable surrogate for DH in the setting of an exacerbation. *Abbreviations*: PFT, pulmonary function test; SVC, slow vital capacity; IC, inspiratory capacity; FRC, functional residual capacity; RV, residual volume; PEFR, peak expiratory flow rate; FVC, forced vital capacity; $FEV_1$, forced expiratory volume in one second; FEF25-75, forced mid-expiratory flow; TLC, total lung capacity; DH, dynamic hyperinflation. *Source*: From Ref. 11.

## A.  Mechanical Consequences of DH

Although DH developing during an exacerbation may serve to optimize expiratory flow rates, it has the deleterious effect of shifting operating lung volumes toward the flattened upper extreme of the respiratory system compliance curve. At operating lung volumes close to TLC, progressive pressure increases result in smaller incremental volume changes; in effect, DH has imposed a "restrictive" mechanical constraint on the respiratory system, and the ability of the tidal volume to expand to meet increased ventilatory demands becomes limited. In essence, the IC represents the true operating limits for tidal volume expansion, and in the setting of an exacerbation, tidal volume is truncated from below because of dynamic increases in EELV and from above as a result of the TLC envelope (20). DH also has the deleterious effect of imposing an inspiratory threshold load (because of the presence of intrinsic positive end-expiratory pressure, $PEEP_i$) on the inspiratory muscles that are already burdened with increased elastic loading (4); this inspiratory threshold load has been measured at 6 to 9 $cmH_2O$ during quiet breathing at rest in clinically stable but hyperinflated COPD patients (21,22) and likely increases during exacerbations. The diaphragm itself may become functionally weakened as a result of shortened muscle fiber length (23). Other factors, such as chronic hypoxemia and hypercapnia, steroid overusage, malnutrition, and electrolyte disturbance may also predispose the respiratory muscles to functional weakness in the face of the already increased mechanical burden (24). Furthermore, tachypnea that develops in the setting of an exacerbation reduces dynamic lung compliance ($C_{DYN}$), which already has exaggerated frequency dependence in COPD (25). These factors, in turn, contribute to an increase in the work of breathing and impart a higher $O_2$ cost to maintain minute ventilation. A summary of the effects of exacerbation on pulmonary mechanics is presented in Figure 3.

## IV.  Effects on Gas Exchange

In the stable state, patients with COPD are usually able to maintain acceptable indices of gas exchange. However, in the setting of acute physiologic stress (e.g., exercise or an exacerbation) the pathophysiologic adaptive mechanisms that serve to maintain adequate oxygenation and alveolar ventilation in the stable state may be quickly overwhelmed, resulting in variable degrees of hypoxemia and hypercarbia. In patients with COPD, the tendency to develop hypercapnia in the face of increased metabolic or ventilatory demands cannot be reliably predicted from baseline (i.e., preexacerbation) PFTs or arterial blood gas analysis, but it follows that patients with more advanced or severe disease have less physiologic reserve and are thus more prone to the development of acute respiratory failure even in the face of a relatively mild insult such as a common cold. Conversely, patients with relatively mild disease may still experience respiratory failure in the setting of severe illness.

   The mechanisms underlying respiratory failure and resulting in hypoxemia and/or hypercarbia in the setting of a COPD exacerbation are several, including worsening of ventilation/perfusion ($V_A/Q$) relationships (26,27), a modest increase in shunt fraction (26), a reduction in mixed venous oxygen tension ($P\bar{v}O_2$) (27), and mechanical effects attributable to tidal volume constraint in the presence of EFL (4,11,28). Using the multiple inert gas elimination technique (MIGET), Barbera and colleagues evaluated 13 patients with severe COPD (mean $FEV_1$ 29% predicted) at the time of acute exacerbation (27). These authors determined that approximately 50% of the observed hypoxemia could be

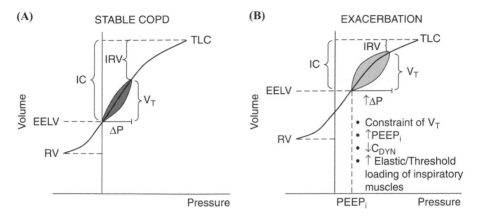

**Figure 3** Schematic illustrating deleterious mechanical effects of exacerbation. Shown are representative pressure-volume plots during stable COPD (*panel A*) and during exacerbation (*panel B*). During exacerbation, there is an increase in both EELV and RV as a consequence of worsening expiratory flow limitation. There are corresponding reductions in IC and IRV, while TLC remains unchanged. As a result, tidal breathing becomes upward-shifted on the compliance curve and essentially becomes constrained from below by the dynamic increase in EELV and from above by the TLC envelope. Mechanically, increased pressures ($\Delta P$) must be generated to maintain VT, representing increased elastic loading of the inspiratory muscles. $C_{DYN}$ is also reduced. At EELV, intrapulmonary pressures during an exacerbation may not return to zero, indicating the presence of PEEP$i$ that in turn imposes an inspiratory threshold load on the inspiratory muscles. *Abbreviations*: COPD, chronic obstructive pulmonary disease; EELV, end-expiratory lung volume; RV, residual volume; IC, inspiratory capacity; IRV, inspiratory reserve volume; TLC, total lung capacity; VT, tidal volume; $C_{DYN}$, dynamic lung compliance; PEEP$i$, intrinsic positive end-expiratory pressure. *Source*: From Ref. 4.

explained on the basis of worsened $V_A/Q$ relationships, compounded further by a reduction in $P\bar{v}O_2$, which was presumably on the basis of increased oxygen consumption by the respiratory muscles. In this study, there was a modest increase in minute ventilation during the exacerbation, and the authors concluded that the observed hypercarbia was the result of worsened $V_A/Q$ relationships as opposed to alveolar hypoventilation. In contrast, it has also been suggested that mechanical factors, notably the constraint of tidal volume expansion imparted by DH, may also contribute significantly to hypercarbia during both exercise (28) and exacerbations (4). In advanced COPD, there is an increase in physiologic dead space (and therefore wasted ventilation) as a consequence of underlying $V_A/Q$ mismatch. During an exacerbation, patients may be forced to adopt a rapid shallow breathing pattern because of the restrictive mechanics that are imposed because of DH and increased elastic and threshold loading of the inspiratory muscles. This further increases the dead space fraction ($V_D/V_T$), resulting in a relative alveolar hypoventilation, despite apparent increases in minute ventilation. In some patients, the use of supplemental oxygen is associated with worsened $CO_2$ retention. Mechanisms that have been postulated to contribute include the loss of hypoxemic vasoconstriction within the lungs, resulting in worsening $V_A/Q$ mismatch (28,29), changes in physiologic dead space (30), and a reduction in central drive to breathe as a result of the loss of hypoxemic ventilatory drive (31). Regardless, the presence of decompensated hypercarbia during an exacerbation has important prognostic considerations, correlating with both short- and long-term mortality (32,33).

In stable COPD, it has been suggested that the use of inhaled $\beta_2$-agonists may have deleterious effects on gas exchange. A study by Khoukaz and Gross (34) demonstrated that in a group of 20 patients with severe COPD (mean $FEV_1$ 43% predicted), administration of either inhaled salbutamol or salmeterol induced a small, but significant, reduction in $PaO_2$ (by 3.45 ± 0.92 and 2.74 ± 0.89 mm Hg, respectively). The small magnitude of change, coupled with a short duration of effect ($PaO_2$ had returned to predose levels after 30 minutes for salbutamol and 90 minutes for salmeterol) and the fact that no patient experienced a decline in $PaO_2$ to less than 59 mm Hg, would certainly question the clinical significance of these findings, at least in stable COPD. Until recently, however, the effects of inhaled $\beta_2$-agonists on gas exchange in the setting of COPD exacerbations, which are already characterized by worsening gas exchange parameters and $V_A/Q$ relationships, was unknown. Polverino and colleagues have since investigated the effects of nebulized salbutamol on spirometry, blood gases, hemodynamics and $V_A/Q$ relationships in patients hospitalized with an exacerbation of COPD (35). Surprisingly, they found that at exacerbation, salbutamol does not worsen the already compromised pulmonary gas exchange, with little effect on $PaO_2$, $PaCO_2$, or $V_A/Q$ mismatch. In contrast, and in keeping with the earlier study by Khoukaz and Gross, administration of nebulized salbutamol to the same patients during convalescence from the exacerbation resulted in small decreases in $PaO_2$ (by 6.7 mm Hg) and $V_A/Q$ mismatch, despite observed bronchodilatory effects. The authors speculated that the reduction in arterial oxygenation in response to salmeterol during convalescence may have been due to increases in blood flow to lower $V_A/Q$ areas, perhaps compounded by a release of hypoxemic vasoconstriction. Nonetheless, these findings are reassuring with regard to the safety of inhaled $\beta_2$-agonists administered during exacerbations and would support current guidelines, which suggest that the dose and frequency of short-acting $\beta_2$-agonists (SABAs) be increased during severe exacerbations (1).

## V.  Cardiovascular Effects

Cardiopulmonary interactions that occur in the setting of COPD are complex and are influenced by the mode of breathing (i.e., spontaneous, negative pressure breathing vs. mechanical ventilation), the phase of the respiratory cycle, lung volumes, and the presence and magnitude of PEEP$i$ that may occur in flow-limited patients (36). In spontaneously breathing COPD patients experiencing an exacerbation, inspiration is associated with an increase in right ventricular end-diastolic volume, suggestive of increased systemic venous return and therefore right ventricular preload (37). However, despite the enhanced return of blood to the right ventricle, patients with COPD often do not exhibit a concomitant increase in right-ventricular ejection fraction (37). It should be noted that at right atrial pressures ($P_{ra}$) that are less than atmospheric, venous return to the right atrium is flow limited, and thus any further increase in negative intrathoracic pressures will not result in further increases in venous return; thus, although patients with COPD suffering an exacerbation can exhibit sizable negative intrapleural inspiratory pressure swings (which are generated in order to overcome the inspiratory threshold load imposed on the inspiratory muscles as a consequence of PEEP$i$), these should not cause further increases to right ventricular preload beyond the point at which $P_{ra}$ becomes subatmospheric. Through the process of ventricular interdependence, however, the diastolic function of the left ventricle may become impaired as a consequence of increasing right ventricular diameter, as the interventricular septum may shift toward the left ventricle during diastole and impair left ventricular filling (38,39).

Mean pulmonary artery pressures ($P_{pa}$) are generally higher at any cardiac output in patients with COPD as compared with healthy subjects, and even patients with normal $P_{pa}$ at rest may demonstrate acute increases in $P_{pa}$ in response to exercise or exacerbations (40–42). The increase in $P_{pa}$ likely occurs as a consequence of emphysematous destruction of vascular beds within the lungs, aggravated by pulmonary alveolar hypoxemia due to relative alveolar hypoventilation and $V_A/Q$ mismatching, and contributes importantly to increases in right ventricular afterload (43,44).

The presence of dynamic hyperinflation during an exacerbation has important consequences to hemodynamics. Pulmonary vascular resistance (PVR) increases progressively at lung volumes above FRC (45), and hence in patients who experience acute DH during an exacerbation or exercise, there may be further increases in PVR (and therefore right ventricular afterload) associated with breathing at lung volumes close to TLC (43,46,47). Although venous return to the right ventricle may be increased during an exacerbation as described above, increases in lung volume may have the opposite effect, by directly resulting in compression of the superior vena cava and right heart (48,49) and indirectly due to increases in $P_{ra}$ (which decreases the gradient for venous return) (50). The application of positive pressure ventilation may be beneficial during an AECOPD in that it may offload the inspiratory muscles (and therefore decrease work of breathing) and provided that the amount of applied (i.e., extrinsic) PEEP is <90% of $PEEP_i$, does not result in further hyperinflation of the lungs, thereby avoiding any further increases in PVR (36,51).

In contrast to left ventricular diastolic function, which may be impaired through the process of ventricular interdependence as described above, left ventricular systolic function is often preserved in COPD in the absence of comorbidities such as ischemic heart disease (46,52). However, in the setting of acute and progressive increases in negative intrathoracic pressure, which may occur during a COPD exacerbation, left ventricular afterload would be expected to increase as a result of the larger imposed transmural pressure gradient (53). In the presence of significant levels of PEEP$i$, or at the upper extremes of the respiratory compliance curve (with DH), these pressures may be substantial and significantly increase the work of the left ventricle to maintain cardiac output.

## VI. Mechanisms of Dyspnea During Exacerbation

Increased perceived respiratory difficulty that persists despite the usual (or increased) bronchodilator therapy is often the dominant symptom of an acute exacerbation. The precise mechanisms of dyspnea in this circumstance are poorly understood and are complex. During an exacerbation, the net effect of airway inflammation, smooth muscle spasm, and sputum inspissation is worsening EFL, while attendant $V_A/Q$ and gas exchange abnormalities increase ventilatory demand. These factors, in turn, result in dynamic pulmonary hyperinflation with increased loading and functional weakness of the inspiratory muscles (54–56). Since the operating lung volumes are shifted upwards on the respiratory system compliance curve, the effort required for tidal inspiration represents a higher fraction of the maximal possible effort that the patient can develop at that lung volume.

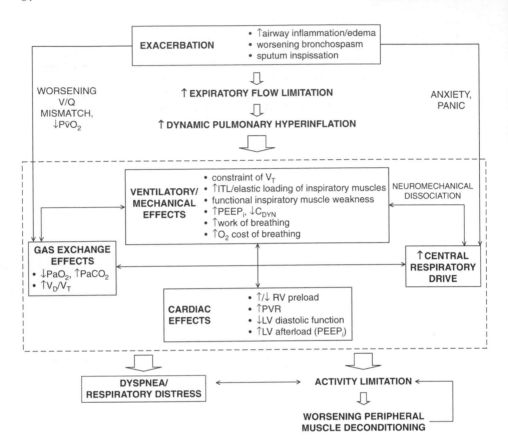

**Figure 4** Schematic illustrating the proposed mechanisms contributing to dyspnea in the setting of a COPD exacerbation. The genesis of dyspnea during exacerbation is complex, related to the interplay between effects on gas exchange, mechanics, central respiratory drive, and cardiovascular function. See text for details. *Abbreviations*: $V_A/Q$, ventilation/perfusion; $P\bar{v}O_2$, mixed venous oxygen tension; $PaO_2$, arterial partial pressure of oxygen; $PaCO_2$, arterial partial pressure of carbon dioxide; $V_D/V_T$, physiologic dead space fraction; VT, tidal volume; ITL, inspiratory threshold loading; PEEP$i$, intrinsic positive end-expiratory pressure; $C_{DYN}$, dynamic pulmonary compliance; RV, right ventricular; PVR, pulmonary vascular resistance; LV, left ventricular.

Beyond a certain threshold, this increased effort may be directly perceived as unpleasant due to increased central motor output and simultaneous central corollary discharge to the somatosensory cortex (57). Central drive to breathe is usually preserved in COPD and actually increases in response to physiologic stressors during an exacerbation (58,59). Neural output to the respiratory muscles may be further stimulated by factors such as arterial hypoxemia, acute hypercarbia, acidosis, fever, or increased sympathetic nervous system activation. As noted already, DH during an exacerbation may constrain tidal volume expansion in the setting of an increase in central drive; this neuromechanical dissociation has been implicated in the genesis of dyspnea during exercise in patients with COPD (60) and in asthmatics during acute bronchoconstriction (61,62). Although definitive data are lacking, it seems logical that similar mechanisms may contribute to the etiology of dyspnea during COPD exacerbations where severe acute DH has been documented. Activation of airway (secondary to mucosal inflammation or dynamic compression during expiration) and cardiovascular mechanosensors (as a result of the effects of hypoxemia and DH) may directly or indirectly induce unpleasant respiratory sensation during an exacerbation. Arterial hypercarbia and critical hypoxemia may directly cause dyspnea, independent of the attendant increased ventilation, by altering chemoreceptor output to the sensory cortex. Respiratory disruption during exacerbations is almost invariably associated with perceived distress or anxiety that in some patients can escalate rapidly to incapacitating panic; in this setting, anxiety results in tachypnea, which further contributes to DH (and thus respiratory distress) in a vicious cycle. This important affective dimension of dyspnea is likely associated with increased limbic and paralimbic system activation (63–66). In elderly patients with more advanced COPD, severe dyspnea during AECOPD can often lead to protracted periods of immobilization with accelerated wasting and deconditioning of the muscles of locomotion. A schematic illustrating the complex interaction of the pathophysiologic changes occurring during an exacerbation, and their proposed relationship to the genesis of dyspnea, is presented in Figure 4.

## VII. Conclusions

Our understanding of the complex pathophysiologic mechanisms that underlie exacerbations of COPD continues to grow. The development of worsening EFL and dynamic pulmonary hyperinflation has important deleterious effects on ventilatory muscles, dynamic mechanics, cardiovascular function, and gas exchange, which collectively contribute to perceived respiratory difficulty during exacerbations. Pharmacologic treatments aimed at reducing lung hyperinflation together with noninvasive mechanical ventilation, which counterbalances the negative effects of acutely increased lung hyperinflation on the ventilatory muscles, should successfully relieve dyspnea and improve outcomes during exacerbations. However, the development of simple and accurate physiologic tests to reliably predict exacerbations, or to provide prognostic information pertaining to their severity, remains an elusive goal. Traditional measures of forced maximal expiratory flow rates and volumes have not consistently proven to be helpful in this regard. It remains to be seen whether indices of pulmonary hyperinflation, such as the IC, provide additional useful information for the clinical evaluation of exacerbations of COPD.

## References

1. O'Donnell DE, Aaron S, Bourbeau J, et al. Canadian Thoracic Society recommendations for management of chronic obstructive pulmonary disease—2007 update. Can Respir J 2007; 14(suppl B):5B–32B.
2. Vincken W, van Noord JA, Greefhorfst APM, et al. Improved health outcomes in patients with COPD during 1 yr's treatment with tiotropium. Eur Respir J 2002; 19:209–216.
3. Poole PJ, Black PN. Oral mucolytic drugs for exacerbations of chronic obstructive pulmonary disease: systematic review. BMJ 2001; 322:1271–1274.
4. O'Donnell DE, Parker CM. COPD Exacerbations. 3: Pathophysiology. Thorax 2006; 61:354–361.

5.  Niewoehner DE, Collins D, Erbland ML. Relation of FEV1 to clinical outcomes during exacerbations of chronic obstructive pulmonary disease. Am J Respir Crit Care Med 2000; 161:1201–1205.

6.  Aaron SD, Vandemheen KJ, Hebert P, et al. Outpatient oral prednisone after emergency treatment of chronic obstructive pulmonary disease. N Engl J Med 2003; 348:2618–2625.

7.  Sachs AP, Koeter GH, Groenier KH, et al. Changes in symptoms, peak expiratory flow, and sputum flora during treatment with antibiotics of exacerbations in patients with chronic obstructive pulmonary disease in general practice. Thorax 1995; 50:758–763.

8.  Davies L, Angus RM, Calverley PMA. Oral corticosteroids in patients admitted to hospital with exacerbations of chronic obstructive pulmonary disease: a prospective randomized controlled trial. Lancet 1999; 354:456–460.

9.  Bhowmik A, Seemungal TAR, Sapsford RJ et al. Relation of sputum inflammatory markers to symptoms and lung function changes in COPD exacerbations. Thorax 2000; 55:114–120.

10. Seemungal TAR, Donaldson GC, Bhowmik A, et al. Time course of recovery of exacerbations in patients with chronic obstructive pulmonary disease. Am J Respir Crit Care Med 1999; 161:1608–1613.

11. Parker CM, Voduc N, Aaron SD, et al. Physiological changes during symptom recovery from moderate exacerbations of COPD. Eur Respir J 2005; 26:420–428.

12. Rodriguez-Roisin R. Towards a consensus definition for COPD exacerbations. Chest 2000; 117 (suppl. 2):398S–401S.

13. Stevenson NJ, Walker PP, Costello RW, et al. Lung mechanics and dyspnea during exacerbations of chronic obstructive pulmonary disease. Am J Respir Crit Care Med 2005; 172:1510–1516.

14. Johnson MK, Birch M, Carter R, et al. Measurement of physiological recovery from exacerbation of chronic obstructive pulmonary disease using within-breath forced oscillometry. Thorax 2007; 62:299–306.

15. Howard P. A long-term follow-up of respiratory symptoms and ventilatory function in a group of working men. Br J Industr Med 1970; 27:326–333.

16. Bates D. The fate of the chronic bronchitic: a report of the 10-year follow-up in the Canadian Department of Veteran's Affairs coordinated study of chronic bronchitis. Am Rev Respir Dis 1973; 108:1043–1065.

17. Kanner RE, Renzetti AD, Klauber MR, et al. Variables associated with changes in spirometry in patients with obstructive lung disease. Am J Med 1979; 67:44–50.

18. Kanner RE, Anthonisen NR, Connett JE. Lower respiratory illnesses promote FEV1 decline in current smokers but not ex-smokers with mild chronic obstructive pulmonary disease. Am J Respir Crit Care Med 2001; 164:358–364.

19. Donaldson GC, Seemungal TAR, Bhowmik A, et al. Relationship between exacerbation frequency and lung function decline in chronic obstructive pulmonary disease. Thorax 2002; 57:847–852.

20. O'Donnell DE, Laveneziana P. Physiology and consequences of lung hyperinflation in COPD. Eur Respir Rev 2006; 15:61–67.

21. Pare PD, Brooks LA, Bates J. Exponential analysis of the lung pressure-volume curve as a predictor of pulmonary emphysema. Am Rev Respir Dis 1982; 126:54–61.

22. Haluszka J, Chartrand DA, Grassino AE, et al. Intrinsic PEEP and arterial pCO2 in stable patients with chronic obstructive pulmonary disease. Am Rev Respir Dis 1990; 141:1194–1197.

23. Sinderby C, Spahija J, Beck J, et al. Diaphragm activation during exercise in chronic obstructive pulmonary disease. Am J Respir Crit Care Med 2001; 163:1637–1641.

24. O'Donnell DE. Exercise limitation and clinical exercise testing in chronic obstructive pulmonary disease. In: Zeballos RJ, Weisman IM, eds. Clinical Exercise Testing: Progress in Respiratory Research. Basel, Switzerland: Karger Series, 2002; 32:138–158.

25. Yan S, Kaminski D, Sliwinski P. Reliability of inspiratory capacity for estimating end-expiratory lung-volume changes during exercise in patients with chronic obstructive pulmonary disease. Am J Respir Crit Care Med 1997; 156:55–59.

26. Calverley PMA. Respiratory failure in chronic obstructive pulmonary disease. Eur Respir J; 2003:22, 26–30.
27. Barbera JA, Roca J, Ferrer A, et al. Mechanisms of worsening gas exchange during acute exacerbations of chronic obstructive pulmonary disease. Eur Respir J 1997; 10:1285–1291.
28. O'Donnell DE, D'Arsigny C, Fitzpatrick M, et al. Exercise hypercapnia in advanced chronic obstructive pulmonary disease. Am J Respir Crit Care Med 2002; 166:663–668.
29. Aubier M, Murciano D, Milic-Emili J, et al. Effects of the administration of O2 on ventilation and blood gases in patients with chronic obstructive pulmonary disease during acute respiratory failure. Am Rev Respir Dis 1980; 122:747–754.
30. Hanson CW, Marshall BE, Frasch HF, et al. Causes of hypercarbia with oxygen therapy in patients with chronic obstructive pulmonary disease. Crit Care Med 1996; 24:23–28.
31. Robinson TD, Freiberg DB, Regnis JA, et al. The role of hypoventilation and ventilation-perfusion redistribution in oxygen-induced hypercapnia during acute exacerbations of chronic obstructive pulmonary disease. Am J Respir Crit Care Med 2000; 161:1524–1529.
32. Seneff MG, Wagner DP, Wagner RP, et al. Hospital and 1-year survival of patients admitted to intensive care units with acute exacerbations of chronic obstructive pulmonary disease. JAMA 1995; 274:1852–1857.
33. Connors AFJ, Dawson NV, Thomas C, et al. Outcomes following acute exacerbations of severe chronic obstructive lung disease. The SUPPORT investigators. Am J Respir Crit Care Med 1996; 154:959–967.
34. Khoukaz G, Gross NJ. Effects of salmeterol on arterial blood gases in patients with stable chronic obstructive pulmonary disease. Am J Respir Crit Care Med 1999; 160:1028–1030.
35. Polverino E, Gomez FP, Manrique H, et al. Gas exchange response to short-acting β2-agonists in chronic obstructive pulmonary disease severe exacerbations. Am J Respir Crit Care Med 2007; 176:350–355.
36. Ranieri VM, Dambrosio M, Brienza N. Intrinsic PEEP and cardiopulmonary interaction in patients with COPD and acute ventilatory failure. Eur Respir J 1996; 9:1283–1292.
37. Dhainaut JF, Brunet F. Phasic changes of right ventricular ejection fraction in patients with acute exacerbation of chronic obstructive pulmonary disease. Intensive Care Med 1987; 12:214–215.
38. Settle HP, Engel PJ, Fowler NO. Echocardiographic study of the paradoxical arterial pulse in chronic obstructive pulmonary disease. Circulation 1980; 62:1297–1307.
39. Jardin F, Gueret P, Prost JF, et al. Two-dimensional echocardiographic assessment of left ventricular function in chronic obstructive pulmonary disease. Am Rev Respir Dis 1984; 129: 135–142.
40. Mahler DA, Brent BN, Loke J, et al. Right ventricular performance and central circulatory hemodynamics during upright exercise in patients with chronic obstructive pulmonary disease. Am Rev Respir Dis 1984; 130:722–729.
41. Lemaire F, Tebul JL, Cinotti L, et al. Acute left ventricular dysfunction during unsuccessful weaning from mechanical ventilation. Anaesthesiology 1988; 69:171–179.
42. Marangoni S, Scalvini S, Schena M, et al. Right ventricular diastolic dysfunction in chronic obstructive lung disease. Eur Respir J; 1992:5, 438–443.
43. Magee F, Wright JL, Wiggs BR, et al. Pulmonary vascular structures and function in chronic obstructive pulmonary disease. Thorax 1988; 43:183–189.
44. Agusti AGN, Barbera JA, Roca J, et al. Hypoxemic pulmonary vasoconstriction and gas exchange during exercise in chronic obstructive pulmonary disease. Chest 1990; 97:268–275.
45. Whittenberger JL, McGregor M, Berglund E. Influence of state of inflation of the lung on pulmonary vascular resistance. J Appl Physiol 1960; 15:878–882.
46. Matthay RA, Berger HJ, Davies RA, et al. Right and left ventricular exercise performance in chronic obstructive pulmonary disease: radionucleotide assessment. Ann Intern Med 1980; 93:234–239.
47. Oswald-Mammosser M, Apprill M, Bachez P, et al. Pulmonary hemodynamics in chronic obstructive pulmonary disease of the emphysematous type. Respiration 1991; 58304–58310.

48. Nakhjaven FK, Palmer WH, McGregor M. Influence of respiration on venous return in pulmonary emphysema. Circulation 1966; 33:8–16.
49. Brookhart JM, Boyd TE. Local differences in intrathoracic pressure and their relation to cardiac filling pressure in the dog. Am J Physiol 1947; 148:434–444.
50. Pinsky MR. Determinants of pulmonary artery flow variation during respiration. J Appl Physiol 1984; 56:1237–1245.
51. Dambrosio M, Cinnella G, Brienza N, et al. Effects of positive end-expiratory pressure on right ventricular function in COPD patients during acute ventilatory failure. Intensive Care Med 1996; 22:923–932.
52. Vizza CD, Lynch JP, Ochoa LL, et al. Right and left ventricular dysfunction in patients with severe pulmonary disease. Chest 1998; 113:576–583.
53. Richard C, Tebul JL, Archambaud F, et al. Left ventricular function during weaning of patients with chronic obstructive pulmonary disease. Intensive Care Med 1994; 20:181–186.
54. Pride NB, Macklem PT. Lung mechanics in disease. In: AP Fishman, ed. Handbook of Physiology, section 3, volume III, part 2: The Respiratory System. Bethesda, MD: American Physiological Society, 1986:659–692.
55. O'Donnell DE, Webb KA. Exercise. In: Calverley PMA, MacNee W, Pride NB, et al., eds. Chronic Obstructive Pulmonary Disease, 2nd ed. London: Arnold, 2003:243–269.
56. Orozco-Levi M. Structure and function of the respiratory muscles in patients with COPD: impairment or adaptation? Eur Respir J 2003; 22(suppl 46):41s–51s.
57. Chen Z, Eldridge FL, Wagner PG. Respiratory-associated thalamic activity is related to the level of respiratory drive. Resp Physiol 1992; 90:99–113.
58. De Troyer A, Leeper JB, McKenzie DK, et al. Neural drive to the diaphragm in patients with severe COPD. Am J Respir Crit Care Med 1997; 155:1335–1340.
59. Sinderby C, Spahija J, Beck J, et al. Diaphragm activation during exercise in chronic obstructive pulmonary disease. Am J Respir Crit Care Med 2001; 163:1637–1641.
60. O'Donnell DE, Chau LKL, Bertley JC, et al. Qualitative aspects of exertional breathlessness in chronic airflow limitation: pathophysiologic mechanisms. Am J Respir Crit Care Med 1997; 155: 109–115.
61. Lougheed MD, Webb K, O'Donnell DE. Breathlessness during induced hyperinflation in asthma: role of the inspiratory threshold load. Am J Respir Crit Care Med 1995; 152:911–920.
62. Lougheed MD, Fisher T, O'Donnell DE. Dynamic hyperinflation during bronchoconstriction in asthma: implications for symptom perception. Chest 2006; 130:1072–1081.
63. Evans KC, Banzett RB, Adams L, et al. BOLD fMRI identifies limbic, paralimbic, and cerebellar activation during air hunger. J Neurophysiol 2002; 88:1500–1511.
64. Liotti M, Brannan S, Egan G, et al. Brain responses associated with consciousness of breathlessness (air hunger). Proc Natl Acad Sci USA 2001; 98:2035–2040.
65. Peiffer C, Poline J, Thivard L, et al. Neural substrates for the perception of acutely induced dyspnea. Am J Respir Crit Care Med 2001; 163:951–957.
66. Banzett RB, Mulnier HE, Murphy K, et al. Breathlessness in humans activates insular cortex. Neuroreport 2000; 11:2117–2120.

# 8
## Systemic Consequences of COPD Exacerbations

**SCOTT S. WAGERS, KARIN GROENEWEGEN, and EMIEL F. WOUTERS**
Department of Respiratory Medicine, University Hospital Maastricht, Maastricht, The Netherlands

## I. Introduction

It is well recognized that the manifestations of chronic obstructive pulmonary disease (COPD) are not limited to the lungs (1), and as an exacerbation is most often defined as an interval of symptomatic deterioration (2), it is not surprising that COPD exacerbations have systemic consequences. However, the systemic consequences of exacerbations of COPD differ from the chronic systemic manifestations of COPD in both mechanism and pathophysiology and are not simply the result of an interval magnification of chronic systemic manifestations. In this chapter, we will review the mechanism and pathophysiology of the systemic consequences of COPD exacerbations, giving special attention to exacerbation-specific aspects. We will begin by describing two consequences of exacerbations, systemic inflammation and oxidative stress, both of which cause and perpetuate most of the other, more specific consequences of exacerbations. We will then describe these other consequences, highlighting their connection with systemic inflammation and oxidative stress (Fig. 1).

## II. Systemic Inflammation and Oxidative Stress

### A. Systemic Inflammation

Along with local pulmonary inflammation, increases in blood concentrations of various inflammatory markers, c-reactive protein (CRP), interleukin (IL)-6, IL-8, LTB4, procalcitonin, copeptin, leptin, ECP, MPO, tumor necrosis factor-$\alpha$ (TNF-$\alpha$), fibrinogen, and markers of neutrophil activation have been reported during exacerbations in multiple studies (3–15). Chronic stable COPD is also characterized by concurrent local pulmonary and systemic inflammation; nonetheless, the direct association between these two compartments has been difficult to elucidate. Vernooy et al. (16) studied both sputum and plasma concentrations of soluble TNF-$\alpha$ receptors (sTNF-$\alpha$R) and IL-8 and found that while both were elevated, there were no direct correlations between sputum and plasma concentrations. Lack of a link between airway inflammation and the systemic inflammatory response in chronic stable disease has also been found by others (17). These studies have led to the notion that systemic and local inflammations are differentially regulated and that

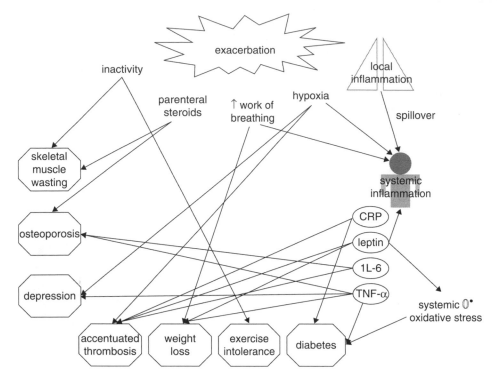

**Figure 1**  Schematic showing systemic consequences of COPD exacerbations. *Abbreviation*: COPD, chronic obstructive pulmonary disease.

invoking "spill over" of local inflammation to explain systemic inflammation is not valid. When it comes to exacerbations, however, such a conclusion is probably not justified. Indeed, Hurst et al. (18) did find significant correlations between lower airway inflammation and the systemic inflammatory response during COPD exacerbations. They found that sputum IL-8 and leukocyte count both correlated with both serum CRP and IL-6, although the correlation coefficients were 0.39 or less. Nonetheless, these correlations do suggest that during an exacerbation, local pulmonary inflammation does spill over into the systemic compartment. This may represent an effect from the increasing degree of pulmonary inflammation, or it could be related to the presence of bacteria or viruses as exacerbations are often associated with infection (1). Hurst et al. (18), in the same study as mentioned above, also found that the presence of pathogenic micro-organisms, bacteria or viruses, in sputum was associated with a significant increase in the systemic inflammatory response, increased concentrations of CRP. Additionally, we know that inducible cell migration is enhanced during respiratory infections consequent to pathogen recognition through receptors such as toll-like receptors (TLRS) (19). This results in the elaboration of chemokines and chemotactic factors, most important of which are IL-8, growth-related oncogene-alpha (GRO-α), monocyte chemoattractant protein (MCP)-1, MCP-2, MCP-3, MCP-4, macrophage inflammatory protein (MIP)-1α, MIP-1β, and RANTES (20–22), which bind to the luminal surface of the vascular endothelium and activate leucocytes (19,20,23,24). Most tissues of the body have resident innate leukocytes such as dendritic cells (DCs), macrophages, and mast cells that are triggered by CCL20-CCR6 receptors, which have recently been shown to have a role in exacerbations (25,26). Thus, it is highly conceivable that the difference between chronic stable COPD and exacerbations, in terms of the local or systemic inflammation link, is the presence of a pathogen, resulting in the marshaling of a system-wide response through the innate immune system.

Hypoxia is a major concern during a COPD exacerbation (27) and may be an additional manner in which local pulmonary inflammation is translated to the systemic compartment. Hypoxia inducible factor-1 (HIF-1) is a transcription factor that is activated in the presence of hypoxia and has a broad array of effects (28,29), including the upregulation of inflammation evidenced by increases in concentrations of TNF-$\alpha$ (30).

### B.  Oxidative Stress

It is in fact difficult to separate systemic inflammation and systemic oxidative stress. Neutrophils are known to produce reactive oxygen species, and in the lung, they have been identified as a major source of superoxide anion (31). As pointed out above, exacerbations do increase neutrophil activation (15), it is therefore easy to see how exacerbations are associated with increased oxidant stress. Rahman et al. (32) demonstrated that Trolox-equivalent antioxidant capacity (TEAC) was low during exacerbations, which is taken to mean that oxidant activity is increased. Subsequently, it was shown that this exacerbation-associated oxidant/antioxidant imbalance returns to normal during the course of exacerbation treatment (13,33). An association between systemic inflammation and systemic oxidative stress during exacerbations has been found (13), suggesting that systemic inflammation is causing and/or perpetuating systemic oxidative stress. However, an association between physical exercise and oxidative stress has also been found (34,35), and when you consider that exacerbations of COPD, at the very least temporarily, can increase the work of breathing even, leading to respiratory failure, it becomes apparent that the muscle strain that comes with a COPD exacerbation may itself be contributing to systemic oxidative stress.

As exacerbations of COPD are of a relatively short duration in comparison to the chronic progressive course of COPD, one has to question what impact exacerbation-associated consequences have on the course of disease. The answer is that systemic inflammation and oxidative stress provoked by an exacerbation are not temporary. Markers of neutrophil activation remain elevated for at least six months following an exacerbation (15). Thus, the impact of exacerbations on other organ systems likely persists longer than the exacerbation itself. In addition, even in terms of symptoms and lung function, approximately a quarter of all exacerbations persist for a month or more (36).

### III.  Skeletal Muscle Wasting

Loss of skeletal muscle, or fat-free mass, has long been established as a feature of chronic stable COPD (37) and has been linked to inflammation, namely circulating concentrations of IL-6 and TNF-$\alpha$ (38). Hopkinson et al. (39) studied a cohort of 64 stable COPD patients prospectively and measured quadriceps strength and fat-free mass. Quadriceps strength did not correlate with exacerbation frequency, whereas when the cohort was separated into exacerbators (>1 exacerbation per year), and nonexacerbators, fat-free mass declined significantly more in the exacerbators. Unlike stable patients, the link with inflammation was less obvious. The authors also found an association between maintenance of steroid use and the decline in fat-free mass, but also pointed out that most of the subjects had received bursts of intermittent steroids, as used in exacerbations, and that there was no association with fat-free mass decline, and therefore suggested that an intermittent burst strategy may be safe in terms of fat-free mass. Nonetheless, there has been at least one study that has found a high correlation ($r = 0.73$) between the presence of a negative nitrogen balance, an indication of muscle wasting, and the dose of methylprednisone used to treat an exacerbation (40). As for inflammation as a causative factor, when skeletal muscle biopsies from the vastus lateralis were taken during an exacerbation, there was no evidence of increase in the inflammatory markers IL-6, IL-8, and TNF-$\alpha$ compared with stable and healthy subjects (41). There was, however, evidence of an increase in markers of disuse (insulin-like growth factor-1 and myogenin), suggesting that disuse was a significant causative factor, and as detailed below in the next section, inactivity or exercise intolerance is clearly a systemic consequence of COPD exacerbations.

## IV. Exercise Intolerance

An individual's activity level decreases when he or she experiences a COPD exacerbation. As a rough measure, Donaldson et al. (42), in a longitudinal study, quantified time spent outdoors and found that frequent exacerbators have a more rapid decline. Prior to an exacerbation, time spent outdoors decreases and remains decreased for up to five weeks, meaning that exacerbations increase an individual's risk for becoming homebound. A more specific quantification of activity can be achieved with ambulatory activity monitoring; and when this was done in COPD patients, the results by Donaldson et al., including the long duration of decreased activity, were confirmed (43). Furthermore, those with a recent exacerbation of less than one year prior, had decreased activity level compared with those who did not, and those with a decreased activity level one month after an exacerbation had an increased risk of being readmitted for an exacerbation. The fact that this decrease in activity results in an increase in exercise intolerance was established by Cote et al. (44) when they examined the effect of exacerbations on the body mass, obstruction, dyspnea, and exercise capacity (BODE) index. They found that the BODE index significantly decreases with an exacerbation and, more importantly, that this decrease was driven the most by decreases in the six-minute walk duration (6MWD). In fact, they found that there is a 75-m deficit in 6MWD up to two years after an exacerbation. Considering the fact that immobilization and disuse results in profound muscle wasting (45)that worsens exercise tolerance, it is clear how muscle wasting and exercise tolerance entwine the patient in a vicious circle that can be initiated by an exacerbation.

## V. Weight Loss

The vicious circle of muscle wasting and exercise tolerance also encompasses weight loss driven mostly by the loss of fat-free mass. However, there are other factors in play that make overall weight loss a consequence of concern. Vermeeren et al. (46) found that prior to admission to the hospital for an exacerbation 41% of patients had experienced involuntary weight loss. All of those admitted had an increase in resting energy expenditure and impaired diet–induced thermogenesis, indicating the presence of a catabolic state. The importance of weight loss is highlighted by the inclusion of body mass index (BMI) in the BODE index (47,48) and by the fact that weight loss has been reported to be a risk factor to hospital admission (49) and readmission (48). The link between TNF-α and weight loss in stable COPD is well established (50,51), and given the exacerbation associated with rise in TNF-α, it is highly conceivable that exacerbations contribute to weight loss in this manner. More specifically, Creutzberg et al. (52) linked elevated concentrations of plasma leptin to the weight loss observed in exacerbations; however, circulating leptin is conventionally thought to be proportional to the amount of adipose tissue in any given individual. This contradiction can be explained by a further association of leptin concentrations with sTNF-α, indicating that leptin is under control of the systemic inflammatory response (52). Leptin exerts most of its energy metabolism effects through effects on the central nervous system, namely the hypothalamic nuclei. These effects include decreases in food intake, increases in energy expenditure, and decreases in metabolic efficiency. In addition, leptin has been shown to influence a wide spectrum of biological functions, including lipid and glucose metabolism, synthesis of glucocorticoids and insulin, regulation of the hypothalamic-pituitary-adrenal axis, maturation of the reproductive system, hematopoiesis, angiogenesis, and fetal development (53–67). It has recently been shown that leptin has a potentiating role in the function of both innate and adaptive immunity (59). Leptin stimulates inflammatory cell chemotaxis (56) and improves oxidative burst (56), phagocytosis (62), and cytokine secretion (60,64). In addition, leptin potentiates T-lymphocytes (60,61,68). So, the weight loss observed in a COPD exacerbation is likely a direct and indirect consequence of an enhanced systemic inflammatory response, with the principal systemic mediators being TNF-α and leptin, which is a process that is further amplified by leptin itself.

## VI. Osteoporosis

Osteoporosis is known to be a major comorbidity for individuals with COPD (69), and there is good reason to believe that exacerbations worsen bone mineral density. TNF-α stimulates leukocytes to secrete factors that facilitate osteoclastic activity and inhibit collagen synthesis (70), while IL-6 can stimulate osteoclasts (71), and both TNF-α and IL-6 are part of the systemic inflammatory response seen in exacerbations. A study of 1004 elderly women examined clinical factors that contributed to the variability seen in bone mineral density and found that body mass was one of the best predictors, whereas activity level only explained 1% to 6% of the variability (72), which is a finding that has been confirmed in a COPD cohort as well (73). Dubois et al. (74) examined the density of the lumbar spine in 86 patients with COPD and found that the osteroporosis was related to a cumulative dose of prednisone greater than 1000 mg, regardless of whether it was dosed intermittently or continuously. Thus, unlike muscle wasting, a steroid burst strategy, as is often used to treat exacerbations, does carry significant risk. Furthermore, steroids have been shown to increase 1,25 dihydroxy vitamin D concentrations in patients with COPD and thereby result in more calcium turnover, resulting in a loss of bone mineral density (75).

## VII.  Diabetes

Rana et al. (76), using the cohort of 103,614 female nurses that comprise the Nurses Health Study, examined the relative risk for the development of diabetes in both patients with asthma and COPD. They found that patients with COPD were at a significantly increased risk (RR 1.8) of developing diabetes compared with those with asthma and those without either. Insulin resistance can be produced by a variety of mechanisms, but perhaps most interesting, in the light of this findings, are those related to the systemic consequences of COPD. CRP, fibrinogen, and TNF-$\alpha$ have all been associated with insulin resistance (77,78). Furthermore, oxidative stress is also considered to be a risk factor for the development of insulin resistance (78), and leptin interferes with insulin secretion (79). Considering these interactions and the knowledge that skeletal muscle is a major site of glucose uptake, it is not surprising that during exacerbations an increased concentration of serum glucose and insulin have been identified and found to subsequently decrease with treatment (52).

## VIII.  Accentuated Thrombosis

One of the most striking systemic consequences of an exacerbation of COPD is the increase in thrombotic events. It is now being recognized that pulmonary emboli (PE) are frequently present during exacerbations. Tillie-Leblond et al. (80), using high resolution computed tomography (CT) scanning to diagnose PEs in patients with an unexplained exacerbation, found a prevalence of 25% of PE. This is in accordance with autopsy studies that have found PEs up to 30% of the time in patients who died during a COPD exacerbation (81). Similarly, a high prevalence of deep venous thrombosis, 10%, has also been reported during COPD exacerbations in multiple studies (81–83). In addition, an association between acute myocardial infarctions and COPD exacerbations has been reported (84); however, there was also an association with ongoing oral steroid use, and the risk abated when the steroids were stopped. Thus, this association may be a consequence of steroid use. A number of factors may be responsible for this thrombotic tendency. Fibrinogen elaboration is promoted by IL-6, and thus fibrinogen concentrations rise with IL-6 during COPD exacerbations (14). Fibrinogen, or more specifically, fibrinopeptide A and B are cleaved by thrombin to form fibrin, which is the major structural component of a thrombosis. Thus, increased concentrations of fibrinogen can result in an accentuated risk of a thrombotic event. Leptin itself is also an independent risk factor for thrombotic disorders because of its promotion of endothelial dysfunction, platelet aggregation, and oxidative stress (85). Platelet aggregation, also an important step in thrombosis formation, has been shown to be enhanced by hypoxemia and thereby may also play a role in these thrombotic consequences (86). Furthermore, CRP has been shown to be a predictive marker of cardiovascular disease (87), and it is not just a marker of inflammation but also contributes directly to the pathogenesis of atherosclerosis (88).

## IX.  Depression

The reported prevalence of depression in individuals with COPD ranges from 20% to 60% (89). Those that have depressive symptoms are more likely to have recently accessed the health care system (90) and are more likely to have been admitted to the hospital (91). Once admitted, the hospital stays of individuals with COPD and depression are generally longer (92), and those that require the use of psychotropic drugs are more likely to be readmitted (93). Thus, exacerbations and depression are associated; however, which is the causative factor is not clear. It can however be pointed out that magnetic resonance imaging (MRI) spectroscopy has revealed alterations in the cerebral cortex of individuals with COPD that resemble those seen in individuals who have been exposed to high altitude hypoxia (94).

## X. Summary

Like chronic stable COPD, the systemic consequences of exacerbations are broad, yet the pathophysiology varies from that seen in stable disease. One also has to take into consideration the impact of an exacerbation, including such factors as acute debilitation, hypoxia, and the effects of steroid use. The consequences of exacerbations can linger long after the exacerbation is symptomatically improved, resulting in more rapid deterioration and more hospital readmissions. Consideration of the systemic consequences of exacerbations of COPD is important not only for management of patients but also if we are to improve our understanding of overall pathogenesis of COPD.

## References

1. Global initiative for chronic obstructive lung disease. Global strategy for the diagnosis, management, and prevention of chronic obstructive pulmonary disease. 2006. Ref Type: Internet Communication (www.goldcopd.com).
2. Hurst JR, Wedzicha JA. The biology of a chronic obstructive pulmonary disease exacerbation. Clin Chest Med 2007; 28(3):525–536, v.
3. Calikoglu M, Sahin G, Unlu A, et al. Leptin and TNF-alpha levels in patients with chronic obstructive pulmonary disease and their relationship to nutritional parameters. Respiration 2004; 71(1):45–50.
4. Dahl M, Vestbo J, Lange P, et al. C-reactive protein as a predictor of prognosis in chronic obstructive pulmonary disease. Am J Respir Crit Care Med 2007; 175(3):250–255.
5. Dentener MA, Creutzberg EC, Schols AM, et al. Systemic anti-inflammatory mediators in COPD: increase in soluble interleukin 1 receptor II during treatment of exacerbations. Thorax 2001; 56(9):721–726.
6. Donaldson GC, Seemungal TA, Patel IS, et al. Airway and systemic inflammation and decline in lung function in patients with COPD. Chest 2005; 128(4):1995–2004.
7. Hurst JR, Donaldson GC, Perera WR, et al. Use of plasma biomarkers at exacerbation of chronic obstructive pulmonary disease. Am J Respir Crit Care Med 2006; 174(8):867–874.
8. Joppa P, Petrasova D, Stancak B, et al. Systemic inflammation in patients with COPD and pulmonary hypertension. Chest 2006; 130(2):326–333.
9. Perera WR, Hurst JR, Wilkinson TM, et al. Inflammatory changes, recovery and recurrence at COPD exacerbation. Eur Respir J 2007; 29(3):527–534.
10. Pinto-Plata V, Toso J, Lee K, et al. Profiling Serum Biomarkers in Patients with COPD: Associations with Clinical Parameters. Thorax 2007; 62(7):595–601.
11. Stolz D, Christ-Crain M, Bingisser R, et al. Antibiotic treatment of exacerbations of COPD: a randomized, controlled trial comparing procalcitonin-guidance with standard therapy. Chest 2007; 131(1):9–19.
12. Stolz D, Christ-Crain M, Morgenthaler NG, et al. Copeptin, C-reactive protein, and procalcitonin as prognostic biomarkers in acute exacerbation of COPD. Chest 2007; 131(4):1058–1067.

13. Tkacova R, Kluchova Z, Joppa P, et al. Systemic inflammation and systemic oxidative stress in patients with acute exacerbations of COPD. Respir Med 2007; 101(8):1670–1676. (Epub 2007, Apr 20.)

14. Wedzicha JA, Seemungal TA, MacCallum PK, et al. Acute exacerbations of chronic obstructive pulmonary disease are accompanied by elevations of plasma fibrinogen and serum IL-6 levels. Thromb Haemost 2000; 84(2):210–215.

15. Groenewegen KH, Dentener MA, Wouters EF. Longitudinal follow-up of systemic inflammation after acute exacerbations of COPD. Respir Med 2007; 101(11):2409–2415.

16. Vernooy JH, Kucukaycan M, Jacobs JA, et al. Local and systemic inflammation in patients with chronic obstructive pulmonary disease: soluble tumor necrosis factor receptors are increased in sputum. Am J Respir Crit Care Med 2002; 166(9):1218–1224.

17. Hurst JR, Wilkinson TM, Perera WR, et al. Relationships among bacteria, upper airway, lower airway, and systemic inflammation in COPD. Chest 2005; 127(4):1219–1226.

18. Hurst JR, Perera WR, Wilkinson TM, et al. Systemic and upper and lower airway inflammation at exacerbation of chronic obstructive pulmonary disease. Am J Respir Crit Care Med 2006; 173 (1):71–78.

19. Laudanna C, Kim JY, Constantin G, et al. Rapid leukocyte integrin activation by chemokines. Immunol Rev 2002; 186:37–46.

20. Iwasaki A, Medzhitov R. Toll-like receptor control of the adaptive immune responses. Nat Immunol 2004; 5(10):987–95.

21. Mantovani A. The chemokine system: redundancy for robust outputs. Immunol Today 1999; 20 (6):254–257.

22. McCurdy JD, Olynych TJ, Maher LH, et al. Cutting edge: distinct Toll-like receptor 2 activators selectively induce different classes of mediator production from human mast cells. J Immunol 2003; 170(4):1625–1629.

23. Hornung V, Rothenfusser S, Britsch S, et al. Quantitative expression of toll-like receptor 1-10 mRNA in cellular subsets of human peripheral blood mononuclear cells and sensitivity to CpG oligodeoxynucleotides. J Immunol 2002; 168(9):4531–4537.

24. Nagase H, Okugawa S, Ota Y, et al. Expression and function of Toll-like receptors in eosinophils: activation by Toll-like receptor 7 ligand. J Immunol 2003; 171(8):3977–3982.

25. Demedts IK, Bracke KR, Van Pottelberge G, et al. Accumulation of dendritic cells and increased CCL20 levels in the airways of patients with chronic obstructive pulmonary disease. Am J Respir Crit Care Med 2007; 175(10):998–1005.

26. Starner TD, Barker CK, Jia HP, et al. CCL20 is an inducible product of human airway epithelia with innate immune properties. Am J Respir Cell Mol Biol 2003; 29(5):627–633.

27. Celli BR, MacNee W. Standards for the diagnosis and treatment of patients with COPD: a summary of the ATS/ERS position paper. Eur Respir J 2004; 23(6):932–946.

28. Semenza GL. HIF-1: mediator of physiological and pathophysiological responses to hypoxia. J Appl Physiol 2000; 88(4):1474–1480.

29. Yu AY, Frid MG, Shimoda LA, et al. Temporal, spatial, and oxygen-regulated expression of hypoxia-inducible factor-1 in the lung. Am J Physiol 1998; 275(4 pt 1):L818–L826.

30. Takabatake N, Nakamura H, Abe S, et al. The relationship between chronic hypoxemia and activation of the tumor necrosis factor-alpha system in patients with chronic obstructive pulmonary disease. Am J Respir Crit Care Med 2000; 161(4 pt 1):1179–1184.

31. Postma DS, Renkema TE, Noordhoek JA, et al. Association between nonspecific bronchial hyperreactivity and superoxide anion production by polymorphonuclear leukocytes in chronic air-flow obstruction. Am Rev Respir Dis 1988; 137(1):57–61.

32. Rahman I, Morrison D, Donaldson K, et al. Systemic oxidative stress in asthma, COPD, and smokers. Am J Respir Crit Care Med 1996; 154(4 pt 1):1055–1060.

33. Rahman I, Skwarska E, MacNee W. Attenuation of oxidant/antioxidant imbalance during treatment of exacerbations of chronic obstructive pulmonary disease. Thorax 1997; 52(6):565–568.

34. Couillard A, Koechlin C, Cristol JP, et al. Evidence of local exercise-induced systemic oxidative stress in chronic obstructive pulmonary disease patients. Eur Respir J 2002; 20(5):1123–1129.
35. van Helvoort HA, Heijdra YF, de Boer RC, et al. Six-minute walking-induced systemic inflammation and oxidative stress in muscle-wasted COPD patients. Chest 2007; 131(2):439–445.
36. Seemungal TA, Donaldson GC, Bhowmik A, et al. Time course and recovery of exacerbations in patients with chronic obstructive pulmonary disease. Am J Respir Crit Care Med 2000; 161 (5):1608–1613.
37. Schols AM, Soeters PB, Dingemans AM, et al. Prevalence and characteristics of nutritional depletion in patients with stable COPD eligible for pulmonary rehabilitation. Am Rev Respir Dis 1993; 147(5):1151–1156.
38. Eid AA, Ionescu AA, Nixon LS, et al. Inflammatory response and body composition in chronic obstructive pulmonary disease. Am J Respir Crit Care Med 2001; 164(8 pt 1):1414–1418.
39. Hopkinson NS, Tennant RC, Dayer MJ, et al. A prospective study of decline in fat free mass and skeletal muscle strength in chronic obstructive pulmonary disease. Respir Res 2007; 8:25.
40. Saudny-Unterberger H, Martin JG, Gray-Donald K. Impact of nutritional support on functional status during an acute exacerbation of chronic obstructive pulmonary disease. Am J Respir Crit Care Med 1997; 156(3 pt 1):794–799.
41. Crul T, Spruit MA, Gayan-Ramirez G, et al. Markers of inflammation and disuse in vastus lateralis of chronic obstructive pulmonary disease patients. Eur J Clin Invest 2007; 37(11):897–904. (Epub 2007, Sep 20.)
42. Donaldson GC, Wilkinson TM, Hurst JR, et al. Exacerbations and time spent outdoors in chronic obstructive pulmonary disease. Am J Respir Crit Care Med 2005; 171(5):446–452.
43. Pitta F, Troosters T, Probst VS, et al. Physical activity and hospitalization for exacerbation of COPD. Chest 2006; 129(3):536–544.
44. Cote CG, Dordelly LJ, Celli BR. Impact of COPD exacerbations on patient-centered outcomes. Chest 2007; 131(3):696–704.
45. Akima H, Kuno S, Suzuki Y, et al. Effects of 20 days of bed rest on physiological cross-sectional area of human thigh and leg muscles evaluated by magnetic resonance imaging. J Gravit Physiol 1997; 4(1):S15–S21.
46. Vermeeren MA, Schols AM, Wouters EF. Effects of an acute exacerbation on nutritional and metabolic profile of patients with COPD. Eur Respir J 1997; 10(10):2264–2269.
47. Celli BR, Cote CG, Marin JM, et al. The body-mass index, airflow obstruction, dyspnea, and exercise capacity index in chronic obstructive pulmonary disease. N Engl J Med 2004; 350 (10):1005–1012.
48. Pouw EM, Ten Velde GP, Croonen BH, et al. Early non-elective readmission for chronic obstructive pulmonary disease is associated with weight loss. Clin Nutr 2000; 19(2):95–99.
49. Hallin R, Koivisto-Hursti UK, Lindberg E, et al. Nutritional status, dietary energy intake and the risk of exacerbations in patients with chronic obstructive pulmonary disease (COPD). Respir Med 2006; 100(3):561–567.
50. Di FM, Barbier D, Mege JL, et al. Tumor necrosis factor-alpha levels and weight loss in chronic obstructive pulmonary disease. Am J Respir Crit Care Med 1994; 150(5 pt 1):1453–1455.
51. Schols AM. TNF-alpha and hypermetabolism in chronic obstructive pulmonary disease. Clin Nutr 1999; 18(5):255–257.
52. Creutzberg EC, Wouters EF, Vanderhoven-Augustin IM, et al. Disturbances in leptin metabolism are related to energy imbalance during acute exacerbations of chronic obstructive pulmonary disease. Am J Respir Crit Care Med 2000; 162(4 pt 1):1239–1245.
53. Bennett BD, Solar GP, Yuan JQ, et al. A role for leptin and its cognate receptor in hematopoiesis. Curr Biol 1996; 6(9):1170–1180.
54. Bornstein SR, Uhlmann K, Haidan A, et al. Evidence for a novel peripheral action of leptin as a metabolic signal to the adrenal gland: leptin inhibits cortisol release directly. Diabetes 1997; 46(7):1235–1238.

55. Bouloumie A, Drexler HC, Lafontan M, et al. Leptin, the product of Ob gene, promotes angiogenesis. Circ Res 1998; 83(10):1059–1066.

56. Caldefie-Chezet F, Poulin A, Vasson MP. Leptin regulates functional capacities of polymorphonuclear neutrophils. Free Radic Res 2003; 37(8):809–814.

57. Harigaya A, Nagashima K, Nako Y, et al. Relationship between concentration of serum leptin and fetal growth. J Clin Endocrinol Metab 1997; 82(10):3281–3284.

58. Koistinen HA, Koivisto VA, Andersson S, et al. Leptin concentration in cord blood correlates with intrauterine growth. J Clin Endocrinol Metab 1997; 82(10):3328–3330.

59. La Cava A, Alviggi C, Matarese G. Unravelling the multiple roles of leptin in inflammation and autoimmunity. J Mol Med 2004; 82:4–11.

60. Loffreda S, Yang SQ, Lin HZ, et al. Leptin regulates proinflammatory immune responses. FASEB J 1998; 12(1):57–65.

61. Martin-Romero C, Santos-Alvarez J, Goberna R, et al. Human leptin enhances activation and proliferation of human circulating T lymphocytes. Cell Immunol 2000; 199(1):15–24.

62. Moore SI, Huffnagle GB, Chen GH, et al. Leptin modulates neutrophil phagocytosis of Klebsiella pneumoniae. Infect Immun 2003; 71(7):4182–4185.

63. Otero M, Lago R, Lago F, et al. Leptin, from fat to inflammation: old questions and new insights. FEBS Lett 2005; 579(2):295–301.

64. Santos-Alvarez J, Goberna R, Sanchez-Margalet V. Human leptin stimulates proliferation and activation of human circulating monocytes. Cell Immunol 1999; 194(1):6–11.

65. Sierra-Honigmann MR, Nath AK, Murakami C, et al. Biological action of leptin as an angiogenic factor. Science 1998; 281(5383):1683–1686.

66. Umemoto Y, Tsuji K, Yang FC, et al. Leptin stimulates the proliferation of murine myelocytic and primitive hematopoietic progenitor cells. Blood 1997; 90(9):3438–3443.

67. Yu WH, Kimura M, Walczewska A, et al. Role of leptin in hypothalamic-pituitary function. Proc Natl Acad Sci U S A 1997; 94(3):1023–1028.

68. Fujita Y, Murakami M, Ogawa Y, et al. Leptin inhibits stress-induced apoptosis of T lymphocytes. Clin Exp Immunol 2002; 128(1):21–26.

69. Ionescu AA, Schoon E. Osteoporosis in chronic obstructive pulmonary disease. Eur Respir J Suppl 2003; 46:64s–75s.

70. Bertolini DR, Nedwin GE, Bringman TS, et al. Stimulation of bone resorption and inhibition of bone formation in vitro by human tumour necrosis factors. Nature 1986; 319(6053):516–518.

71. Manolagas SC, Jilka RL. Bone marrow, cytokines, and bone remodeling. Emerging insights into the pathophysiology of osteoporosis. N Engl J Med 1995; 332(5):305–311.

72. Gerdhem P, Ringsberg KA, Akesson K, et al. Influence of muscle strength, physical activity and weight on bone mass in a population-based sample of 1004 elderly women. Osteoporos Int 2003; 14(9):768–772.

73. Incalzi RA, Caradonna P, Ranieri P, et al. Correlates of osteoporosis in chronic obstructive pulmonary disease. Respir Med 2000; 94(11):1079–1084.

74. Dubois EF, Roder E, Dekhuijzen PN, et al. Dual energy X-ray absorptiometry outcomes in male COPD patients after treatment with different glucocorticoid regimens. Chest 2002; 121(5): 1456–1463.

75. Bikle DD, Halloran B, Fong L, et al. Elevated 1,25-dihydroxyvitamin D levels in patients with chronic obstructive pulmonary disease treated with prednisone. J Clin Endocrinol Metab 1993; 76(2):456–461.

76. Rana JS, Mittleman MA, Sheikh J, et al. Chronic obstructive pulmonary disease, asthma, and risk of type 2 diabetes in women. Diabetes Care 2004; 27(10):2478–2484.

77. Hotamisligil GS, Arner P, Caro JF, et al. Increased adipose tissue expression of tumor necrosis factor-alpha in human obesity and insulin resistance. J Clin Invest 1995; 95(5):2409–2415.

78. Rosen P, Nawroth PP, King G, et al. The role of oxidative stress in the onset and progression of diabetes and its complications: a summary of a Congress Series sponsored by UNESCO-MCBN,

the American Diabetes Association and the German Diabetes Society. Diabetes Metab Res Rev 2001; 17(3):189–212.

79. Seufert J. Leptin effects on pancreatic beta-cell gene expression and function. Diabetes 2004; 53 (suppl 1):S152–S158.

80. Tillie-Leblond I, Marquette CH, Perez T, et al. Pulmonary embolism in patients with unexplained exacerbation of chronic obstructive pulmonary disease: prevalence and risk factors. Ann Intern Med 2006; 144(6):390–396.

81. Ambrosetti M, Ageno W, Spanevello A, et al. Prevalence and prevention of venous thromboembolism in patients with acute exacerbations of COPD. Thromb Res 2003; 112(4):203–207.

82. Erelel M, Cuhadaroglu C, Ece T, et al. The frequency of deep venous thrombosis and pulmonary embolus in acute exacerbation of chronic obstructive pulmonary disease. Respir Med 2002; 96 (7):515–518.

83. Schonhofer B, Kohler D. Prevalence of deep-vein thrombosis of the leg in patients with acute exacerbation of chronic obstructive pulmonary disease. Respiration 1998; 65(3):173–177.

84. Huiart L, Ernst P, Ranouil X, et al. Oral corticosteroid use and the risk of acute myocardial infarction in chronic obstructive pulmonary disease. Can Respir J 2006; 13(3):134–138.

85. Beltowski J. Leptin and atherosclerosis. Atherosclerosis 2006; 189(1):47–60.

86. Wedzicha JA, Syndercombe-Court, Tan KC. Increased platelet aggregate formation in patients with chronic airflow obstruction and hypoxaemia. Thorax 1991; 46(7):504–507.

87. Ridker PM, Hennekens CH, Buring JE, et al. C-reactive protein and other markers of inflammation in the prediction of cardiovascular disease in women. N Engl J Med 2000; 342(12):836–843.

88. Bisoendial RJ, Kastelein JJ, Stroes ES. C-reactive protein and atherogenesis: From fatty streak to clinical event. Atherosclerosis 2007; 195(2):e10–e18. (Epub 2007, Jul 31.)

89. Norwood R. Prevalence and impact of depression in chronic obstructive pulmonary disease patients. Curr Opin Pulm Med 2006; 12(2):113–117.

90. Coultas DB, Edwards DW, Barnett B, et al. Predictors of depressive symptoms in patients with COPD and health impact. COPD 2007; 4(1):23–28.

91. Egede LE. Major depression in individuals with chronic medical disorders: prevalence, correlates and association with health resource utilization, lost productivity and functional disability. Gen Hosp Psychiatry 2007; 29(5):409–416.

92. Ng TP, Niti M, Tan WC, et al. Depressive symptoms and chronic obstructive pulmonary disease: effect on mortality, hospital readmission, symptom burden, functional status, and quality of life. Arch Intern Med 2007; 167(1):60–67.

93. Cao Z, Ong KC, Eng P, et al. Frequent hospital readmissions for acute exacerbation of COPD and their associated factors. Respirology 2006; 11(2):188–195.

94. Mathur R, Cox IJ, Oatridge A, et al. Cerebral bioenergetics in stable chronic obstructive pulmonary disease. Am J Respir Crit Care Med 1999; 160(6):1994–1999.

# 9

# Mechanisms of Respiratory Failure in COPD Exacerbations

**BORJA G. COSIO**
Department of Respiratory Medicine, Hospital Universitario Son Dureta, Palma de Mallorca, Spain
**ROBERTO RODRÍGUEZ-ROISIN**
Department of Pneumology, Hospital Clínic, University of Barcelona, Barcelona, Spain

## I. Introduction

Respiratory failure is a common and important event that is frequently associated with severe exacerbations of chronic obstructive pulmonary disease (COPD) (1). Despite the definition of COPD exacerbation being based mainly on clinical outcomes, episodes of exacerbations are commonly characterized by worsening of pulmonary gas exchange, which results in moderate-to-severe hypoxemia with or without hypercapnia. This may represent a worsening in the patient's premorbid condition or, alternatively, these changes may occur for the first time in someone with less severe COPD who develops a different cause for deterioration, e.g., lobar pneumonia or acute pulmonary edema. In either case, the physiological abnormality is invariably the development of a significant degree of hypoxemia ($<$60 mm Hg) with a variable risk of carbon dioxide retention ($>$45 mm Hg) (2).

As a consequence, acute or acute-on-chronic respiratory failure is a common cause for hospital admission in this subset of patients, and somehow hypoxemia is linked to hospitalization that underprescription of oxygen has been shown to be associated with the risk of hospitalization and readmission (3,4). In fact, it has been clearly shown that chronic hypercapnic respiratory insufficiency and pulmonary hypertension are predictive factors of hospitalization for exacerbations in COPD patients (5). Also, respiratory failure is one of the factors strongly related to mortality, along with $FEV_1$, cardiac status, body mass index or serum albumin, during COPD exacerbations (6). Hospital mortality of patients admitted for a hypercapnic COPD exacerbation is approximately 10% and the long-term outcome is poorer. Mortality reaches 40% at one year in those needing mechanical support, and all-cause mortality is even higher (up to 49%) three years after hospitalization for a COPD exacerbation (1).

Since about 10% of all hospitalizations are directly or indirectly attributable to COPD and respiratory failure is a common finding during exacerbations (6), it seems relevant to understand the mechanisms underlying this medical condition. The major function of the lung is to exchange physiological (respiratory) gases, namely oxygen ($O_2$) and carbon dioxide ($CO_2$). Only when the lungs fail as a gas exchanger, arterial hypoxemia or hypercapnia or both appear and respiratory failure ensues. In this chapter, a review of the intrapulmonary and the extrapulmonary factors governing pulmonary gas exchange and the effects of different therapeutic interventions will be revisited.

## II. Mechanisms of Hypoxemia and Hypercapnia

The ultimate goal of the respiratory system is to exchange $O_2$ and $CO_2$ to meet the metabolic needs of the body. In order to effectively transfer both gases, ventilation and blood flow must be adequately apportioned and matched within the lungs. This important function is altered in COPD and can be severely disrupted during exacerbations of the disease. Of the four classical mechanisms determining abnormal arterial blood respiratory gases, i.e., alveolar hypoventilation, impaired alveolar-to-endcapillary diffusion to $O_2$, increased intrapulmonary shunt, and ventilation-perfusion ($\dot{V}_A/\dot{Q}$) mismatching—the last is by far the most common cause of impaired pulmonary gas exchange in stable and acute COPD (7). All the abnormalities alluded to above except alveolar hypoventilation may be viewed as intrapulmonary determinants of pulmonary gas exchange. Other key extrapulmonary factors governing respiratory blood gases include the fractional concentration of $O_2$ in the inspired gas, the hemodynamic circulatory state (cardiac output), and the metabolic demands ($O_2$ consumption) of the body.

### A. Intrapulmonary Factors

Worsening of pulmonary gas exchange during exacerbations is primarily produced by further $\dot{V}_A/\dot{Q}$ worsening, namely increased perfusion to poorly ventilated areas with low $\dot{V}_A/\dot{Q}$ ratios, compounded by a decreased mixed-venous $O_2$ tension that results from an increased $O_2$ consumption, presumably because of increased work of the respiratory muscles. Interestingly, the increased cardiac output only partially counterbalances the effect of greater $O_2$ consumption on mixed-venous $PO_2$.

Classical physiological analyses of the changes in arterial blood gas tensions during episodes of respiratory failure in COPD have always underlined the role of alveolar ventilation to pulmonary perfusion imbalance together with other non-$\dot{V}_A/\dot{Q}$ related mechanisms, such as relative alveolar hypoventilation.

More modern techniques using the multiple inert gas elimination technique (MIGET) have confirmed and extended these findings and shown that individuals with a relatively large dead space and a preponderance of ventilation being sent to alveolar units of the lung with a high ratio of ventilation to perfusion are initially hypercapnic (7).

It is important to stress that other non-$\dot{V}_A/\dot{Q}$ related mechanisms also play an important role in the development of hypercapnia (8). There are three major causes of pump failure leading to hypercapnia during an exacerbation (2). Firstly, when working under excessive inspiratory load, the inspiratory muscles may become fatigued, i.e., they become unable to continue to generate an adequate pleural pressure despite an appropriate central respiratory drive and an intact chest wall. Secondly, severe lung hyperinflation, with flat diaphragm and reduced mechanical action of the inspiratory muscles is one of the most common causes of impaired mechanical performance of the inspiratory muscles. And finally, although not less important in this context of elderly pluri-medicated patients, the output of the respiratory center controlling the muscles may be inadequate (anesthesia, drug overdose), resulting in a central respiratory drive that is insufficient for the demand, or the respiratory center may reflexively modify its output in order to prevent respiratory muscle injury and avoid or postpone fatigue.

Respiratory, more specifically inspiratory, muscle function is altered in COPD (8,9). Many of these alterations are secondary to a mechanical disadvantage related to lung hyperinflation. Other factors, including glucocorticosteroid therapy and nutritional depletion, are also deleterious to muscle function. In addition, the load imposed on the respiratory muscles is increased in COPD. Along with the altered respiratory muscle function, this increase induces important changes in respiratory muscle drive and recruitment.

## B. Extrapulmonary Factors

Patients with COPD exacerbation may show different values of arterial partial pressure of oxygen ($PaO_2$) for a given degree of $\dot{V}_A/\dot{Q}$ inequalities because extrapulmonary determinants (i.e., total ventilation, cardiac output and oxygen consumption ($\dot{V}O_2$), as the three most vital factors) contribute to govern the final value of arterial blood gases by modulating the impact of $\dot{V}_A/\dot{Q}$ inequality (7). The increase in alveolar ventilation shifts the distribution of blood flow towards areas with higher $\dot{V}_A/\dot{Q}$ ratios thus increasing its mean $\dot{V}_A/\dot{Q}$ ratio. Lung units with higher $\dot{V}_A/\dot{Q}$ ratios have a higher alveolar $PO_2$ and lower $PCO_2$, and the increased perfusion in these areas offsets the deleterious impact on $PaO_2$ of the blood flow in areas with low $\dot{V}_A/\dot{Q}$ ratios. The effects of the breathing pattern on gas exchange are particularly relevant during the episodes of exacerbation (7). Cardiac output may modify gas exchange basically through its effect on the $O_2$ content of mixed-venous blood. A decrease in cardiac output will reduce mixed-venous oxygen tension and $PaO_2$ will rise and fall following the increases and decreases of the mixed-venous $PO_2$. This important role of cardiac output on gas exchange has been clearly shown during exacerbations of COPD (7), where an increase in cardiac output contributed to compensate for the deleterious effect of an increased $O_2$consumption by the respiratory muscles on mixed-venous $PO_2$.

Another important issue is the crucial role of both cardiac output and ventilatory pattern in influencing gas exchange when patients are discontinued from mechanical ventilation or are treated with noninvasive mechanical ventilation. During weaning (10), while cardiac output increases considerably because of the abrupt increase in venous return (following the reduction of intrathoracic pressure) and total ventilation is maintained, tidal volume is reduced and respiratory frequency increases and becomes less efficient. As a result, both the dispersion of alveolar ventilation and the overall $\dot{V}_A/\dot{Q}$ heterogeneity increases resulting in further $\dot{V}_A/\dot{Q}$ mismatch. Interestingly, there is only a small non-significant increase in intrapulmonary shunt from mechanical ventilation to spontaneous breathing (from 3% to 9% of cardiac output) despite the substantial increases in cardiac output and mixed-venous $PO_2$. This is at variance with the well-known, although poorly understood, strong linear relationship between increase in pulmonary blood flow and intrapulmonary shunt, commonly observed in patients with acute lung injury.

Another striking finding during weaning from mechanical ventilation is that respiratory blood gases remain unaltered despite increases in mixed-venous $PO_2$ and $O_2$ delivery (arterial $O_2$ content times cardiac output). In other words, the potentially beneficial effect of the increased cardiac output on $PaO_2$ is offset by the deleterious influence of the change in ventilatory pattern on $PaO_2$. Despite these problems, weaning in these patients is successful. When patients were removed from the ventilator in this study, $O_2$ consumption (calculated according to the Fick principle) did not change (10). Subsequently, the effects of positive end-expiratory pressure (PEEP) and those of intrinsic PEEP ($PEEP_i$) on $\dot{V}_A/\dot{Q}$ imbalance in mechanically ventilated patients with chronic airflow obstruction have been investigated

(11), the rationale being that low levels of PEEP can improve rather than impair lung mechanics as PEEP can replace $PEEP_i$. It was shown that the application of PEEP equivalent to 50% of the initial $PEEP_i$ improved pulmonary gas exchange without deleterious any effect on lung mechanics nor on hemodynamics. Moreover, the use of "controlled hypoventilation" (or permissive hypercapnia) in conjunction with low $PEEP_i$ values significantly reduced alveolar pressure, while increasing cardiac output and systemic $O_2$ delivery, could be recommended during exacerbations.

The acute effects of noninvasive mechanical ventilation (Fig. 1), a progressively demanding therapeutic approach for acute respiratory failure within the context of acute

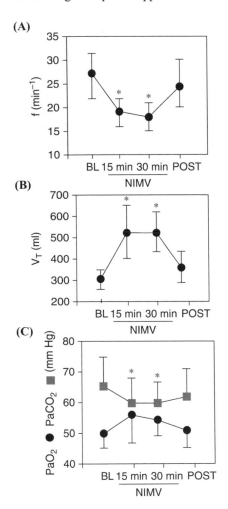

**Figure 1**   Individual time courses of (**A**) breathing frequency (*f*), (**B**) tidal volume (VT) and (**C**) arterial $PaO_2$ (*closed circles*) and $PaCO_2$ (*closed squares*) at baseline (BL), 15 and 30 min during noninvasive ventilation (NIMV), and 15 minutes after its withdrawal (POST). Horizontal bars represent mean values at each time point. *Source*: Modified from Ref. 12.

COPD, with an undoubtedly cost-benefit outcome, have been also been investigated in our environment (12). It was clearly demonstrated that the beneficial effect on pulmonary gas exchange, namely the combination of decreased hypercapnia, increased $PaO_2$ and increased pH (improvement), was essentially due to a more optimal ventilatory pattern, i.e., less shallow and less rapid breathing, without any beneficial influence on the underlying $\dot{V}_A/\dot{Q}$ inequalities. It is of note that the significant decrease in cardiac output during the application of mechanical support, because of increased intrathoracic pressure, did not result in any detrimental effect on arterial oxygenation.

## III.  Natural History of Hypoxemic Respiratory Failure

We have shown that the severity of $\dot{V}_A/\dot{Q}$ abnormalities and their patterns during episodes of exacerbation of COPD may improve substantially over a period of few weeks of adequate treatment (7,13). In this sequential study of patients with mild hypercapnic respiratory failure not needing mechanical ventilation (7), there was a decrease in $PaO_2$ and an increase in $PaCO_2$ due to further $\dot{V}_A/\dot{Q}$ worsening during exacerbations, with negligible increases in intrapulmonary shunt (less than 5% of cardiac output). The latter did not contribute significantly to arterial hypoxemia in COPD, probably because these patients do not completely occlude their airways or because they develop an efficient collateral ventilation, or both. One month after the onset of study, all spirometric and gas exchange indices had improved substantially. Thus, while $PaO_2$ increased and $PaCO_2$ decreased some distributions of $\dot{V}_A/\dot{Q}$ inequalities became unimodal. These data suggest that part of the $\dot{V}_A/\dot{Q}$ abnormalities during exacerbations are related to partially reversible pathophysiological abnormalities of airway narrowing, such as mucus plugging, bronchial wall edema, bronchoconstriction, increased $PEEP_i$ and/or air trapping and acute-on-chronic lung hyperinflation.

Additional studies of COPD patients needing mechanical support for exacerbation of the disease have shown essentially similar qualitatively $\dot{V}_A/\dot{Q}$ patterns, although quantitatively more severe, to those observed in patients with acute COPD breathing spontaneously (10,11). The main difference was the presence of intrapulmonary shunt, which was always slightly increased (range, 4–10% of cardiac output). This suggests that some airways were completely occluded, possibly by inspissated bronchial secretions. However, if a patient with COPD shows a substantial increase in intrapulmonary shunt despite a normal chest X ray, excluding atelectasis, pneumonia, lung collapse or pulmonary edema, then the possibility of a reopening of the *foramen ovale* because of an increase in right atrial pressure should be borne in mind. Under these circumstances, $PaO_2$ fails to increase substantially (>300–350 mm Hg) while breathing 100% $O_2$.

## IV.  Effects of Oxygen Breathing

The response to high $O_2$ concentrations in patients with COPD is broadly similar irrespective of the clinical severity of the disease. With little $\dot{V}_A/\dot{Q}$ mismatch, $PaO_2$ rises almost linearly, as the inspired $O_2$ is increased. As the severity of $\dot{V}_A/\dot{Q}$ inequality worsens, the rate of rise of $PaO_2$ is reduced and becomes more curvilinear. We have shown in patients with COPD and acute respiratory failure needing mechanical ventilation that full nitrogen washout of alveolar units, even in patients with poorly ventilated alveolar units with low or very low $\dot{V}_A/\dot{Q}$ ratios, is rapid and that steady-state conditions are easily reached even before 30 minutes (14). The coexistence of a modest increased intrapulmonary shunt, however, further decreases the elevation of $PaO_2$. In clinical practice, however, physicians administrate low inspired $O_2$ concentrations (either 0.24 or 0.28) delivered through high flow masks to patients with COPD and acute respiratory failure not needing ventilatory support. This provides modest but effective increases in $PaO_2$, of the order of 10 to 15 mm Hg, without inducing detrimental $CO_2$ retention, to optimise $O_2$ delivery to peripheral tissues.

Although $\dot{V}_A/\dot{Q}$ inequality is no longer a barrier to $O_2$ exchange when 100% $O_2$ is breathed, hyperoxic mixtures always deteriorate $\dot{V}_A/\dot{Q}$ mismatch, as assessed by a significant increase in the dispersion of blood flow, without changes in intrapulmonary shunt nor in the dispersion of alveolar ventilation; in contrast, pulmonary arterial pressure and pulmonary vascular resistance remain essentially unchanged (14). The impairment in $\dot{V}_A/\dot{Q}$ relationships indicates release or inhibition of hypoxic pulmonary vasoconstriction. The total absence of further increases in intrapulmonary shunt suggests that reabsorption atelectasis does not take place, suggesting that either collateral ventilation is very efficient or regional airway obstruction is never complete, or both. This response indicates the absence of critical alveolar units (with low inspired $\dot{V}_A/\dot{Q}$ ratios) that become unstable and vulnerable to high $O_2$ concentrations over time. These units tend to easily collapse, hence leading to the development of reabsorption atelectasis. When there is no release of hypoxic vasoconstriction, the amount of shunt is always greater, irrespective of the inspired $O_2$ fraction. The contention is that alveolar units with poorly ventilated $\dot{V}_A/\dot{Q}$ ratios are not able to redistribute blood flow if their pulmonary vascular resistance remains unaltered. Alternatively, it has been shown, in patients with COPD, that breathing high inspired $O_2$ concentrations reduces the degree of airways resistance. This should tend to improve the distribution of ventilation, other factors being equal, thus reducing the amount of areas with low $\dot{V}_A/\dot{Q}$ ratios and, consequently, the dispersion of pulmonary blood flow.

Using traditional gas exchange measurements, such as the Bohr's dead space in patients with COPD on acute-on-chronic respiratory insufficiency, the administration of 100% $O_2$ breathing spontaneously resulted in a remarkable increase in $PaCO_2$. Since the respiratory muscles maintained ventilation at nearly the same level as when breathing room air, it is suggested that the increase in $PaCO_2$ is mainly attributed to an increased dead space; additional mechanisms included a small reduction in both tidal volume together with the Haldane effect, namely the changes in the $CO_2$ dissociation curve facilitating the release of $CO_2$ from bicarbonate and also from that directly bound as carbamate during 100% $O_2$. We have also shown an increase in $PaCO_2$ during 100% $O_2$ breathing in COPD patients needing mechanical support (14). Conceivably, the increased dead space and the experimental evidence that increased $\dot{V}_A/\dot{Q}$ disturbances can worsen not only the $O_2$ transfer but also $CO_2$ exchange are behind this increase. Notwithstanding, the Haldane effect could also enhance the ratio of $PCO_2$ to blood $CO_2$ content. We estimated however that the hyperoxia-induced increments of $PaCO_2$ in this subset of patients could be attributed almost entirely to the simultaneous increased dead space, thereby indicating a marginal role of the Haldane effect. This was further supported by the persistence of hypercapnia when maintenance inspired $PO_2$ was re-started. The increased dead space suggests redistribution of pulmonary blood flow from high $\dot{V}_A/\dot{Q}$ ratios to poorly but still ventilated units (low $\dot{V}_A/\dot{Q}$ ratios).

It has also been found that in hyperoxia-induced $CO_2$, retaining patients with COPD during exacerbations ventilation fell by an average of 20% and the dispersion of alveolar ventilation, a reflection of an inert gas measurement of alveolar dead space, increased by about 25% when breathing 100% $O_2$ (8). Likewise, patients who were $CO_2$ retainers showed a significant increase in alveolar dead space, indicating a higher $CO_2$ retention, perhaps related to bronchodilation. Moreover, there was an increase in the dispersion of pulmonary blood flow (i.e., areas with low $\dot{V}_A/\dot{Q}$ ratios) due to the release of hypoxic vasoconstriction, irrespective of the presence or absence of $CO_2$ retention.

## V. Response to Bronchodilators

The specific effects of the different bronchodilators on $\dot{V}_A/\dot{Q}$ relationships depend on their pharmacologic group and on the route of administration. The review of the different studies of bronchodilators on pulmonary gas exchange in acute COPD shows that as in asthma, both short-acting $\beta_2$-agonists (SABAs) and long-acting ones may induce small decreases in oxygen saturation that can be easily removed by conventional $O_2$ therapy (13,15,16). These mild-to-moderate deleterious effects on gas exchange (a decrease in $PaO_2$ of the order of 5 mm Hg as a mean in the vast majority of studies, although in a few cases these decrements can be more prominent) are subclinical and well tolerated. As a general rule, the fall in $PaO_2$ is shown essentially within the first 30 minutes following the administration of the agents, and it is always transient and more conspicuous in patients with relatively well-preserved $PaO_2$. We have, however, shown that during severe COPD exacerbation, salbutamol does not aggravate pulmonary gas exchange abnormalities (13). When in convalescence, however, baseline lung function improvement was associated with a detrimental gas exchange response to salbutamol, resulting in further $\dot{V}_A/\dot{Q}$ imbalance and small decreases in $PaO_2$ compounded by small increases in cardiac output and $O_2$ consumption (Fig. 2). Contrary to the original hypothesis of the latter study (i.e., the interplay between intrapulmonary and extrapulmonary factors governing arterial blood gases during exacerbations would be more influential than while at convalescence), pulmonary gas exchange abnormalities after salbutamol remained essentially unvaried. It is most likely that the lack of gas exchange response to salbutamol suggests a weaker (or even absent) hypoxic pulmonary vascular response related more to acutely severe alveolar hypoxia than to a permanent structural derangement of the pulmonary vasculature. Moreover, the high dosage of SABAs usually given during the most critical days of exacerbation may facilitate an underlying vasodilatory state of the pulmonary vasculature. However, there remains the potential of SABA-induced inhibitory effects on the postcapillary bronchial venoconstriction and airway microvascular leakage, possibly amplified by their potent relaxant effect on conducting airways, which cannot be overlooked. Likewise, SABAs can minimize the subsequent release of other inflammatory mediators into the pulmonary circulation, with vasodilator effects during COPD exacerbations that can disturb the underlying $\dot{V}_A/\dot{Q}$ imbalance. The latter two effects could offset further $\dot{V}_A/\dot{Q}$ inequality, thus reinforcing hypoxic pulmonary vasoconstriction. It may also be plausible that both collateral ventilation and hypoxic vasoconstriction can be more effective, hence maximizing a more adequate $\dot{V}_A/\dot{Q}$ balance. Notwithstanding, salbutamol caused further $\dot{V}_A/\dot{Q}$ worsening and hypoxemia, compounded by increases in both cardiac output and $\dot{V}O_2$, while at convalescence. Increased cardiac output can increase the amount of blood flow diverted to areas with low $\dot{V}_A/\dot{Q}$ ratio, reflected in increases in the regions of low $\dot{V}_A/\dot{Q}$ ratio. Conceivably, arterial hypoxemia is amplified by the parallel increase in $\dot{V}O_2$ that decreases mixed-venous $PO_2$. However, this

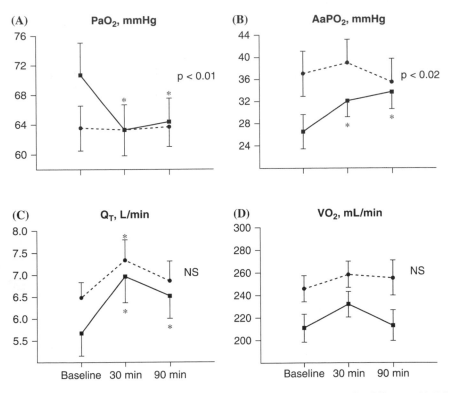

**Figure 2**  Mean (±SEM) values for (**A**) $PaO_2$, (**B**) alveolar-to-arterial $PO_2$ difference ($AaPO_2$), (**C**) cardiac output ($\dot{Q}_T$), and (**D**) oxygen consumption ($\dot{V}O_2$), before (baseline) and at 30 and 90 minutes after salbutamol, during exacerbation (*closed circles* and *dashed lines*) and while at convalescence (*open squares* and *solid lines*) for paired measurements. *Source*: Modified from Ref. 13.

situation is not sufficiently counterbalanced by the simultaneous increase in mixed-venous $PO_2$ induced by a high cardiac output, the net effect being a small decrease in PaO2.

The effects of intravenous aminophylline on $\dot{V}_A/\dot{Q}$ relationships have been studied in patients recovering from an exacerbation of COPD (17). Aminophylline increased FVC and $FEV_1$, but it did not produce changes in blood gases or in $\dot{V}_A/\dot{Q}$ relationships. Although therapeutic doses of aminophylline can increase $\dot{V}_A/\dot{Q}$ inequality in some patients, in general the effect is moderate and of little clinical significance.

## VI.  Response to Glucocorticoids

Systemic glucocorticoids are often used to treat exacerbations of COPD necessitating hospitalisation for respiratory failure. In an inpatient study, it has been shown that these agents improve $PaO_2$, alveolar-arterial gradient, $FEV_1$ and peak expiratory flow more rapidly than placebo and more effectively in a 10-day course than in a 3-day course (18). Nebulized budesonide may be an effective and safe alternative to systemic glucocorticoids with similar improvements in arterial oxygen tension for the treatment of exacerbations of COPD (19,20). These studies have shown that either treatment with systemic cortico-steroids or nebulized budesonide improve arterial blood gases faster than control, with $PaO_2$ improvements within the first 24 hours of treatment compared with, at least, 72 hours for the placebo group. The mechanisms for improving lung function and arterial blood gases and the patients most likely to benefit from steroid treatment during exacerbations remain contentious. No clinical, biochemical, or functional markers can clearly identify which patients will respond better to steroid treatment. Although no effects on airway cytokines have been found in patients with stable COPD, several studies have reported reductions in airway eosinophilic inflammatory markers and in serum C-reactive protein after two weeks of treatment with oral steroids (21) The beneficial response to glucocorticoids during exacerbations suggests that enhanced airway inflammation and edema and systemic inflammation are reduced, or that the inflammatory pattern is sensitive to corticosteroids. It is plausible that glucocorticoids have a rapid anti-inflammatory effect that improves $\dot{V}_A/\dot{Q}$ mismatch, thereby resulting in a faster recovery of acute COPD-induced arterial blood gas abnormalities.

## VII. Conclusion

In summary, taken altogether all these findings point to the view that respiratory gas disturbances (arterial hypoxemia and hypercapnia) are the integrative end-point of $\dot{V}_A/\dot{Q}$ abnormalities plus the interaction of extrapulmonary factors governing gas exchange, namely total alveolar ventilation, cardiac output, and $O_2$ consumption. All in all, the interplay of these determinants governing arterial blood gases should be borne in mind to make a much comprehensive pathophysiologic approach to the management of acute respiratory failure during exacerbations of COPD (21).

## References

1. Rabe KF, Hurd S, Anzueto A, et al. Global strategy for the diagnosis, management, and pre-vention of chronic obstructive pulmonary disease: GOLD executive summary. Am J Respir Crit Care Med 2007; 176(6):532–555.
2. Calverley PMA. Respiratory failure in chronic obstructive pulmonary disease. Eur Respir J 2003; 22: (suppl 47):S26–S30.
3. Garcia-Aymerich J, Monso E, Marrades RM, et al. Risk factors for hospitalization for a chronic obstructive pulmonary disease exacerbation. EFRAM study. Am J Respir Crit Care Med 2001; 164:1002–1007.
4. Garcia-Aymerich J, Farrero E, Felez MA, et al. Risk factors of readmission to hospital for a COPD exacerbation: a prospective study. Thorax 2003; 58:100–105.
5. Kessler R, Faller M, Fourgaut G, et al. Predictive factors of hospitalization for acute exacer-bation in a series of 64 patients with chronic obstructive pulmonary disease. Am J Respir Crit Care Med 1999; 159:158–164.
6. Gunen H, Hacievliyagil SS, Kosar F, et al. Factors affecting survival of hospitalised patients with COPD. Eur Respir J 2005; 26:234–241.
7. Barbera JA, Roca J, Ferrer A, et al. Mechanisms of worsening gas exchange during acute exacerbations of chronic obstructive pulmonary disease. Eur Respir J 1997; 10:1285–1291.

8.   Robinson TD, Freiberg DB, Regnis JA, et al. The role of hypoventilation and ventilation-perfusion redistribution in oxygen-induced hypercapnia during acute exacerbations of chronic obstructive pulmonary disease. Am J Respir Crit Care Med 2000; 161:1524–1529.

9.   Ottenheijm CAC, Heunks LMA, Dekhuijzen PNR. Diaphragm muscle fiber dysfunction in chronic obstructive pulmonary disease toward a pathophysiological concept. Am J Respir Crit Care Med 2007; 175:1233–1240.

10.  Torres A, Reyes A, Roca J, et al. Ventilation-perfusion mismatching in chronic obstructive pulmonary disease during ventilator weaning. Am Rev Respir Dis 1989; 140:1246–1250.

11.  Rossi A, Santos C, Roca J, et al. Effects of PEEP on VA/Q mismatching in ventilated patients with chronic airflow obstruction. Am J Respir Crit Care Med 1994; 149:1077–1084.

12.  Diaz O, Iglesia R, Ferrer M, et al. Effects of noninvasive ventilation on pulmonary gas exchange and hemodynamics during acute hypercapnic exacerbations of chronic obstructive pulmonary disease. Am J Respir Crit Care Med 1997; 156:1840–1845.

13.  Polverino E, Gomez FP, Manrique H, et al. Gas exchange response to short-acting beta2-agonists in COPD severe exacerbations. Am J Respir Crit Care Med 2007; 176(4):350–355.

14.  Santos C, Ferrer M, Roca J, et al. Pulmonary gas exchange response to oxygen breathing in acute lung injury. Am J Respir Crit Care Med 2000; 161:26–31.

15.  Viegas CA, Ferrer A, Montserrat JM, et al. Ventilation-perfusion response after fenoterol in hypoxemic patients with stable COPD. Chest 1996; 110(1):71–77.

16.  Karpel JP, Pesin J, Greenberg D, et al. A comparison of the effects of ipratropium bromide and metaproterenol sulfate in acute exacerbations of COPD. Chest 1990;98:835–839.

17.  Barbera JA, Reyes A, Roca J, et al. Effect of intravenously administered aminophylline on ventilation/perfusion inequality during recovery from exacerbations of chronic obstructive pulmonary disease. Am Rev Respir Dis 1992; 145:1328–1333.

18.  Sayiner A, Aytemur ZA, Cirit M, et al. Systemic glucocorticoids in severe exacerbations of COPD. Chest 2001; 119:726–730.

19.  Maltais F, Ostinelli J, Bourbeau J, et al. Comparison of nebulized budesonide and oral prednisolone with placebo in the treatment of acute exacerbations of chronic obstructive pulmonary disease: a randomized controlled trial. Am J Respir Crit Care Med 2002; 165:698–703.

20.  Gunen H, Hacievliyaquil SS, Yetkin O, et al. The role of nebulised budesonide in the treatment of exacerbations of COPD. Eur Resp J 2007; 29(4):660–667.

21.  Rodríguez-Roisin R. COPD exacerbations 5: management. Thorax 2006; 61:535–544.

# 10
## Role of Respiratory Viral Infection at Exacerbation

**J. K. QUINT** and **JADWIGA A. WEDZICHA**
Academic Unit of Respiratory Medicine, University College London, London, U.K.

### I. Introduction

Exacerbations of chronic obstructive pulmonary disease (COPD) are a major cause of morbidity and mortality worldwide and have important consequences for patients and health care providers. They are predominantly triggered by infection and viruses are thought to be an increasingly important cause, with up to 64% of exacerbations associated with symptomatic colds (Fig. 1). The presence of cold symptoms at exacerbation increases the severity of an exacerbation, lengthens the recovery time (1) (Fig. 2), and in polymerase chain reaction (PCR)-confirmed colds, is associated with higher levels of airway inflammatory markers (2).

As many as 78% of hospitalized COPD exacerbations have a virus and/or bacteria detected—30% bacterial, 23% viral, and 25% coinfection (3). Exacerbations caused by viral infection are more likely to lead to hospitalization and viral infection has been identified in up to 47% of COPD patients with very severe exacerbations requiring intubation and mechanical ventilation (4). Viral exacerbations are more common in the winter months when temperatures are colder (5) and when there are more respiratory viral infections present in the community.

Respiratory viruses have also been detected in stable COPD, suggesting that chronic viral infection may occur; however, the exact impact of this on the course of disease and exacerbations has not yet been established. Nonetheless, prevention of viral infection would have a significant effect on morbidity in COPD and improve quality of life.

The major viruses associated with COPD exacerbations include human rhinovirus, coronavirus, influenza A and B, parainfluenza, adenovirus, and respiratory syncytial virus (RSV). *Human metapneumovirus* (hMPV) has also been found at exacerbation in some studies. This chapter will cover the changes in virus pattern detection with improvement in detection techniques, the effect of viral infection on inflammation and the role of these viruses at exacerbation and in the stable state.

### II. Detection of Viruses

Historically, detection of viruses has been by culture and serology of the virus from respiratory secretions. This is difficult, however, as samples need to contain live virus. Immunochemical techniques for the detection of viruses have lower sensitivity and

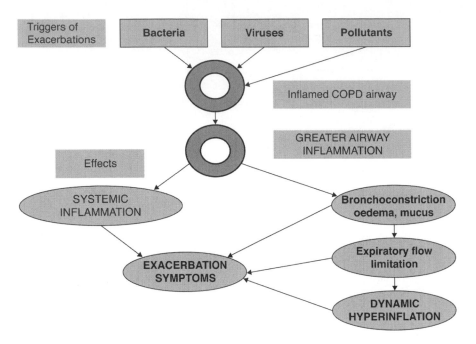

**Figure 1**   Exacerbation triggers in COPD. *Abbreviation*: COPD, chronic obstructive pulmonary disease.

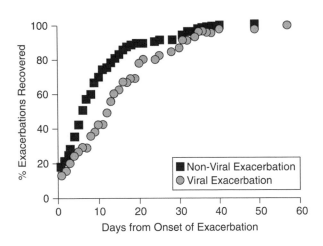

**Figure 2**   Viral exacerbations take longer to recover than nonviral exacerbations.

specificity. Serological techniques are also limited, as they rely on the host's immune response. Additionally, sensitivity of a technique is only useful if sound methods of sample collection have been used; and, in the case of viral detection, sputum is more sensitive than nasal samples (6). Prevention of sample contamination is also important.

PCR has enabled a more detailed evaluation for the role of viruses, particularly rhinovirus (7). Studies evaluating the use of reverse transcription (RT) and amplification of viral nucleic acid by PCR have shown superior sensitivity and specificity than culture or antigen detection methods (8). PCR techniques are not uniformly sensitive however, and this may explain some of the disparity in prevalence of viruses (particularly RSV) found in similar populations (7,9,10,11).

It is also important to remember that COPD is a heterogeneous disease, and exacerbations heterogeneous events. Therefore reasons for disparity in virus detection in studies not only include variable sensitivity of techniques used, but geographical differences may also account for some of the variation given that viral epidemics appear to be local rather than national or global (6).

Conventional PCR relies on a qualitative visualization of amplified target product at the end of the reaction, and the sensitivity of standard PCR can be increased with a nested PCR. Quantitative or real-time PCR is based on detection of a fluorescent signal produced during amplification of a PCR product. By measuring the amplification product in the exponential phase of the reaction, differences in the quantities of starting viral gene copies can be detected, and the initial concentration can be calculated.

With PCR, up to 40% of COPD exacerbations have been shown to be associated with viral infection (7). In one study using PCR, rhinovirus was detected in 39 of 66 (59%) viral exacerbations, coronovirus in 7 of 66 (10.6%), influenza A in 6 of 66 (9%) and B in 3 of 66 (4.5%), and parainfluenza and adenovirus each detected at one exacerbation (1.5%). RSV, although detected in 19 of 66 (28.8%) exacerbations was also seen in a significant number of patients in the stable state, unlike the other viruses detected at exacerbation (7) (Fig. 3). PCR has also allowed multiple viruses to be detected more easily at a single exacerbation. In a study of 81 exacerbations, 88 viral infections were identified (10). Although serologic methods identified 57% of these, RT-PCR assays identified an additional 38 viruses, with rhinovirus the most common infection and the most frequent identified only by RT-PCR.

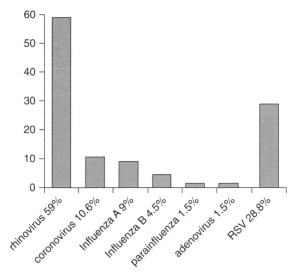

**Figure 3** Percentage of each virus detected at viral exacerbation.

### III. Mechanisms of Virus-Induced Exacerbations and Host Response

A number of mechanisms may be involved in the etiology of viral exacerbations. The innate component of the host response to an infecting virus is fully functional before the virus even enters the host airway epithelium (12). An adaptive component then develops in response to the presence of the virus and has memory, specificity, and diversity (13) and involves T and B cells. The components of innate immunity include the barrier provided by the epithelium, natural killer cells, intraepithelial lymphocytes, polymorphonuclear neutrophils, monocytes, and macrophages that are recruited to the site of infection. The innate response then generates cytokines that initiate both a local and a systemic response.

#### A. Airway Inflammation

Experimental rhinoviral infection has been shown to increase sputum IL-6 and IL-8 in normal and asthmatic subjects (14–16). In COPD, exacerbations associated with the presence of rhinovirus in induced sputum had larger increases in airway IL-6, (7) IL-8 and myeloperoxidase (MPO) (17) levels compared with exacerbations where rhinovirus was not detected.

Viral infections have also been associated with increased oxidative stress at exacerbation (18). Rhinovirus can replicate in the lower airway, and activates NF-κB thus upregulating pro-inflammatory mediators in the airway (19). Through their chemotactic effect on neutrophils (via IL-8, ENA-78, and LTB4), lymphocytes, and monocytes (RANTES) and the upregulation of adhesion molecules (such as TNF-α), these mediators increase inflammation that is characteristically seen at exacerbation.

Viral infections can also induce the expression of stress response genes, such as heme-oxygenase-1 and genes encoding antioxidant enzymes. These antioxidant enzymes may be important in protecting against virally mediated inflammation at exacerbation. Endothelin-1, an important bronchoconstrictor, which is pro-inflammatory and mucogenic, has also been implicated in the pathogenesis of virally mediated inflammation. Levels increase in the airway and systemically at exacerbation (20).

#### B. Systemic Inflammation

Plasma fibrinogen and IL-6 increase at exacerbation (21) and plasma fibrinogen is higher in the presence of a cold and with detection of respiratory viral infection at exacerbation (7,21). This suggests that viral exacerbations are associated with an increased systemic inflammatory response and may predispose to increased vascular disease.

### IV. Susceptibility to Viral Infection

Whether COPD patients are more susceptible to viral infection compared with normal subjects is strongly debated. Factors thought to be important in susceptibility to viral infection include upper and lower airway inflammation, cigarette smoking, airway bacterial colonization, possible viral persistence, coinfection, and seasonality. One study suggests that infection with *Hemophilus influenzae* increases intercellular adhesion molecule-1 (ICAM-1) and Toll-like receptor 3 (TLR3) expressions in airway epithelial cells, thus increasing the potential for rhinovirus binding and subsequent cytokine responses (22).

Frequent exacerbators of COPD, i.e., those individuals that have three or more exacerbations per year, have more episodes of naturally occurring colds than infrequent exacerbators, suggesting that frequent exacerbators are particularly susceptible to viral infection (23). In one study, 64% of patients had at least one virus detected at exacerbation, and these patients had a higher exacerbation frequency than those in whom no virus was detected at exacerbation. Patients colonized with bacteria are thought to be more susceptible to developing viral associated exacerbations, and this may account for the fact that frequent exacerbators have a higher incidence of bacterial colonization (24). Cigarette smoke is also thought to play a role, increasing susceptibility to viral infections possibly via alteration of immune responses (25).

## V. Rhinovirus

Rhinovirus, most commonly responsible for the common cold, is currently thought to be the most important trigger of COPD exacerbations. A member of the *picornavirus* group of ribonucleic acid (RNA) viruses, it has over 100 serotypes making detection by culture and serologic methods very difficult. It is spread from person to person by infected respiratory secretions. The major group of rhinovirus attaches to airway epithelium through ICAM-1, inducing its expression, thus promoting inflammatory cell recruitment and activation (26). Latent expression of adenoviral E1A protein in alveolar epithelial cells may increase ICAM-1 expression, and this may be a potential mechanism for increased rhinoviral susceptibility in COPD (27).

Using viral culture and serology, 27% of COPD exacerbations have been shown to be associated with viral infection as opposed to 44% of acute respiratory illness in control subjects (28). In the COPD population, 43% of the viral infection was attributable to rhinovirus, thus making it responsible for about 12% of the total exacerbations. The lower percentage of virus seen in COPD patients compared with controls may be due to detection methods.

In other studies, rhinovirus has been detected in up to 23% of patients during exacerbations but in less than 1% of stable patients. Studies have illustrated (17) a synergistic effect of viral and bacterial infections in that inflammatory and lung function changes are more pronounced in proven rhinoviral infections, measured with sputum IL-6. The presence of virus may indirectly increase bacterial load in addition to direct viral effects. Rhinoviral infection increases susceptibility to bacterial adherence to airway epithelial cells.

In a pilot study, mild COPD patients were infected with the minimal amount of rhinovirus to induce clinical colds. All of the first four patients exposed to the lowest dose experienced cold symptoms and lower respiratory tract symptoms, including shortness of breath, wheeze, cough, and increased sputum production (29). This study showed that COPD patients developed colds and exacerbations with 100- to 1000-fold lower doses of viruses than used in previous studies on normal and asthmatics. Also, there was a three- to four-day gap between the peak of cold symptoms and the peak of lower respiratory symptoms.

## VI. Coronavirus

Coronaviruses are enveloped RNA viruses and are the second most frequent cause of the common cold (30). They also occasionally can cause pneumonia in elderly and immunocompromised patients (31). There are two human strains—HCoVs 229E and OC43 in two antigenic groups.

Use of RT-PCR has improved coronavirus detection. In a large Asian study of acute exacerbations of COPD, coronavirus OC43 was detected in 4.9% of exacerbations (32). Other studies have detected coronavirus at similar levels, i.e., 4.2% of exacerbations (7).

## VII.  Influenza and Parainfluenza

Because of the introduction of influenza immunization in patients with chronic lung disease, influenza has become a less common cause of exacerbations, but is still likely to be important in times of epidemics, and some studies (9) have shown influenza to be associated with as many as 25% of COPD exacerbations. Patients who have not been vaccinated against influenza have twice the hospitalization rate in the influenza season compared with the noninfluenza season, and influenza vaccination is associated with a lower risk of death. (33).

Serological evidence of a past infection with influenza virus has been detected in 5% to 28% of patients following an exacerbation, but is present in only 6% of patients who have not had an exacerbation. The prevalent strain of influenza has some effect on exacerbation frequency and severity. An American study carried out over four consecutive winters noted that when the dominant strain of influenza was H1N1, hospital admission for influenza-related chest infections were low. In contrast, when H3N2 influenza was prevalent (a more virulent strain), admissions for chest infections and related deaths were significantly raised (34).

Parainfluenza viruses have been associated with a lower percentage of exacerbations— 3% in one study (28)—and are usually seen in the summer months.

## VIII.  Adenovirus

A double-strand DNA virus, adenovirus has more than 40 known serotypes that are responsible for a wide range of human infection, including infection in the upper and lower airways. Types 4 (group E), 7 (group B), and 1, 2, 5 (group C) cause the most frequent respiratory disease in adults and have an incubation period of five to eight days.

Adenovirus adheres to the cell surface through its fiber protein and penton base and is internalized by receptor-mediated endocytosis. After it has entered the cell, it is translocated to the nucleus and transcribed in early and late groups of genes. The first early gene to be expressed is the E1A gene, which generally activates the cell thus allowing the virus to gradually take over host cell protein generation to manufacture viral particles and initiate production of other molecules that contribute to host cell defense. Viral E1A protein has been shown to continue to be expressed in lung epithelial cells long after the virus has stopped replicating and clinical signs of infection have cleared. The latently infected cells continue to produce viral proteins without replicating a complete virus and the host response to them includes an increase in CD8+ T cells (35).

Infections usually occur in the first year of life, and in adults with COPD, it is detected in 0.5% to 1.5% of exacerbations. In a study of 136 COPD patients seen at exacerbation, 10 exacerbated patients were positive for the adenovirus hexon gene (capsular protein) and only 2 were positive for adenovirus 5 E1A DNA in epithelial cells (36).

## IX. Respiratory Syncytial Virus

RSV, a negative-stranded RNA virus of the *Paramyxoviridae* family, is predominantly recognized as a pediatric pathogen, but is also becoming recognized as an important adult pathogen. RSV is implicated as a cause of acute exacerbations, and the normal seasonal variation of acute RSV is linked to frequencies of COPD hospitalizations (37).

RSV enters its host's respiratory epithelium by cell surface fusion, and replication triggers an inflammatory response that may be modulated by the virus itself. The non-structural proteins antagonize IFN-$\alpha$, IFN-$\beta$, and IFN-$\lambda$ responses, which may impair antiviral immunity and contribute to persistence of the virus. The virus can also avoid early termination of infection via inhibition of apoptosis in host cells.

Serological studies have indicated that RSV infection has been associated with up to 6% of exacerbations of COPD, although studies have reported that 11.4% of hospital admissions for COPD could be accounted for by the presence of RSV, when diagnosed using serology, RT-PCR, and viral culture (38).

In addition to the interest in the role of RSV in acute exacerbations, recent studies have led to the suggestion that the virus may persist in some cases, and it may contribute to pathogenesis of stable disease.

## X. Human Metapneumovirus

In 2001, van den Hoogen et al. (39) reported the discovery of hMPV, which has subsequently been described by many others worldwide. It is similar to other paramyxoviruses, has a seasonal distribution, and has been predominantly identified in winter and early spring in North America. It has been isolated in adults with upper and lower respiratory tract infections and is associated with acute onset of wheeze. hMPV infection is most likely due to reinfection as most individuals are seropositive by the age of 5 to 10 years. As with RSV and parainfluenza, the degree of protective immunity may decrease with time. hMPV isolates segregate into two distinct genotypes, and it is possible that infection with one hMPV genotype may not confer complete protective immunity against other strains (40).

hMPV in one study was identified in 6 out of 50 hospitalized COPD exacerbations (12%) (39). Patients with hMPV were more frequently febrile during hospitalization and also had change in cough, sputum production, and dyspnea. Three of six patients positive for hMPV had evidence of a lower respiratory tract infection as the presence of a new infiltrate on chest X ray and did not test positive for bacterial infection. Other investigators have found hMPV in 5.5% patients having a COPD exacerbation when no other pathogen could be identified. Other studies have shown no evidence of MPV in 194 respiratory illnesses in 96 patients over a four-year study period. This may be due to temporal or geographical factors, and it is unknown if hMPV affects COPD patients in other climates at other times of the year.

## XI. Viruses in Stable COPD

Respiratory viruses have been detected in stable COPD patients—7.3% rhinoviruses and 5.9% coronaviruses—but the most common is RSV. In some studies, more patients had RSV detected in the stable state than at exacerbation (7). Chronic viral infection is thought to be important in CD8+ recruitment to the airways. This CD8+ T lymphocytosis driven inflammation can further damage lungs leading to COPD progression. COPD patients with repeated RSV in sputum over two years have faster lung function decline over that time (41). RSV may persist in many cases of COPD and may contribute to pathogenesis of stable disease in a manner similar to latent adenovirus. Patients with RSV found in more than 50% of sputum samples had a mean decline in $FEV_1$ of 101.4 mL/yr as compared with 51.2 mL/yr in patients with RSV in 50% of samples or less (41).

Latent adenoviral infections may also be important in COPD. E1A has the ability to initiate a cycle of viral replication that results in either cell lysis of the host cell with release of a large number of viral particles to infect other cells, or the shedding of viral particles from the surface of a living host cell (35). Low levels of viral replication allow the virus to establish a persistent infection that can last long after the virus has cleared. Viral persistence after an acute infection can also occur if viral DNA forms a plasmid within the host cell or integrates into the host cell genome. During a latent infection, viral proteins are produced without replication of a complete virus, and there is evidence this type of infection can influence the inflammatory response to stimuli in COPD. These principles may be applied to other latent viral infections.

## XII. Summary

Viruses are recognized as an increasingly important cause of COPD exacerbations, and new techniques leading to increased sensitivity of viral detection will no doubt allow for increased detection of virus in COPD both in the stable and exacerbating state. In the future, viruses are likely to be found to play an even greater role in this disease.

### References

1. Seemungal TAR, Donaldson GC, Bhowmik A, et al. Time course and recovery of exacerbations in patients with chronic obstructive pulmonary disease. Am J Respir Crit Care Med 2000; 161:1608–1613.
2. Bhowmik A, Seemungal TAR, Sapsford RJ, et al. Relation of sputum inflammatory markers to symptoms and physiological changes at COPD exacerbations. Thorax 2000; 55:114–200.
3. Papi A, Bellettato CM, Braccioni F, et al. Infections and airway inflammation in chronic obstructive pulmonary disease severe exacerbations. Am J Respir Crit Care Med 2006; 173: 1114–1121.
4. Qui Y, Zhu J, Bandi V, et al. Biopsy neutrophilia, neutrophil chemokine and receptor gene expression in severe exacerbations of chronic obstructive pulmonary disease. Am J Respir Crit Care Med 2003; 168:968–975.
5. Donaldson GC, Seemungal TAR, Jeffries DJ, et al. Effect of environmental temperature on symptoms, lung function and mortality in COPD patients. Eur Respir J 1999; 13:844–849.
6. Anderson LRJM, Hendry LT, Pierik C, et al. Multicenter study of strains of respiratory syncytial virus. J Infect Dis 1991; 163:687–692.
7. Seemungal TAR, Harper-Owen R, Bhowmik A, et al. Respiratory viruses, symptoms and inflammatory markers in acute exacerbations and stable chronic obstructive pulmonary disease. Am J Respir Crit Care Med 2001; 164:1618–1623.
8. Freymuth F, Vabret A, Cuvillon-Nimal D, et al. Comparison of multiplex PCR assays and conventional techniques for the diagnostic of respiratory virus infections in children admitted to hospital with an acute respiratory illness. J Med Virol 2006; 78(11):1498–1504.

9. Rohde G, Wiethege A, Borg I, et al. Respiratory viruses in exacerbations of chronic obstructive pulmonary disease requiring hospitalisation: a case-control study. Thorax 2003; 58(1):37–42.
10. Beckham JD, Cadena A, Lin J, et al. Respiratory viral infections in patients with chronic, obstructive pulmonary disease. J Infect 2005; 50(4):322–330.
11. Borg I, Rohde G, Löseke S, et al. Evaluation of a quantitative real-time PCR for the detection of respiratory syncytial virus in pulmonary diseases. Eur Respir J 2003; 21(6):944–951.
12. Medzhitov R, Janeway CA. Innate immunity: the virtues of a non-clonal system or recognition. Cell 1997; 91:295–298.
13. Abbas AK, Lichtman AH, Pober JS. Effector mechanisms of cell-mediated immunity. In: Abbas AK, Lichtman AH, Pober JS, eds. Cellular and Molecular Immunology. 4th ed. Philadelphia, PA: WB Saunders, 2000:291–308.
14. Fraenkel DJ, Bardin PG, Sanderson G, et al. Lower airways inflammation during rhinovirus colds in normal and in asthmatic subjects. Am J Respir Crit Care Med 1995; 151:879–886.
15. Grunberg K, Smits HH, Timmers MC, et al. Experimental rhinovirus 16 infection: effects on cell differentials and soluble markers in sputum of asthmatic subjects. Am J Respir Crit Care Med 1997; 156:609–616.
16. Fleming HE, Little EF, Schnurr D, et al. Rhinovirus-16 colds in healthy and asthmatic subjects. Am J Respir Crit Care Med 1999; 160:100–108.
17. Wilkinson TM, Hurst JR, Perera WR, et al. Effect of interactions between lower airway bacterial and rhinoviral infection in exacerbations of COPD. Chest 2006; 129:317–324.
18. Rahman I, Skwarska E, MacNee W. Attenuation of oxidant/antioxidant imbalance during treatment of exacerbations of chronic obstructive pulmonary disease. Thorax 1997; 52:565–568.
19. Biagioli MC, Kaul P, Singh I, et al. The role of oxidative stress in rhinovirus induced elaboration of IL-8 by respiratory epithelial cells. Free Radic Biol Med 1999; 26:454–462.
20. Wedzicha JA. Role of viruses in exacerbations of chronic obstructive pulmonary disease. Proc Am Thorac Soc 2004; 1:115–120.
21. Wedzicha JA, Seemungal TAR, MacCallum PK, et al. Acute exacerbations of chronic obstructive pulmonary disease are accompanied by elevations of plasma fibrinogen and serum IL-6 levels. Thromb Haemost 2000; 84:210–215.
22. Sajjan US, Jia Y, Newcomb DC, et al. H. influenzae potentiates airway epithelial cell responses to rhinovirus by increasing ICAM-1 and TLR3 expression. FASEB J 2006; 20:E1419–E1429.
23. Hurst JR, Donaldson GC, Wilkinson TM et al. Epidemiological relationships between the common cold and exacerbation frequency in COPD. Eur Respir J 2005; 26(5):846–52.
24. Patel IS, Seemungal TAR, Wilks M, et al. Relationship between bacterial colonisation and the frequency, character and severity of COPD exacerbations. Thorax 2002; 57:759–764.
25. Robbins CS, Dawe DE, Goncharova SI, et al. Cigarette smoke decreases pulmonary dendritic cells and impacts antiviral immune responsiveness. Am J Respir Cell Mol Biol 2004; 30:202–211.
26. Papi A, Johnston SL, Moric I, et al. Rhinovirus infection induces expression of its own receptor ICAM-1 via increased NFκB mediated transcription. J Biol Chem 1999; 274:9707–9720.
27. Retmales I, Elliott WM, Meshi B, et al. Amplification of inflammation in emphysema and its association with latent adenoviral infection. Am J Respir Crit Care Med 2001; 164:469–473.
28. Greenberg SB, Allen M, Wilson J, et al. Respiratory viral infections in adults with and without chronic obstructive pulmonary disease. Am J Respir Crit Care Med 2000; 162:167–173.
29. Mallia P, Message SD, Kebadze T, et al. An experimental model of rhinovirus induced chronic obstructive pulmonary disease exacerbations: a pilot study. Respir Res 2006; 7:116.
30. Makela MJ, Puhakka T, Ruuskanen O, et al. Viruses and bacteria in the etiology of the common cold. J Clin Microbiol 1998; 36:539–542.
31. van Elden LJR, van Loon AM, van Alphen F, et al. Frequent detection of human Coronaviruses in clinical specimens from patients with respiratory tract infection by use of a Novel Real-Time reverse-transcriptase polymerase chain reaction. J Infect Dis 2004; 189:652–657.

32. Ko FWS, Ip M, Chan PKS, et al. Viral etiology of acute exacerbations of COPD in Hong Kong. Chest 2007; 132:900–908.

33. Nichol KL, Baken L, Nelson A. Relation between influenza vaccination and outpatients visits, hospitalisation and mortality in elderly persons with chronic lung disease. Ann Intern Med 1999; 130:397–403.

34. Centres for Disease Control and Prevention. Influenza. A season summary. 2005. Available at: http://www cdc gov/flu/weekly/fluactivity/htm.

35. Hogg JC. Role of latent viral infections in chronic obstructive pulmonary disease and asthma. Am J Respir Crit Care Med 2001; 164:S71–S75.

36. McManus TE, Coyle PV, Kidney JC. Childhood respiratory infections and hospital admissions for COPD. Respir Med 2006; 100(3):512–518.

37. McManus TE, Marley AM, Baxter N et al. Acute and latent adenovirus in COPD. Respir Med 2007; 101:2084–2090.

38. Falsey AR, Hennessey PA, Formica MA, et al. Respiratory syncytial virus infection in elderly and high-risk adults. N Engl J Med 2005; 352:1749–59.

39. van den Hoogen BG, de Jong JC, Groen J, et al. A newly discovered human pneumovirus isolated from young children with respiratory tract disease, Nat Med 2001; 6:719–724.

40. Martinello RA, Esper F, Weibel C, et al. Human metapneumovirus and exacerbations of chronic obstructive pulmonary disease. J Infect 2006; 53(4):248–254.

41. Wilkinson TM, Donaldson GC, Johnston SL, et al. Respiratory syncytial virus, airway inflammation, and FEV1 decline in patients with chronic obstructive pulmonary disease. Am J Respir Crit Care Med 2006; 173:871–876.

# 11
## Do Airway Bacteria Cause COPD Exacerbations?

**HIMANSHU DESAI**
Division of Pulmonary, Critical Care, and Sleep Medicine, Department of Medicine and University of Buffalo, State University of New York, Buffalo, New York, U.S.A.

**SANJAY SETHI**
Division of Pulmonary, Critical Care, and Sleep Medicine, Department of Medicine, Veterans Affairs Western New York Health Care System, and University of Buffalo, State University of New York, Buffalo, New York, U.S.A.

## I. Introduction

Although noninfectious stimuli are capable of stimulating airway inflammation in chronic obstructive pulmonary disease (COPD) and contributing to exacerbations, infectious agents, including bacteria, viruses, and atypical pathogens are currently implicated in up to 80% of acute exacerbations, with bacteria likely playing a role in 50% of exacerbations (1). However, the precise role of bacterial infection in COPD has been a source of controversy for several decades (2,3). Opinion has ranged from a pre-eminent role (along with mucus hypersecretion) as embodied in the British hypothesis in the 1950s and 1960s to bacterial infection being regarded as a mere epiphenomenon in the 1970s and 1980s. In the last two decades, enhanced knowledge of microbial pathogenesis and application of new research tools have transformed our understanding of the role of infections in COPD, especially bacterial infections.

## II. Pathogenesis of Infectious COPD Exacerbations

A considerable amount of empirical evidence supports the concept that exacerbations are acute inflammatory events superimposed on the chronic inflammation that is characteristic of COPD (4,5). Several inflammatory cells and molecules in exhaled breath, sputum, bronchoalveolar lavage, or bronchial biopsy have been found to be elevated during exacerbations. Furthermore, systemic inflammation has been described during exacerbations (6). A normal tracheobronchial tree has excellent defense mechanisms to maintain sterility in the face of repeated exposure to microbial pathogens. These innate defense mechanisms appear to be compromised in the inflamed airway of COPD, allowing establishment and proliferation of microbial pathogens. These proliferating microbial pathogens induce an inflammatory response, which is associated with increased secretions in the airway, bronchospasm, and mucosal edema. These pathologic changes lead to worsening of ventilation-perfusion mismatch and hyperinflation. The clinical consequences of these pathophysiologic changes are the cardinal symptoms of an exacerbation, including new onset of or worsening of dyspnea, cough, sputum production, and sputum purulence (7). In addition, this inflammatory process in the airways could have systemic effects, resulting in clinical manifestations of fever and fatigue.

## III.   Role of Airway Bacteria in COPD Exacerbation

Bacteria are isolated from sputum in 40% to 60% of acute exacerbations of COPD (8). The three predominant bacterial species isolated are nontypeable *Haemophilus influenzae*, *Moraxella catarrhalis*, and *Streptococcus pneumoniae*. Other less frequently isolated potential pathogens include *Pseudomonas aeruginosa*, gram-negative enterobacteria, *Staphylococcus aureus*, *Haemophilus parainfluenzae*, and *Haemophilus hemolyticus* (9). Whether isolation of a potential pathogen from sputum represents infection of the lower airway causing the exacerbation has been a controversial issue for several decades. This controversy can be related to results of studies examining sputum bacteriology, immune response to bacterial pathogens, and benefit of antibiotics in exacerbations. Sputum bacteriology was expected to reveal an increased incidence of bacterial pathogen isolation during exacerbation than during stable state, but failed to do so (10). Immune studies were expected to demonstrate development of specific responses to bacteria following exacerbations. However, the results of these studies were confusing and contradictory. Antibiotics were beneficial as compared to placebo in some but not all trials, and the magnitude of benefit was small. Changes in bacterial concentration (or load) in the airways were then proposed to explain how bacteria cause exacerbations in the face of chronic colonization (11). However, there was no clear evidence that such changes in bacterial load are sufficient by itself to explain the occurrence of exacerbations. This lack of clear evidence of the bacterial etiology of exacerbations led many to doubt their role in causing exacerbations, often withholding appropriate antibiotic treatment on that basis (12).

### A.   Proposed Model for Bacterial Exacerbation Pathogenesis

A recent study investigated the role of bacterial load in COPD exacerbation pathogenesis, taking into account new strain acquisition (see below). Among pre-existing strains, sputum concentrations of potential bacterial pathogens were either no different or significantly lower during exacerbations as compared to stable periods. Among new strains of *H. influenzae* and *M. catarrhalis*, increased concentrations were seen during exacerbations; however, the differences were small. These results demonstrated that change in bacterial load is unlikely to be an important mechanism for exacerbations (13). A new model of bacterial exacerbation pathogenesis has been proposed on the basis of recent studies that investigated the pathogenesis of exacerbations with newer molecular and immunologic techniques (Fig. 1) (14). Acquisition of new strains from the environment of nontypeable *H. influenzae*, *S. pneumoniae*, and *M. catarrhalis* appears to be the predominant initiating event for an exacerbation. In the absence of lung disease, the natural course of infection with these pathogens is colonization of the upper respiratory tract. However, in patients

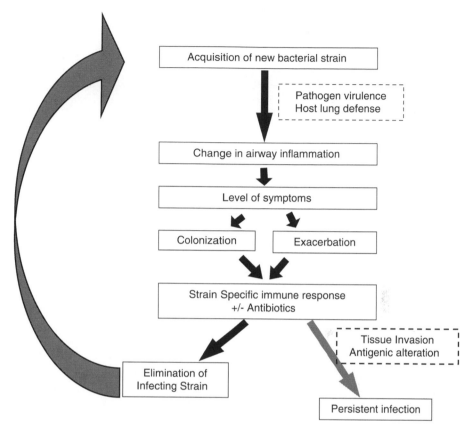

**Figure 1** Proposed model of bacterial infection in COPD. *Abbreviation*: COPD, chronic obstructive pulmonary disease. *Source*: From Ref. 14.

with an abnormal tracheobronchial tree, these bacteria infect both the upper and lower respiratory tracts and cause mucosal and, occasionally, systemic infections.

## B. Acquisition of New Bacterial Strains

Variation in the antigenic structure among strains of a bacterial species is now understood to be a major mechanism for the evasion of the human immune response and causation of bacterial infection (15). Therefore, simply culturing and enumerating colony counts of pathogens from bodily fluids are inadequate in understanding this infectious process. In a recent longitudinal COPD cohort study, strains of potential respiratory pathogens isolated from sputum were characterized by molecular techniques, to identify when new strains were acquired by a patient and when those strains were cleared from the respiratory tract. Using this approach, acquisition of new strains of certain bacterial species has been shown to be clearly associated with a greater than twofold increased risk of exacerbation of COPD (Fig. 2, Table 1). The time frame of increased risk appears to be up to four to eight weeks

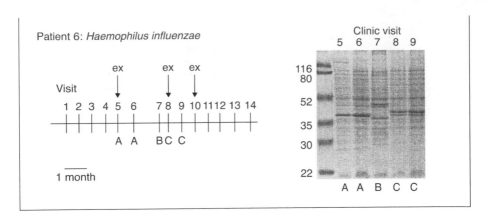

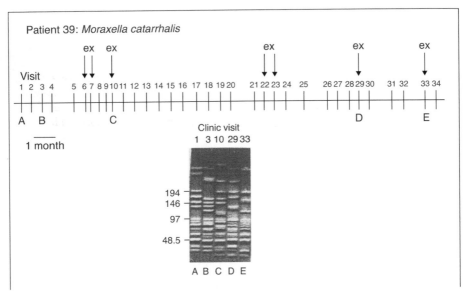

**Figure 2** Time lines and molecular typing for patients with COPD. The horizontal line is a time line, with each number indicating a clinic visit. The arrows indicate exacerbations. Isolates of *Haemophilus influenzae* and *Moraxella catarrhalis* were assigned types on the basis of sodium dodecyl sulfate-polyacrylamide gel and pulsed field gel electrophoresis, respectively (**A–E**). Molecular mass standards are noted on the left of the gels. *Abbreviation*: COPD, chronic obstructive pulmonary disease. *Source*: From Ref. 15.

after acquisition of a new strain. Specifically by pathogen, the increased risk of exacerbations with new strain acquisition was seen for *H. influenzae*, *M. catarrhalis*, and *S. pneumoniae*. New strain acquisition is not related to exacerbation for *P. aeruginosa* and *H. hemolyticus*, and its role in exacerbations associated with *H. parainfluenzae*, *S. aureus*, and *Enterobacteriaceae* has not been elucidated (9).

**Table 1** Isolation of New Strains of Bacterial Pathogens
Increasing the Risk of Exacerbation of COPD

| New strain | Relative risk of exacerbation | 95% CI of relative risk |
|---|---|---|
| *Any pathogen* | 2.15[a] | 1.83–2.53 |
| *Haemophilus influenzae* | 1.69[a] | 1.37–2.09 |
| *Moraxella catarrhalis* | 2.96[a] | 2.39–3.67 |
| *Streptococcus pneumoniae* | 1.77[a] | 1.14–2.75 |
| *Pseudomonas aeruginosa* | 0.61 | 0.21–1.82 |

[a]Statistically significant increase in risk of exacerbation.
*Abbreviation*: COPD, chronic obstructive pulmonary disease.
*Source*: From Ref. 15.

## C. Host-Pathogen Interaction

Whether a new bacterial strain acquisition in COPD leads to an exacerbation is likely to be determined by a complex host-pathogen interaction in the airways. Therefore, it is not surprising that not every new strain acquisition of bacterial pathogens is associated with exacerbation. The balance between host defense and pathogen virulence determines the level of airway inflammation, which in turn determines the level of symptoms in the patient (Fig. 2).

### Pathogen Virulence

Putative pathogen virulence factors for respiratory bacterial pathogens include adhesion to and invasion of airway epithelial cells, inactivation of host defense mechanisms, and elicitation of inflammatory mediators from airway cells. Chin et al. demonstrated that *H. influenzae* strains isolated during exacerbations induced greater airway neutrophil recruitment in a mouse pulmonary clearance model than colonizing strains (16). Furthermore, exacerbation strains adhered in significantly higher numbers to and elicited more interleukin-8 (IL-8) from primary human airway epithelial cells. Fernaays et al. with a genomics approach found that a specific combination of genes was related to exacerbation inducing potential in *H. influenzae* strains (17). One of these genes was an immunoglobulin A (IgA) protease, suggesting that inactivation of host defenses is an important determinant of disease expression among bacterial strains. However, our understanding of pathogen virulence with relevance to COPD is still in its infancy and additional observations are needed.

### Host Defense

Failure of innate defense mechanisms in COPD leads to adaptive immune responses to control and eradicate the infection. When immune responses to new strains of *M. catarrhalis* associated with COPD exacerbation and colonization were compared, a mucosal IgA response to the infecting strain was more common and vigorous with colonization, while a systemic IgG immune response was more common and vigorous with exacerbations (18). Therefore, the host immune response could dictate the clinical expression of a bacterial strain acquisition in COPD. A vigorous mucosal immune response could "exclude" the bacteria from interacting with the epithelial mucosa, resulting in less airway inflammation and therefore favoring colonization. Abe et al. demonstrated that having diminished peripheral blood mononuclear cell proliferation on exposure to a *H. influenzae* antigen, outer membrane protein P6, was associated with a history of exacerbations with *H. influenzae* (19). This suggests that an adequate cellular response to *H. influenzae* antigens suppresses newly acquired strains of this pathogen and therefore prevents exacerbations.

Several studies have clearly shown that the frequency of exacerbations increases with worsening severity of COPD. Furthermore, the proportion of exacerbations related to viruses declines, while purulent sputum (presumably bacterial) exacerbations increase as the underlying disease worsens (20,21). Furthermore, more opportunistic pathogens such as gram-negative bacteria become more prevalent during exacerbations with worsening COPD (22). All these pieces of evidence point toward a worsening innate and possibly adaptive host defense system in the lung allowing more bacterial persistence and acute infection as COPD progresses.

### Airway Inflammation

The inflammatory process in exacerbations is not uniform and is related to the etiology of the exacerbation. Exacerbations associated with bacterial pathogens exhibit significantly more neutrophilic inflammation than nonbacterial episodes (23). The intensity of neutrophilic inflammation in bacterial exacerbations is related to airway bacterial concentrations and their clinical severity (23,24). The major molecular mediators of this neutrophilic inflammation in bacterial exacerbations are IL-8, LTB4 (leukotriene B4), and TNF-α (tumor necrosis factor-alpha), and the damaging effects are likely related to release of neutrophil elastase and MMPs (matrix metalloproteinases). Clinical resolution of symptoms of exacerbation is associated with a consistent decrease in neutrophilic airway inflammation (24). Furthermore, a more marked reduction in airway inflammation is seen when such clinical resolution is accompanied by bacteriologic eradication of the offending pathogen, compared to when bacterial pathogens persist in the airway in spite of clinical resolution.

### Strain-Specific Immune Response

Development of an adaptive immune response is strong evidence of an infective process. Previous studies that examined the humoral immune response to bacterial pathogens following exacerbations had methodological limitations, and, therefore, the results were contradictory and confusing. Recent studies with homologous (infecting) strains as the antigen, paired serum samples, and immunoassays specific for antibodies that bind to surface antigens of the bacterial pathogen have clearly demonstrated the development of antibodies following exacerbations to *H. influenzae, M. catarrhalis,* and *S. pneumoniae* (18,25,26). In the case of *H. influenzae,* these bactericidal antibodies display a strong degree of strain specificity (25). Development of adaptive immune responses following exacerbation with these respiratory bacterial pathogens supports the pathogenic role of these organisms in the lower airway. The strain specificity of these immune responses accounts for the recurrent exacerbations seen in COPD.

### D.  Other Potential Mechanisms of Bacterial Exacerbations

*P. aeruginosa* is prevalent in exacerbations, usually with underlying severe airflow obstruction. However, an association between exacerbations and new strain isolation was not identified for *P. aeruginosa* in COPD and in cystic fibrosis, suggesting the existence of alternative mechanisms (15,27). *P. aeruginosa* forms biofilms in the airways in cystic fibrosis, and a change from this biofilm state to a free-floating planktonic state has been associated with exacerbations of this disease. A similar mechanism may exist among patients with COPD. Alternative mechanisms include increased bacterial load or reinfection from an endogenous site. Other gram-negative *Enterobacteriaecae* and *S. aureus* are often isolated from sputum and from bronchoscopy samples. However, their etiologic role in exacerbations and the mechanisms of such exacerbations is unclear. Whether increased bacterial load could cause exacerbations with these pathogens has not been examined. In studies of atypical bacteria in exacerbations, those with rigorous methodology show that *M. pneumoniae* is a rare cause of exacerbation and the incidence of *C. pneumoniae* is 4% to 5% (28). Again, little is known mechanistically about exacerbations related to the atypical pathogens.

## IV.  Conclusions

Substantial progress has been made in the understanding of the role of airway bacteria in COPD exacerbations. Availability of animal models of smoking-induced airway disease that could be infected with the respiratory pathogens that cause exacerbations will substantially accelerate research in this area. The complexity of the host-pathogen interaction that determines the onset and course of exacerbations needs to be explored further. Examination of cellular and molecular mechanisms in human subjects will add to our knowledge regarding infectious exacerbations. Understanding the virulence determinants of pathogens in the airway and their interaction with airway epithelial cells and macrophages would be invaluable. Insight into the mechanisms and pathophysiology of exacerbations should eventually lead to novel methods of treatment and prevention.

### References

1.  Sethi S. New developments in the pathogenesis of acute exacerbations of chronic obstructive pulmonary disease. Curr Opin Infect Dis 2004; 17(2):113–119.
2.  Murphy TF, Sethi S. Bacterial infection in chronic obstructive pulmonary disease. Am Rev Respir Dis 1992; 146:1067–1083.
3.  Tager I, Speizer FE. Role of infection in chronic bronchitis. N Engl J Med 1975; 292(11): 563–571.
4.  White AJ, Gompertz S, Stockley RA. Chronic obstructive pulmonary disease. 6: The aetiology of exacerbations of chronic obstructive pulmonary disease. Thorax 2003; 58(1):73–80.
5.  Papi A, Bellettato CM, Braccioni F, et al. Infections and airway inflammation in chronic obstructive pulmonary disease severe exacerbations. Am J Respir Crit Care Med 2006; 173(10): 1114–1121.
6.  Hurst JR, Donaldson GC, Perera WR, et al. Use of plasma biomarkers at exacerbation of chronic obstructive pulmonary disease. Am J Respir Crit Care Med 2006; 174(8):867–874.

7.  Anthonisen NR, Manfreda J, Warren CPW, et al. Antibiotic therapy in exacerbations of chronic obstructive pulmonary disease. Ann Intern Med 1987; 106:196–204.
8.  Sethi S. Infectious etiology of acute exacerbations of chronic bronchitis. Chest 2000; 117: 380S–385S.
9.  Murphy TF, Brauer AL, Sethi S, et al. Haemophilus haemolyticus: a human respiratory tract commensal to be distinguished from Haemophilus influenzae. J Infect Dis 2007; 195(1):81–89.
10. Gump DW, Phillips CA, Forsyth BR, et al. Role of infection in chronic bronchitis. Am Rev Respir Dis 1976; 113:465–473.
11. Rosell A, Monso E, Soler N, et al. Microbiologic determinants of exacerbation in chronic obstructive pulmonary disease. Arch Intern Med 2005; 165(8):891–897.
12. Hirschmann JV. Do bacteria cause exacerbations of COPD? Chest 2000; 118:193–203.
13. Sethi S, Sethi R, Eschberger K, et al. Airway bacterial concentrations and exacerbations of chronic obstructive pulmonary disease. Am J Respir Crit Care Med 2007; 176(4):356–361.
14. Veeramachaneni SB, Sethi S. Pathogenesis of bacterial exacerbations of COPD. COPD 2006; 3:109–115.
15. Sethi S, Evans N, Grant BJB, et al. Acquisition of a new bacterial strain and occurrence of exacerbations of chronic obstructive pulmonary disease. N Engl J Med 2002; 347(7):465–471.
16. Chin CL, Manzel LJ, Lehman EE, et al. Haemophilus influenzae from patients with chronic obstructive pulmonary disease exacerbation induce more inflammation than colonizers. Am J Respir Crit Care Med 2005; 172(1):85–91.
17. Fernaays MM, Lesse AJ, Sethi S, et al. Differential genome contents of nontypeable Haemophilus influenzae strains from adults with chronic obstructive pulmonary disease. Infect Immun 2006; 74(6):3366–3374.
18. Murphy TF, Brauer AL, Grant BJ, et al. Moraxella catarrhalis in chronic obstructive pulmonary disease: burden of disease and immune response. Am J Respir Crit Care Med 2005; 172(2): 195–199.
19. Abe Y, Murphy TF, Sethi S, et al. Lymphocyte proliferative response to P6 of Haemophilus influenzae is associated with relative protection from exacerbations of chronic obstructive pulmonary disease. Am J Respir Crit Care Med 2002; 165(7):967–971.
20. Greenberg SB, Allen M, Wilson J, et al. Respiratory viral infections in adults with and without chronic obstructive pulmonary disease. Am J Respir Crit Care Med 2000; 162:167–173.
21. Donaldson GC, Seemungal TA, Patel IS, et al. Longitudinal changes in the nature, severity and frequency of COPD exacerbations. Eur Respir J 2003; 22(6):931–936.
22. Eller J, Ede A, Schaberg T, et al. Infective exacerbations of chronic bronchitis: relation between bacteriologic etiology and lung function. Chest 1998; 113:1542–1548.
23. Sethi S, Muscarella K, Evans N, et al. Airway inflammation and etiology of acute exacerbations of chronic bronchitis. Chest 2000; 118(6):1557–1565.
24. Gompertz S, O'Brien C, Bayley DL, et al. Changes in bronchial inflammation during acute exacerbations of chronic bronchitis. Eur Respir J 2001; 17(6):1112–1119.
25. Sethi S, Wrona C, Grant BJB, et al. Strain-specific immune response to Haemophilus influenzae in chronic obstructive pulmonary disease. Am J Respir Crit Care Med 2004; 169:448–453.
26. Bogaert D, van der Valk P, Ramdin R, et al. Host-pathogen interaction during pneumococcal infection in patients with chronic obstructive pulmonary disease. Infect Immun 2004; 72(2): 818–823.
27. Aaron SD, Ramotar K, Ferris W, et al. Adult cystic fibrosis exacerbations and new strains of Pseudomonas aeruginosa. Am J Respir Crit Care Med 2004; 169(7):811–815.
28. Blasi F, Legnani D, Lombardo VM, et al. Chlamydia pneumoniae infection in acute exacerbations of COPD. Eur Respir J 1993; 6:19–22.

# 12

## Interactions of Airway Pathogens and Inflammatory Processes

**MARCO CONTOLI, GAETANO CARAMORI, BRUNILDA MARKU, and ALBERTO PAPI**
Department of Clinical and Experimental Medicine, Research Center on Asthma and COPD,
University of Ferrara, Ferrara, Italy

**ANITA PANDIT**
Royal Glamorgan Hospital, Llantrisant, U.K.

## I. Introduction

The clinical history of chronic obstructive pulmonary disease (COPD) is punctuated by recurrent episodes of increases in dyspnea, cough, or sputum production named exacerbations. In addition to increasing COPD-associated morbidity and mortality, exacerbations contribute to loss of lung function and impaired health status in COPD patients (1).

Although it is often assumed that exacerbations are associated with increased airway inflammation, there is little information on the nature of the acute-on-chronic inflammation that characterizes these episodes. Most of the data currently available refer to soluble indirect markers of airway inflammation rather than inflammatory cell infiltration per se (2).

Infections of the tracheobronchial tree, together with air pollution, are considered the most common causes of COPD exacerbations (1). Whether different patterns of airway inflammation correspond to different etiologies is largely unknown. Better understanding of these relationships and of the underlying pathophysiological mechanisms would give the opportunity to identify relevant targets (pathogens and inflammation) for the treatment and prevention of COPD exacerbations.

Many exacerbations are associated with symptoms of infection of the tracheobronchial tree, and bacteria have been considered the main infective cause of exacerbations (1). Determining the contribution of bacteria to exacerbations is difficult, as COPD patients are often colonized with bacteria even when clinically stable (3). The proportion of patients with positive bacterial cultures and a high bacterial load increases during exacerbations in most, although not in all, studies (4–6). Newer molecular techniques have recently shown that colonization is not a static condition and there is a frequent turnover of different strains of bacteria evoking specific host responses (7). Thus, it is likely that a change in the strain but not the organism may be responsible for the exacerbations. Therefore, previous studies lacking in the molecular characterization of bacterial strains may have missed evidence of a new infection. Indeed, it has been documented that the acquisition of a new strain of colonizing bacteria increases the risk of an exacerbation (8).

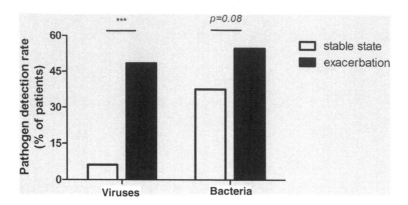

**Figure 1**  Pathogen detection rate in COPD patients at stable state versus exacerbation. *Source*: From Ref. 5.

In the last few decades, the use of highly sensitive diagnostic methods, such as polymerase chain reaction (PCR), to evaluate the association between respiratory virus infections and COPD exacerbations has shown that viruses are responsible for a much higher proportion of exacerbations than was previously realized. In a study of the East London COPD cohort, respiratory viruses were detected in 39% of exacerbations, the most common being rhinoviruses that accounted for 58% of viruses (9). A respiratory virus was detected in around 50% of patients with severe COPD exacerbation admitted to hospitals in Germany and Italy, with rhinovirus again being the most common (5,10). In patients with very severe COPD exacerbations requiring intubation and mechanical ventilation, viruses were identified in 47% of patients (11). At variance with bacterial infections, the respiratory viruses more commonly found at exacerbations were virtually absent in stable state (5,12), suggesting that they play a relevant role in the etiology of the acute episodes.

A recent study has addressed the relative importance of viral versus bacterial infections to the etiology of severe (hospitalized) COPD exacerbations. Viral and/or bacterial infection was detected in 78% of COPD exacerbations, with viruses in 48.4% (6.2% when stable), and bacteria in 54.7% (37.5% when stable) (Fig. 1). The more severe exacerbations were those in which viral and bacterial coinfection was detected (5). Similar results have also been found in studies of COPD exacerbations in outpatients (13); if both bacteria and symptom of common cold were present, then the sputum inflammatory markers were higher and lung function impairment was greater.

## II.  Pathogens and Inflammation

### A.  Inflammatory Responses During Bacteria-Associated COPD Exacerbations

Enhanced neutrophilic inflammation and sputum purulence have been considered for many years markers of bacterial etiology of COPD exacerbations. The traditional association of sputum purulence with bacterial infection is supported by the higher rate of isolation of bacterial pathogens in individuals with purulent sputum at presentation, with one study identifying a positive bacterial culture in 84% of purulent sputum compared with 38%, if sputum was mucoid (14). Self-reported assessment of sputum purulence has also been investigated: bacterial cultures performed on sputum samples and protected brush specimens showed that self-reported sputum purulence was associated with a high yield of potentially pathogenic microorganisms with a positive predictive value of 77% (15). Gompertz et al. have shown that when purulent sputum exacerbations are treated with antibiotics, resolution of exacerbations is associated with progressive reduction of neutrophilic airway inflammation (16). A number of studies documented that higher bacterial loads were more frequently associated with increased sputum neutrophils, supporting the concept that when bacteria are present at exacerbation, airway inflammation is higher in those samples where bacterial load is higher (6,13). IL-8 and TNF-$\alpha$ are potent neutrophilic chemoattractant chemokines with increased levels in sputum supernatants during COPD exacerbations. Although not in all studies, bacterial exacerbation has been associated with higher levels of sputum IL-8 and TNF-$\alpha$, leading to enhanced neutrophil recruitment and activation (17,18).

Virtually all the studies that have found a relationship between bacterial infection and increased markers of neutrophilic inflammation in sputum samples and/or increased sputum purulence during exacerbation did not take into account viral and/or viral/bacterial coinfections. Whether enhanced neutrophilic inflammation in the airways of COPD patients during exacerbation is a marker of bacterial infection has been debated in the last few years. Indeed, in experimental condition rhinovirus infection induces peripheral blood and sputum netrophilia in smokers and COPD subjects (19). A recent study showed increased number of neutrophils in sputum during exacerbations and the neutrophilic response occurred irrespective of the pathogen detected (bacteria vs. viruses vs. coinfection viruses + bacteria). The same study documented that purulent sputum at exacerbation was more frequent in infective exacerbations as compared with noninfective exacerbations, but no difference was found between viral versus bacterial infections (5). Intriguingly, a very recent study found that COPD exacerbations associated with acquisition of new strains of bacteria, specifically *Haemophilus influenzae*, *Streptococcus pneumoniae*, *Moraxella catarrhalis*, and *Pseudomonas aeruginosa*, were associated with a more intense neutrophilic inflammatory response in the airway, as well as more intense systemic inflammation, compared with exacerbations not associated with new strain acquisition (20).

One of the future major tasks in the field of exacerbation will be to identify inflammatory or specific biological markers able to tell us whether bacteria are in fact responsible for the ongoing exacerbation. This would be extremely helpful in addressing an appropriate use of antibiotic treatments. With this aim, several specific markers of bacterial infections have been tested in the last few years. A promising role of procalcitonin to define patients with a COPD exacerbation with a higher likelihood of bacterial infection has been recently suggested. Procalcitonin is a small (13 kDa) protein normally undetectable in plasma that increases markedly in bacterial infections (21). Data from a single-center, cluster-randomized, single-blind study suggest that procalcitonin-guided therapy can be safely used to reduce antibiotic use in patients admitted to the hospital with COPD exacerbation at a low likelihood of bacterial infection (22).

## B. Mechanisms of Bacteria-Induced Airway Inflammation

Several mechanisms have been proposed to explain how bacterial infection can affect airway inflammation, leading to COPD exacerbations. These include induction of mucus hypersecretion (23), reduction of ciliary beat frequency (24), and enhancement of neu-trophilic inflammation (25). In particular, *H. influenzae* can cause direct epithelial damage and its endotoxin has been shown to increase epithelial expression of the proinflammatory cytokines IL-6, IL-8, and TNF-α in vitro, providing potential mechanisms to upregulate inflammation and specifically neutrophilic inflammation (25). This is in line with in vivo data showing that COPD patients with a positive bacterial culture of potential pathogenic microbes have higher concentrations of TNF-α and increased neutrophils in the airways (17,26).

Activated neutrophils degranulate, resulting in the release of elastases, oxidants, and proteases. Proteases and oxidants can damage the epithelium, reduce ciliary beat frequency, stimulate mucus secretion by mucus-secreting cells, and increase the permeability of the bronchial mucosa. These changes, especially in the small airways, may increase airflow obstruction, leading to increased dyspnea, as well as increased mucus secretion and sputum purulence. In addition, neutrophil elastase and oxidants have been shown to increase epi-thelial mucin mRNA and protein gene expression in vitro. Neutrophil elastase is a major driver of lung injury, thus elevated levels of this enzyme seen in bacterial exacerbations could contribute significantly to the loss of lung function seen in COPD (27).

Bacterial components, such as lipopolysaccharide (LPS), through their interaction with toll-like receptors can activate nuclear transcription factor κB (NF-κB) (28). Acti-vation of NF-κB leads to the production of several cytokines, chemokines, and adhesion molecules involved in the inflammatory cascade that characterizes COPD exacerbation (29). Interestingly, a recent study found increased NF-κB activation in sputum macrophages during COPD exacerbations (30).

Although in vitro models can provide important insights into the molecular mecha-nisms of inflammatory and immune responses to bacterial infection, the in vitro data require validation in in vivo models. Unfortunately, despite bacterial infections being considered the most important cause of COPD exacerbations, there is still no in vivo model of bacteria-induced COPD exacerbation.

### C. Inflammatory Responses During Virus-Associated COPD Exacerbations

Few studies have investigated the role of respiratory virus infection in COPD exacerbations, and very few have looked at the relationship between viral infections and airway inflam-mation at exacerbations.

One study found increased sputum IL-6 in virus-associated acute episodes as compared with nonviral exacerbations (12). Intriguingly, and only recently, it has been documented that plasma fibrinogen levels, a marker of systemic inflammation and a recognized independent risk factor for cardiovascular disease, are higher in virus-associated COPD exacerbation (31). This indicates that respiratory viral infections are associated with an increased systemic inflammation and might predispose to an increased risk of cardiovascular disease. Bacterial and virus infection can synergistically interact to increase the severity of inflammatory response. Indeed, it has been shown that rhinovirus and *H. influenzae* coinfection at exacer-bations is associated with increased levels of serum IL-6 (13). In this situations, i.e., viral and bacterial coinfection, exacerbations are more severe both in term of clinical and lung function parameters (5,13). Similarly, levels of endothelin (ET)-1, a potent vasoconstrictor and bron-choconstrictor peptide with important proinflammatory activities in the airways, tend to be higher during COPD exacerbation associated with viral or chlamydial infection both in sputum and plasma (32).

A recent study investigated the relative importance of viral and bacterial infection in COPD exacerbations and their relationship with airway inflammation (5). At variance with neutrophils, sputum eosinophils were significantly elevated at exacerbation only in the subgroups with viral infections (Fig. 2). In this study, sputum eosinophils at exacerbation could predict a positive viral detection in sputum, with a sensitivity of 0.82 and a specificity of 0.77 for eosinophil counts of $1.68 \times 10^6$/g or greater (best cut-off point). Similarly, sputum eosinophil count increases from stable conditions to exacerbation of $0.3 \times 10^6$/g or more predicted a virus-associated COPD exacerbation with a sensitivity of 0.87 and a specificity of 0.81. Sputum eosinophilic cationic protein (ECP) levels in the supernatant of samples obtained from exacerbations associated with viral infection, either with or without a bacterial coinfection, were significantly higher as compared with virus-free exacerbations.

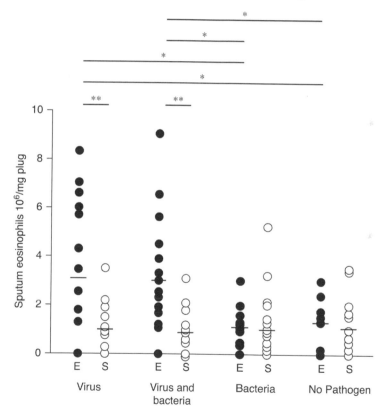

**Figure 2** Sputum eosinophil counts in patients with COPD during severe exacerbation requiring hospitalization (E) and during stable convalescence (S). Subjects were grouped according to the presence of respiratory viruses alone (Virus), bacteria alone (Bacteria), both viruses and bacteria (Virus and Bacteria), or no pathogen (No Pathogens) in the sputum during exacerbation. Airway eosinophil counts are only increased during COPD exacerbations associated with virus detection. *Note*: *$p < 0.05$; **$p < 0.01$. *Source*: From Ref. 5.

These data suggest that sputum eosinophilia and not sputum neutrophilia can be a marker of viral infection during COPD exacerbations (5). Previous studies reported a prominent airway eosinophilia at exacerbation with a 30-fold increase in the number of eosinophils in the exacerbated group compared with the stable patients (33,34).

Taken together, these data indicate that noninvasive measurements could be used in clinical practice to provide clinically relevant etiological information. Further studies are required to confirm and extend this pivotal observation.

Interestingly, increased sputum CD8+ T lymphocytes have been reported during COPD exacerbations, with a relative reduction in the ratio of interferon (IFN)-γ/IL-4 expressing CD8+ T lymphocyte (35). Thus, a switch toward a T helper (Th)-2-like immunophenotype during COPD exacerbations could trigger recruitment of eosinophils and might be activated by the immune response to some microbial pathogens.

### D. Mechanisms of Virus-Associated Airway Inflammation

Despite growing clinical evidence for a role of respiratory viral infections in the pathogenesis of COPD exacerbations, the precise mechanisms of interactions between respiratory virus and lower airway inflammation and of host resistance against respiratory viruses are poorly understood (29). Most of the data available relate to rhinovirus, i.e., the respiratory virus that appears to be more frequently involved in COPD exacerbations (5,10,36).

The major group of rhinoviruses (accounting for 90% of total rhinovirus types) attaches to airway epithelium through intercellular adhesion molecule 1 (ICAM-1) (37). Interestingly, rhinovirus infection induces expression of its own receptor (ICAM-1) (38), which might promote inflammatory cell recruitment and activation. Indeed, since ICAM-1 is overexpressed in the bronchial mucosa of patients with stable chronic bronchitis (39), one of the possible mechanisms for increased susceptibility to infections and for increased airway inflammation is rhinovirus-induced ICAM-1 upregulation in bronchial epithelial cells.

Several studies document that in vitro experimental rhinovirus infection of bronchial epithelial cells induces proinflammatory mediators, including cytokines, chemokines, and adhesion molecules able to induce both neutrophilc (i.e. CXCL8, GM-CSF) and eosinophilic (i.e. eotaxin, CCL5) inflammation. These in vitro experimental data are in line with clinical observations showing that neutrophilic and eosinophilic inflammatory responses can occur in vivo following rhinovirus infection (29). Interestingly, bronchial eosinophilia has been described some years ago in bronchial biopsies of healthy subjects experimentally infected with rhinovirus (40).

In vitro rhinovirus infection of human bronchial epithelial cells increases their MUC5AC (one of the major mucins in the sputum) synthesis and release (41). This could be relevant to explain the increased amount of sputum observed in some patients during COPD exacerbations.

Rhinovirus infection induces increased production of oxidants (i.e. superoxide anion) in bronchial epithelial cells, and this event is a crucial step for the activation of NF-κB and the following production of proinflammatory cytokines, chemokines, and adhesion molecules (42). Reducing agents inhibit both rhinovirus-induced oxidant generation and inflammatory mediator production and release (42). These data suggest that the inhibition of intracellular oxidative stress may be a potential therapeutic target for the treatment of virus-induced COPD exacerbations.

It has been recently shown that early activation of mitogen-activated protein (MAP) kinase p38 is a key regulatory event of rhinovirus-induced proinflammatory transcription factor activation and cytokine/chemokine transcription both in bronchial epithelial cells, monocytes and macrophages (43,44). These mechanisms could be a target for inhibition of airway inflammation associated with rhinovirus infection.

To validate in vitro observations, the development of an in vivo model is necessary. Thus the recent development of a human experimental model of rhinovirus-induced COPD exacerbations represents an innovative tool that will offer the opportunity to deeply elucidate the inflammatory and immunological mechanisms that lead COPD patients to exacerbate after respiratory virus infections and to identify novel possible pharmacological targets (45). This model shows that experimental rhinovirus infection in COPD patients induces symptoms, lung function changes, increased peripheral blood total leukocyte count, increased peripheral neutrophil, and increased sputum neutrophil number (19,45) similar to that observed in naturally occurring exacerbations. In COPD, this is so far the only scenario in which a specific etiology has been experimentally proven to induce an exacerbation.

## III.  Conclusion

COPD is a major health problem worldwide, with rising prevalence and mortality. The major morbidity, mortality, and health care costs of COPD are due to exacerbations (1).

Thanks to the development of highly sensitive diagnostic tools, the interaction between respiratory viruses and bacteria has emerged as a leading cause of COPD exacerbations (5,13). However, the mechanisms responsible for the interaction between these airway pathogens and the inflammatory processes in causing COPD exacerbations are still largely unknown (29). Only recently, researchers have started to identify specific inflammatory markers that can distinguish among different pathogens involved in COPD exacerbations.

The recent development of the first human model of virus-induced COPD exacerbation is rapidly advancing our knowledge on these interactions (45). Improved understanding of the host-pathogen interaction in the lower airways in COPD patients will undoubtedly facilitate the identification of novel pharmacological targets that will provide opportunities to develop new treatments for COPD exacerbations.

## References

1. Global Initiative for Chronic Obstructive Lung Disease (GOLD). National Institute of Health, National Heart Lung, and Blood Institute. Global strategy for the diagnosis, management and prevention of chronic obstructive pulmonary disease. NHLBI/WHO Workshop report. NIH Publication No 2701A, March 2001. Last update 2007.
2. Papi A, Luppi F, Franco F, et al. Pathophysiology of exacerbations of chronic obstructive pulmonary disease. Proc Am Thorac Soc 2006; 3:245–251.
3. Sethi S, Maloney J, Grove L, et al. Airway inflammation and bronchial bacterial colonization in chronic obstructive pulmonary disease. Am J Respir Crit Care Med 2006; 173:(9):991–998.
4. Monso E, Ruiz J, Rosell A, et al. Bacterial infection in chronic obstructive pulmonary disease. A study of stable and exacerbated outpatients using the protected specimen brush. Am J Respir Crit Care Med 1995; 152(4 pt 1):1316–1320.
5. Papi A, Bellettato CM, Braccioni F, et al. Infections and airway inflammation in chronic obstructive pulmonary disease severe exacerbations. Am J Respir Crit Care Med 2006; 173(10):1114–1121.

6.  White AJ, Gompertz S, Stockley RA. Chronic obstructive pulmonary disease. 6: The aetiology of exacerbations of chronic obstructive pulmonary disease. Thorax 2003; 58:73–80.
7.  Sethi S, Wrona C, Grant BJ, et al. Strain-specific immune response to Haemophilus influenzae in chronic obstructive pulmonary disease. Am J Respir Crit Care Med 2004; 169(4):448453.
8.  Sethi S, Evans N, Grant BJ, et al. New strains of bacteria and exacerbations of chronic obstructive pulmonary disease. N Engl J Med 2002; 347(7):465–471.
9.  Seemungal T, Harper-Owen R, Bhowmik A, et al. Respiratory viruses, symptoms, and inflammatory markers in acute exacerbations and stable chronic obstructive pulmonary disease. Am J Respir Crit Care Med 2001; 164(9):1618–1623.
10. Rohde G, Wiethege A, Borg I, et al. Respiratory viruses in exacerbations of chronic obstructive pulmonary disease requiring hospitalisation: a case-control study. Thorax 2003; 58(1):37–42.
11. Qiu Y, Zhu J, Bandi V, et al. Biopsy neutrophilia, neutrophil chemokine and receptor gene expression in severe exacerbations of chronic obstructive pulmonary disease. Am J Respir Crit Care Med 2003; 168(8):968–975.
12. Seemungal TA, Harper-Owen R, Bhowmik A, et al. Detection of rhinovirus in induced sputum at exacerbation of chronic obstructive pulmonary disease. Eur Respir J 2000; 16(4):677–683.
13. Wilkinson TM, Hurst JR, Perera WR, et al. Effect of interactions between lower airway bacterial and rhinoviral infection in exacerbations of COPD. Chest 2006; 129(2):317324.
14. Stockley RA, O'Brien C, Pye A, et al. Relationship of sputum color to nature and outpatient management of acute exacerbations of COPD. Chest 2000; 117:1638–1645.
15. Soler N, Augusti C, Angrill J, et al. Bronchoscopic validation of the significance of sputum purulence in severe exacerbations of chronic obstructive pulmonary disease (COPD). Thorax 2007; 62:29–35.
16. Gompertz S, O'Brien C, Bayley DL, et al. Changes in bronchial inflammation during acute exacerbations of chronic bronchitis. Eur Respir J 2001; 17(6):1112–1119.
17. Sethi S, Muscarella K, Evans N, et al. Airway inflammation and etiology of acute exacerbations of chronic bronchitis. Chest 2000; 118(6):1557–1565.
18. Aaron SD, Angel JB, Lunau M, et al. Granulocyte inflammatory markers and airway infection during acute exacerbation of chronic obstructive pulmonary disease. Am J Respir Crit Care Med 2001; 163(2):349–355.
19. Mallia P, Message S, Contoli M, et al. An Experimental Model of Virus-Induced COPD Exacerbation. Thorax 2006; 61:S076.
20. Sethi S, Wrona C, Eschberger K, et al. Inflammatory profile of new bacterial strain exacerbations of chronic obstructive pulmonary disease. Am J Respir Crit Care Med 2007; Dec 13 (epub ahead of print).
21. Simon L, Gauvin F, Amre DK, et al. Serum procalcitonin and C-reactive protein levels as markers of bacterial infection: a systematic review and meta-analysis. Clin Infect Dis 2004; 39(2):206–217.
22. Stolz D, Christ-Crain M, Bingisser R, et al. Antibiotic treatment of exacerbations of COPD: a randomized, controlled trial comparing procalcitonin-guidance with standard therapy. Chest 2007; 131(1):9–19.
23. Adler KB, Hendley DD, Davis GS. Bacteria associated with obstructive pulmonary disease elaborate extracellular products that stimulate mucin secretion by explants of guinea pig airways. Am J Pathol 1986; 125(3):501–514.
24. Wilson R, Roberts D, Cole P. Effect of bacterial products on human ciliary function in vitro. Thorax 1985; 40(2):125–131.
25. Read RC, Wilson R, Rutman A, et al. Interaction of nontypable Haemophilus influenzae with human respiratory mucosa in vitro. J Infect Dis 1991; 163(3):549–558.
26. Tumkaya M, Atis S, Ozge C, et al. Relationship between airway colonization, inflammation and exacerbation frequency in COPD. Respir Med 2007; 101(4):729–737.

27. Quint JK, Wedzicha JA. The neutrophil in chronic obstructive pulmonary disease. J Allergy Clin Immunol 2007; 119(5):1065–1071.
28. Carmody RJ, Chen YH. Nuclear factor-kappaB: activation and regulation during toll-like receptor signaling. Cell Mol Immunol 2007; 4(1):31–41.
29. Mallia P, Contoli M, Caramori G, et al. Exacerbations of asthma and chronic obstructive pulmonary disease (COPD). Focus on virus induced exacerbations. Curr Pharm Des 2007; 13:73–97.
30. Caramori G, Romagnoli M, Casolari P, et al. Nuclear localisation of p65 in sputum macrophages but not in sputum neutrophils during COPD exacerbations. Thorax 2003; 58(4):348–351.
31. Wedzicha JA, Seemungal TAR, MacCallum PK, et al. Acute exacerbations of chronic obstructive pulmonary disease are accompanied by elevations of plasma fibrinogen and serum IL-6 levels. Thromb Haemost 2000; 84:210–215.
32. Roland M, Bhowmik A, Sapsford RJ, et al. Sputum and plasma endothelin-1 levels in exacerbations of chronic obstructive pulmonary disease. Thorax 2001; 56(1):30–35.
33. Saetta M, Di Stefano A, Maestrelli P, et al. Airway eosinophilia in chronic bronchitis during exacerbations. Am J Respir Crit Care Med 1994; 150(6 pt 1):1646–1652.
34. Zhu J, Qiu YS, Majumdar S, et al. Exacerbations of Bronchitis: bronchial eosinophilia and gene expression for interleukin-4, interleukin-5, and eosinophil chemoattractants. Am J Respir Crit Care Med 2001; 164(1):109–116.
35. Tsoumakidou M, Tzanakis N, Chrysofakis G, et al. Changes in sputum T-lymphocyte subpopulations at the onset of severe exacerbations of chronic obstructive pulmonary disease. Respir Med 2005; 99(5):572–579.
36. Donaldson GC, Seemungal TA, Patel IS, et al. Longitudinal changes in the nature, severity and frequency of COPD exacerbations. Eur Respir J 2003; 22(6):931–936.
37. Greve JM, Davis G, Meyer AM, et al. The major human rhinovirus receptor is ICAM-1. Cell 1989; 56(5):839–847.
38. Papi A, Johnston SL. Rhinovirus infection induces expression of its own receptor intercellular adhesion molecule 1 (ICAM-1) via increased NF-kappaB-mediated transcription. J Biol Chem 1999; 274(14):9707–9720.
39. Vignola AM, Campbell AM, Chanez P, et al. HLA-DR and ICAM-1 expression on bronchial epithelial cells in asthma and chronic bronchitis. Am Rev Respir Dis 1993; 148(3):689–694.
40. Fraenkel DJ, Bardin PG, Sanderson G, et al. Lower airways inflammation during rhinovirus colds in normal and in asthmatic subjects. Am J Respir Crit Care Med 1995; 151:879–886.
41. Inoue D, Yamaya M, Kubo H, et al. Mechanisms of mucin production by rhinovirus infection in cultured human airway epithelial cells. Respir Physiol Neurobiol 2006; 154(3):484–499.
42. Papi A, Papadopoulos NG, Stanciu LA, et al. Reducing agents inhibit rhinovirus-induced upregulation of the rhinovirus receptor intercellular adhesion molecule-1 (ICAM-1) in respiratory epithelial cells. Faseb J 2002; 16(14):1934–1936.
43. Griego SD, Weston CB, Adams JL, et al. Role of p38 mitogen-activated protein kinase in rhinovirus-induced cytokine production by bronchial epithelial cells. J Immunol 2000; 165(9):5211–5220.
44. Hall DJ, Bates ME, Guar L, et al. The role of p38 MAPK in rhinovirus-induced monocyte chemoattractant protein-1 production by monocytic-lineage cells. J Immunol 2005; 174(12):8056–8063.
45. Mallia P, Message SD, Kebadze T, et al. An experimental model of rhinovirus induced chronic obstructive pulmonary disease exacerbations: a pilot study. Respir Res 2006; 7:116.

# 13
## Comorbidity at Exacerbation of COPD

**DAVID MCALLISTER, JOHN MACLAY, WILLIAM MACNEE, and ROBERTO RABINOVICH**
ELEGI/Colt Research Laboratories, MRC/University of Edinburgh Centre for Inflammation Research, Queens Medical Research Institute, Edinburgh, U.K.

## I. Introduction

As a result of the ageing population, and the fact that several chronic conditions have common risk factors, comorbidity is common in patients with chronic obstructive pulmonary disease (COPD) (1). Consequently, the management of patients with complex comorbidity, which was previously the concern of the geriatrician, has become an issue of concern for most physicians treating respiratory disease today.

There is no consensus definition of comorbidity. Clearly, a comorbid condition must be distinct from the main condition of interest, in this case, exacerbation of chronic obstructive pulmonary disease (ECOPD). However, it is not always clear whether a coexisting disease is most accurately described as incidental (e.g., osteoarthritis in a patient with Crohn's disease), complicating (e.g., deep venous thrombosis in a patient with pneumonia), or as a distinct disease that nonetheless impacts on the patient's condition (e.g., heart failure in a patient with COPD). Here we pragmatically define a comorbid condition as any disease that may exert an additional or synergistic effect on the morbidity or mortality arising from ECOPD. To this end, we review several respiratory, cardiovascular, and other conditions that commonly coexist with ECOPD.

## II. Respiratory CoMorbidity

### A. Pulmonary Embolism

Patients hospitalized with ECOPD may have an increased risk of pulmonary thromboembolism (PE) as a result of sedentarism, age, and acute infection. COPD patients have raised levels of $\beta$-thromboglobulin (a marker of platelet activation) and thrombin-antithrombin III complexes (a marker of a hypercoagulable state), which may act to increase their risk of DVT/PE (2). Schonhofer and Kohler performed Doppler ultrasound on 196 patients with COPD and found DVT in 10%, almost four times higher than the general hospital population (3).

The diagnosis of PE is difficult in the general population. Moreover, since PE causes acute dyspnea and can occur without chest pain, it is likely to be more difficult to detect clinically in the context of ECOPD. Tillie-Leblond et al. published a high-profile study examining 197 patients with COPD attending hospital with exacerbation of "unknown origin," i.e., no evidence of increased sputum purulence or volume or systemic symptoms of infection (4). In this highly selected population (29% had concurrent malignancy), 25% of patients had PE on CT pulmonary angiogram (CTPA). However, Rutschmann et al. studied a serial sample of 123 consecutive patients admitted to hospital with primary diagnosis of ECOPD and found that PE was far less common (5). In this group, 39% had clinical features suggestive of PE—chest pain, syncope, and hypoxemia ($pO_2 < 8$ kPa), 77% had a raised D-dimer, but only 3.3% had confirmed DVT or PE (Doppler ultrasound and CTPA, respectively). Nevertheless, of those patients with clinical features suggestive of PE, 6.2% of cases were confirmed. As such, PE remains an important differential diagnosis in ECOPD (6).

### B.  Pneumothorax

Pneumothorax (PTX) in COPD carries a fourfold increased risk of death (7). COPD is the commonest cause of secondary PTX, and patients with bullae/hyperinflation may be at even higher risk. On a background of respiratory compromise, losing partial or complete ventilation of one lung has potentially catastrophic consequences. PTX may mimic ECOPD. Giant bullae and reduced lung markings in COPD make PTX difficult to diagnose on chest X ray (8). CT scanning is definitive but is costly and involves significant exposure to radiation. Secondary spontaneous PTX recurs in 40% to 50% of patients who do not undergo a definitive preventative procedure (9), and aggressive early intervention is recommended in patients with COPD (10).

### C.  Pneumonia

Pneumonia, which is associated with increased mortality in patients with underlying lung disease, may complicate ECOPD (11). The burden of pneumonia in COPD is considerable. Results of retrospective observational studies of patients admitted to hospital have shown that 10% of COPD patients have pneumonia, 30% of pneumonia patients have underlying COPD, and patients with both conditions have increased mortality and prolonged admissions (11,12).

## III.  Cardiovascular CoMorbidity

COPD and coronary heart disease (CHD) commonly occur in middle and later life and therefore coexist in an ageing population (1). Both conditions share common causes and risk factors, including cigarette smoke exposure, poor diet, and low socioeconomic status (13,14), and airflow limitation is related to cardiovascular risk independent of age, sex, smoking, cholesterol, and blood pressure (15).

Several features of ECOPD such as tachycardia, hypoxia, reduced venous return, systemic inflammation, and oxidative stress may increase the likelihood of COPD patients experiencing the effects of underlying CHD (16). Additionally, other comorbidities in ECOPD, such as hyperglycemia and anemia, may also have a role in precipitating cardiovascular events in patients with ECOPD (Fig. 1).

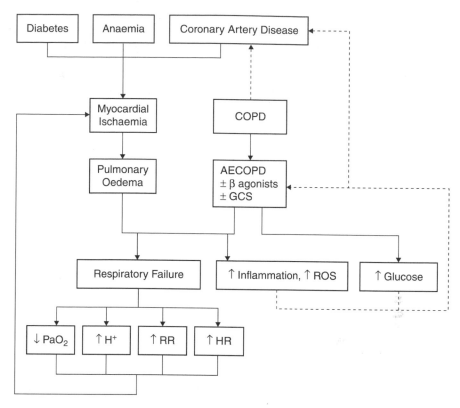

**Figure 1**   Interaction of comorbidity at exacerbation of COPD. Dashed line represents putative association.

## A.   Treatment of ECOPD and Cardiovascular Risk

During ECOPD, systemic steroids improve $FEV_1$ and hypoxia and reduce length of hospital stay (17), and are thus a recommended treatment (18). However, steroids are also associated with an increased risk of myocardial infarction, heart failure, and atrial fibrillation (AF) (19–21). Steroid use, as a marker of ECOPD, has also been associated with an increased risk of cardiovascular events (22).

Similarly, inhaled β-agonists improve symptoms, airflow limitation, and gas exchange, and are recommended for the management of ECOPD (18). However, β-receptor *antagonists* effectively treat heart failure, AF, and myocardial infarction, and there has therefore been concern regarding β-agonist in comorbid CHD/COPD. Indeed, the American Heart Association (AHA) recommend avoiding β-agonists in patients with "bronchospastic disease" who develop AF (23). However, β-agonist use among patients with ECOPD remains controversial (24,25) and is beyond the scope of this chapter.

### B.  Atrial Fibrillation

AF is common in COPD and is associated with worse survival (26). The joint AHA/ACC guidelines on the management of AF recommend that during ECOPD acidosis and hypoxia should be corrected and that a calcium channel blocker may be used for rate control. Anticoagulation should be used as for uncomplicated AF, and β-blockers and adenosine are not recommended (23).

### C.  Heart Failure

Heart failure is common among patients with ECOPD (20–40%) (27). However, determining the true prevalence of pulmonary edema during ECOPD is problematic because of difficulties identifying pulmonary edema alongside ECOPD with which it shares a number of common pathophysiological and symptomatic features (27). Although pulmonary edema has characteristic features on chest X ray, these are not usually seen until lung water increases by more than 30% (28), and patients with COPD might be expected to experience symptoms with less severe edema. Transthoracic echocardiography, used to diagnose heart failure, is technically difficult in the presence of emphysema, and transesophageal is invasive (28). Amino terminal pro-brain natriuretic peptide (NT-proBNP) is a circulating marker of pulmonary edema, and Abroug et al. (29) recently showed that this marker could distinguish severe ECOPD complicated by pulmonary edema from uncomplicated ECOPD.

Although β-blocker therapy improves survival and quality of life, there is a reluctance to use β-blockers in patients with stable COPD and heart failure despite evidence that cardioselective β-blocking agents are safe (30). Nonetheless, there is no data supporting safety in ECOPD wherein β-blockers remain contraindicated.

Noninvasive ventilation (NIV) is a safe, effective, widely used therapy for the treatment of respiratory failure in ECOPD (31), and several systematic reviews have found no difference in mortality or need for intubation between NIV and continuous positive airway pressure for pulmonary edema (32). It seems reasonable therefore to use NIV for the treatment of respiratory failure in patients with both conditions, although the optimal inspiratory/expiratory pressures have yet to be established.

### D.  Myocardial Ischemia

Because cardiovascular risk is increased in COPD, and because chest pain is common in exacerbations (5), clinicians are faced with a significant diagnostic problem. Such chest pain could be myocardial, respiratory (e.g., secondary to hyperinflation), or unrelated to either.

Discerning the cause of chest pain is problematic because although raised troponin (a marker of cardiac myocyte damage) is associated with a worse outcome in ECOPD (33), its *diagnostic* significance is not known (33). Moreover, even in the presence of raised troponin and evidence of ischemia on serial electrocardiograms (ECGs), it is difficult to determine whether such ischemia is due to hypoxia on a background of coronary artery disease (34), or whether patients are having true thrombo-occlusive coronary disease, which may require revascularization. Further research is needed to address these diagnostic and therapeutic problems.

## IV. Anemia and Hyperglycemia

Seventeen percent of patients with COPD seen in secondary care have anemia, which is independently associated with dyspnea, but not death (35). In patients on long-term oxygen therapy, hospital admission and length of stay are inversely related to the hematocrit level. COPD patients with anemia have higher circulating inflammatory markers than those without, suggesting that the anemia seen in COPD is one example of the "anemia of chronic disease" seen in several inflammatory conditions (36). Similarly, hyperglycemia is common in ECOPD, occurring in upward of 30% of patients admitted to hospital (17). The acute-phase response, high prevalence of diabetes (37), and the frequent use of oral steroids have been implicated. A recent retrospective study found an association between hyperglycemia and mortality/increased length of stay (composite endpoint) in ECOPD (38), and tight control of glucose homeostasis (target glucose 80–110 mg/dL) improves mortality in the surgical ICU setting (39). However, for both anemia and hyperglycemia, the role of aggressive treatment in ECOPD remains unknown.

## V. Conclusion

The 2003 British Thoracic Society/Royal College of Physicians National COPD Audit found that the 90-day mortality for hospital-admitted ECOPD was 15%, and that 70% of patients had at least one comorbid condition (37). Future strategies targeting comorbidity in ECOPD may therefore have the potential to improve mortality and morbidity. However, most translational and clinical research is targeted at single diseases, with patients with comorbidity being excluded to reduce variation and make interpretation easier. Therefore, clinician scientists need to consider how best to study comorbid disease, and consumers of research also need to think carefully about how to apply findings obtained studying single-disease subjects to the complex populations they treat.

Moreover, clinicians will need to be alert to comorbidity, and changes in the organization of acute health care may also be needed to facilitate this. It may also be necessary to consider how chronic-disease care is organized, with a need for clinicians to ensure close cooperation, particularly between respiratory and cardiology specialists.

### References

1. Soriano JB, Visick GT, Muellerova H, et al. Patterns of comorbidities in newly diagnosed COPD and asthma in primary care. Chest 2005; 128(4):2099–2107.
2. Ashitani J, Mukae H, Arimura Y, et al. Elevated plasma procoagulant and fibrinolytic markers in patients with chronic obstructive pulmonary disease. Intern Med 2002; 41(3):181–185.
3. Schonhofer B, Kohler D. Prevalence of deep-vein thrombosis of the leg in patients with acute exacerbation of chronic obstructive pulmonary disease. Respiration 1998; 65:173–177.
4. Tillie-Leblond I, Marquette CH, Perez T, et al. Pulmonary embolism in patients with unexplained exacerbation of chronic obstructive pulmonary disease: prevalence and risk factors. Ann Intern Med 2006; 144(6):390–396.
5. Rutschmann OT, Cornuz J, Poletti PA, et al. Should pulmonary embolism be suspected in exacerbation of chronic obstructive pulmonary disease? Thorax 2007; 62(2):121–125.

6.  Sohne M, Kruip MJ, Nijkeuter M, et al. Accuracy of clinical decision rule, D-dimer and spiral computed tomography in patients with malignancy, previous venous thromboembolism, COPD or heart failure and in older patients with suspected pulmonary embolism. J Thromb Haemost 2006; 4(5):1042–1046.

7.  Videm V, Pillgram-Larsen J, Ellingsen O, et al. Spontaneous pneumothorax in chronic obstructive pulmonary disease: complications, treatment and recurrences. Eur J respir Dis 1987; 71(5):365–371.

8.  Light RW, O'Hara VS, Moritz TE, et al. Intrapleural tetracycline for the prevention of recurrent spontaneous pneumothorax. Results of a Department of Veterans Affairs cooperative study. JAMA 1990; 264(17):2224–2230.

9.  Henry M, Arnold T, Harvey J, et al. BTS guidelines for the management of spontaneous pneumothorax. Thorax 2003; 58(suppl 2):ii39–ii52.

10. Baumann MH, Strange C, Heffner JE, et al. Management of spontaneous pneumothorax: an American College of Chest Physicians Delphi consensus statement. Chest 2001; 119(2): 590–602.

11. Restrepo MI, Mortensen EM, Pugh JA, et al. COPD is associated with increased mortality in patients with community-acquired pneumonia. Eur Respir J 2006; 28(2):346–351.

12. Chen Y, Stewart P, Dales R, et al. In a retrospective study of chronic obstructive pulmonary disease inpatients, respiratory comorbidities were significantly associated with prognosis. J Clin Epidemiol 2005; 58(11):1199–1205.

13. Chapman KR, Mannino DM, Soriano JB, et al. Epidemiology and costs of chronic obstructive pulmonary disease. Eur Respir J 2006; 27(1):188–207.

14. Doyle JT, Dawber TR, Kannel WB, et al. Cigarette smoking and coronary heart disease. Combined experience of the Albany and Framingham studies. N Engl J Med 1962; 26:796–801.

15. Hole DJ, Watt GC, Davey-Smith G, et al. Impaired lung function and mortality risk in men and women: findings from the Renfrew and Paisley prospective population study. BMJ 1996; 313 (7059):711–715.

16. O'Donnell DE, Parker CM. COPD exacerbations 3: Pathophysiology. Thorax 2006; 61(4): 354–361.

17. Wood-Baker RR, Gibson PG, Hannay M, et al. Systemic corticosteroids for acute exacerbations of chronic obstructive pulmonary disease. Cochrane Database Syst Rev 2005;(1):CD001288.

18. Rabe KF, Hurd S, Anzueto A, et al. Global strategy for the diagnosis, management, and prevention of chronic obstructive pulmonary disease: GOLD executive summary. Am J Respir Crit Care Med 2007; 176(6):532–555.

19. Souverein PC, Berard A, Van Staa TP, et al. Use of oral glucocorticoids and risk of cardiovascular and cerebrovascular disease in a population based case-control study. Heart 2004; 90 (8):859–865.

20. van der Hooft CS, Heeringa J, Brusselle GG, et al. Corticosteroids and the risk of atrial fibrillation. Arch Intern Med 2006; 166(9):1016–1020.

21. Wei L, MacDonald TM, Walker BR. Taking glucocorticoids by prescription is associated with subsequent cardiovascular disease. Ann Intern Med 2004; 141(10):764–770.

22. Huiart L, Ernst P, Ranouil X, et al. Oral corticosteroid use and the risk of acute myocardial infarction in chronic obstructive pulmonary disease. Can Respir J 2006; 13(3):134–138.

23. Fuster V, Ryden LE, Cannom DS, et al. ACC/AHA/ESC 2006 guidelines for the management of patients with atrial fibrillation. Circulation 2006; 114(7):e257–e354.

24. Au DH, Udris EM, Curtis JR, et al. Association between chronic heart failure and inhaled beta-2-adrenoceptor agonists. Am Heart J 2004; 148(5):915–920.

25. Salpeter SR, Ormiston TM, Salpeter EE. Cardiovascular effects of beta-agonists in patients with asthma and COPD: a meta-analysis. Chest 2004; 125(6):2309–2321.

26. Fuso L, Incalzi RA, Pistelli R, et al. Predicting mortality of patients hospitalized for acutely exacerbated chronic obstructive pulmonary disease. Am J Med 1995; 98(3):272–277.

27. Le Jemtel TH, Padeletti M, Jelic S. Diagnostic and therapeutic challenges in patients with coexistent chronic obstructive pulmonary disease and chronic heart failure. J Am Coll Cardiol 2007; 49(2):171–180.

28. Ware LB, Matthay MA. Clinical practice. Acute pulmonary edema. N Engl J Med 2005; 353 (26):2788–2796.

29. Abroug F, Ouanes-Besbes L, Nciri N, et al. Association of left-heart dysfunction with severe exacerbation of chronic obstructive pulmonary disease: diagnostic performance of cardiac bio-markers. Am J Respir Crit Care Med 2006; 174(9):990–996.

30. Egred M, Shaw S, Mohammad B, et al. Under-use of beta-blockers in patients with ischaemic heart disease and concomitant chronic obstructive pulmonary disease. QJM 2005; 98(7): 493–497.

31. Baudouin S, Blumenthal S, Cooper B, et al. Non-invasive ventilation in acute respiratory failure. Thorax 2002; 57(3):192–211.

32. Monnet X, Teboul JL, Richard C. Cardiopulmonary interactions in patients with heart failure. Curr Opin Crit Care 2007; 13(1):6–11.

33. Baillard C, Boussarsar M, Fosse JP, et al. Cardiac troponin I in patients with severe exacerbation of chronic obstructive pulmonary disease. Intensive Care Med 2003; 29(4):584–589.

34. ACC/AHA 2007 Guidelines for the Management of Patients With Unstable Angina/Non ST-Elevation Myocardial Infarction. Circulation 2007; 116(7):e148–e304.

35. Cote C, Zilberberg MD, Mody SH, et al. Haemoglobin level and its clinical impact in a cohort of patients with COPD. Eur Respir J 2007; 29(5):923–929.

36. Similowski T, Agusti A, Macnee W, et al. The potential impact of anaemia of chronic disease in COPD. Eur Respir J 2006; 27(2):390–396.

37. Anstey K, Lowe D, Roberts M, et al. Report of the 2003 National COPD Audit. Royal College of Physicians and the British Thoracic Society; September 2004. Available at: http://www.rcplondon. ac.uk/clinical-standards/ceeu/Current-work/Pages/copd-audit.aspx. Accessed October 1, 2007.

38. Baker EH, Janaway CH, Philips BJ, et al. Hyperglycaemia is associated with poor outcomes in patients admitted to hospital with acute exacerbations of chronic obstructive pulmonary disease. Thorax 2006; 61(4):284–289.

39. Van den Berghe G, Wouters P, Weekers F, et al. Intensive insulin therapy in critically ill patients. N Engl J Med 2001; 345(19):1359–1367.

# 14

# Environmental Causes of Exacerbations

**FANNY WS KO and DAVID SC HUI**
Department of Medicine and Therapeutics, The Chinese University of Hong Kong, Prince of Wales Hospital, Hong Kong

## I. Introduction

Environmental factors such as changes in the composition, temperature and humidity of inspired air, and air pollution (outdoor and indoor) can potentially increase airway inflammation and result in acute exacerbations of chronic obstructive pulmonary disease (AECOPD). Other factors such as infection, social factors, and drug treatment may modify the response of patients with COPD to the surrounding stimuli.

## II. Environmental Factors Associated with AECOPD

### A. Outdoor Air Pollution

*Association Between Outdoor Air Pollution and AECOPD*

Air pollution is associated with increase in morbidity and mortality in patients with respiratory and cardiac diseases (1–10). Major outdoor air pollutants include nitrogen dioxide ($NO_2$), ozone ($O_3$), sulphur dioxide ($SO_2$), particulate matters (PMs), and carbon monoxide (CO). The major sources of $NO_2$, $SO_2$, PMs, and CO are due to fuel combustion from motor vehicles, power stations, and factories. $O_3$, a major constituent of photochemical smog, is formed by a series of complicated photochemical reactions of oxygen, nitrogen oxides, and volatile organic compounds in the presence of sunlight and warm temperature. PM is a mixture of solid, liquid, or solid and liquid particles suspended in the air. PM with an aerodynamic diameter of less than 10 μm ($PM_{10}$) is considered within the respirable range and can penetrate the lower respiratory tract. Fine particulates in the air are generally measured by $PM_{2.5}$, whereas coarse particulates are measured by $PM_{2.5-10}$. There are also ultrafine PMs with particulate size less than 100 nm. It is believed that $PM_{2.5}$ and ultrafine PM are able to penetrate deeper in the airway upon inhalation than the coarse particles because of their smaller sizes.

Large-scale studies in the United States and Europe have observed a significant association between outdoor air pollution and COPD admissions (1–5). In Asia, large-scale studies are lacking, but the Health Effects Institute has published in a Web-based summary report that all-cause mortality was associated with increases in ambient $PM_{10}$, total suspended particles (TSP), and $SO_2$ levels. However, COPD admissions or mortality were not separately addressed in this study (6). An intervention study has shown that following restriction of sulfur content in fuel oil to less than 0.5% by weight in Hong Kong since July 1990, the intervention led to an immediate fall in ambient $SO_2$, with a significant decline in the average annual trend in deaths of all causes (2.1%) and respiratory (3.9%) and cardiovascular diseases (2.0%) over the subsequent 12 months (11). Another study in Hong Kong focused specifically on the effect of air pollutants on AECOPD hospitalization and found a significant association between AECOPD admissions and the levels of $SO_2$, $NO_2$, $O_3$, $PM_{10}$, and $PM_{2.5}$ (7). Examples of the effect of air pollution on COPD admissions are summarized in Table 1.

Apart from increased hospitalization rates for AECOPD, higher levels of air pollutants were associated with more emergency department visits for AECOPD (8) and more daily general practice consultations for asthma and other lower respiratory diseases (not

**Table 1**　Association Between Outdoor Pollutants and AECOPD Admissions

| Pollutants | Author/groups | Increase in concentration of pollutants | RR (%) | | Lag (days) | Remarks |
|---|---|---|---|---|---|---|
| $PM_{10}$ | U.S. multicity (Medina-Ramon et al., 2006) (3) | 10 $\mu g/m^3$ | 1.47 | 0.93–2.01[a] | Lag 1 | Warm season only |
| | APHEA 2 (Atkinson et al., 2001) (4) | 10 $\mu g/m^3$ | 1.0 | 0.4–1.5[b] | n/a | |
| | U.S. multicity (Zanobetti et al., 2000) (1) | 10 $\mu g/m^3$ | 2.5 | 1.8–3.3[a] | Lag 0–5 | |
| | HK (Ko et al., 2007) (7) | 10 $\mu g/m^3$ | 1.02 | 1.02–1.03[a] | Lag 0–5 | |
| $PM_{2.5}$ | NMMAPS (Dominici et al., 2007) (2) | 10 $\mu g/m^3$ | ~0.9 | ~0.2–1.9[b] | Lag 1 | |
| | HK (Ko et al., 2007) (7) | 10 $\mu g/m^3$ | 1.03 | 1.03–1.04[a] | Lag 0–5 | |
| TSP | APHEA (Anderson et al., 1997) (5) | 50 $\mu g/m^3$ | 1.02 | 1.00–1.05[a] | Lag 1–3 | |
| O3 | U.S. multicity (Medina-Ramon, et al., 2006) (3) | 5 ppb | 0.27 | 0.08–0.47[a] | Lag 0–1 | Warm season only |
| | APHEA (Anderson et al., 1997) (5) | 50 $\mu g/m^3$ | 1.04 | 1.02–1.07[a] | Lag 1–3 | |
| | HK (Ko et al., 2007) (7) | 10 $\mu g/m^3$ | 1.04 | 1.03–1.04[a] | Lag 0–5 | |
| $NO_2$ | APHEA (Anderson et al., 1997) (5) | 50 $\mu g/m^3$ | 1.02 | 1.00–1.05[a] | Lag 1–3 | |
| | HK (Ko et al., 2007) (7) | 10 $\mu g/m^3$ | 1.03 | 1.02–1.03[a] | Lag 0–3 | |
| $SO_2$ | APHEA (Anderson et al., 1997) (5) | 50 $\mu g/m^3$ | 1.02 | 0.98–1.06[a] | Lag 1–3 | |
| | HK (Ko et al., 2007) (7) | 10 $\mu g/m^3$ | 1.01 | 1.00–1.01[a] | Lag 0 | |

[a]95% CI.
[b]range.
*Abbreviations*: na, not available; ppb, parts per billion; NMMAPS, National Morbidity, Mortality, and Air Pollution Study; APHEA, Air Pollution on Health: a European Approach 2; HK, Hong Kong.

specific for COPD) (9). Air pollution is also associated with increased COPD mortality (10). However, it is uncertain whether the associated mortality is secondary to AECOPD or other factors such as cardiovascular events or pneumonia.

### Mechanisms

Pollutant exposure with resulting AECOPD is likely due to the harmful effects of pollutants on the respiratory epithelium. Studies in healthy human adults have shown that exposure to elevated concentrations of $O_3$ increases cellular and biochemical inflammatory changes in the lungs. For example, the bronchoalveolar lavage (BAL) of healthy adults with experimental exposure to $O_3$ showed elevated numbers of netrophils and levels of immunoreactive elastase, albumin, protein, and immunoglobulin G, when compared with subjects that were exposed to filtered air (12). Epithelial permeability is also altered after $O_3$ exposure (13).

Exposure to $NO_2$ might enhance the recruitment of macrophages and T lymphocytes to the airway, as reflected by increased CD45RO+ lymphocytes, B cells, and natural killer cells in the BAL fluid of healthy volunteers (14). For particulate pollutants, it appears that respirable PMs of different sizes all have damaging effect on the respiratory epithelium. In a mass basis, the proportion of fine PMs being deposited to the pulmonary tree is three times larger than the proportion of coarse PMs (15). The increased sensitivity to a C5a chemotactic gradient could make the ultrafine PM-exposed macrophages more likely to be retained in the lungs and thus allowing the dose to accumulate (16). On the other hand, the cytokine production of the macrophages was especially enhanced by the bacterial endotoxin content of coarse PM (17). Oxidative stress-induced DNA damage appears to be an important mechanism of action of urban particulate air pollution. Previous studies have shown that in both outdoor and indoor environment, guanine oxidation in DNA correlated with exposure to $PM_{2.5}$ and ultrafine particles (18). $SO_2$ is very soluble in the upper respiratory tract and thus may produce an immediate irritant effect on the respiratory mucosa (7). There is also evidence that low levels of CO may increase oxidative stress, with competition for intracellular binding sites, which increases the steady state levels of nitric oxide and allows generation of peroxynitrite by endothelium (19).

Furthermore, exposure to air pollutants has systemic effects. The cytokines produced in the lungs are capable of stimulating the bone marrow to produce leukocytosis and thrombocytosis and stimulate the liver to produce acute-phase proteins such as C-reactive protein (CRP) and fibrinogen (20). An episode of acute air pollution could increase the circulating levels of IL-1$\beta$ and IL-6 (21). These acute-phase proteins and inflammatory cytokines may increase blood coagulability, which is a predictor of total cardiovascular morbidity and mortality in large population studies (20).

### B.  Indoor Air Pollution

#### Association Between Indoor Air Pollution and AECOPD

Cigarette smoking is the most important risk factor for COPD in developed countries. Both active smoking and environmental tobacco smoke (ETS) exposures are harmful to COPD patients, whereas subjects with tobacco smoke exposure have increased respiratory symptoms (22). Similar observation was found in those pipe and cigar smokers. Data from the Lung Health Study over a period of five years showed that among the smokers with mild to moderate COPD, subjects who had stopped smoking experienced an improvement in $FEV_1$ in the year after quitting, and the subsequent rate of decline in $FEV_1$ was half the rate when compared with the continuing smokers. The rate of decline in lung function in these sustained quitters was comparable to the never smokers (23). Among patients with COPD, exposure to ETS is also associated with more respiratory symptoms, decreased lung function, and impaired health status (24,25). All these point to the fact that smoking (either active or ETS) is harmful to COPD patients with possibly more exacerbations.

Biomass exposure is associated with the development of COPD. It is estimated that around 50% of the world's population (about 3 billion people) uses biomass as their primary energy source for domestic cooking, heating, and lighting. The use of biomass as energy source occurs rarely in industrialized countries; however, its use is more than 80% in China, India, and sub-Saharan Africa and about 50% to 70% in Latin America (26). The burning of wood, animal dung, crop residues, and coal, typically in open fires or poorly functioning stoves, may lead to very high levels of indoor air pollution, especially with high levels of PM in indoor air. Women are affected to a greater extent than men as they spend more time cooking and staying indoor. Women with domestic exposure to biomass developed COPD with clinical characteristics, quality of life, and increased mortality similar in degree to that of tobacco smokers (27).

### Mechanisms

Cigarette smoke is a complex mixture of more than 4700 chemical compounds of which free radicals and other oxidants are present in high quantity. ETS, produced by tobacco combustion, contains over 4500 compounds in both vapor and particle phases, whereas many of them are known carcinogens and irritants. Biomass smoke, on the other hand, contains a wide range of chemicals that are known or suspected human carcinogens (28).

In fact, tobacco smoke, ETS, and combustion of biomass for heating or cooking are the main determinants of elevated indoor PM levels. Previous studies have shown that indoor $PM_{2.5}$ level was significantly higher in smoking households and that was associated with higher levels of endotoxin and $NO_2$ (29). $PM_{2.5}$ was significantly associated with increased respiratory symptoms, with a greater effect for current smokers (29). Endotoxin, on the other hand, is a major proinflammatory agent and is significantly associated with symptoms and reduced lung function among asthmatics, likely through its inflammatory effect on the airway (30). It has been suggested that $NO_2$ and ETS interact to increase the risk of respiratory symptoms among children (31).

Chronic cigarette smoking can increase the circulating leukocyte numbers, including the immature neutrophils, with high levels of myeloperoxidase and $\alpha1$-antitrypsin (32,33). The production of these natural inhibitors of serine proteases could lead to alveolar wall damage. In addition, both ETS and direct smoking may increase airway permeability, causing increased IgE levels and enhanced allergic sensitization to airborne antigens (22,34). Thus, ETS and cigarette smoking could cause airway damage through increase in both bronchial hyperresponsiveness and airway inflammation. Oxidative stress markers and DNA damage were increased in both patients' groups with smoking- and biomass-related COPD when compared with healthy controls (28).

### C.  Effect of Climate

Changes in temperature can have an effect on AECOPD. A study in East London noted that fall in outdoor or bedroom temperature was associated with increased frequency of

AECOPD and decline in lung function over a period of 12 months (35). It appears that the effect of cold temperature varies in different places. In the Eurowinter study, the warmer the average temperature, the greater the mortality was noted in the cold weather. For example, increased mortality per degree centigrade below 18°C fell from 2.15% in Athens to 0.27% in southern Finland (36).

Heat may also have impact on AECOPD. A previous study has reported heat-related increases in emergency admissions for respiratory disease in the 75+ age group, though this study was not specific for COPD subjects (37). The mechanisms on the effect of temperature on AECOPD are not fully understood. This may be related in part to increased susceptibility to upper respiratory tract virus infections in cold weather.

## D. Other Factors

Drugs and infectious agents are exogenous factors that may have protective or harmful effects on COPD patients. Drugs such as bronchodilators, inhaled corticosteroids, and vaccinations would help decrease AECOPD, whereas infection and withdrawal of medications may increase AECOPD. These will be discussed in other chapters.

## E. Interactions Among Different Factors

### Air Pollutants May Interact with Infectious Agents

Environmental agents may modify the course of respiratory viral infections, and ambient pollutant levels have been proposed to play a role in modulating disease severity and health outcome in exposed individuals. A cell culture study indicated that the oxidant pollutants of $NO_2$ and $O_3$ could amplify the generation of proinflammatory cytokines by rhinovirus 16–infected cells, suggesting that virus-induced inflammation in upper and lower airways might be exacerbated by concurrent exposure to ambient levels of oxidants (38).

Particulates such as $PM_{10}$ could induce oxidative stress and, in vitro, this led to activation of nuclear factor-kappa B (NF-κB), histone acetylation, and increased expression of CXCL8 (39). A previous cell culture study observed that these inflammatory responses were enhanced by adenoviral early region 1A (40).

### Air Pollutants Interacting with Temperature and Air-Conditioning

Air pollutants interact with temperature. Previous studies found an increased risk of admissions for respiratory diseases, including COPD and pneumonia, associated with ambient $O_3$ and $PM_{10}$ levels predominantly in the warm season (3,5). $O_3$ concentrations are in general higher during the summer. As $O_3$ is a very reactive compound, its concentrations are much lower indoor than outdoor. A study in Hong Kong, in contrast, showed that $O_3$ was associated with AECOPD more in winter (7). It is likely that individual time spent outdoor determines the amount of ambient air pollutants exposure. In countries with cold winter, people are exposed to outdoor pollutants more in summer. For cities such as Hong Kong where the winter season is too mild to require central heating, windows are often opened in winter for ventilation purposes whereas most people spend more time indoor with air-conditioning during summer. Air-conditioned homes have lower air exchange rates than homes with windows opened for ventilation, (41) and thus subjects living in home with central air conditioning are less exposed to outdoor air pollutants, resulting in attenuation of the association between ambient air pollution and health effects (42).

### Effect of Social Factors

There are conflicting data on the interaction between social factors and the response to air pollution. Some studies noted that individuals with a lower household education and income levels had increased adverse vulnerability health outcomes to air pollution (43,44). Other studies noted low –educational attainment and high manufacturing employment in the living zones significantly and positively modified the acute mortality effects of air pollution exposure (45). In contrast, a study from Sao Paulo, Brazil, found that persons in districts with higher, rather than lower, socioeconomic characteristics were slightly more susceptible to air pollution effects (46). Figure 1 illustrates the complex interaction between these factors.

### F.  Effects of Intervention

Interventions such as ban of coal sales in Dublin and restrictions on sulphur content of fuel in Hong Kong are effective in improving air quality and reducing respiratory and cardiac deaths in the community (11,47). A study in Xuanwei in China assessed 20,453 people born into homes with unvented coal stoves. After 16,606 (81.2%) people subsequently changing to stoves with chimneys, the incidence of COPD decreased markedly after installation of chimney on formerly unvented coal stoves (48).

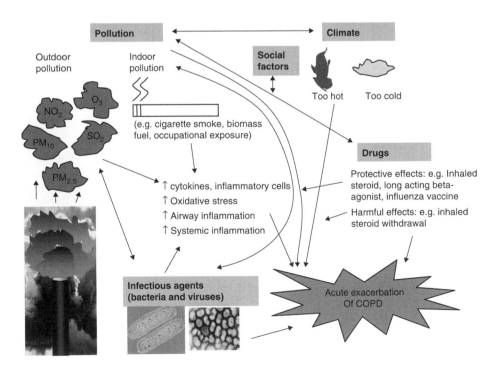

**Figure 1**  An illustration of the complex interaction between the different environmental factors for acute exacerbation of COPD. *Abbreviation*: COPD, chronic obstructive pulmonary disease.

## III. Summary

Outdoor and indoor air pollutants are major environmental triggers for AECOPD, whereas climate changes may also play a contributory role. These factors may interact with other components such as airway infection, drugs, and social factors, leading to AECOPD. Interventions to improve indoor and outdoor air quality are important nonpharmacological measures to reduce the morbidity and mortality of patients with this disabling condition.

## References

1. Zanobetti A, Schwartz J, Dockery DW. Airborne particles are a risk factor for hospital admissions for heart and lung disease. Environ Health Perspect 2000; 108(11):1071–1077.
2. Dominici F, Peng RD, Bell ML, et al. Fine particulate air pollution and hospital admission for cardiovascular and respiratory diseases. JAMA 2006; 295(10):1127–1134.
3. Medina-Ramon M, Zanobetti A, Schwartz J. The effect of ozone and PM10 on hospital admissions for pneumonia and chronic obstructive pulmonary disease: a national multicity study. Am J Epidemiol 2006; 163(6):579–588.
4. Atkinson RW, Anderson HR, Sunyer J, et al. Acute effects of particulate air pollution on respiratory admissions: results from APHEA 2 project. Air Pollution and Health: a European Approach. Am J Respir Crit Care Med 2001; 164(10 pt 1):1860–1866.
5. Anderson HR, Spix C, Medina S, et al. Air pollution and daily admissions for chronic obstructive pulmonary disease in 6 European cities: results from the APHEA project. Eur Respir J 1997; 10(5):1064–1071.
6. Health Effects Institute. Health Effects of Outdoor Air Pollution in Developing Countries of Asia. Special Report 15. April 2004. Available at: http://pubs.healtheffects.org/getfile.php?u=13.
7. Ko FW, Tam W, Wong TW, et al. Temporal relationship between air pollutants and hospital admissions for chronic obstructive pulmonary disease in Hong Kong. Thorax 2007; 62(9): 780–785.
8. Sunyer J, Anto JM, Murillo C, et al. Effects of urban air pollution on emergency room admissions for chronic obstructive pulmonary disease. Am J Epidemiol 1991; 134(3):277–286 (discussion 87–89).
9. Hajat S, Haines A, Goubet SA, et al. Association of air pollution with daily GP consultations for asthma and other lower respiratory conditions in London. Thorax 1999; 54(7):597–605.
10. Aga E, Samoli E, Touloumi G, et al. Short-term effects of ambient particles on mortality in the elderly: results from 28 cities in the APHEA2 project. Eur Respir J Suppl 2003; 40:28s–33s.
11. Hedley AJ, Wong CM, Thach TQ, et al. Cardiorespiratory and all-cause mortality after restrictions on sulphur content of fuel in Hong Kong: an intervention study. Lancet 2002; 360(9346): 1646–1652.
12. Koren HS, Devlin RB, Graham DE, et al. Ozone-induced inflammation in the lower airways of human subjects. Am Rev Respir Dis 1989; 139(2):407–415.
13. Foster WM, Stetkiewicz PT. Regional clearance of solute from the respiratory epithelia: 18–20 h postexposure to ozone. J Appl Physiol 1996; 81(3):1143–1149.
14. Blomberg A, Krishna MT, Bocchino V, et al. The inflammatory effects of 2 ppm $NO_2$ on the airways of healthy subjects. Am J Respir Crit Care Med 1997; 156(2 pt 1):418–424.
15. Venkataraman C, Kao AS. Comparison of particle lung doses from the fine and coarse fractions of urban PM-10 aerosols. Inhal Toxicol 1999; 11(2):151–169.
16. Renwick LC, Brown D, Clouter A, et al. Increased inflammation and altered macrophage chemotactic responses caused by two ultrafine particle types. Occup Environ Med 2004; 61(5): 442–447.

17. Becker S, Fenton MJ, Soukup JM. Involvement of microbial components and toll-like receptors 2 and 4 in cytokine responses to air pollution particles. Am J Respir Cell Mol Biol 2002; 27(5): 611–618.

18. Risom L, Moller P, Loft S. Oxidative stress-induced DNA damage by particulate air pollution. Mutat Res 2005; 592(1–2):119–137.

19. Thom SR, Xu YA, Ischiropoulos H. Vascular endothelial cells generate peroxynitrite in response to carbon monoxide exposure. Chem Res Toxicol 1997; 10(9):1023–1031.

20. van Eeden SF, Yeung A, Quinlam K, et al. Systemic response to ambient particulate matter: relevance to chronic obstructive pulmonary disease. Proc Am Thorac Soc 2005; 2(1):61–67.

21. van Eeden SF, Tan WC, Suwa T, et al. Cytokines involved in the systemic inflammatory response induced by exposure to particulate matter air pollutants (PM(10)). Am J Respir Crit Care Med 2001; 164(5):826–830.

22. Janson C, Chinn S, Jarvis D, et al. Effect of passive smoking on respiratory symptoms, bronchial responsiveness, lung function, and total serum IgE in the European Community Respiratory Health Survey: a cross-sectional study. Lancet 2001; 358(9299):2103–2109.

23. Scanlon PD, Connett JE, Waller LA, et al. Smoking cessation and lung function in mild-to-moderate chronic obstructive pulmonary disease. The Lung Health Study. Am J Respir Crit Care Med 2000; 161(2 pt 1):381–390.

24. Simoni M, Jaakkola MS, Carrozzi L, et al. Indoor air pollution and respiratory health in the elderly. Eur Respir J Suppl 2003; 40:15s–20s.

25. Sippel JM, Pedula KL, Vollmer WM, et al. Associations of smoking with hospital-based care and quality of life in patients with obstructive airway disease. Chest 1999; 115(3):691–696.

26. Bruce N, Perez-Padilla R, Albalak R. Indoor air pollution in developing countries: a major environmental and public health challenge. Bull World Health Organ 2000; 78(9):1078–1092.

27. Ramirez-Venegas A, Sansores RH, Perez-Padilla R, et al. Survival of patients with chronic obstructive pulmonary disease due to biomass smoke and tobacco. Am J Respir Crit Care Med 2006; 173(4):393–397.

28. Ceylan E, Kocyigit A, Gencer M, et al. Increased DNA damage in patients with chronic obstructive pulmonary disease who had once smoked or been exposed to biomass. Respir Med 2006; 100(7):1270–1276.

29. Osman LM, Douglas JG, Garden C, et al. Indoor air quality in homes of patients with chronic obstructive pulmonary disease. Am J Respir Crit Care Med 2007; 176(5):465–472.

30. Michel O, Ginanni R, Duchateau J, et al. Domestic endotoxin exposure and clinical severity of asthma. Clin Exp Allergy 1991; 21(4):441–448.

31. Emenius G, Pershagen G, Berglind N, et al. NO2, as a marker of air pollution, and recurrent wheezing in children: a nested case-control study within the BAMSE birth cohort. Occup Environ Med 2003; 60(11):876–881.

32. Corre F, Lellouch J, Schwartz D. Smoking and leucocyte-counts. Results of an epidemiological survey. Lancet 1971; 2(7725):632–634.

33. Chan-Yeung M, Abboud R, Buncio AD, et al. Peripheral leucocyte count and longitudinal decline in lung function. Thorax 1988; 43(6):462–466.

34. Oryszczyn MP, Annesi-Maesano I, Charpin D, et al. Relationships of active and passive smoking to total IgE in adults of the Epidemiological Study of the Genetics and Environment of Asthma, Bronchial Hyperresponsiveness, and Atopy (EGEA). Am J Respir Crit Care Med 2000; 161(4 pt 1): 1241–1246.

35. Donaldson GC, Seemungal T, Jeffries DJ, et al. Effect of temperature on lung function and symptoms in chronic obstructive pulmonary disease. Eur Respir J 1999; 13(4):844–849.

36. Cold exposure and winter mortality from ischaemic heart disease, cerebrovascular disease, respiratory disease, and all causes in warm and cold regions of Europe. The Eurowinter Group. Lancet 1997; 349(9062):1341–1346.

37. Kovats RS, Hajat S, Wilkinson P. Contrasting patterns of mortality and hospital admissions during hot weather and heat waves in Greater London, UK. Occup Environ Med 2004; 61(11): 893–898.
38. Spannhake EW, Reddy SP, Jacoby DB, et al. Synergism between rhinovirus infection and oxidant pollutant exposure enhances airway epithelial cell cytokine production. Environ Health Perspect 2002; 110(7):665–670.
39. Gilmour PS, Rahman I, Donaldson K, et al. Histone acetylation regulates epithelial IL-8 release mediated by oxidative stress from environmental particles. Am J Physiol Lung Cell Mol Physiol 2003; 284(3):L533–L540.
40. Gilmour PS, Rahman I, Hayashi S, et al. Adenoviral E1A primes alveolar epithelial cells to PM (10)-induced transcription of interleukin-8. Am J Physiol Lung Cell Mol Physiol 2001; 281(3): L598–L606.
41. Wallace L. Indoor particles: a review. J Air Waste Manag Assoc 1996; 46(2):98–126.
42. Janssen NA, Schwartz J, Zanobetti A, et al. Air conditioning and source-specific particles as modifiers of the effect of PM(10) on hospital admissions for heart and lung disease. Environ Health Perspect 2002; 110(1):43–49.
43. Cakmak S, Dales RE, Judek S. Respiratory health effects of air pollution gases: modification by education and income. Arch Environ Occup Health 2006; 61(1):5–10.
44. Laurent O, Bard D, Filleul L, et al. Effect of socioeconomic status on the relationship between atmospheric pollution and mortality. J Epidemiol Community Health 2007; 61(8):665–675.
45. Jerrett M, Burnett RT, Brook J, et al. Do socioeconomic characteristics modify the short term association between air pollution and mortality? Evidence from a zonal time series in Hamilton, Canada. J Epidemiol Community Health 2004; 58(1):31–40.
46. Gouveia N, Fletcher T. Time series analysis of air pollution and mortality: effects by cause, age and socioeconomic status. J Epidemiol Community Health 2000; 54(10):750–755.
47. Clancy L, Goodman P, Sinclair H, et al. Effect of air-pollution control on death rates in Dublin, Ireland: an intervention study. Lancet 2002; 360(9341):1210–1214.
48. Chapman RS, He X, Blair AE, et al. Improvement in household stoves and risk of chronic obstructive pulmonary disease in Xuanwei, China: retrospective cohort study. BMJ 2005; 331 (7524):1050.

# 15

# Exacerbations in Alpha-1-Antitrypsin Deficiency

**R. A. STOCKLEY**
Queen Elizabeth Hospital, Edgbaston, Birmingham, U.K.

## I.  Introduction

Exacerbations of chronic obstructive pulmonary disease (COPD) are a major cause of morbidity and mortality. They are well recognized in usual COPD to be a determinant of health status (1), and recurrent exacerbations relate to the decline in lung function (2). However, despite a multitude of studies measuring a variety of inflammatory mediators in exacerbations of COPD, the exact mechanism responsible for the cause of lung function decline remains uncertain.

## II.  Potential Role of the Neutrophil

Neutrophilic inflammation has been implicated in the pathophysiology of COPD for many reasons. Firstly, serine proteinases are recognized to have the ability to reproduce all of the features of COPD (3). Neutrophil elastase and cathepsin G can cause bronchial disease, mucous gland hyperplasia (4), and both are major secretagogues (5). Neutrophil elastase released by migrating neutrophil has been shown to stimulate mucous gland secretion via its effect on the epidermal growth factor (EGF) receptor (6). Neutrophil elastase has also been shown to effect ciliary beat frequency (7) and damage bronchial epithelium (8), again features of COPD. Proteinase 3 (9) and neutrophil elastase (4) have also been shown to cause pathological changes typical of pulmonary emphysema.

All these proteinases are present within the same granule and are released by activation. Neutrophil elastase and proteinase 3 in particular have been shown to colocate with the cell surface (10) and be resistant to inhibition by surrounding proteinase inhibitors (11). However, in addition, exocytosis of granules is associated with the release of high concentrations of these proteinases into the microenvironment around the neutrophil. As these proteinases diffuse away from the azurophil granule, their concentration drops but initially remains too high to be inhibited by the normal concentrations of the surrounding inhibitors, and an area of obligate proteolysis therefore exists. As the proteinases diffuse away, eventually the concentration drops sufficiently for the surrounding proteinase inhibitors to inactivate them (12).

More recent elegant studies (13) have tracked the process of elastase release as cells migrate through endothelial tissue. The proteinase colocalizes to the leading edge of the migrating cell, and as the cell passes, it leaves a portion of neutrophil elastase behind. This may explain the relationship of the amount of neutrophil elastase seen immunohistologically in emphysematous tissues of varying severity (14).

In the airway, the major inhibitor of neutrophil elastase and cathepsin G is secretory leukoproteinase inhibitor (SLPI); however, in the presence of neutrophilic inflammation and the release of neutrophil elastase, SLPI concentrations drop (15) further, enabling the activity of these proteinases to persist over a wider area. Once neutrophils die, they can undergo secondary necrosis particularly in the presence of bacteria (16), releasing even more proteinases with the potential for further damage.

Neutrophils are present in the airway of smokers and in particular in those with COPD (17). Neutrophilia is also a feature of patients with bacterial colonization and increases greatly in the presence of exacerbations (18) related to an increase in bacterial numbers (19). This change takes place as the airway secretions turn from mucoid to purulent, and there is a clear relationship between the degree of purulence and the neutrophil numbers, inflammatory cytokines, and particular neutrophil elastase activity (15). Some of these changes are demonstrated in Figure 1, also indicating that these changes are associated with a fall in the local inhibitor of neutrophil serine proteinases, SLPI.

At the same time, there is inflammation with an increase in protein leakage into the airway, including alpha-1-antitrypsin. However, the compensatory increase in this inhibitor still remains insufficient to control the increased amount of released elastase.

Although it can be seen that this is a normal response to a bacterial challenge in the lung, it does however have some implications. First, there would be increased neutrophil traffic, and as indicated above, this would cause a degree of collateral damage due to proteinases released either onto the cell surface or in high concentrations in the microenvironment close to the neutrophil. The free elastase activity that is detectable also has a pro-inflammatory effect in that neutrophil elastase has been shown to increase IL-8 (20) and probably LTB4 (21) release from airway epithelium and macrophages, which can lead to enhanced and further neutrophil recruitment. In addition, neutrophil elastase has been shown to cleave the important opsinophagocytic receptor C3bi from the surface of the cell (22) and also cleave immunoglobulins (23), decreasing the efficiency of opsinophagocytosis. Finally, neutrophil elastase not only damages bronchial epithelium but can reduce ciliary beat frequency (7), again having a major effect on important host defences. These changes can actually lead to a perpetuation of bacterial colonization and reduce the ability for the host response to resolve the episode. This is summarized in Figure 2.

## III.  Proteinase Cascade

Although neutrophil elastase has clearly been shown to cause all the features that we recognise as part of COPD, other proteinases of different classes have also been implicated. For instance, metalloproteinases have been suggested as an important cause of emphysema, largely on the basis of the protection that occurs in metalloproteinase knockout mice (24). In addition, other proteinases such as cathepsin B, which is a cysteine proteinase, have also been shown to produce changes typical of chronic bronchitis (25) and emphysema (26), again in animal models.

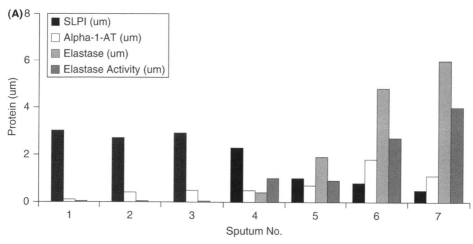

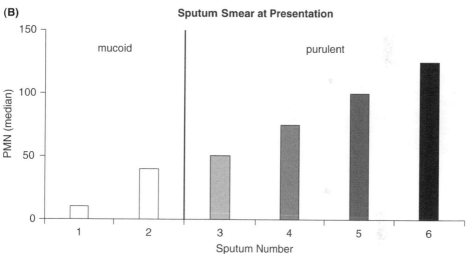

**Figure 1** (**A**) The relationship of mediator concentrations to sputum purulence, using an extended colour range with results >3, indicating increased purulence. Note SLPI decreases in the presence of purulence as alpha-1-antitrypsin increases because of protein leakage. The elastase content also rises, and its activity is only partially inhibited. (**B**) The number of neutrophils seen or high-power field on sputum smears related to the colour determined by comparison with a colour chart (BronkoTest UK, Middlesex, U.K.). Mucoid samples are to the left of the line and increasing purulence to the right. *Abbreviation*: SLPI, secretory leukoproteinase inhibitor.

Nevertheless, this probably represents a very integrated and mutually dependent proteinase and antiproteinase cascade. For instance, neutrophil elastase has been shown to inactivate the natural tissue inhibitors of metalloproteinases (TIMPS), at the same time neutrophil elastase can activate metalloproteinase proenzymes, leading to their persistent activity. The same process also applies to cysteine proteinases where neutrophil elastase

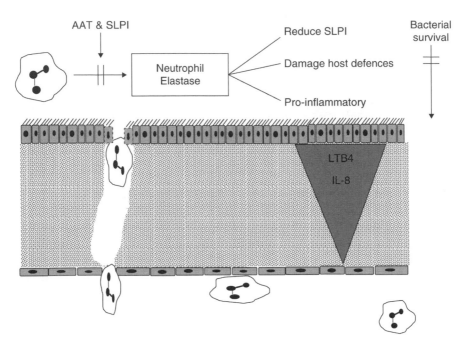

**Figure 2**  Schematic representation of perpetual cycle of inflammation in the airways in AATD. Circulating neutrophils are recruited to the lung, causing tissue destruction. Elastase released in the airways is incompletely inactivated and perpetuates its activity by decreasing the release of its local inhibitor SLPI. Damage to the airway host defences facilitates bacterial colonization, resulting in further neutrophil recruitment. In addition the pro-inflammatory effects of elastase releasing IL-8 and LTB4 from epithelium cells and macrophages, respectively, amplify the neutrophil recruitment. *Abbreviations*: AATD, alpha-1-antitrypsin deficiency; SLPI, secretory leukoproteinase inhibitor.

reduces the function of the important cathepsin B inhibitor cystatin C while at the same time activating the proenzyme form of cathepsin B into the active form. These other proteinases themselves can inactivate the natural proteinase inhibitors of serine proteinases, thereby also amplifying the activity of this class of enzymes (27).

On the basis of all these changes therefore, it is relatively easy to understand how exacerbations may lead to excessive lung damage, resulting in decline of lung function. However, since exacerbations of COPD that are not associated with increased bacterial load are also not associated with inflammation (18) and in particular neutrophilic inflammation, it is more likely that these episodes would not influence lung function decline, although careful studies will be necessary to confirm this hypothesis.

## IV.  Alpha-1-Antitrypsin Deficiency

It can be seen from the above evidence that an acute bacterial exacerbation of COPD is associated with several changes that are important in controlling proteolytic activity within the lung. First, there is an acute-phase response that increases the alpha-1-antitrypsin levels,

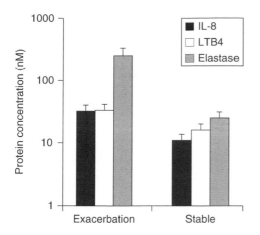

**Figure 3** The average sputum concentrations ($\pm$SE) are shown for IL-8, LTB4, and elastase activity at the start of an exacerbation and in the stable state. These data are greater than seen in usual COPD. *Abbreviation*: COPD, chronic obstructive pulmonary disease. *Source*: From Ref. 29.

and this together with increased inflammation in the airway results in a rise in the local levels of alpha-1-antitrypsin (28). This counterbalances the reciprocal fall in the local inhibitor in neutrophil elastase (SLPI), but despite these changes, free elastase activity is still detectable (29) with all the potential effects on host defences mentioned previously. In patients with alpha-1-antitrypsin deficiency, however, not only is the circulating level of alpha-1-antitrypsin low, the acute-phase response does not occur (29), and although airway inflammation leads to an increase in airways' alpha-1-antitrypsin levels, this is far less than in usual COPD (29). The result therefore is an even greater imbalance between proteinases and antiproteinases in the airway and an increased inflammatory response. These data are shown for comparison in Figure 3 together with increase in other pro-inflammatory cytokines such as IL-8 and particularly LTB4. As the episode resolves, these processes reverse and neutrophil elastase activity falls; but it will be seen from Figure 3 that even in the stable clinical state, free neutrophil elastase activity can be detected in airway secretions from deficient patients. Therefore, patients with deficiency continue to have free enzyme activity in the airway, with all its potential subsequent effects on host defences. It might be expected therefore that such patients would be more susceptible to exacerbations together with a greater degree of inflammation and potential lung damage.

During exacerbations, a variety of other cytokines will increase, although few have been measured to date. Defensins are increased in the stable state and further changes occur during exacerbations (Fig. 4). These small molecular weight proteins have the ability both to kill bacteria as well as damage host cells. Studies in the past have indicated that alpha-1-antitrypsin can abrogate this effect (30), and this should be confirmed in patients who are on augmentation therapy for comparison with those who are not. Systemic markers of inflammation also change in line with that seen in usual COPD with a rise in C-reactive protein and an increase in neutrophil activation as indicated by the change in plasma calprotectin levels (Fig. 5). It should be noted that as with the airways inflammation calprotectin levels do not return to normal following an exacerbation in alpha-1-antitrypsin deficiency (AATD).

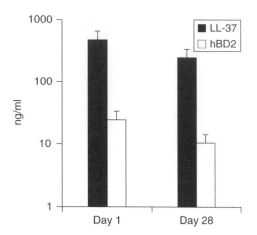

**Figure 4**  The average concentrations of defensins in sputum samples from AATD patients at the start of an exacerbation and in the stable state are shown. Both LL37 and HbD2 are significantly raised ($p < 0.01$) at the start of the exacerbations. *Abbreviation*: AATD, alpha-1-antitrypsin deficiency. *Source*: Samples assayed by R. Bals, Marburg, Germany.

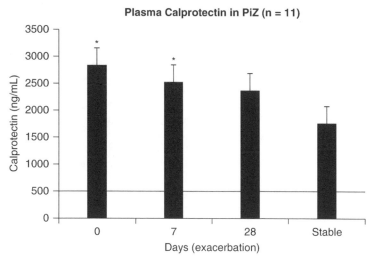

*p < 0.05 vs stable

**Figure 5**  Plasma calprotectin levels (a marker of neutrophil activation) are shown for AATD subjects during an exacerbation and in the stable state. The horizontal line represents the average value for normal subjects. *Abbreviation*: AATD, alpha-1-antitrypsin deficiency.

The evidence so far suggests that although patients with alpha-1-antitryspsin deficiency have exacerbations, they are not particularly more frequent than in usual COPD (31). The episodes occur throughout the year with a tendency for a greater number in the wintertime. The nature of the episodes appear to be predominantly classified as Anthonisen

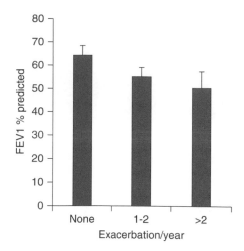

**Figure 6** The average $FEV_1$ is shown for subjects with 0, 1 to 2, or >2 exacerbations each year. *Abbreviation*: $FEV_1$, forced expiratory volume in one second. *Source*: From Ref. 31.

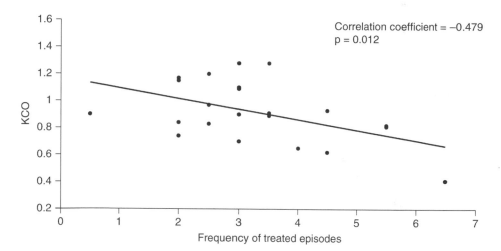

**Figure 7** Diary card data taken from AATD subjects over 24 to 30 months. Each point is the average number of exacerbations/yr for an individual patient related to absolute gas transfer (mmol/min/kPa/L). *Abbreviation*: AATD, alpha-1-antitrypsin deficiency.

type I; however, when compared with usual COPD, the episodes do appear to last longer (29), suggesting that alpha-1 antitrypsin plays a role in resolution of the episode.

There is some relationship of exacerbation frequency to forced expiratory volume in one second ($FEV_1$), but overall the relationship is weak (Fig. 6). Indeed, in AATD the relationship of gas transfer to frequency is much stronger (Fig. 7). Patients with a history of chronic bronchitis are more susceptible to exacerbations, and data have indicated that the episodes relate to progressive loss of lung function, with particular reference to slow vital

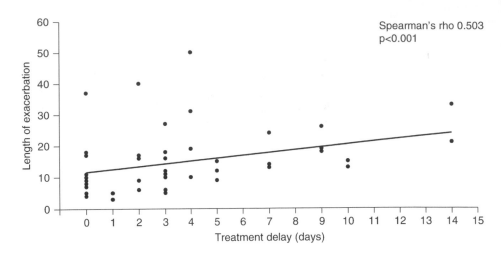

**Figure 8** Relationship between the length of exacerbation and the delay from onset to instigation of therapy.

capacity and diffusing capacity of the lung for carbon monoxide (DLco) (32). These data suggest that the major impact of the inflammation of exacerbations in AATD is at the small airways level.

More recent evidence has explored the nature of the exacerbations in AATD in more detail. As in usual COPD, patients not only have symptomatic changes that lead them to increase their therapy but also have similar episodes recorded in a daily diary card where they do not increase their therapy. This is analogous to the reported and unreported exacerbations described by others in usual COPD (1). Evidence suggests that one of the key components that differentiate these two types of exacerbation, however, is general well-being. Patients who feel generally unwell in addition to their increased respiratory symptoms usually wait for several days before making a decision about new therapy, and if the feeling of unwellness settles within that period, patients do not often seek extra therapy, allowing the episode to resolve itself (33). Whether these episodes (which are also associated with purulent sputum) should be treated and whether this would have an impact on long-term progression need to be explored.

Studies show that the number of episodes recorded on the diary card relate to the gas transfer (Fig. 7), which is an indicator of the degree of emphysema. Also as in usual COPD (34), the length of the episode relates to the delay in commencing therapy (Fig. 8), and the presence of preceding "coryzal-like" illness makes it more likely that the episode will be treated (35).

## V. Management

At present the management of exacerbations in AATD should be in line with current guidelines for usual COPD. For patients with recurrent exacerbations, particularly with moderate-to-severe airflow obstruction, appropriate preventative therapies including inhaled corticosteroids (36), long-acting $\beta_2$ agonists (37), and anticholinergic agents (38) are all likely to reduce the overall frequency of such episodes. The neutrophilic inflammatory response to bacteria is more excessive in patients with AATD, which is particularly relevant to the release of neutrophil elastase into the airway, and such episodes should be treated promptly. As with usual COPD, these episodes would be recognized by the development or increase of sputum purulence (39).

It remains unknown whether alpha-1-antitrypsin augmentation therapy decreases the incidence or modifies the nature of exacerbations in alpha-1 antitrypsin deficiency. A retrospective study by Lieberman (40) suggested that at least recall of the number of episodes classified as exacerbations decreased in patients on augmentation therapy. Whether that is true remains to be proven, but it seems logical that augmentation would at least reduce the severity of the inflammation and hence the quantity of elastase activity present in the airways more in line with that seen in usual COPD. The results of the EXACTLE (EXAcerbations and CT as Lung Endpoints) trial in AATD should at least answer in part some of these questions.

## References

1. Seemungal TA, Donaldson GC, Paul EA, et al. Effect of exacerbation on quality of life in patients with chronic obstructive pulmonary disease. Am J Respir Crit Care Med 1998; 157(5 pt 1): 1418–1422.
2. Donaldson GC, Seemungal TA, Bhowmik A, et al. Relationship between exacerbation frequency and lung function decline in chronic obstructive pulmonary disease. Thorax 2002; 57(10):847–852.
3. Stockley RA. Neutrophils and the pathogenesis of COPD. Chest 2002; 121(5 suppl):151S–155S.
4. Snider GL, Lucey EC, Christensen TG, et al. Emphysema and bronchial secretory cell metaplasia induced in hamsters by human neutrophil products. Am Rev Respir Dis 1984; 129(1):155–160.
5. Sommerhoff CP, Nadel JA, Basbaum GB, et al. Neutrophil elastase and cathepsin G stimulate secretion from cultured bovine airway gland serous cells. J Clin Invest 1990; 85(3):682–689.
6. Lee HM, Malm L, Dabbagh K, et al. Epidermal growth factor receptor signaling mediates regranulation of rat nasal goblet cells. J Allergy Clin Immunol 2001; 107(6):1046–1050.
7. Smallman LA, Hill SL, Stockley RA. Reduction of ciliary beat frequency in vitro by sputum from patients with bronchiectasis: a serine proteinase effect. Thorax 1984; 39(9):663–667.
8. Amitani R, Wilson R, Rutman A, et al. Effects of human neutrophil elastase and Pseudomonas aeruginosa proteinases on human respiratory epithelium. Am J Respir Cell Mol Biol 1991; 4(1): 26–32.
9. Kao RC, Wehner NG, Skubitz KM, et al. Proteinase 3. A distinct human polymorphonuclear leukocyte proteinase that produces emphysema in hamsters. J Clin Invest 1988; 82(6):1963–1973.
10. Owen CA, Campbell MA, Sannes PL, et al. Cell surface-bound elastase and cathepsin G on human neutrophils: a novel, non-oxidative mechanism by which neutrophils focus and preserve catalytic activity of serine proteinases. J Cell Biol 1995; 131(3):775–789.
11. Owen CA, Campbell EJ. Angiotensin II generation at the cell surface of activated neutrophils: novel cathepsin G-mediated catalytic activity that is resistant to inhibition. J Immunol 1998; 160(3): 1436–1443.
12. Liou TG, Campbell EJ. Quantum proteolysis resulting from release of single granules by human neutrophils: a novel, nonoxidative mechanism of extracellular proteolytic activity. J Immunol 1996; 157(6):2624–2631.
13. Cepinskas G, Sandig M, Kvietys PR. PAF-induced elastase-dependent neutrophil transendothelial migration is associated with the mobilization of elastase to the neutrophil surface and localization to the migrating front. J Cell Sci 1999; 112(pt 12):1937–1945.
14. Damiano VV, Tsang A, Kucich U, et al. Immunolocalization of elastase in human emphysematous lungs. J Clin Invest 1986; 78(2):482–493.

15. Hill AT, Campbell EJ, Hill SL, et al. Association between airway bacterial load and markers of airway inflammation in patients with stable chronic bronchitis. Am J Med 2000; 109(4):288–295.

16. Naylor EJ, Bakstad D, Biffen M, et al. Haemophilus influenzae induces neutrophil necrosis: a role in chronic obstructive pulmonary disease? Am J Respir Cell Mol Biol 2007; 37(2):135–143.

17. Confalonieri M, Mainardi E, Della Porta R, et al. Inhaled corticosteroids reduce neutrophilic bronchial inflammation in patients with chronic obstructive pulmonary disease. Thorax 1998; 53(7): 583–585.

18. Gompertz S, O'Brien C, Bayley DL, et al., Changes in bronchial inflammation during acute exacerbations of chronic bronchitis. Eur Respir J 2001; 17(6):1112–1119.

19. White AJ, Gompertz S, Bayley DL, et al. Resolution of bronchial inflammation is related to bacterial eradication following treatment of exacerbations of chronic bronchitis. Thorax 2003; 58(8):680–685.

20. Van Wetering S, Mannesse-Lazeroms SP, Dijkman JH, et al. Effect of neutrophil serine proteinases and defensins on lung epithelial cells: modulation of cytotoxicity and IL-8 production. J Leukoc Biol 1997; 62(2):217–226.

21. Hubbard RC, Fells G, Gadek J, et al. Neutrophil accumulation in the lung in alpha 1-antitrypsin deficiency. Spontaneous release of leukotriene B4 by alveolar macrophages. J Clin Invest 1991; 88(3):891–897.

22. Berger M, Sorensen RU, Tosi MF, et al. Complement receptor expression on neutrophils at an inflammatory site, the Pseudomonas-infected lung in cystic fibrosis. J Clin Invest 1989; 84(4): 1302–1313.

23. Solomon A. Possible role of PMN proteinases in immunogloulin degradation and amyloid formation. In: Havemann K, Janoff A, eds. Neutrophil Proteinases of Human Polymorphonuclear Leukocytes. Baltimore: Urban and Schwarzenberg, 1978:423–438.

24. Hautamaki RD, Kobayashi DK, Senior RM, et al. Requirement for macrophage elastase for cigarette smoke-induced emphysema in mice. Science 1997; 277(5334):2002–2004.

25. Cardozo C, Padilla ML, Choi HS, et al. Goblet cell hyperplasia in large intrapulmonary airways after intratracheal injection of cathepsin B into hamsters. Am Rev Respir Dis 1992; 145(3):675–679.

26. Lesser M, Padilla ML, Cardozo C. Induction of emphysema in hamsters by intratracheal instillation of cathepsin B. Am Rev Respir Dis 1992; 145(3):661–668.

27. Sullivan A, Stockley RA, Proteinases in COPD. In: Hansel TT, Barnes PJ. Eds., Recent Advances in the Pathophysiology of COPD. Basel, Switzerland: Birkhauser Verlag, 2004:75–99.

28. Stockley RA, Burnett D. Alpha-antitrypsin and leukocyte elastase in infected and noninfected sputum. Am Rev Respir Dis 1979; 120(5):1081–1086.

29. Hill AT, Campbell EJ, Bayley DL, et al. Evidence for excessive bronchial inflammation during an acute exacerbation of chronic obstructive pulmonary disease in patients with alpha(1)-antitrypsin deficiency (PiZ). Am J Respir Crit Care Med 1999; 160(6):1968–1975.

30. Spencer LT, Paone G, Krein PM, et al. Role of human neutrophil peptides in lung inflammation associated with alpha1-antitrypsin deficiency. Am J Physiol Lung Cell Mol Physiol 2004; 286(3): L514–L520. [Epub 2003, Oct 31].

31. Needham M, Stockley RA. Exacerbations in {alpha}1-antitrypsin deficiency. Eur Respir J 2005; 25(6):992–1000.

32. Dowson LJ, Guest PJ, Stockley RA. Longitudinal changes in physiological, radiological, and health status measurements in alpha(1)-antitrypsin deficiency and factors associated with decline. Am J Respir Crit Care Med 2001; 164(10 pt 1):1805–1809.

33. Vijayasaratha K, Stockley RA. "Reported" and "Unreported" exacerbations of COPD—Analysis by diary cards. Chest 2008; 133(1):34–41. [Epub 2007, Nov 7].

34. Wilkinson TM, Donaldson GC, Hurst JR, et al. Early therapy improves outcomes of exacerbations of chronic obstructive pulmonary disease. Am J Respir Crit Care Med 2004; 169(12):1298–1303.

35. Seemungal, T, Harper-Owen R, Bhowmik A, et al. Respiratory viruses, symptoms, and inflammatory markers in acute exacerbations and stable chronic obstructive pulmonary disease. Am J Respir Crit Care Med 2001; 164(9):1618–1623.
36. Paggiaro PL, Dahle R, Bakran I, et al. Multicentre randomised placebo-controlled trial of inhaled fluticasone propionate in patients with chronic obstructive pulmonary disease. International COPD Study Group. Lancet 1998; 351(9105):773–780.
37. Stockley RA, Chopra N, Rice L. Addition of salmeterol to existing treatment in patients with COPD: a 12 month study. Thorax 2006; 61(2):122–128.
38. Dusser D, Bravo ML, Iacono P. The effect of tiotropium on exacerbations and airflow in patients with COPD. Eur Respir J 2006; 27(3):547–555.
39. Stockley RA, O'Brien C, Pye A, et al. Relationship of sputum color to nature and outpatient management of acute exacerbations of COPD. Chest 2000; 117(6):1638–1645.
40. Lieberman J. Augmentation therapy reduces frequency of lung infections in antitrypsin deficiency: a new hypothesis with supporting data. Chest 2000; 118(5):1480–1485.

# 16
## Animal Models of COPD—Current Status of an Evolving Field

**PAUL J. CHRISTENSEN**
Pulmonary and Critical Care Medicine Section, Medical Service, Department of Veterans Affairs Health System and the Division of Pulmonary and Critical Care Medicine, Department of Internal Medicine, University of Michigan Health System, Ann Arbor, Michigan, U.S.A.

**W. BRADLEY FIELDS and CHRISTINE M. FREEMAN**
Division of Pulmonary and Critical Care Medicine, Department of Internal Medicine, University of Michigan Health System, Ann Arbor, Michigan, U.S.A.

**JEFFREY L. CURTIS**
Pulmonary and Critical Care Medicine Section, Medical Service, Department of Veterans Affairs Health System and the Division of Pulmonary and Critical Care Medicine, Department of Internal Medicine and the Graduate Program in Immunology, University of Michigan Health System, Veterans Administration Medical Center, Ann Arbor, Michigan, U.S.A.

## I. Introduction

Robust animal models of human disease serve several salutary ends: they allow mechanistic analysis of pathogenesis, permit preclinical testing of proposed therapies, and foster the generation of hypotheses that can be examined for relevance to the corresponding human disease. Animal models come in two overall varieties, spontaneous and induced, both of which have their experimental strengths. Ideally, animal models of a given disease should be available in a variety of species, including the mouse, the premier mammalian species for genetic and immunological manipulation (1), as well as in larger species to facilitate toxicological and physiological studies. The generation of animal model systems that faithfully mimic human diseases, although neither obligatory nor in all cases possible, is one of the surest means of developing treatments and cures.

At present, chronic obstructive pulmonary disease (COPD) has no practical, universally accepted animal model. This fact should not be surprising, as there is likewise no single pathological finding common to all COPD patients. No nonhuman species spontaneously develops the range of pathological findings and the symptoms of progressive dyspnea, cough, and sputum production that characterize human COPD. Indeed, it has been argued, on the basis of the marked differences between the respiratory system of rodents and humans, that the task is pointless (2). On the basis of the great potential benefit to be derived from ethical animal experimentation in this disabling disease, we believe that this viewpoint is excessively nihilistic, even given the current limited success of the endeavor.

Considerable strides have been made in the last decade, especially using mice, in producing systems that permit studies on the development of emphysema, the effects of cigarette smoke exposure (CSE) on the innate and adaptive immune systems, and some aspects of airways diseases. These subjects have been reviewed previously (3–11). This article will focus primarily on recent developments in modeling COPD via tobacco smoke exposure and by genetic approaches, especially in mice. Several excellent reviews cover the induction of anatomic emphysema by installation of proteases (10,12,13), animal models of allergic airways inflammation more relevant to asthma (14–18), and inflammatory airway disease of horses ("heaves") (19,20), a spontaneously occurring condition sometimes considered relevant to COPD. These topics will not be considered here.

## II.  Murine Models of COPD

In industrialized nations, COPD is chiefly caused by firsthand exposure to cigarette smoke (CS). The observation that only a minority of smokers ever develop COPD is believed to reflect the complex interaction between genetic and environmental factors. Mice are a highly convenient species in which to study gene-environment interactions in tightly controlled experiments. Their small size and rapid breeding cycle keep the cost of housing and care comparatively low. Antibodies against murine antigens are the most widely available of any species. Probably, the greatest strength of this species as an experimental model is the well-characterized genome of the mouse, with many markers available for locus identification, together with the ability to perform transgenic manipulation.

As in all animal modeling, extrapolation from findings in the mouse to human pathobiology often suffers from interspecies differences. The murine respiratory system has important anatomical differences from the human respiratory system. Mice are obligate nose breathers with large nasal chambers, which may provide more particulate clearance than that occurs in human smokers. Mice have a shorter and strikingly more simplified respiratory tree than humans, with only six to eight branch points to reach the terminal bronchiole (vs. up to 23–27 in human lungs). Murine airways also contain much less extensive bronchial submucosal glands, have less well-developed cilia, and lack respiratory bronchioles and goblet cells. These last features are at present a major limitation in developing model systems directly relevant to humans. Yet, despite these differences, mice remain the most popular and arguably the most powerful species in which to investigate the inflammatory and oxidative stress cascades putatively involved in the pathogenesis of COPD (21).

### A.  Murine Model Systems Involving CSE in Wild-Type Mice

Several groups have shown that wild-type mice exposed to CS for at least 5 day/wk for three to six months will exhibit mild emphysema characterized by airspace enlargement and alveolar wall destruction (22–24). These findings are significant, considering that review articles published as recently as 1989 stated that convincing evidence of CS-induced emphysema was lacking in animal models (5). Unfortunately, comparison of data from different laboratories is limited by the staggering variability in model design. Sources of variability include important differences in the type of cigarette used, in the method [mainstream vs. mainstream plus sidestream smoke (25)], and in the intensity and duration of exposure.

Reference cigarettes manufactured at the University of Kentucky Tobacco Research and Development Center (UKTRDC), Lexington, Kentucky, U.S. are the most widely cited in the English-language literature, in part because they are tax free to American investigators. Three cigarette models have been reported in murine studies: 1R3F (the most commonly reported but no longer produced), 2R1, and 2R4F (26). Several commercial brands have also been studied, but concrete comparison data to the UKTRDC reference cigarettes are lacking. Each brand varies in its content of tar and nicotine, making toxicological comparisons problematic (27). The source of cigarettes used in a given experiment is a crucial variable that should always be reported. Importantly, however, regardless of brand, and even in studies reported from the tobacco industry itself (28), most studies report inflammatory cell recruitment after acute exposures and discernable airspace enlargement with chronic exposure. It is important to note, however, that no protocol of CSE in the wild-type mouse produces the degree of severe bullous changes seen in some humans with advanced emphysema.

The intensity of exposure reported in various studies also varies dramatically. In acute models, almost any intensity appears capable of inducing detectable pulmonary inflammation. Castro et al. exposed C57BL/6J mice to 10 mL of CS (1 puff) daily for one to seven days (29). They showed a dose-dependent increase of macrophages in the bron-choalveolar lavage fluid (BAL), beginning after the first treatment. By contrast, Vlahos et al. gave the same strain of mice between three and nine cigarettes daily over one to four days (30). Their method was also well tolerated and likewise produced dose-dependent increases in inflammatory cell number and protease activity in lavage fluid. Thus, very short-term murine CSE models are clearly feasible and can rapidly produce interesting data.

Chronic exposure models also vary in the intensity of exposure. In his seminal work on protease dependence of murine emphysema (22), Shapiro popularized a now widely used technique originally developed for use in guinea pigs (31) and modified for use in rats (32). Mice underwent nose-only exposure to mainstream CS from two cigarettes daily, 6 day/wk for up to six months. Inflammatory cell recruitment increased over time, and airspace enlargement was noted at three months. March et al. exposed female A/J mice at a slightly higher concentration of smoke and demonstrated significant emphysema as early as 10 weeks (33). Maes et al. exposed mice to 20 cigarettes daily, a dose that was also well tolerated for up to six months and which resulted in changes characteristic of emphysema (34). Hence, despite variation in protocols, almost all groups have shown a degree of airspace enlargement in wild-type mice after months of CSE.

These examples, which will be amplified in later sections, illustrate the importance of considering the uses and limitations of murine models. By providing mechanistic information about the earliest genetic and epigenetic changes induced by CSE, acute models may provide novel insights on the reason only some smokers develop COPD. However, because the effects of chronic CSE differ from those of acute CSE, especially on parameters related to innate immunity, models of more prolonged exposures are also necessary to investigate progression.

Several methods have been used in an attempt to standardize exposures in murine systems. Shapiro et al. reported murine carboxyhemoglobin levels of 10% to 14% after exposure (22), similar to levels found in human tobacco users. These data, which have been reproduced by these and other investigators (35,36), strengthen extrapolation to human exposure and argue that findings are unlikely to be simply the consequence of hypoxemia. Reporting the concentration of smoke generated may also encourage reproducibility. Several groups dilute their product with medical air, with exposure expressed as a smoke-to-air ratio. Ratios of smoke to air of 1:12 are most frequently reported (24,34). More specifically, the smoke concentration may also be quantified by the wet weight of total particulate matter (TPM) and expressed as milligrams (mg) $TPM/m^3$. This determination allows for different dosages to be tightly manipulated and compared directly. The method has been described in both acute (37) and chronic models (38). Concentrations of 240 to 400 mg $TPM/m^3$ are most commonly reported.

The issue of murine strain variation in susceptibility to CSE-induced pathology is crucial for investigators interested in using the genetic approaches described below. Guerassimov et al. studied five strains of inbred mice exposed to identical doses of CS for up to six months, measuring airspace enlargement as determined by Lm (mean linear intercept) and lung elastance. They identified the AKR/J strain as supersusceptible to the development of emphysema, the C57BL/6J, A/J and SJ/L strains as mildly susceptible, and the NZWLac/J strain as resistant (39). Strain variation was also noted in a study contrasting DBA mice with C57BL/6 mice, which shows a relative deficiency in $\alpha_1$-antitrypsin serum levels as compared with other strains (40). By contrast, after exposure of mice to smoke generated from three, six, and nine cigarettes/day for four days, gene expression profiles in whole lung and in alveolar macrophages of BALB/c mice and C57BL/6 mice were very similar, except for MMP-12, which was lower in C57BL/6 mice (30). The differences between the results of these studies emphasize the importance of considering duration of exposure in interpreting studies using various murine models.

Although CSE-induced models of pulmonary inflammation and emphysema have so far been used principally to study mechanisms of pathogenesis, these models can also be used to explore interventions. Treatment of mice in an acute setting with the oral phosphodiesterase 4 ($PDE_4$) inhibitor cilomilast before smoke exposure significantly reduced numbers of inflammatory cells recoverable by BAL (41). By contrast, another $PDE_4$ inhibitor, roflumilast, at a dose of 5 mg/kg/day blocked induction of emphysema in a chronic CSE model (3 cigarettes/day for 7 months), as assessed by mean linear intercept, internal surface alveolar area, and desmosine content (42). In a 16-week smoke dose–response study in A/J mice, some experimental cohorts were concurrently treated with the antioxidants $N$-acetylcysteine or polyphenol epigallocatechin gallate, which produced no differences in alveolar damage (33). An orally active small molecule inhibitor of CXCR2 reduced neutrophil influx to the lungs of mice exposed to CS (37). Collectively, these results show how even the currently imperfect murine models can be useful in preclinical testing of proposed therapies.

## B.   Analysis of Immune Effects of CSE in Murine Models

Murine models have also been used to study the effects of CSE on the immune system, a subject with direct relevance to acute exacerbations of chronic obstructive pulmonary disease (AECOPD). Importantly, the effects appear to differ both with the duration of exposure and with the specific immune parameter being measured. Acute exposures induce distinct evidence of inflammation. One hour after exposure of C57BL/6J mice to one puff of mainstream CS, alveolar macrophages (AMø) showed increased DNA-binding activity of nuclear factor-κB (NF-κB) (29). Acute exposures to CS for up to a week induced elevated lung concentrations of the macrophage attractant chemokine CCL2 and dose-dependent increases in AMø numbers that were reduced by inhibition of IL-1β (29). In another study of acute CSE, CCL2 was also induced, along with CCL3, TNF-α, and net neutrophil chemoattractant activity, in wild-type mice, but not in mice lacking both p55 and p75 TNF-α receptors (43). Elimination of neutrophils abolished detection of desmosine and hydroxyproline, markers of the breakdown of elastin and collagen, respectively, which were otherwise detectable after a single exposure to CS (44). MMP-12 was necessary for release of TNF-α and increases in lung concentration of the leukocyte adhesion molecule CD62E (E-selectin) in response to short-term CSE (45). Thus, murine studies disclose striking changes induced by even very short smoke exposures.

By contrast, chronic exposures to CS have more complex effects, which in the aggregate adversely effect the host immune system. Early studies documented the ability of chronic CSE to depress bacterial clearance in vivo and the phagocytic and bactericidal activities of murine AMø in vitro (46). Exposure for five weeks induced increases in numbers of neutrophils, macrophages, and lymphocytes in the lungs. Development of emphysema in this study did not depend on cells of the adaptive immune system, as there was no difference between wild-type mice and *scid* mice (47). Inflammatory cell recruitment in response to smoke exposure depends in part on TLR4, as shown by the reductions seen in C3H/HeJ mice, which have a mutated TLR4 (34). Induction of emphysema, lung inflammatory cell infiltration, and peribronchial lymphoid follicles by CSE were also partially attenuated by genetic deficiency of the chemokine receptors CCR6 (48) and CCR5 (49).

Differing effects of CSE on dendritic cell (DC) numbers and function have been found, again likely due to differences in the specific exposure protocol. In a study using chronic, relatively low-dose mainstream exposures (2 1R1 or 1R3 reference cigarettes/day, 5 day/wk for 3, 6, or 10 months), CSE decreased the number of DCs in lung tissue, with a striking decrease on their expression of the costimulatory molecule CD80 (50). This exposure protocol also decreased pulmonary clearance of a replication-deficient adenovirus and was associated with reduced adenovirus-specific antibody titers (50). However, more prolonged and intense CSE induced increases in lung DC number and activation state (24). These differences not only emphasize the importance of tailoring the interpretation of an experimental model system to the question being studied but also illustrate the complexity of the problem of studying COPD progression in animal models.

Probably the most promising avenue for development of robust models of AECOPD is the combination of additional stimuli, especially infection, to CSE. Mice exposed chronically to CS showed reduced pulmonary clearance of *Pseudomonas aeruginosa*, with an increase in associated morbidity and weight loss (51). AMø from the smoke-exposed mice in that study produced less TNF-α and IL-6 in response to LPS than did AMø from nonexposed mice. Both of these differences were seen only with viable bacteria, but not with inactive bacteria, suggesting the primacy of the clearance defect in determining the outcome of infection in this model. It will be important to study multiple pulmonary pathogens in these types of model systems, as the net effect of CSE on host responses may vary. For example, a study of high-dose experimental infection with influenza virus by the same group found that chronic CSE increased lung inflammation, lung cytokine (TNF-α, IL-6, type 1 interferon) levels, and mortality, without a change in viral clearance (52).

## C.  Analysis of Sex Disparities in COPD Using Murine Models

The rapidly increasing prevalence of women with COPD indicates that sex disparities is a highly significant subject for analysis in animal model systems. Since the year 2000, women surpassed men in the number of individuals dying annually from COPD in the United States (53). Much of the increased prevalence of COPD in women has been attributed to increased use of tobacco products in women over the 20th century. In 1923, women consumed only 5% of all cigarettes sold in the United States (54). In the United States in 1965, 35% of women smoked, as compared to 50% of men. Women may also be at greater risk of smoking-induced lung function impairment than men for the same level of tobacco exposure (54). A systematic review and meta-analysis of population-based cohort studies showed that female current smokers had a significantly faster annual decline in lung function with increasing age compared with male current smokers (55).

There are several plausible explanations for a sex difference in tobacco susceptibility. The lungs and airways of women are smaller, so each cigarette represents a proportionately greater exposure. Secondhand smoke exposure and differences in cigarette brand preferences could also play a role. Other possible etiologies include hormonal effects on lung development, airway size, and differences in β-adrenergic and acetylcholine receptors (56,57). Women may have different biological responses to chronic tobacco exposure than men. Recent analysis of data from the National Emphysema Treatment Trial demonstrated less severe overall emphysema in women, particularly in the periphery of the lung. Morphometric examination of resected lung tissue revealed significantly thicker airway walls and smaller lumens in female subjects, suggesting that men and women respond differently in type and location of lung damage with tobacco exposure (58). Previous studies have suggested that chronic bronchitis is more prevalent in women, whereas emphysema is more prevalent in men (59). These phenotypic tendencies raise intriguing mechanistic questions that are best answered using a relevant animal model.

To date, few studies have addressed the effect of sex in murine models of smoke exposure. March et al. exposed male and female mice to CS for 10, 16, or 22 weeks. At the most concentrated exposure, female mice more rapidly developed evidence of emphysema (10 weeks vs. 16 weeks in male mice). Airflow obstruction and increased pulmonary compliance were not observed until 22 weeks; decreased elasticity was likely the major contributor to airflow obstruction, as remodeling of the conducting airways, beyond mild mucous cell hyperplasia, was lacking (33). These data are similar to those from other murine models, in which prolonged CSE induces emphysema with only minor changes in airway mucus or inflammation.

Sex disparities also need to be considered when additional stimuli are combined with CSE. The results of Mitchell and Gershwin, who examined the effects of progesterone on allergic airway disease in the setting of environmental tobacco smoke exposure (60), are a relevant example. In this study, female mice were ovariectomized and implanted with time-release progesterone pellets (or controls) and then housed so that they were exposed to environmental tobacco smoke with or without allergen. Serum total IgE levels were significantly greater in progesterone-treated mice that were also exposed to allergen, as compared with nonprogesterone-treated mice. Environmental CSE also enhanced total IgE levels. Lung cells from antigen/progesterone-treated groups produced significantly more IL-4 compared with antigen-exposed groups not treated with progesterone and had higher eosinophilia in lavage than all other groups. These results not only imply that progesterone levels exacerbate the allergic airway phenotype, but are evidence for an interaction between sex hormones and environmental CSE. Given the broad ranging effects of sex hormone throughout development, these issues merit increased investigation in models that involve multiple stimuli.

Animal models have the potential to address experimentally some of the major remaining questions on the genesis of sex disparities in COPD. One is the effect of difference in lung development. In humans, pathological changes in both the bronchioles and lung parenchyma contribute to airflow obstruction in COPD (61). Even from birth, the female lungs tend to be smaller than the male lungs (62). In both boys and girls, lung parenchyma appears to develop independently of the airways, a phenomenon termed "dysanapsis." The adult female lung results from the proportional growth at all ages of airways relative to parenchyma, whereas more rapid growth of the airways after puberty in males leads to the greater relative size of airways to lungs in men (63). By adulthood, Mead commented, the "airways of men were approximately 17% larger in diameter than the airways of women," speculating that "the adult sex difference in airway size develops relatively late in the growth phase" (63). Even after correcting for body size, adult men have larger volumes and flow rates than do women (64). Thus, simply on the basis of anatomic differences, one might hypothesize that physiological differences would exist in men and women with COPD. Animal models, especially conditional transgenic murine systems, could allow this hypothesis to be tested. A second question is the contribution of airways hyperresponsiveness (AHR) to COPD progression. In the Lung Health Study, AHR, presumably an early result of airway inflammation, appeared to identify a population at risk for cigarette-induced lung damage and was more common in women (65,66). Our laboratory has found minimal effects on either AHR or lung inflammation in male mice exposed to CS alone (unpublished data), but neither we nor others have published on the effect of either smoke or a combined stimuli in female mice. These and other questions illustrate the importance of continued work to develop reproducible, faithful animal model systems to increase the understanding of sex on physiological and pathological changes in human COPD.

## III. Genetic Models of Emphysema

Most attempts to produce animal models of COPD by genetic approaches have focused on the pathogenesis of emphysema. The slow and usually inexorable pace of this process in COPD patients makes experimental analysis in an animal model system particularly attractive. Model systems can be divided conceptually into those due to spontaneous loss-of-function mutations and transgenic approaches that involve either loss or gain of function.

The choice of genes to be targeted in these murine models has reflected the competing schools of thought regarding the pathogenesis of emphysema in humans. Hence, early models followed the protease imbalance theory, in which emphysema is thought to result from extracellular matrix degradation due either to excessive protease activity or to inadequate antiprotease activity (67,68). This theory has been examined primarily via overexpression systems. More recently, an alternative theory has highlighted the importance of apoptosis of structural cells in emphysema pathogenesis (69–71). This theory, which is not entirely contradictory to the protease imbalance theory, particularly lends itself to study in loss-of-function systems ("knockouts"), although it also appears to be unexpectedly relevant to the interpretation of findings in overexpression systems.

## A. Loss-of-Function Mutations and Genetic Models of Accelerated Aging as Models of Emphysema

Airspace enlargement was recognized to occur in several naturally occurring murine mutants (Table 1). In the *tightskin* mutant (72), in which airspace enlargement is detectable shortly after birth, the process clearly appears to be developmental rather than degenerative. Mutation of the fibrillin-1 gene in the tightskin mutation leads to a broad spectrum of pathological changes throughout the body. Emphysema develops more slowly in mice bearing the blotchy (onset at 4–6 months) and pallid (onset at 10–12 months) mutations (73). These particular spontaneous loss-of-function murine mutants have been felt to be more relevant to sporadic emphysema in humans with generalized defects of connective tissue than as models of human COPD resulting from exposure to CS or other oxidant injuries (8). However, pallid mice have been shown to develop accelerated emphysema when chronically exposed to CS (74).

An interesting recent finding is age-related emphysema in several mutant mouse strains, either spontaneous or induced transgenically, that display accelerated aging (Table 1). These strains show normal fetal and neonatal lung development, an important distinction from the strains cited above, but then show progressive emphysema starting,

**Table 1** Murine Loss-of-Function Mutants Associated with Airspace Enlargement

| Common name | Gene name | Additional features | References |
|---|---|---|---|
| Spontaneous mutations associated with defective alveolarization | | | |
| blotchy | Menkes disease gene | Prenatal death of males | 138 |
| pallid | Syntaxin 13 | Serum $\alpha_1$-antitrypsin activity deficiency (mild) | 139,140 |
| tightskin | Fibrillin-1 | Prenatal death of homozygotes; heterozygous mice: platelet storage pool defect, pigment dilution, kidney lysosomal enzyme elevation, serum $\alpha_1$-antitrypsin activity deficiency (mild), and abnormal otolith formation | 72,141,142 |
| Induced mutations associated with defective alveolarization | | | |
| Ltbp-3- | Latent transforming growth factor-binding protein-3 | Craniofacial malformation, osteopetrosis, and osteoarthritis | 143 |
| Spontaneous mutations associated with accelerated senescence | | | |
| SAM strain P1 | unknown | | 83 |
| Induced mutations associated with accelerated senescence | | | |
| *klotho* | *klotho* | Accelerated atherosclerosis, osteoporosis, ectopic calcification, skin atrophy, infertility | 144,145 |
| Fibroblast growth factor 23 | FGF23 | Accelerated atherosclerosis, osteoporosis, ectopic calcification, skin atrophy, infertility | 76 |
| Senescence marker protein 30 | regucalcin | | 81 |

*Abbreviation*: SAM, senescence-accelerated mice.

e.g., at four weeks of age in mice with the *klotho* mutation. *Klotho* is a single-pass trans-membrane product with β-glycosidase activity, found mainly in the kidney and not expressed in the lungs. However, the cleaved extracellular fragment of *klotho* is also found in the serum, and the protein was recently shown to contribute to systemic calcium homeostasis (75). Emphysema also develops in mice lacking function of fibroblast growth factor-23 (FGF-23), a regulator of phosphate homeostasis (76). Recent studies imply that both *klotho* and FGF-23 interact in the same pathway, inducing their very similar phenotype of accelerated aging via elevated 1,25-$(OH)_2$ vitamin D. The life span in both mutants can be extended by reducing 1,25-$(OH)_2$ vitamin D levels (77–79). An important insight from the *klotho* strain is that lung activity of MMP-9 and TIMP-1 is normal at two weeks of age, but abnormal at five weeks, with increased MMP-9 and decreased TIMP-1 (80). Thus, these two strains appear to be examples of proteolysis-dependent emphysema.

As part of a similarly accelerated aging process, mice lacking senescence marker 30 (SMP30) not only develop spontaneous emphysema (81) but are also hypersensitive to the effects of CSE (82). SMP30 is a 34 kD protein that protects cells throughout the body from oxidative stress and from apoptosis resulting from increased intracellular concentrations of calcium ions. Spontaneous emphysema with increased sensitivity to CSE is also seen in the senescence-accelerated mouse (SAM) strains, which were produced by selective breeding rather than transgenic manipulation (83). Importantly, antioxidant therapy of the SAM strains with lycopene-containing tomato juice reduced the lung damage caused by smoking and was associated with decreased alveolar cell apoptosis and increased lung expression of vascular endothelial growth factor (VEGF) (84). Besides providing support for the alternative theory of emphysema pathogenesis, this study illustrates the value of animal model systems in testing both biological mechanisms and potential therapies.

Knockout approaches have been used to provide evidence for the importance of both specific proteases and of apoptosis in emphysema development. Mice lacking MMP-12 (macrophage elastase) are completely protected against CS (22). By contrast, induction of emphysema by CSE is exaggerated in mice lacking Nrf2 (nuclear factor, erythroid-derived 2), a redox-sensitive basic leucine zipper protein transcription factor that regulates multiple detoxification and antioxidant genes (85). Emphysema also develops in mice conditionally deprived of pulmonary expression of VEGF by intratracheal delivery of an adeno-associated *cre* recombinase virus (AAV/Cre) to VEGF*loxP* mice (86).

## B. Transgenic Murine Models Involving Overexpression

Transgenic overexpression systems allow examination of the effect of single gene products in vivo and are thus a powerful tool that continues to be used actively (Table 2). Systems that permit inducible gene expression in the adult mouse are the most useful, as they largely circumvent the criticism that transgene expression during development induces airspace enlargement simply by preventing alveolarization rather than degrading formed alveoli, as occurs in COPD. However, as mentioned below, even tissue-specific inducible systems require careful controls and cautious interpretation.

Overexpression of IFN-γ, TNF-α, or IL-1β under the control of inducible lung-specific promoters caused changes characteristic of COPD, including lung inflammation and airspace enlargement (87–89). These results are in keeping with findings from human pathological specimens, which have shown increased expression of these inflammatory cytokines and a generally type 1 immunological response (90,91). However, similar changes were seen in mice

**Table 2** Transgenic Overexpressing Mice with Associated Emphysema Phenotypes

| Gene ID | Airspace enlargement? | Inflammatory cell infiltrate | MMP production | Additional features | References |
|---|---|---|---|---|---|
| Human Collagenase-1 (MMP-1) | Yes | No infiltrate | Not done | | 94 |
| TNF-α | Yes | B-cells, CD4+, and CD8+ T cells | MMP-12 | Upregulated cathepsin K; presence of lymphoid nodules adjacent to airways and within the lung parenchyma; some fibrotic lesions; increased CXCL13, CXCL12, CCL7, and CCL8 | 88 |
| IFN-γ | Yes | Neutrophils and mononuclear cells | MMP-12 | Augmented cathepsins B, D, H, and S; inhibits the antiprotease SLPI; epithelial cell apoptosis | 87,102 |
| IL-13 | Yes | Eosinophils and mononuclear cells | MMP-9, MMP-12 | Augmented cathepsins B, H, D, and S; mucus metaplasia; airway fibrosis; epithelial cell apoptosis; inhibits $\alpha_1$-antitrypsin | 92 |
| Human IL-1β | Yes | Neutrophils and macrophages | MMP-9, MMP-12 | Mucus metaplasia, airway fibrosis, enhanced production of CXCL1 and CXCL2 in the lungs | 89 |

*Abbreviation*: SLPI, secretory leukocyte proteinase inhibitor.

with inducible overexpression of IL-13, a cytokine more characteristic of type 2 immunological responses (92). This finding is open to several interpretations, since IL-13 also has profibrotic properties, and evidence for a type 2, particularly Tc2 phenotype of intracellular cytokine production, rather than type 1 phenotype, has recently been identified in humans with COPD (93). Nevertheless, these systems clearly illustrate the utility of this experimental approach.

Important experimental support for the protease imbalance theory came from an early model system overexpressing collagenase (94). Likewise, all four inducible transgenic mouse strains produced by the Elias laboratory (IFN-γ, IL-13, TNF-α, and IL-1β) displayed enhanced MMP-12 production relative to control mice. The IL-1β and IL-13 transgenic mice also had increased MMP-9 production (87–89,92). Cathepsin S, a cysteine protease expressed in an exaggerated fashion in the lungs of human smokers, was similarly augmented in the lungs of both the IFN-γ and IL-13 transgenic mice (95). Cathepsin K was increased in the lungs of the TNF-α transgenic mice (88). Further evidence to support the protease/antiprotease theory was seen in transgenic mice overexpressing human IL-1β. The lungs of these mice contained decreased elastin, an important component of the lung extracellular matrix, although it is unclear whether this finding resulted from impaired elastin deposition or destruction via the increased production of elastolytic enzymes (89,96). This model has particular relevance to human emphysema, as BAL fluid from smokers contains elevated levels of IL-1β that correlate with impairment in lung function (97). Hence, several transgenic murine models support both the protease imbalance theory and the capacity of inflammatory cytokines known to be abundant in the lungs of COPD patients to induce lung destruction by activating MMPs in vivo.

The theory that emphysema derives from excessive apoptosis or inadequate repair (70,98–101) also finds support from transgenic overexpression systems. Both IFN-γ and IL-13 overexpression models displayed increased levels of epithelial cell apoptosis (92,102). In fact, inhibition or genetic ablation of caspase-3, an effector molecule common to apoptosis due to many types of stimuli, caused a 50% to 60% decrease in IFN-γ-induced emphysema. This finding suggests that epithelial cell apoptosis is indeed a critical event in pathogenesis in this model system. Endothelial cell apoptosis induced by CSE was reduced by lung-specific overexpression of prostacyclin (103). In a subsequent study, crossbreeding of IFN-γ transgenic mice with mice expressing a defective mutant MMP-12 gene resulted in a significant decrease in emphysema, but no effect on epithelial cell apoptosis (95). This result implies that although apoptosis contributes, at least in the IFN-γ overexpression model, emphysema can be driven by both apoptosis-dependent and apoptosis-independent pathways. TNF-α, which is upregulated in patients with COPD as compared with healthy smokers and nonsmokers, also has the potential to act on resident lung cells and to induce apoptosis, although apoptosis of lung parenchymal cells has not yet been reported in the TNF-α overexpression model (88).

On a cautionary note, it is important to be sure that the phenotype of the transgenic mouse is due solely to the overexpressed gene and not an off-target effect of the expression system itself (104). One of the most popular means of temporally regulating transgene expression is via tetracycline-based externally regulatable (Tet-based) systems, which, depending on their design, can either induce or suppress specific transgenes. Zhu et al. have described ways of eliminating baseline "leakiness" of transgene expression, in the absence of doxycycline administration in Tet-based systems, by crossbreeding in an additional transgene, containing the tetracycline-controlled transcriptional silencer (tTS) (105,106). However, Sisson and colleagues observed an increase in lung compliance, total lung capacity, and alveolar size in control mice that received the reverse tetracycline trans-activator (rtTA) construct alone, with or without doxycycline exposure (107). The mechanism for this airspace enlargement, also previously reported in CCSP-rtTA mouse lines (108), is unknown. The potential influence of rtTA, and similar as yet unknown artifacts in other inducible expression systems, must be considered in designing and interpreting studies using transgenic manipulation. Although translation of the insights from transgenic mice will require careful interpretation, increasingly more sophisticated methods of genetic engineering hold the promise for model systems that will more faithfully recapitulate COPD in humans.

## IV.  Autoimmune and Other Murine Models not Involving CSE

Although the technique of inducing autoimmune emphysema originated in a rat model system described below (109), emphysema has been induced in normal mice by transfer of serum from immune rats (110). Data supporting the potential relevance of autoimmune models have subsequently come from studies in COPD patients (111). Studying autoimmune emphysema in animal models assumes special importance due to the recent finding that significant emphysema can be detected by computed tomography in the absence of airflow obstruction in a sizeable fraction of human smokers (112). Smoking has also been implicated in over a dozen epidemiological studies [summarized in (113)] as a risk factor for one of the quintessential autoimmune diseases, rheumatoid arthritis.

Emphysema has also been modeled in mice without the use of CSE by treatments that increase apoptosis of lung parenchymal cells. Enlargement of the airspaces in mice followed the induction of transient alveolar wall apoptosis by intratracheal installation of caspase-3 using a protein transfection agent, or of the pro-apoptotic serine/threonine kinase inhibitor nodularin (114). Another productive model results from inhibition of receptors for VEGF (115,116).

Probably the most crucial step in developing animal models of AECOPD would be to have a system mimicking chronic bronchitis in humans, even if it did not depend on CSE. Unfortunately, mice have proven to be relative resistant to infection with a variety of bacterial pathogens relevant to AECOPD. Mice very rapidly clear their lungs of nontypeable *Haemophilus influenzae* (117,118) by a process that depends on TLR4 (119). Interestingly, the speed of this clearance is reduced in transgenic mice lacking murine β-defensin (120), an example of how the genetic manipulations possible in the mouse can be exploited to study pathogenesis of even difficult-to-model organisms. To retard bacterial clearance and thereby develop more persistent models, some groups have impregnated bacteria into agarose beads, which lodge in distal airways after intratracheal delivery. Although bacterial survival is prolonged within the beads, in our opinion, these models currently are more relevant to cystic fibrosis (the usual intent of the authors) than to AECOPD.

## V.  COPD Models in Nonmurine Species

### A.  Rat Models

Despite the unchallenged merits of mice, their very small size does complicate some types of invasive physiological measurements, especially of the cardiovascular system. Progress is being made in miniaturizing instrumentation for use in mice, but the larger size of rats clearly facilitates physiological monitoring. Rats have also historically been used more broadly in toxicological studies. Early studies showed that the F344 strain of rats develop airspace enlargement in response to exposure to mainstream CS (2R1 cigarettes, 6 hr/day, 5 day/wk for 7 or 13 months) (23), although not as severely as similarly exposed B6C3F1 mice (23). Previous studies in rats implied that this level of exposure (250 mg TPM/m$^3$) approximated a human smoking three packs per day (121).

Rats have been used in a variety of model systems that have led to seminal discoveries germane to COPD pathogenesis. Chronic inhibition of the VEGF receptor 2 (KDR/Flk-1) in rats using the chemical inhibitor SU5416 resulted in both increased alveolar size and septal cell apoptosis, unaccompanied by inflammatory cell influx (122,123). Evidence for a potential autoimmune induction of emphysema was first derived from studies in which rats were immunized with human umbilical vein–derived endothelial cells or human airway smooth muscle cells, in either case in adjuvant (109). Use of rats would undoubtedly grow if the ease of their transgenic manipulation could be increased to that of the mouse (124,125).

## B. Guinea Pig Models

Guinea pig models of CSE-induced emphysema show some pathophysiological similarities to human COPD. Short-term or acute CSE leads to airflow obstruction and an increase in inflammatory cells in peripheral blood and BAL fluid. Chronic exposure greater than three months causes secretory cell metaplasia and airspace enlargement that exceed what is typically seen in mice with similar exposures (126). Cytokine and chemokine levels in the CS-exposed guinea pigs also have some similarity to those in human COPD. Increased messenger ribonucleic acid (mRNA) expression of TNF-$\alpha$, IL-1$\beta$, IL-8, and MCP-1 resulted from acute CS exposure, while elevated MCP-1 and IL-8 mRNA levels were detected in the chronic phase, and this correlated to the accumulation of macrophages and neutrophils in lavage fluid (127).

On the basis of the observations that DNA from the adenoviral early transcription gene, E1A, is increased in lung samples from patients with COPD (128) and that E1A protein is expressed in human bronchial epithelial cells (129), Vitalis and colleagues used a guinea pig model to test the effects of latent adenoviral infection and CSE (130). Latent adenoviral infection alone of guinea pigs induced an increase in B cells, CD4+, and CD8+ lymphocytes, monocytes, and macrophages in the lung parenchyma. The combination of adenoviral infection with a single dose of CS led to an increase in the volume of macrophages and T-helper cells (130). Likewise, chronic CSE over 13 weeks produced excess inflammation and lung destruction. There was an additive effect of infection and CSE on neutrophils and macrophages, but not on CD4+ and CD8+ cells. Rather, CD4+ cells increased exclusively because of CSE, whereas CD8 cells increased only in the presence of latent adenoviral infection (131).

More recently, this dual stimulus model system has been used to examine the molecular consequence of smoking cessation and to test whether latent infection might be responsible for steroid resistance (132). In the guinea pig model, smoking cessation was associated with an increase in lung surface area and surface area-to-volume ratio. Smoking cessation was also associated with decreases in lung neutrophils and CD4+ cells and reductions in mRNA concentrations of IL-8, CCL5, and IFN-$\gamma$ to control levels. Steroid treatment significantly lowered neutrophils, eosinophils, and IFN-$\gamma$ mRNA expression;

although adenoviral infection did not alter these steroid-induced changes, it independently increased airway wall infiltration by neutrophils and CD8+ cells (132). Thus, despite the relative paucity of specific reagents, guinea pigs continue to be used productively to investigate COPD pathogenesis.

## VI. Summary and Future Directions

Given both the known heterogeneity of pathological changes in COPD and the relative immaturity of our understanding of its fundamental basis, it should not be surprising that the perfect animal model of COPD so far eludes the scientific community. However, as this review illustrates, many useful advances have been made recently. More sophisticated transgenic approaches are becoming available that allow genes to be expressed or deleted for defined time periods. Murine models of smoke exposure that benefited recently from automated systems of smoke delivery that permit exposure of larger numbers of mice and from recent improvements in the measurement of pulmonary function. This field is ripe for analysis by state-of-the-art imaging techniques that are increasingly available for small animals (133). That COPD has different features in men and women (58,134–136) is an important recent observation, which should also be further explored in animal model systems (33,137).

CSE clearly leads to pulmonary inflammation and air space enlargement in normal mice. Although no murine model to date has shown all the relevant features of the human disease, these models have generated significant information about the pulmonary response to CS. The disparity between results in mice and humans may relate to species-specific difference in lung anatomy, generation of inflammatory responses, and how the smoke is delivered to the lungs. Even though a variety of protocols have been used to expose mice to smoke, none of them mimic the exposure in humans. Because of the variability in CSE methodologies, it is important for investigators in this field to define the exposure protocols, including the method of smoking, the environment generated (e.g., wet particulate weight or CO in ppm), and estimates of the exposure dosage (e.g., carboxyhemoglobin concentration), so that different methods may be compared at least qualitatively. With these caveats in mind, murine models of CSE will continue to play an important role in elucidating COPD pathogenesis and in testing potential therapies.

Progress in developing animal systems that faithfully reproduce the pathological findings of human COPD has been much greater in models of emphysema than of chronic bronchitis. Considering the greater prevalence of the latter process among COPD patients and the uncontested role of AECOPD in driving health care costs and reduced pulmonary function and health status (considered elsewhere in this issue), development of practical animal models of chronic bronchitis is an important unmet goal. On the basis of the anatomic consideration reviewed in this article, it is also likely to be a more difficult challenge than investigating emphysema. We predict that animal models of chronic bronchitis will best be achieved by combining three ingredients: carefully defined CSE; transgenic approaches targeting the innate and adaptive immune system and mucus production; and infection with specific pathogens, especially those native to the animal species being studied. The potential of such combined approaches to produce workable animal models of AECOPD fully justifies continued support of ethical animal experimentation.

## References

1. Shapiro SD. Mighty mice: transgenic technology "knocks out" questions of matrix metalloproteinase function. Matrix Biol 1997; 15(8–9):527–533.
2. Canning BJ. Modeling asthma and COPD in animals: a pointless exercise? Curr Opin Pharmacol 2003; 3(3):244–250.
3. Karlinsky JB, Snider GL. Animal models of emphysema. Am Rev Respir Dis 1978; 117(6): 1109–1133.
4. Reid LM. Needs for animal models of human diseases of the respiratory system. Am J Pathol 1980; 101(3 suppl):S89–S101.
5. Thomas RD, Vigerstad TJ. Use of laboratory animal models in investigating emphysema and cigarette smoking in humans. Regul Toxicol Pharmacol 1989; 10(3):264–271.
6. Campbell EJ. Animal models of emphysema: the next generations. J Clin Invest 2000; 106(12): 1445–1446.
7. Nikula KJ, Green FH. Animal models of chronic bronchitis and their relevance to studies of particle-induced disease. Inhal Toxicol 2000; 12(suppl 4):123–153.
8. Dawkins PA, Stockley RA. Animal models of chronic obstructive pulmonary disease. Thorax 2001; 56(12):972–977.
9. Fehrenbach H. Animal models of chronic obstructive pulmonary disease: some critical remarks. Pathobiology 2002; 70(5):277–283.
10. Tuder RM, McGrath S, Neptune E. The pathobiological mechanisms of emphysema models: what do they have in common? Pulm Pharmacol Ther 2003; 16(2):67–78.
11. Vlahos R, Bozinovski S, Gualano RC, et al. Modelling COPD in mice. Pulm Pharmacol Ther 2006; 19(1):12–17.
12. Mahadeva R, Shapiro SD. Chronic obstructive pulmonary disease-3: experimental animal models of pulmonary emphysema. Thorax 2002; 57(10):908–914.
13. Brusselle GG, Bracke KR, Maes T, et al. Murine models of COPD. Pulm Pharmacol Ther 2006; 19(3):155–165.
14. Pauluhn J, Mohr U. Experimental approaches to evaluate respiratory allergy in animal models. Exp Toxicol Pathol 2005; 56(4–5):203–234.
15. Corry DB, Irvin CG. Promise and pitfalls in animal-based asthma research: building a better mousetrap. Immunol Res 2006; 35(3):279–294.
16. Shapiro SD. Animal models of asthma: pro: allergic avoidance of animal (model[s]) is not an option. Am J Respir Crit Care Med 2006; 174(11):1171–1173.
17. Wenzel S, Holgate ST. The mouse trap: it still yields few answers in asthma. Am J Respir Crit Care Med 2006; 174(11):1173–1176.
18. Zosky GR, Sly PD. Animal models of asthma. Clin Exp Allergy 2007; 37(7):973–988.
19. Herszberg B, Ramos-Barbon D, Tamaoka M, et al. Heaves, an asthma-like equine disease, involves airway smooth muscle remodeling. J Allergy Clin Immunol 2006; 118(2): 382–388.
20. Couetil LL, Hoffman AM, Hodgson J, et al. Inflammatory airway disease of horses. J Vet Intern Med 2007; 21(2):356–361.
21. Shapiro SD. Transgenic and gene-targeted mice as models for chronic obstructive pulmonary disease. Eur Respir J 2007; 29(2):375–378.
22. Hautamaki RD, Kobayashi DK, Senior RM, et al. Requirement for macrophage elastase for cigarette smoke-induced emphysema in mice. Science 1997; 277(5334):2002–2004.
23. March TH, Barr EB, Finch GL, et al. Cigarette smoke exposure produces more evidence of emphysema in B6C3F1 mice than in F344 rats. Toxicol Sci 1999; 51(2):289–299.
24. D'Hulst AI, Vermaelen KY, Brusselle GG, et al. Time course of cigarette smoke-induced pulmonary inflammation in mice. Eur Respir J 2005; 26(2):204–213.

25. Edwards K, Braun KM, Evans G, et al. Mainstream and sidestream cigarette smoke condensates suppress macrophage responsiveness to interferon gamma. Hum Exp Toxicol 1999; 18(4): 233–240.

26. Sullivan S. The Reference and Research Cigarette Series. Lexington, KY: University of Kentucky Printing Services, 1984.

27. Roemer E, Stabbert R, Rustemeier K, et al. Chemical composition, cytotoxicity and mutagenicity of smoke from US commercial and reference cigarettes smoked under two sets of machine smoking conditions. Toxicology 2004; 195(1):31–52.

28. Hodge-Bell KC, Lee KM, Renne RA, et al. Pulmonary inflammation in mice exposed to mainstream cigarette smoke. Inhal Toxicol 2007, 19(4), 361–376.

29. Castro P, Legora-Machado A, Cardilo-Reis L, et al. Inhibition of interleukin-1beta reduces mouse lung inflammation induced by exposure to cigarette smoke. Eur J Pharmacol 2004; 498 (1–3):279–286.

30. Vlahos R, Bozinovski S, Jones JE, et al. Differential protease, innate immunity, and NF-kappaB induction profiles during lung inflammation induced by subchronic cigarette smoke exposure in mice. Am J Physiol Lung Cell Mol Physiol 2006; 290(5):L931–L945.

31. Simani AS, Inoue S, Hogg JC. Penetration of the respiratory epithelium of guinea pigs following exposure to cigarette smoke. Lab Invest 1974; 31(1):75–81.

32. Sekhon HS, Wright JL, Churg A. Cigarette smoke causes rapid cell proliferation in small airways and associated pulmonary arteries. Am J Physiol 1994; 267(5 pt 1):L557–L563.

33. March TH, Wilder JA, Esparza DC, et al. Modulators of cigarette smoke-induced pulmonary emphysema in A/J mice. Toxicol Sci 2006; 92(2):545–559.

34. Maes T, Bracke KR, Vermaelen KY, et al. Murine TLR4 Is Implicated in cigarette smoke-induced pulmonary inflammation. Int Arch Allergy Immunol 2006; 141(4):354–368.

35. Houghton AM, Quintero PA, Perkins DL, et al. Elastin fragments drive disease progression in a murine model of emphysema. J Clin Invest 2006; 116(3):753–759.

36. Elliott MK, Sisson JH, Wyatt TA. Effects of cigarette smoke and alcohol on ciliated tracheal epithelium and inflammatory cell recruitment. Am J Respir Cell Mol Biol 2007; 36(4):452–459.

37. Thatcher TH, McHugh NA, Egan RW, et al. Role of CXCR2 in cigarette smoke-induced lung inflammation. Am J Physiol Lung Cell Mol Physiol 2005; 289(2):L322–L328.

38. Valenca SS, Castro P, Pimenta WA, et al. Light cigarette smoke-induced emphysema and NFkappaB activation in mouse lung. Int J Exp Pathol 2006; 87(5):373–381.

39. Guerassimov A, Hoshino Y, Takubo Y, et al. The development of emphysema in cigarette smoke-exposed mice is strain dependent. Am J Respir Crit Care Med 2004; 170(9):974–980.

40. Bartalesi B, Cavarra E, Fineschi S, et al. Different lung responses to cigarette smoke in two strains of mice sensitive to oxidants. Eur Respir J 2005; 25(1):15–22.

41. Leclerc O, Lagente V, Planquois JM, et al. Involvement of MMP-12 and phosphodiesterase type 4 in cigarette smoke-induced inflammation in mice. Eur Respir J 2006; 27(6):1102–1109.

42. Martorana PA, Beume R, Lucattelli M, et al. Roflumilast fully prevents emphysema in mice chronically exposed to cigarette smoke. Am J Respir Crit Care Med 2005; 172(7):848–853.

43. Churg A, Dai J, Tai H, et al. Tumor necrosis factor-alpha is central to acute cigarette smoke-induced inflammation and connective tissue breakdown. Am J Respir Crit Care Med 2002; 166(6):849–854.

44. Dhami R, Gilks B, Xie C, et al. Acute cigarette smoke-induced connective tissue breakdown is mediated by neutrophils and prevented by alpha1-antitrypsin. Am J Respir Cell Mol Biol 2000; 22(2):244–252.

45. Churg A, Wang RD, Tai H, et al. Macrophage metalloelastase mediates acute cigarette smoke-induced inflammation via tumor necrosis factor-alpha release. Am J Respir Crit Care Med 2003; 167(8):1083–1089.

46. Thomas WR, Holt PG, Keast D. Cigarette smoke and phagocyte function: effect of chronic exposure in vivo and acute exposure in vitro. Infect Immun 1978; 20(2):468–475.

47. D'Hulst AI, Maes T, Bracke KR, et al. Cigarette smoke-induced pulmonary emphysema in scid-mice. Is the acquired immune system required? Respir Res 2005; 6:147.
48. Bracke KR, D'Hulst AI, Maes T, et al. Cigarette smoke-induced pulmonary inflammation and emphysema are attenuated in CCR6-deficient mice. J Immunol 2006; 177(7):4350–4359.
49. Bracke KR, D'Hulst AI, Maes T, et al. Cigarette smoke-induced pulmonary inflammation, but not airway remodelling, is attenuated in chemokine receptor 5-deficient mice. Clin Exp Allergy 2007; 37(10):1467–1479.
50. Robbins CS, Dawe DE, Goncharova SI, et al. Cigarette smoke decreases pulmonary dendritic cells and impacts antiviral immune responsiveness. Am J Respir Cell Mol Biol 2004; 30(2): 202–211.
51. Drannik AG, Pouladi MA, Robbins CS, et al. Impact of cigarette smoke on clearance and Inflammation following *Pseudomonas aeruginosa* infection. Am J Respir Crit Care Med 2004; 170(11):1164–1171.
52. Robbins CS, Bauer CM, Vujicic N, et al. Cigarette smoke impacts immune inflammatory responses to influenza in mice. Am J Respir Crit Care Med 2006; 174(12):1342–1351.
53. Mannino D, Homa D, Akinbami L, et al. Chronic obstructive pulmonary disease surveillance—United States, 1971 to 2000. MMWR 2002; 51(SS-6):1–16.
54. Chapman KR. Chronic obstructive pulmonary disease: are women more susceptible than men? Clin Chest Med 2004; 25(2):331–341.
55. Gan WQ, Man SFP, Postma DS, et al. Female smokers beyond the perimenopausal period are at increased risk of chronic obstructive pulmonary disease: a systematic review and meta-analysis. Respir Res 2006; 7:52.
56. Becklake MR, Kauffmann F. Gender differences in airway behaviour over the human life span. Thorax 1999; 54(12):1119–1138.
57. Tan KS, McFarlane LC, Lipworth BJ. Paradoxical down-regulation and desensitization of beta2-adrenoceptors by exogenous progesterone in female asthmatics. Chest 1997; 111(4):847–851.
58. Martinez FJ, Curtis JL, Sciurba F, et al. Sex differences in severe pulmonary emphysema. Am J Respir Crit Care Med 2007; 176(3):243–252.
59. Burrows B, Bloom JW, Traver GA, et al. The course and prognosis of different forms of chronic airways obstruction in a sample from the general population. N Engl J Med 1987; 317(21): 1309–1314.
60. Mitchell VL, Gershwin LJ. Progesterone and environmental tobacco smoke act synergistically to exacerbate the development of allergic asthma in a mouse model. Clin Exp Allerg 2007; 37(2): 276–286.
61. Barnes PJ. Chronic obstructive pulmonary disease. N Engl J Med 2000; 343(4):269–280.
62. Thurlbeck WM. Postnatal human lung growth. Thorax 1982; 37(8):564–571.
63. Mead J. Dysanapsis in normal lungs assessed by the relationship between maximal flow, static recoil, and vital capacity. Am Rev Respir Dis 1980; 121(2):339–342.
64. Society. AT. Lung function testing: selection of reference values and interpretative strategies. Am Rev Respir Dis 1991; 144(5):1202–1218.
65. Tashkin DP, Altose MD, Bleecker ER, et al. The lung health study: airway responsiveness to inhaled methacholine in smokers with mild to moderate airflow limitation. The Lung Health Study Research Group. Am Rev Respir Dis 1992; 145(2 pt 1):301–310.
66. Tashkin DP, Altose MD, Connett JE, et al. Methacholine reactivity predicts changes in lung function over time in smokers with early chronic obstructive pulmonary disease. The Lung Health Study Research Group. Am J Respir Crit Care Med 1996; 153(6 pt 1):1802–1811.
67. Shapiro SD. Proteolysis in the lung. Eur Respir J Suppl 2003; 44:30s–32s.
68. Churg A, Wright JL. Proteases and emphysema. Curr Opin Pulm Med 2005; 11(2):153–159.
69. Majo J, Ghezzo H, Cosio MG. Lymphocyte population and apoptosis in the lungs of smokers and their relation to emphysema. Eur Respir J 2001; 17(5):946–953.
70. Calabrese F, Giacometti C, Beghe B, et al. Marked alveolar apoptosis/proliferation imbalance in end-stage emphysema. Respir Res 2005; 6:14.

71. Demedts IK, Demoor T, Bracke KR, et al. Role of apoptosis in the pathogenesis of COPD and pulmonary emphysema. Respir Res 2006; 7:53.
72. Martorana PA, van Even P, Gardi C, et al. A 16-month study of the development of genetic emphysema in tight-skin mice. Am Rev Respir Dis 1989; 139(1):226–232.
73. Lucattelli M, Cavarra E, de Santi MM, et al. Collagen phagocytosis by lung alveolar macrophages in animal models of emphysema. Eur Respir J 2003; 22(5):728–734.
74. Takubo Y, Guerassimov A, Ghezzo H, et al. Alpha1-antitrypsin determines the pattern of emphysema and function in tobacco smoke-exposed mice: parallels with human disease. Am J Respir Crit Care Med 2002; 166(12 pt 1):1596–1603.
75. Imura A, Tsuji Y, Murata M, et al. alpha-Klotho as a regulator of calcium homeostasis. Science 2007; 316(5831):1615–1618.
76. Lanske B, Razzaque MS. Premature aging in klotho mutant mice: cause or consequence? Ageing Res Rev 2007; 6(1):73–79.
77. Tsujikawa H, Kurotaki Y, Fujimori T, et al. Klotho, a gene related to a syndrome resembling human premature aging, functions in a negative regulatory circuit of vitamin D endocrine system. Mol Endocrinol 2003; 17(12):2393–2403.
78. Razzaque MS, Sitara D, Taguchi T, et al. Premature aging-like phenotype in fibroblast growth factor 23 null mice is a vitamin D-mediated process. FASEB J 2006; 20(6):720–722.
79. Sato A, Hirai T, Imura A, et al. Morphological mechanism of the development of pulmonary emphysema in klotho mice. Proc Natl Acad Sci U S A 2007; 104(7):2361–2365.
80. Funada Y, Nishimura Y, Yokoyama M. Imbalance of matrix metalloproteinase-9 and tissue inhibitor of matrix metalloproteinase-1 is associated with pulmonary emphysema in Klotho mice. Kobe J Med Sci 2004; 50(3–4):59–67.
81. Mori T, Ishigami A, Seyama K, et al. Senescence marker protein-30 knockout mouse as a novel murine model of senile lung. Pathol Int 2004; 54(3):167–173.
82. Sato T, Seyama K, Sato Y, et al. Senescence marker protein-30 protects mice lungs from oxidative stress, aging, and smoking. Am J Respir Crit Care Med 2006; 174(5):530–537.
83. Takeda T. Senescence-accelerated mouse (SAM): a biogerontological resource in aging research. Neurobiol Aging 1999; 20(2):105–110.
84. Kasagi S, Seyama K, Mori H, et al. Tomato juice prevents senescence-accelerated mouse P1 strain from developing emphysema induced by chronic exposure to tobacco smoke. Am J Physiol Lung Cell Mol Physiol 2006; 290(2):L396–L404.
85. Rangasamy T, Cho CY, Thimmulappa RK, et al. Genetic ablation of Nrf2 enhances susceptibility to cigarette smoke-induced emphysema in mice. J Clin Invest 2004; 114(9):1248–1259.
86. Tang K, Rossiter HB, Wagner PD, et al. Lung-targeted VEGF inactivation leads to an emphysema phenotype in mice. J Appl Physiol 2004; 97(4):1559–1566.
87. Wang Z, Zheng T, Zhu Z, et al. Interferon gamma induction of pulmonary emphysema in the adult murine lung. J Exp Med 2000; 192(11):1587–1600.
88. Vuillemenot BR, Rodriguez JF, Hoyle GW. Lymphoid tissue and emphysema in the lungs of transgenic mice inducibly expressing tumor necrosis factor-alpha. Am J Respir Cell Mol Biol 2004; 30(4):438–448.
89. Lappalainen U, Whitsett JA, Wert SE, et al. Interleukin-1beta causes pulmonary inflammation, emphysema, and airway remodeling in the adult murine lung. Am J Respir Cell Mol Biol 2005; 32(4):311–318.
90. Majori M, Corradi M, Caminati A, et al. Predominant TH1 cytokine pattern in peripheral blood from subjects with chronic obstructive pulmonary disease. J Allergy Clin Immunol 1999; 103 (3 pt 1):458–462.
91. Saetta M, Mariani M, Panina-Bordignon P, et al. Increased expression of the chemokine receptor CXCR3 and its ligand CXCL10 in peripheral airways of smokers with chronic obstructive pulmonary disease. Am J Respir Crit Care Med 2002; 165(10):1404–1409.

92. Zheng T, Zhu Z, Wang Z, et al. Inducible targeting of IL-13 to the adult lung causes matrix metalloproteinase- and cathepsin-dependent emphysema. J Clin Invest 2000; 106(9):1081–1093.
93. Barcelo B, Pons J, Fuster A, et al. Intracellular cytokine profile of T lymphocytes in patients with chronic obstructive pulmonary disease. Clin Exp Immunol 2006; 145(3):474–479.
94. D'Armiento J, Dalal SS, Okada Y, et al. Collagenase expression in the lungs of transgenic mice causes pulmonary emphysema. Cell 1992; 71(6):955–961.
95. Elias JA, Kang MJ, Crouthers K, et al. State of the art. Mechanistic heterogeneity in chronic obstructive pulmonary disease: insights from transgenic mice. Proc Am Thorac Soc 2006; 3(6): 494–498.
96. Kuang PP, Goldstein RH. Regulation of elastin gene transcription by interleukin-1 beta-induced C/EBP beta isoforms. Am J Physiol Cell Physiol 2003; 285(6):C1349–C1355.
97. Ekberg-Jansson A, Andersson B, Bake B, et al. Neutrophil-associated activation markers in healthy smokers relates to a fall in DL(CO) and to emphysematous changes on high resolution CT. Respir Med 2001; 95(5):363–373.
98. Kasahara Y, Tuder RM, Cool CD, et al. Endothelial cell death and decreased expression of vascular endothelial growth factor and vascular endothelial growth factor receptor 2 in emphysema. Am J Respir Crit Care Med 2001; 163(3 pt 1):737–744.
99. Tuder RM, Petrache I, Elias JA, et al. Apoptosis and emphysema: the missing link. Am J Respir Cell Mol Biol 2003; 28(5):551–554.
100. Yokohori N, Aoshiba K, Nagai A. Increased levels of cell death and proliferation in alveolar wall cells in patients with pulmonary emphysema. Chest 2004; 125(2):626–632.
101. Wright JL, Churg A. Current concepts in mechanisms of emphysema. Toxicol Pathol 2007; 35(1): 111–115.
102. Zheng T, Kang MJ, Crothers K, et al. Role of cathepsin S-dependent epithelial cell apoptosis in IFN-gamma-induced alveolar remodeling and pulmonary emphysema. J Immunol 2005; 174(12): 8106–8115.
103. Nana-Sinkam SP, Lee JD, Sotto-Santiago S, et al. Prostacyclin prevents pulmonary endothelial cell apoptosis induced by cigarette smoke. Am J Respir Crit Care Med 2007; 175(7):676–685.
104. Whitsett JA, Perl AK. Conditional control of gene expression in the respiratory epithelium: a cautionary note. Am J Respir Cell Mol Biol 2006; 34(5):519–520.
105. Zhu Z, Zheng T, Lee CG, et al. Tetracycline-controlled transcriptional regulation systems: advances and application in transgenic animal modeling. Semin Cell Dev Biol 2002; 13(2): 121–128.
106. Zhu Z, Ma B, Homer RJ, et al. Use of the tetracycline-controlled transcriptional silencer (tTS) to eliminate transgene leak in inducible overexpression transgenic mice. J Biol Chem 2001; 276(27):25222–25229.
107. Sisson TH, Hansen JM, Shah M, et al. Expression of the reverse tetracycline-transactivator gene causes emphysema-like changes in mice. Am J Respir Cell Mol Biol 2006; 34(5):552–560.
108. Perl AK, Wert SE, Loudy DE, et al. Conditional recombination reveals distinct subsets of epithelial cells in trachea, bronchi, and alveoli. Am J Respir Cell Mol Biol 2005; 33(5):455–462.
109. Taraseviciene-Stewart L, Scerbavicius R, Choe KH, et al. An animal model of autoimmune emphysema. Am J Respir Crit Care Med 2005; 171(7):734–742.
110. Taraseviciene-Stewart L, Douglas IS, Nana-Sinkam PS, et al. Is alveolar destruction and emphysema in chronic obstructive pulmonary disease an immune disease? Proc Am Thorac Soc 2006; 3(8):687–690.
111. Lee SH, Goswami S, Grudo A, et al. Antielastin autoimmunity in tobacco smoking-induced emphysema. Nat Med 2007; 13(5):567–569.
112. Omori H, Nakashima R, Otsuka N, et al. Emphysema detected by lung cancer screening with low-dose spiral CT: prevalence, and correlation with smoking habits and pulmonary function in Japanese male subjects. Respirology 2006; 11(2):205–210.

113. Stolt P, Bengtsson C, Nordmark B, et al. Quantification of the influence of cigarette smoking on rheumatoid arthritis: results from a population based case-control study, using incident cases. Ann Rheum Dis 2003; 62(9):835–841.

114. Aoshiba K, Yokohori N, Nagai A. Alveolar wall apoptosis causes lung destruction and emphysematous changes. Am J Respir Cell Mol Biol 2003; 28(5):555–562.

115. Petrache I, Natarajan V, Zhen L, et al. Ceramide upregulation causes pulmonary cell apoptosis and emphysema-like disease in mice. Nat Med 2005; 11(5):491–498.

116. Petrache I, Fijalkowska I, Zhen L, et al. A novel antiapoptotic role for alpha1-antitrypsin in the prevention of pulmonary emphysema. Am J Respir Crit Care Med 2006; 173(11):1222–1228.

117. Foxwell AR, Kyd JM, Cripps AW. Characteristics of the immunological response in the clearance of non-typeable *Haemophilus influenzae* from the lung. Immunol Cell Biol 1998; 76(4):323–331.

118. Foxwell AR, Kyd JM, Cripps AW. Kinetics of inflammatory cytokines in the clearance of non-typeable *Haemophilus influenzae* from the lung. Immunol Cell Biol 1998; 76(6):556–559.

119. Wang X, Moser C, Louboutin JP, et al. Toll-like receptor 4 mediates innate immune responses to *Haemophilus influenzae* infection in mouse lung. J Immunol 2002; 168(2):810–815.

120. Moser C, Weiner DJ, Lysenko E, et al. beta-Defensin 1 contributes to pulmonary innate immunity in mice. Infect Immun 2002; 70(6):3068–3072.

121. Finch GL, Lundgren DL, Barr EB, et al. Chronic cigarette smoke exposure increases the pulmonary retention and radiation dose of $^{239}$Pu inhaled as $^{239}$PuO$_2$ by F344 rats. Health Phys 1998; 75(6):597–609.

122. Kasahara Y, Tuder RM, Taraseviciene-Stewart L, et al. Inhibition of VEGF receptors causes lung cell apoptosis and emphysema. J Clin Invest 2000; 106(11):1311–1319.

123. Tuder RM, Zhen L, Cho CY, et al. Oxidative stress and apoptosis interact and cause emphysema due to vascular endothelial growth factor receptor blockade. Am J Respir Cell Mol Biol 2003; 29(1):88–97.

124. Tesson L, Cozzi J, Menoret S, et al. Transgenic modifications of the rat genome. Transgenic Res 2005; 14(5):531–546.

125. Melo EO, Canavessi AM, Franco MM, et al. Animal transgenesis: state of the art and applications. J Appl Genet 2007; 48(1):47–61.

126. Wright JL, Churg A. A model of tobacco smoke-induced airflow obstruction in the guinea pig. Chest 2002; 121(5 suppl):188S–191S.

127. Kubo S, Kobayashi M, Masunaga Y, et al. Cytokine and chemokine expression in cigarette smoke-induced lung injury in guinea pigs. Eur Respir J 2005; 26(6):993–1001.

128. Matsuse T, Hayashi S, Kuwano K, et al. Latent adenoviral infection in the pathogenesis of chronic airways obstruction. Am Rev Respir Dis 1992; 146(1):177–184.

129. Elliott WM, Hayashi S, Hogg JC. Immunodetection of adenoviral E1A proteins in human lung tissue. Am J Respir Cell Mol Biol 1995; 12(6):642–648.

130. Vitalis TZ, Kern I, Croome A, et al. The effect of latent adenovirus 5 infection on cigarette smoke-induced lung inflammation. Eur Respir J 1998; 11(3):664–669.

131. Meshi B, Vitalis TZ, Ionescu D, et al. Emphysematous lung destruction by cigarette smoke. The effects of latent adenoviral infection on the lung inflammatory response. Am J Respir Cell Mol Biol 2002; 26(1):52–57.

132. Milot J, Meshi B, Taher Shabani Rad M, et al. The effect of smoking cessation and steroid treatment on emphysema in guinea pigs. Respir Med 2007; 101(11):2327–2335.

133. Olsson LE, Lindahl M, Onnervik PO, et al. Measurement of MR signal and T2* in lung to characterize a tight skin mouse model of emphysema using single-point imaging. J Magn Reson Imaging 2007; 25(3):488–494.

134. Dransfield MT, Washko GR, Foreman MG, et al. Gender differences in the severity of CT emphysema in COPD. Chest 2007; 132(2):464–470.

135. Fan VS, Ramsey SD, Giardino ND, et al. Sex, depression, and risk of hospitalization and mortality in chronic obstructive pulmonary disease. Arch Intern Med 2007; 167(21):2345–2353.
136. Han MK, Postma D, Mannino D, et al. Gender and COPD: why it matters. Am J Respir Crit Care Med 2007; 176(12):1179–1184.
137. Card JW, Carey MA, Bradbury JA, et al. Gender differences in murine airway responsiveness and lipopolysaccharide-induced inflammation. J Immunol 2006; 177(1):621–630.
138. Mercer JF, Grimes A, Ambrosini L, et al. Mutations in the murine homologue of the Menkes gene in dappled and blotchy mice. Nat Genet 1994; 6(4):374–378.
139. Martorana PA, Brand T, Gardi C, et al. The pallid mouse. A model of genetic alpha 1-antitrypsin deficiency. Lab Invest 1993; 68(2):233–241.
140. Huang L, Kuo YM, Gitschier J. The pallid gene encodes a novel, syntaxin 13-interacting protein involved in platelet storage pool deficiency. Nat Genet 1999; 23(3):329–332.
141. Szapiel SV, Fulmer JD, Hunninghake GW, et al. Hereditary emphysema in the tight-skin (Tsk/+) mouse. Am Rev Respir Dis 1981; 123(6):680–685.
142. Keil M, Lungarella G, Cavarra E, et al. A scanning electron microscopic investigation of genetic emphysema in tight-skin, pallid, and beige mice, three different C57 BL/6J mutants. Lab Invest 1996; 74(2):353–362.
143. Colarossi C, Chen Y, Obata H, et al. Lung alveolar septation defects in Ltbp-3-null mice. Am J Pathol 2005; 167(2):419–428.
144. Kuro-o M, Matsumura Y, Aizawa H, et al. Mutation of the mouse klotho gene leads to a syndrome resembling ageing. Nature 1997; 390(6655):45–51.
145. Suga T, Kurabayashi M, Sando Y, et al. Disruption of the klotho gene causes pulmonary emphysema in mice. Defect in maintenance of pulmonary integrity during postnatal life. Am J Respir Cell Mol Biol 2000; 22(1):26–33.

# 17
# Comparison of Asthma and COPD Exacerbations

**JOSEPH FOOTITT, ANNEMARIE SYKES, PATRICK MALLIA, and SEBASTIAN L. JOHNSTON**
Department of Respiratory Medicine, National Heart and Lung Institute, Imperial College, London, U.K.

## I. Introduction

Although difficult to define, acute exacerbations of both chronic obstructive pulmonary disease (AECOPD) and asthma are well recognized by both patients and clinicians. They present a significant health burden, causing enormous morbidity and significant mortality, and they represent a major drain on health care resources. An estimated 70% of the total expenditure on COPD is attributed to exacerbations (1), and hospital admissions alone account for 50% of total spending in asthma (2).

Despite differences in the underlying etiology and pathology of both diseases, there are many similarities in the clinical nature of exacerbations. This may reflect considerable overlap in the etiology; however, significant heterogeneity does exist both between and within both the conditions. In asthma, allergen-induced exacerbations can produce different inflammatory cell profiles to those caused by infection, and in COPD, bacterial exacerbations may be different from viral.

Both prevention and treatment of exacerbations remain suboptimal, and a better understanding of underlying mechanisms and specific etiology may lead to urgently needed new therapies. Finally, although traditionally regarded as clearly defined and discrete episodes, exacerbations can have long-lasting effects with faster decline in lung function being related to exacerbation frequency. This is particularly true for COPD, but there is emerging evidence that this may be the case in asthma as well (3).

## II. Epidemiology of Exacerbations

Epidemiological studies show seasonal factors have a striking impact on exacerbation frequencies in both asthma and COPD (4). A peak in asthma exacerbations around mid- to late September, strongly correlating with return to school, is seen in children and younger adults (4). A peak in COPD exacerbations, and in older asthmatics, follows weeks later in December. A strong correlation between Christmas holidays and COPD exacerbations is seen in every Northern Hemisphere country studied (4).

These trends are likely to reflect a complex combination of many causative factors; however, the leading cause of exacerbations in both asthma and COPD is respiratory virus infection (5–7), particularly with rhinovirus. The peak in asthma exacerbations correlates with the highest incidence of rhinovirus infections in the community (5) and may be aggravated by less use of controller medication during the summer (8). The asthma peak starts in younger children (6 years old) and then spreads to older age groups. The delay in COPD exacerbations may reflect the delay of virus transmission through the community; however, more work is needed as the role of viruses in the Christmas epidemic is presently unknown (4).

COPD patients have been reported to experience exacerbations at an average frequency of 0.1 per patient per month (9), but this reflects a wide range between individual patients and the severity of underlying disease. Recent national surveillance data for asthma from the United States have shown that 55% of patients experienced one or more attacks in the previous year (10) and 5% to 10% were hospitalized. Factors associated with an increased risk of hospital admission for COPD exacerbations included forced expiratory volume in one second ($FEV_1$), patient age, degree of mucus secretion, and comorbidities, (11), but it is acknowledged that admission criteria vary widely between different institutions and countries. Risk of hospitalization in asthmatics was increased in those exposed to tobacco smoke, from a low household income group, or previously hospitalized with asthma (12). Mortality was increased in those with worse lung function, older patients, and in African-American and Hispanic groups who also had higher hospitalization rates (12).

An Australian study documenting hospital admissions and outcomes for all airway diseases over 10 years showed a general fall in asthma-related admissions and mortality, but an increase in COPD admissions. Of particular concern was increasing mortality among women with COPD, not seen in their male counterparts (13). Improved asthma outcomes are likely the result of increased use of inhaled corticosteroids, whereas increasing rates of COPD exacerbations likely reflect limitations in treatment and increasing smoking rates, particularly in women.

## III.   Etiology of Exacerbations

Infection, predominately viral, is the major cause of exacerbations in both asthma and COPD. Controversy remains regarding the precise role of bacteria, particularly in COPD exacerbations, as many patients' airways are colonized when stable (14). Other potential triggers have been identified, including allergens, atmospheric changes, and pollution; these are likely to be of greater significance in asthmatics.

### A.   Allergy

The incidence of allergy within industrialized populations is increasing at a rate that makes it unlikely that genetic factors are responsible, so interest has focused on environmental factors (15).

Interaction between allergen sensitization, allergen exposure, and virus infection has been detected in asthmatics during acute exacerbations. Synergy between these factors has been demonstrated in both adults (16) and children (17).

This is supported by experimental models of rhinovirus infection, which demonstrated increased airway inflammation and hyperresponsiveness with evidence of synergy between viral infection and allergens (18,19).

Elevated immunoglobulin E (IgE) levels are found in atopic asthmatics and are associated with sputum eosinophilia. IgE inhibitors reduce eosinophilia and in some groups improve symptoms and reduce exacerbation frequency (20). In an experimental infection study, IgE has been shown to be a marker of severity (20), as asthmatics with higher IgE had elevated markers of inflammation prior to infection and experienced both earlier and more severe symptoms.

Specific triggers for allergic asthma are often inhaled. These aeroallergens include pollen, fungal spores, dust mites, feces, and animal allergens. The role of allergic triggers in AECOPD is less well understood, but they may play a significant part.

## B. Air Pollution

The relative importance of air pollution, aeroallergens, and climatic factors in the etiology of exacerbations of airway disease is difficult to quantify. There is a close association between these factors, and they may act synergistically to worsen asthma exacerbations (15). An observational study in asthmatic children demonstrated an association between exposure to nitrogen dioxide and the severity of virus-induced exacerbations (22). A variety of possible mechanisms have been suggested, including increased susceptibility to viral infection by damage to the airway epithelium, changes in inflammatory mediators, or upregulation of intercellular adhesion molecule (ICAM)-1, the adhesion molecule that acts as receptor for over 90% of rhinoviruses. Finally, a recent crossover study exposing asthmatics to environments of both high and low levels of diesel fumes demonstrated an increase in biomarkers of neutrophilic airway inflammation and falls in $FEV_1$, which were greater following exposure to areas of high pollution (23).

Epidemiological studies have demonstrated a link between atmospheric conditions, air pollution, and the number of hospital admissions due to both COPD and asthma. A recent study by Elliott et al. showed an association with air pollution, specifically sulfur dioxide and black smoke and long-term mortality in the United Kingdom (24); this supports previous studies demonstrating harmful effects of short-term pollution exposure. The link between urban living and worsening of airway disease has been most strikingly demonstrated in asthma, especially in the pediatric population. Data based on observational studies demonstrated wheeze in children living in close proximity to roads and worsening symptoms at periods of high ozone levels; conversely, there are fewer exacerbations during periods of reduced traffic or during factory closures (25). The role of particulate matter from diesel engines is also an area of interest as levels have increased significantly. Normal subjects exposed to diesel fumes have increased airway inflammation (26), and in asthmatic subjects, airway hyperresponsiveness and sputum levels of IL-6 are increased (27).

The mechanisms of pollution in exacerbations of airway diseases is not yet clear and interventional studies in this area are difficult to perform; however, it appears that pollution is probably an important factor in exacerbations of both asthma and COPD.

## C. Infection

### Viruses

An association between viruses and exacerbations has long been recognized, but the availability of polymerase chain reaction (PCR), a more sensitive detection method, has shown that viruses are responsible for a much higher proportion than previously realized. Studies in a range of severities of COPD exacerbations have detected viruses in 40% to 60% of cases (7,28). In asthma, the percentage is higher, between 80% to 85% in children (6,29) and 75% to 80% in adults (30,31), with rhinovirus accounting for up to two-thirds of viruses identified.

A human experimental rhinovirus infection model of acute exacerbations has been developed in asthmatics (32), and one is under development for COPD (18). These models will enable detailed study and improved understanding of the mechanisms and patho-physiology of exacerbations; also, characterized, homogeneous populations can be studied at baseline and during an exacerbation with a single-defined etiological agent. The record of symptoms and physiological and pathological changes cannot be recorded in the same way during naturally occurring exacerbations.

Interest has focused on whether patients with airways disease are more susceptible to viral infections. A longitudinal cohort study found that asthmatics were not at an increased risk of developing rhinoviral infection but did develop longer-lasting and more severe lower respiratory tract symptoms than healthy controls (33). Recent studies suggest that antiviral immunity is reduced in asthmatic subjects compared with nonasthmatics. Peripheral blood monocytes from asthmatics exposed to rhinovirus were deficient in production of interferon-$\gamma$ (IFN-$\gamma$) and IL-12 compared with normal subjects (34). An experimental infection study has also demonstrated deficient induction of Th-1 cytokines and IL-10 and augmented induction of Th-2 cytokines in asthma (32); furthermore, the model also demonstrated deficient levels of IFN-$\gamma$ in primary bronchial epithelial cells and alveolar macrophages, which correlated with the severity of exacerbation and viral load (35). Bronchial epithelial cells from asthmatics have previously been shown to support increased rhinovirus replication (36), associated with impaired apoptosis of infected cells and a deficiency of the antiviral cytokine IFN-$\beta$ and subsequent proinflammatory response. Replacement of IFN-$\beta$ resulted in a restoration of viral defence. Similar mechanisms may apply in COPD, but further study in this area is required.

### Bacteria

The role of bacteria in both asthma and COPD exacerbations remains controversial. In COPD, bacteria have traditionally been regarded as a major etiological factor and are isolated in approximately 50% of episodes of exacerbation. However, the relationship between host and bacteria is complex as 30% to 40% patients with chronic mucus production are colonized in the stable state (37).

Older studies did not differentiate between bacterial strains, and more recent work has found that isolation of new strains of bacteria are associated with an increased risk of exacerbation, supporting a causative role for bacteria in exacerbations (38) In addition, a Cochrane review (39) in 2005 found that overall antibiotic use was beneficial in exacerbations where significant symptoms of infection were present. Patients likely to benefit from antibiotic therapy can be identified by sputum characteristics, according to one study (40), further supporting a role for antibiotic therapy in selected patients. Procalcitonin has also been used to guide treatment in exacerbations (41), resulting in significantly fewer antibiotic prescriptions (reduced from 72% to 40%) compared with a control group, reinforcing the importance of correctly indentifying which patients to treat with antibiotics and the potential benefit of a biomarker for this.

Antibiotic treatment for acute asthma remains contentious with little randomized data in the current literature. Three decades ago, antibiotic use was widespread, but present guidelines do not support the routine use of antibiotics. However, emerging data have rekindled interest, particularly in the role of atypical bacteria in the pathogenesis of asthma exacerbations.

### Atypical Bacterial Infection

There is increasing evidence to support an association between *Mycoplasma pneumoniae* and *Chlamydophila pneumoniae* and exacerbations of airway disease. The evidence is stronger in asthma than COPD as although several serological studies demonstrated elevated antibody titres, suggesting atypical bacteria play a part in AECOD, this was not supported by PCR analysis of sputum taken during an exacerbation (42). In asthma, the literature remains conflicting, but the majority of studies performed in both adults and children have supported a pathogenical role for atypical infection (30,43). Acute and chronic infection has been implicated in asthma. Chronic infection with *C. pneumoniae,* but not *M. pneumoniae,* was associated with worse asthma symptoms in children (44). However, atypical infection was not identified in other studies, particularly three groups of hospitalized asthmatics whose exacerbations were predominately viral (16).

The Telithromycin, Chlamydophila, and Asthma (TELICAST) study was a placebo-controlled double-blind trial that investigated use of the ketolide antibiotic, telithromycin, in acute asthma (45). Treatment resulted in improved symptoms and lung function in the treated group, but the mechanisms for this are unclear. Further studies are required to investigate if this treatment effect extends to macrolide or other antibiotics.

### Coinfection

Bacterial and viral coinfection may act synergistically (46). Coinfection is associated with increased severity of symptoms, lung function impairment, and airway inflammation in COPD exacerbations and is present in 25% of COPD exacerbations (14). The interaction between bacteria and virus in the lower airway in COPD is not well understood. Work is required to characterize this further.

## IV.  Mechanisms of Exacerbations

Lower airway viral infection causes inflammation; however, the cellular mechanisms of this remain unclear. In addition to direct cell necrosis, there is immune-mediated damage and release of cytokines causing epithelial damage.

### A.  Cellular Mechanisms

The cellular response to exacerbations in asthmatic subjects is heterogeneous. Viral infection produces an influx of leukocytes into the airway. Elevated levels of both neutrophils and eosinophils have been found (30). It is likely that cellular mechanisms of inflammation differ between stable asthma and during exacerbations. This may reflect not only the success of inhaled corticosteroids in the treatment of stable disease but also their relative ineffectiveness during exacerbations. COPD studies of airway inflammation have demonstrated conflicting results. A bronchial biopsy study showed a 30-fold increase in eosinophils with smaller increases in neutrophils and T lymphocytes (47), whereas in another study bronchoalveolar lavage (BAL) fluid demonstrated neutrophilia and eosinophilia, but a more marked increase in neutrophils (48). Noninvasive studies examining sputum are easier to perform, but again results are inconsistent, reporting no change in cell number (49) or increases in lymphocytes, neutrophils, and eosinophils (50). Recently, neutrophilia was shown to be related to exacerbation severity independent of etiology, while eosinophilia was a good predictor of viral exacerbations (14). The mixed picture reflects the heterogeneity of exacerbations and partly explains the variable response to inhaled steroids in COPD exacerbations.

## B.  Cellular Inflammation

Characteristic inflammatory changes, with high levels of macrophages and lymphocytes, are seen in the airways of smokers. These are enhanced in patients with COPD, and this may represent an exaggerated normal response to an inhaled toxin. The cellular pattern of inflammation changes between the stable and exacerbated state in both asthma and COPD. Eosinophilic inflammation is classically associated with asthmatic airways (51,52) and is the predominant cell type in all states of asthma. However, recently, neutrophilic-based inflammation has been identified in the airways of more severe asthmatics (53), and this appears to predominate during exacerbations. It has been suggested that this more severe neutrophil-predominant group responds less well to traditional inhaled corticosteroid therapy than those with eosinophilic inflammation. Neutrophils and macrophages predominate in COPD, and their levels rise with disease severity and still further during exacerbations, this is in contrast to asthma where macrophages are not thought to play a role. Lymphocytic inflammation is being recognized as increasingly important in COPD with elevated levels of CD-8 plus T lymphocytes (54); increased levels are associated with more severe disease, and markers associated with Th-1 cells (55) predominate, and this differs from asthma where Th-2 cells predominates.

The chronic and progressive nature of this cell damage is driven by inflammatory genes and these are in turn controlled by transcription factors, such as nuclear factor-κB (NF-κB), which is found to be activated in COPD.

## C.  Molecular Mechanisms

It is essential to understand the inflammatory mechanisms underlying airway disease to identify new approaches to treatment and eventually improve our management of these conditions. Although clearly distinct, similarities exist in cellular inflammation of COPD and asthma. There are many inflammatory genes that are active in the lung, and focus on the mechanisms controlling these has led to an interest in the role of histones and the enzymes controlling them. Work in the field of epigenetics, the process by which cells can alter genetic expression without changing the underlying DNA sequence, is presently expanding and may provide further insights into inflammatory lung diseases.

### Histones

Initially regarded simply as packing material for DNA, histones have a major function in gene regulation. By altering the amount of DNA exposed for transcription, histones can up-

or downregulate the inflammatory response in COPD and asthma. This process is controlled, at least partially, by the acetylation of histones, which allows DNA exposure and inflammatory genes to be activated. The enzymes that control histone acetylation are histone acetyltransferases (HAT), and in contrast, histone deacetylases (HDAC) deacetylate the histone and reduce the inflammatory response.

Levels of HAT have been found to be higher in bronchial biopsies from asthmatic patients, and there is a slight reduction in HDAC levels, which is exaggerated in those asthmatics who smoke (56). These changes are also seen in macrophages obtained from BAL but not in cells from peripheral blood, suggesting that this effect maybe localized to the airways. Corticosteroid therapy is highly effective in stable asthma, and in those subjects receiving inhaled steroid therapy, the levels of HAT returned to normal.

Histone acetylation is also increased in COPD, and the degree of acetylation correlates with disease severity; however, in contrast to asthma, this is a result of marked reductions in HDAC levels found in bronchial biopsies from COPD patients (57). Although this study investigated different severities of COPD, no work has yet been done on HDAC activity during exacerbations of COPD. However, activation of NF-κB and reduction in HDAC activity have been demonstrated following infection in bronchial epithelial cells with *Moraxella catarrhalis* (58), an important pathogen in COPD exacerbations.

### Transcription Factor NF-κB

The role of NF-κB as a transcription factor common to many pathways is well established. Levels were increased synergistically, via two distinct pathways, following infection of cells with *Haemophilus inflenzae* and exposure to tumor necrosis factor-α (TNF-α) (59). Rhinoviral infection elevates levels of TNF-α via NK-κB, giving an insight into how exaggerated inflammatory responses in infection are likely to have on many diverse promoters (60). Studies on NF-κB in COPD and asthma during exacerbations are limited. In one study of COPD exacerbation (61), levels of both TNF-α and IL-8 were elevated, and a challenge study in asthma (6) demonstrated a rise in TNF-α, indicating further study is merited.

### Cytokines

In vitro and in vivo studies in asthmatics have demonstrated induction of inflammatory mediators following viral infection. The proinflammatory cytokine IL-6 and the neutrophil chemokine IL-8 have been found in nasal (62) and lower airway samples (63) during experimental viral infection. It is not clear if the response to viral infection differs quantitatively or qualitatively compared with normal subjects as there have been conflicting reports in the literature. Inflammatory cell products, such as neutrophil elastase and eosinophil cationic protein, also contribute to the process, and in a sputum study of children with exacerbations, these were found to be elevated compared with the baseline (64). In COPD exacerbations, many proinflammatory mediators have been implicated in the inflammation, including TNF-α, leukotriene B4 (LTB4), epithelial-derived neutrophil attractant-78 (ENA-78), and IL-8. Again, there are conflicting reports regarding their individual roles, but ENA-78 and IL-8 appear to be central to the process.

## V.  Pathophysiology of Exacerbations

### A.  Bronchoconstriction

In the stable state, reversibility of bronchoconstriction is the hallmark of asthma, and although traditionally thought to be less in COPD, it is now acknowledged that a degree of reversibility is often present. During an exacerbation of asthma the reversibility is reduced, and bronchoconstriction contributes significantly to symptoms.

In the stable state, the differing underlying etiology of asthma and COPD result in differences in the mechanisms of bronchoconstriction. In asthma, there is significant smooth muscle hypertrophy, and this is predominately in the larger airways. Smooth muscle enlargement is more significant in the smaller airways in COPD. There are changes in the basement membrane, with hyaline thickening, in asthma, which are not seen in COPD, but the activity of proteases and other cytokines causes more parenchymal destruction in COPD. It is not known if these factors influence airway responsiveness during an exacerbation.

In comparison to asthma, the changes in lung function during exacerbations of COPD are generally smaller and inconsistent, making them less reliable as markers for severity or exacerbation diagnosis. A fall in $FEV_1$ and peak expiratory flow (PEF) reported during COPD exacerbations found a greater recovery in $FEV_1$ when patients were treated with prednisolone compared with placebo (65). Lung volume has been shown to fall during exacerbations as has transfer factor in a group of more severe patients (14); however, several studies have reported no change in $FEV_1/FVC$ ratio during exacerbations, suggesting that falls in $FEV_1$ are due to loss of lung volume rather than increased obstruction (66,67). It is postulated that airway obstruction is present early in mild exacerbations and may lead to air trapping and hyperinflation in more severe exacerbations.

### B.  Dynamic Hyperinflation

Hyperexpansion, and associated diaphragm weakness, is well recognized in COPD patients and is a major contributor to symptoms in the stable state. This has been less clearly investigated in patients with asthma but is likely to play a significant role in disease severity, particularly during acute attacks. A recent study showed dynamic hyperinflation contributed to dyspnea in asthma and was significant even with modest changes in $FEV_1$ (68). Work looking at respiratory muscle training has been shown to reduce residual volume and improve symptoms in both conditions. Air trapping is a major feature of COPD and asthma, where it leads to progressive restriction. Air hunger and difficult inspiration are recognized in asthmatic subjects.

### C.  Mucus Hypersecretion

In comparison to bronchoconstriction and inflammation, mucus hypersecretion is under-recognized as a pathological mechanism in airway disease. Few therapies specifically target this, but it contributes to the pathophysiology of both asthma and COPD (69). Increased sputum production and goblet cell hyperplasia are seen in both conditions. However, the mucus in asthmatic subjects is more viscous with subsequent mucus plugging, which is not seen in patients with COPD. It has been suggested that this difference occurs as a result of intrinsic differences in mucin production. Rhinovirus has been shown to increase expression of mucin genes and so stimulate mucus production. This has been demonstrated in vitro (70) and in vivo (71) and may represent an important mechanism of virus-induced exacerbations.

## VI. Conclusion

Exacerbations in asthma and COPD have similar etiology, with viral infection as the major contributor. Despite some similarities in the pathophysiology and mechanisms of exacerbations, there are significant differences that remain poorly understood. Finally, treatment strategies for exacerbations remain suboptimal and reflect a major unmet need in health care provision. We hope that a better understanding of the mechanisms driving exacerbations will lead to development of better treatment approaches.

### References

1. Seemungal Terence AR, Donaldson Gavin C, Paul Elizabeth A, et al. Effect of exacerbation on quality of life in patients with chronic obstructive pulmonary disease. Am J Respir Crit Care Med 1998; 157:1418–1422.
2. Smith David H, Malone Daniel C, Lawson Kenneth A, et al. A national estimate of the economic costs of asthma. Am J Respir Crit Care Med 1997; 156:787–793.
3. Rennard SI, Farmer SG. Exacerbations and progression of disease in asthma and chronic obstructive pulmonary disease. Proc Am Thorac Soc 2004; 1:88–92.
4. Johnston NW. The similarities and differences of epidemic cycles of chronic obstructive pulmonary disease and asthma exacerbations. Proc Am Thorac Soc 2007; 4:591–596.
5. Johnston SL, Pattemore PK, Sanderson G, et al. The relationship between upper respiratory infections and hospital admissions for asthma: a time-trend analysis. Am J Respir Crit Care Med 1996; 154:654–660.
6. Johnston SL, Pattemore PK, Sanderson G, et al. Community study of role of viral infections in exacerbations of asthma in 9-11 year old children. BMJ 1995; 310:1225–1229.
7. Rohde G, Wiethege A, Borg I, et al. Respiratory viruses in exacerbations of chronic obstructive pulmonary disease requiring hospitalisation: a case-control study. Thorax 2003; 58:37–42.
8. Johnston N, Johnston S, Duncan J, et al. The september epidemic of asthma exacerbations in children: a search for etiology (see comment). J Allergy Clin Immunol 2005; 115:132–138.
9. Fabbri L, Beghe B, Caramori G, et al. Similarities and discrepancies between exacerbations of asthma and chronic obstructive pulmonary disease. Thorax 1998; 53:803–808.
10. Moorman JE, Rudd RA, Johnson CA, et al. National surveillance for asthma—United States, 1980 to 2004. MMWR Surveill Summ 2007; 56:1–54.
11. Miravitlles M, Guerrero T, Mayordomo C, et al. Factors associated with increased risk of exacerbation and hospital admission in a cohort of ambulatory COPD patients: a multiple logistic regression analysis. The EOLO Study Group. Respiration 2000; 67:495–501.
12. Boudreaux ED, Emond SD, Clark S, et al. Acute asthma among adults presenting to the emergency department: the role of race/ethnicity and socioeconomic status. Chest 2003; 124:803–812.
13. Wilson DH, Tucker G, Frith P, et al. Trends in hospital admissions and mortality from asthma and chronic obstructive pulmonary disease in Australia, 1993–2003. Med J Aust 2007; 186:408–411.
14. Papi A, Bellettato CM, Braccioni F, et al. Infections and airway inflammation in chronic obstructive pulmonary disease severe exacerbations. Am J Respir Crit Care Med 2006; 173:1114–1121.

15. D'Amato G, Liccardi G, D'Amato M, et al. Environmental risk factors and allergic bronchial asthma. Clin Exp Allergy 2005; 35:1113–1124.
16. Green RM, Custovic A, Sanderson G, et al. Synergism between allergens and viruses and risk of hospital admission with asthma: case-control study. BMJ 2002; 324:763.
17. Murray CS, Poletti G, Kebadze T, et al. Study of modifiable risk factors for asthma exacerbations: virus infection and allergen exposure increase the risk of asthma hospital admissions in children. Thorax 2006; 61:376–382.
18. Lemanske RF, Vrtis RF, Busse WW, et al. Rhinovirus upper respiratory infection increases airway hyperreactivity and late asthmatic reactions. J Clin Invest 1989; 83:1–10.
19. Calhoun W, Dick EE, Schwartz L, et al. A common cold virus, rhinovirus 16, potentiates airway inflammation after segmental antigen bronchoprovocation in allergic subjects. J Clin Invest 1994; 94:2200–2208.
20. Chanez P. Immunological intervention with anti-immunoglobulin-E antibody to prevent asthma exacerbations. Eur Respir J 2001; 18:249–250.
21. Zambrano J, Carper H, Rakes G, et al. Experimental rhinovirus challenges in adults with mild asthma: response to infection in relation to IgE. J Allergy Clin Immunol 2003; 111:1008–1016.
22. Chauhan AJ, Inskip HM, Linaker CH, et al. Personal exposure to nitrogen dioxide ($NO_2$) and the severity of virus-induced asthma in children. Lancet 2003; 361:1939–1944.
23. McCreanor J, Cullinan P, Nieuwenhuijsen MJ, et al. Respiratory effects of exposure to diesel traffic in persons with asthma. N Engl J Med 2007; 357:2348–2358.
24. Elliott P, Shaddick G, Wakefield JC, et al. Long-term associations of outdoor air pollution with mortality in Great Britain. Thorax 2007; 62:1088–1094.
25. Byrd RS, Joad JP. Urban asthma. Curr Opin Pulm Med 2006; 12:68–74.
26. Nightingale JA, Maggs R, Cullinan P, et al. Airway inflammation after controlled exposure to diesel exhaust particulates. Am J Respir Crit Care Med 2000; 162:161–166.
27. Nordenhall C, Pourazar J, Ledin MC, et al. Diesel exhaust enhances airway responsiveness in asthmatic subjects. Eur Respir J 2001; 17:909–915.
28. Seemungal TA, Harper-Owen R, Bhowmik A, et al. Detection of rhinovirus in induced sputum at exacerbation of chronic obstructive pulmonary disease. Eur Respir J 2000; 16:677–683.
29. Kling S, Donninger H, Williams Z, et al. Persistence of rhinovirus RNA after asthma exacerbation in children. Clin Exp Allergy 2005; 35:672–678.
30. Wark PAB, Johnston SL, Moric I, et al. Neutrophil degranulation and cell lysis is associated with clinical severity in virus-induced asthma. Eur Respir J 2001; 19:68–75.
31. Grissell TV, Powell H, Shafren DR, et al. Interleukin-10 gene expression in acute virus-induced asthma. Am J Respir Crit Care Med 2005; 172:433–439.
32. Message SD, Laza-Stanca V, Mallia P, et al. Rhinovirus induced lower respiratory illness is increased in asthma and related to virus load and Th1/2 cytokine and IL-10 production. Proc Natl Acad Sci U.S.A. 2008, in press.
33. Corne JM, Marshall C, Smith S, et al. Frequency, severity, and duration of rhinovirus infections in asthmatic and non-asthmatic individuals: a longitudinal cohort study. Lancet 2002; 359:831–834.
34. Papadopoulos NG, Stanciu LA, Papi A, et al. A defective type 1 response to rhinovirus in atopic asthma. Thorax 2002; 57:328–332.
35. Contoli M, Message SD, Laza-Stanca V, et al. Role of deficient type III interferon-lambda production in asthma exacerbations. Nat Med 2006; 12:1023–1026.
36. Wark PA, Johnston SL, Bucchieri F, et al. Asthmatic bronchial epithelial cells have a deficient innate immune response to infection with rhinovirus. J Exp Med 2005; 201:937–947.
37. Monso E, Ruiz J, Rosell A, et al. Bacterial infection in chronic obstructive pulmonary disease. A study of stable and exacerbated outpatients using the protected specimen brush. Am J Respir Crit Care Med 1995; 152:1316–1320.
38. Sethi S, Evans N, Grant BJB, et al. New strains of bacteria and exacerbations of chronic obstructive pulmonary disease. N Engl J Med 2002; 347:465–471.

39. Ram FS, Rodriguez-Roisin R, Granados-Navarrete A, et al. Antibiotics for exacerbations of chronic obstructive pulmonary disease. Cochrane Database Syst Rev 2006; 2:CD004403.
40. Stockley RA, O'Brien C, Pye A, et al. Relationship of sputum color to nature and outpatient management of acute exacerbations of COPD. Chest 2000; 117:1638–1645.
41. Stolz D, Christ-Crain M, Bingisser R, et al. Antibiotic treatment of exacerbations of COPD: a randomized, controlled trial comparing procalcitonin-guidance with standard therapy. Chest 2007; 131:9–19.
42. Diederen BMW, van der Valk PDLPM, Kluytmans JAWJ, et al. The role of atypical respiratory pathogens in exacerbations of chronic obstructive pulmonary disease. Eur Respir J 2007; 30:240–244.
43. Johnston SL, Martin RJ. Chlamydophila pneumoniae and mycoplasma pneumoniae: a role in asthma pathogenesis? Am J Respir Crit Care Med 2005; 172:1078–1089.
44. Cunningham AF, Johnston SL, Julious SA, et al. Chronic chlamydia pneumoniae infection and asthma exacerbations in children. Eur Respir J 1998; 11:345–349.
45. Johnston SL, Blasi F, Black PN, et al. The effect of telithromycin in acute exacerbations of asthma. N Engl J Med 2006; 354:1589–1600.
46. Wilkinson TMA, Hurst JR, Perera WR, et al. Effect of interactions between lower airway bacterial and rhinoviral infection in exacerbations of COPD. Chest 2006; 129:317–324.
47. Saetta M, Di Stefano A, Maestrelli P, et al. Airway eosinophilia in chronic bronchitis during exacerbations. Am J Respir Crit Care Med 1994; 150:1646–1652.
48. Balbi B, Bason C, Balleari E, et al. Increased bronchoalveolar granulocytes and granulocyte/macrophage colony-stimulating factor during exacerbations of chronic bronchitis. Eur Respir J 1997; 10:846–850.
49. Bhowmik A, Seemungal TAR, Sapsford RJ, et al. Relation of sputum inflammatory markers to symptoms and lung function changes in COPD exacerbations. Thorax 2000; 55:114–120.
50. Fujimoto K, Yasuo M, Urushibata K, et al. Airway inflammation during stable and acutely exacerbated chronic obstructive pulmonary disease. Eur Respir J 2005; 25:640–646.
51. Djukanovic R, Roche WR, Wilson JW, et al. Mucosal inflammation in asthma. Am Rev Respir Dis 1990; 142:434–457.
52. Bousquet J, Chanez P, Lacoste JY, et al. Eosinophilic inflammation in asthma. N Engl J Med 1990; 323:1033–1039.
53. Wenzel SE, Schwartz LB, Langmack EL, et al. Evidence that severe asthma can be divided pathologically into two inflammatory subtypes with distinct physiologic and clinical characteristics. Am J Respir Crit Care Med 1999; 160:1001–1008.
54. Lams BE, Lee TH, Sousa AR, et al. Subepithelial immunopathology of the large airways in smokers with and without chronic obstructive pulmonary disease. Eur Respir J 2000; 15:512–516.
55. Grumelli S, Green L, Bag R, et al. An immune basis for lung parenchymal destruction in chronic obstructive pulmonary disease and emphysema. PLoS Med 2004; 1:e8. (Epub 2004, Oct 19.)
56. Ito K, Caramori G, Lim S, et al. Expression and activity of histone deacetylases in human asthmatic airways. Am J Respir Crit Care Med 2002; 166:392–396.
57. Ito K, Ito M, Elliott WM, et al. Decreased histone deacetylase activity in chronic obstructive pulmonary disease. N Engl J Med 2005; 352:1967–1976.
58. Slevogt H, Schmeck B, Jonatat C, et al. Moraxella catarrhalis induces inflammatory response of bronchial epithelial cells via MAPK and NF-{kappa}B activation and histone deacetylase activity reduction. Am J Physiol Lung Cell Mol Physiol 2006; 290:L818–L826.
59. Watanabe T, Jono H, Han J, et al. Synergistic activation of NF-{kappa}B by nontypeable Haemophilus influenzae and tumor necrosis factor {alpha}. Proc Natl Acad Sci U S A 2004; 101:3563–3568.
60. Laza-Stanca V, Stanciu LA, Message SD, et al. Rhinovirus replication in human macrophages induces NF-{kappa}B-dependent tumor necrosis factor alpha production. J Virol 2006; 80:8248–8258.

61. Aaron SD, Angel JB, Lunau M, et al. Granulocyte inflammatory markers and airway infection during acute exacerbation of chronic obstructive pulmonary disease. Am J Respir Crit Care Med 2001; 163:349–355.

62. Fleming HE, Little FF, Schnurr D, et al. Rhinovirus-16 colds in healthy and in asthmatic subjects: similar changes in upper and lower airways. Am J Respir Crit Care Med 1999; 160: 100–108.

63. Grunberg K, Smits Hermelijn H, Timmers Mieke C, et al. Experimental rhinovirus 16 infection. Effects on cell differentials and soluble markers in sputum in asthmatic subjects. Am J Respir Crit Care Med 1997; 156:609–616.

64. Norzila MZ, Fakes K, Henry RL, et al. Interleukin-8 secretion and neutrophil recruitment accompanies induced sputum eosinophil activation in children with acute asthma. Am J Respir Crit Care Med 2000; 161:769–774.

65. Davies L, Angus RM, Calverley PM. Oral corticosteroids in patients admitted to hospital with exacerbations of chronic obstructive pulmonary disease: a prospective randomised controlled trial. Lancet 1999, (354), 456–460.

66. Parker CM, Voduc N, Aaron SD, et al. Physiological changes during symptom recovery from moderate exacerbations of COPD. Eur Respir J 2005; 26:420–428.

67. Stevenson NJ, Walker PP, Costello RW, et al. Lung mechanics and dyspnea during exacerbations of chronic obstructive pulmonary disease. Am J Respir Crit Care Med 2005; 172:1510–1516.

68. Lougheed MD, Fisher T, O'Donnell DE. Dynamic hyperinflation during bronchoconstriction in asthma: implications for symptom perception. Chest 2006; 130:1072–1081.

69. Rogers DF. Airway mucus hypersecretion in asthma: an undervalued pathology? Curr Opin Pharmacol 2004; 4:241–250.

70. Inoue D, Yamaya M, Kubo H, et al. Mechanisms of mucin production by rhinovirus infection in cultured human airway epithelial cells. Respir Physiol Neurobiol 2006; 154:484–499.

71. Yuta A, Ali M, Van Deusen M, et al. Rhinovirus infection induces mucus hypersecretion. Am J Physiol 1998; 274:L1017–L1023.

# 18

## Risk Factors for Hospital Admission

**JUDITH GARCIA-AYMERICH**

Centre for Research in Environmental Epidemiology (CREAL), Institut Municipal d'Investigació Mèdica (IMIM), Barcelona, Spain

## I. Methodological Introduction

### A. Hospital Admission as Surrogate of COPD Exacerbation

An exacerbation of chronic obstructive pulmonary disease (COPD) may appear in a wide range of presentations from increased symptoms to hospitalizations, respiratory failure, and death (1). Accordingly, the definition of exacerbations both for clinical purposes and in research has been controversial (2). Because identification of exacerbations may be difficult and costly, many epidemiological studies have used hospital admissions due to COPD exacerbations as a surrogate of exacerbation.

However, one should keep in mind that "a hospital admission for a COPD exacerbation" is not strictly equivalent to "a COPD exacerbation." First, it is likely that only the severe COPD exacerbations need hospitalization. Actually, it has been reported that patients only seek medical attention in half of their exacerbations (3). Second, the hospitalization could be subjected to factors not related to the severity of the exacerbation, mainly those related to accessibility to hospital care. Third, there are several limitations when hospital admissions are obtained from administrative databases, such as the need of validating diagnoses and the need of taking into account readmissions by counting as a unique admission other admissions that occurred in a short period of time (e.g., less than 14 days) (4). Finally, it is likely that new schemes to manage exacerbations, such as hospital at home, make necessary a change in the identification of COPD exacerbations from health care databases.

Despite the mentioned limitations, many interventional and observational studies have used hospital admissions to investigate the determinants of COPD exacerbation. One of the advantages of this approach is that, although validity should always be tested, information from databases is not subjected to patients' criteria (as in a symptoms diary) and usually involves a medical diagnosis. Thus, it is less likely to produce misclassification. Moreover, the hospital admission is a relevant event in the evolution of COPD both for the patient and the health services. Finally, it is a practical, unambiguous, and cheap approach to identify exacerbations (2).

## B.  The Concept of Risk Factor

A risk factor of a given outcome is defined as a factor that is statistically associated with an increased frequency of the outcome, being such association not explained by confounding, bias, or chance (5). Broadly speaking, the term risk factor can be used for factors non-causally or (directly or indirectly) causally associated with the outcome (6,7).

In the study of hospital admissions for a COPD exacerbation, the term "risk factor" is used for any individual characteristic (environmental, social, clinical, functional, health services related, or other) that has been statistically associated with an increased probability or frequency of COPD hospital admissions. For some of the described risk factors, such as many functional variables, a causal association with the exacerbation is biologically plausible. For other factors (e.g., quality of life or anxiety), the observed association is likely mediated by a higher probability of admission, given the same severity of exacerbation. It is also possible that some risk factors, such as comorbidities, may act through an increase in both the risk of the exacerbation and the probability of being admitted.

"Modifiability" of the risk factors is another important concept, where "modifiable" refers both to the factor and the risk). Some of the factors reviewed below, specifically those related to lifestyle, should be considered amenable to modification, and therefore their identification is very useful both for the patient and the health services, given the potential benefit of their modification.

## C.  Methodological Issues in the Studies of Risk Factors for COPD Admission

Although a large body of literature on COPD exacerbations is available, the number of studies aimed to assess which are the risk factors of hospital admission for an exacerbation is relatively small. The present chapter excludes factors that, although likely related to the risk of admission for a COPD exacerbation, have been covered in depth elsewhere in this volume: air pollutants, respiratory infections, and health services–related factors (influenza and pneumococcal vaccination, long-term oxygen therapy, respiratory rehabilitation, health education, alternative models of COPD care, and pharmacological treatment). Studies about risk factors for relapse (a readmission within a short period of time after an index admission) have also been excluded. Table 1 summarizes the studies finally included. Some of their main characteristics are discussed below to facilitate the interpretation of results.

### Research Objective

Most of the studies in Table 1 have aimed to assess the effect of a single factor on hospital admission for a COPD exacerbation on the basis of a priori hypotheses. These single factors include nutritional status (8–10), quality of life (11,12), muscle force (13), anxiety and depression (14), physical activity (15,16), and exercise tolerance (17). Strength of this kind of studies relies on the fact that they were hypothesis based, so they were theoretically designed to optimally answer their specific research question. However, because a multi-factorial view of the exacerbation was generally not considered, the associated variables could be surrogates of the true risk factors. Additionally, results could have been biased because of the lack of adjustment for potential confounders not included in the studies.

A second group of studies was designed specifically with the aim of explaining what the risk factors of hospital admission for a COPD exacerbation are, through the study of a

**Table 1** Studies of Sociodemographic, Clinical, Functional, and Lifestyle Risk Factors of Hospital Admission for a COPD Exacerbation, After Excluding Studies Concerning Factors Covered in Depth in Other Chapters (Air Pollution, Infections, and Health Services–Related Factors)

| Ref. | Author year, journal | Design | Study population | Risk factors of interest (potential confounders considered)[a] |
|---|---|---|---|---|
| Research objective: single factor approach | | | | |
| 8 | Braun 1984, Chest | Cohort, 6 mo follow-up | 39 COPD patients from outpatient clinic, U.S.A. | Weight, **triceps skin fold**, midarm muscle circumference (sex, age, dyspnea, $FEV_1$, daily caloric intake) |
| 11 | Osman 1997, Thorax | Cohort, 1 yr follow-up | 266 COPD patients from hospital, U.K. | **Quality of life** (sex, age, smoking, $FEV_1$, FVC) |
| 13 | Decramer 1997, Eur Respir J | Case-control (admitted/not admitted previous 1 yr) | 57 (23 cases and 34 controls) male COPD patients from outpatient clinic, Belgium | MIP, MEP, QF ($FEV_1$, $TL_{CO}$, FRC, dyspnea, serum electrolytes, blood gases, walking distance) |
| 12 | Fan 2002, Chest | Cohort, 1 yr follow-up | 3282 COPD patients from primary care centres, U.S.A. | **Quality of life** (**age**, distance to hospital, working status, smoking, **steroids use**, comorbidities, **previous COPD admission**) |
| 9 | Chailleux 2003, Chest | Cohort, 7.5 yr follow-up | 4088 patients with chronic bronchitis or emphysema and LTOT treatment from a LTOT database, France | **BMI** (age, sex, $FEV_1$, $FEV_1/VC$, **VC**, **$PaO_2$**) |
| 10 | Ringbaek 2004, Chron Respir Dis | Cohort, 6 yr follow-up | 221 COPD patients with LTOT treatment from a LTOT database, Denmark | **BMI, oral corticosteroids** (inhaled corticosteroids, smoking, ECG, weight, height, $FEV_1$, **blood gases, outdoor activity, performance status**) |
| 14 | Gudmunsson 2005, Eur Respir J | Cohort, 1 yr follow-up | 406 COPD patients from hospitals, Iceland, Sweden, Denmark, Finland, and Norway | **Anxiety and depression, quality of life** (**age**, sex, smoking, education, cohabitation, **previous COPD hospitalizations, $FEV_1$**, FVC, LTOT, comorbidities, medications ($β_2$-agonists, anticholinergics, methilxanthines, inhaled and oral corticosteroids)) |

*(Continued)*

**Table 1** Studies of Sociodemographic, Clinical, Functional, and Lifestyle Risk Factors of Hospital Admission for a COPD Exacerbation, After Excluding Studies Concerning Factors Covered in Depth in Other Chapters (Air Pollution, Infections, and Health Services–Related Factors) (*Continued*)

| Ref. | Author year, journal | Design | Study population | Risk factors of interest (potential confounders considered)[a] |
|---|---|---|---|---|
| 15 | Garcia-Aymerich 2006, Thorax | Cohort, 20 yr follow-up | 2386 COPD subjects from the general population, Denmark | **Physical activity** (**age**, gender, education, marital status, cohabitation, income, dyspnea, **sputum**, chest pain, leg pain, intermittent claudication, asthma, **ischemic heart disease**, myocardial infarction, stroke, diabetes, **smoking**, alcohol, **visits to doctor**, blood pressure, plasma cholesterol, glucose, body mass index, **FEV₁**, FVC) |
| 16 | Pitta 2006, Chest | Cohort, 1 yr follow-up | 17 COPD patients from a hospital, Belgium | **Physical activity** (sex, age, BMI, FFM, FEV₁, FVC, FRC, TLC, DLco, MIP, MEP, QF, PaO₂, PaCO₂, **walking distance**) |
| 17 | Emtner 2007, Respir Med | Cohort, 1 yr follow-up | 21 COPD patients from a hospital, Sweden | **Walking distance** (age, sex, smoking status, FEV₁, BMI, LTOT, **quality of life, SpO₂ at rest, SpO₂ at exercise**) |

Research objective: multiple factors (comprehensive) approach

| Ref. | Author year, journal | Design | Study population | Risk factors of interest (potential confounders considered)[a] |
|---|---|---|---|---|
| 18 | Kessler 1999, Am J Respir Crit Care Med | Cohort, 2.5 yr follow-up | 64 COPD patients from outpatient clinic, France | Age, smoking status, comorbidities, BMI, dyspnea, walking distance, VC, FEV₁, PaO₂, **PaCO₂**, ***Ppa at rest***, *Ppa* at exercise, CT score emphysema, LTOT. |
| 19 | Miravitlles 2000, Respiration | Cross-sectional, admissions previous 1 yr | 713 COPD patients from primary care centers, Spain | Age, sex, BMI, **FEV₁**, smoking, sputum, **comorbidities** |

| # | Reference | Design | Patients | Factors |
|---|---|---|---|---|
| 20 | Garcia-Aymerich 2001, Am J Respir Crit Care Med | Case-control (admitted/stable) | 172 (86 cases and 86 controls) COPD patients from hospitals, Spain | Sex, age, marital status, working activity, education, socioeconomic status, cohabitation, **previous COPD admissions, FEV$_1$, FEV$_1$/FVC, PaO$_2$, PaCO$_2$**, comorbidities, BMI, reformed primary care, **cared by a generalist or respiratory specialist**, medication ($\beta_2$-agonists, **anticholinergics**, methilxanthines, inhaled and oral corticosteroids, and antibiotics), influenza and pneumococcal vaccination, respiratory rehabilitation, **LTOT appropriateness**, adherence to medication, correctness in the inhaler, **smoking**, alcohol consumption, sedatives consumption, **usual physical activity**, quality of life, difficulty to take medication, social support. |
| 21 | Garcia-Aymerich 2003, Thorax | Cohort, 2 yr follow-up | 340 COPD patients from hospital, Spain | |
| 22 | Roberts 2002, Thorax | Cohort, 3 mo follow-up | 1400 COPD patients from 38 hospitals, U.K. | Sociodemographic data[b], symptoms[b], management[b], **previous COPD admissions, FEV$_1$, performance status, medications**[b] |

[a] In **bold:** factors independently associated with COPD admission, according to multivariate analysis of each study.
[b] Not detailed in the original paper.

*Abbreviations*: LTOT, long-term oxygen therapy; FEV$_1$, forced expiratory volume in 1 second; FVC, forced vital capacity; MIP, maximal inspiratory pressure; MEP, maximal expiratory pressure; QF, quadriceps force; TL$_{CO}$, transfer factor of the lungs for carbon monoxide; FRC, functional residual capacity; BMI, body mass index; VC, vital capacity; PaO$_2$, arterial oxygen pressure; ECG, electrocardiogram; FFM, fat-free mass; TLC, total lung capacity; DL$_{CO}$, carbon monoxide diffusion capacity; PaCO$_2$, arterial carbon dioxide pressure; SpO$_2$, oxygen saturation; $P$pa, pulmonary artery pressure; CT, computerized tomography.

(narrower or wider) range of potential risk factors. First, a hospital sample of 64 COPD patients was followed for 2.5 years, with a special focus on pathophysiological characteristics (18). Another study in the primary care setting compared, retrospectively, several clinical characteristics between 713 admitted and nonadmitted COPD patients (19). The Study of the Risk Factors of COPD Exacerbation (EFRAM study) included a case control (*n* = 172) and a follow-up (*n* = 340) of COPD patients and a very wide range of potential risk factors of COPD admission (20,21). An audit from the United Kingdom also aimed at identifying risk factors for COPD admission in 1400 COPD patients followed for three months, driven by the need of identifying deficiencies in the process of care (22). These studies, in general, provided a better control for confounders than the previous group. In many cases, the inclusion of potential risk factors was based on a revision of the literature and clear a priori hypotheses about plausibility of the associations with COPD admission. However, other potential risk factors were suggested by experts, despite lack of previous evidence, so the associations, if found, should had been interpreted as "hypothesis generating" that would need replication.

### Design

All the studies alluded to above are observational, most of them being cohort studies. Those with a cross-sectional (19) or case-control (13,20) design should be interpreted with caution, given that whether the presence of the risk factor preceded or followed the exacerbation cannot be established.

### Study Population

Patients in these studies have been recruited from a broad range of sources: general population (15), primary care (12,19), outpatient clinics (8,13,18), hospitals (11,14,16,17,20–22), or oxygen national databases (9,10). It is likely that many characteristics of the patients, including severity of COPD, vary from one setting to another. Therefore, a given risk factor could yield different results among settings when, for instance, its distribution in a specific setting leads to a small proportion of subjects in the level of exposure that is associated with the admission and when the study does not have enough statistical power.

## II. Risk Factors of Hospital Admission for a COPD Exacerbation

### A. Sociodemographic Factors

#### Age

Among the several effects of the aging process, likely the most relevant for COPD patients is lung function decline (23). Thus, it could be expected that age is associated with COPD progression, including increased risk of COPD admission for an exacerbation. However, most of the above-mentioned studies found no relation between age and the risk of COPD admission (8–11,16–21), and only three of them found an increased risk with increasing age (12,14,15). One possible explanation for these controversial findings is that all studies have considered lung function as a risk factor for COPD admission. Thus, if the role of age is supposedly mediated by lung function, the joint inclusion of both factors in a multivariate model would drop age from the model. Another plausible explanation is that hospital-based samples may have a more limited range of age than primary care– or population-based samples. Thus, when the age range is narrow, it is not possible to find statistical differences even when the differences exist, and also the clinical decision to hospitalize may be more related to other individual characteristics than the differences in age. In the population-based samples with a wide range of most individual characteristics, even after controlling for lung function, age may still be associated with the admission either because it acts as a marker of unknown pathophysiological risk factors or influences the clinical decision.

### Sex

Females showed a higher risk of hospital admission for COPD in the 7 to 16 years of follow-up of two population-based samples in Denmark ($n = 13897$) (24) after adjusting for smoking. However, since this study included subjects from the general population, it is likely that the observed data reflect an association between sex and COPD development in the general population rather than between sex and COPD admission in COPD subjects. Actually, none of the reported studies in COPD patients found an association between sex and COPD admission (8–12,14–22).

### Socieconomic Status

Education and income were first described as associated with COPD hospital admission in the 17 years of follow-up of the population-based ($n = 14223$ subjects) Copenhagen City Heart Study (25). Authors suggested that the link could be multifactorial, including housing conditions, air pollution, diet, or other lifestyle factors (26). Again, this association could reflect socioeconomic differences in the risk of COPD development, rather than differences in the risk of admission. In fact, neither socioeconomic status, education, and cohabitation nor working activity were related to the risk of hospital admission for a COPD exacerbation in the studies restricted to COPD patients (12,14,15,20–22). Despite the fact that an association with admission has so far not been found, it is important to keep in mind the difficulty of measuring socioeconomic status and the relevance of contextual factors, such as health care availability, that are usually not addressed in individual studies.

### B. Clinical Factors

#### Respiratory Symptoms

Most of the studies did not find associations between the several symptoms explored (dyspnea, sputum, chest pain) and COPD admission (8,13,18,19,22), with the only exception being of sputum in a population-based study (15). These controversial results suggest that in samples of COPD subjects with a wide range of severity, and predominance of mild forms of the disease, symptoms may discriminate the severity of COPD with respect to events in the prognosis. However, when samples include mainly clinically ill patients, the associations disappear because of the limited variability in symptoms and/or because, in advanced stages of the disease, other factors play a more important role.

#### Health-Related Quality of Life

Poor health-related quality of life was related to increased risk of COPD admission in several studies using different methods in different populations and different geographical areas (11,12,14,17), after adjusting for lung function, comorbidities, drug treatment, prior hospitalizations, anxiety and depression, or exercise tolerance. It is interesting to note that in all cases the associations were observed both in the summary score and in the different subscales and that the strongest associations were found for the activity dimensions (12,14). Additionally, both the case-control and cohort components of the EFRAM study found an association between quality of life and COPD admission, although only in the univariate analysis (20,21). Interestingly, quality of life dropped from the multivariate models when physical activity was included, in agreement with the mentioned strongest associations with the activity scales of the quality of life scores. Regarding the mechanism, it is likely that for the same severity of the exacerbation, differences in quality of life may modulate clinical decisions and use of resources.

### Depression and Anxiety

Although psychological status is important in COPD patients (1), only one study has assessed the role of these factors in COPD admission. A strong independent association between anxiety and COPD hospitalization was found, although it was restricted to the subsample with poor quality of life (14). It is plausible that, faced with an exacerbation, anxiety may influence the decision of hospitalization.

### Nutritional Status

Despite the large body of knowledge about the relation between nutritional status and risk of mortality in COPD, the information for hospitalization is scarce. A study considering several measures of nutritional status found only triceps skin fold related to the risk of COPD admission (8). Two studies restricted to COPD patients using long-term oxygen therapy (LTOT) found that low body mass index (BMI) was an independent risk factor for hospitalization (9,10). Another study found this association only in the univariate analysis (18). Most of the remaining studies have considered this factor, but no statistical association has been found after adjustment for other variables (15–17,19–21). It is likely that studies with severely ill patients, such as those using LTOT, include a larger proportion of mal-nourished patients than other type of samples. Then, in the lack of enough variability, differences cannot be statistically detected even if they exist. It is also likely that BMI does not capture the appropriate nutritional information potentially related to the COPD admission, and further studies using body composition measures will provide new results. Actually, low fat-free mass has been related to muscle fatigue (27), which could contribute to the physiological response to an exacerbation and/or to the decision of admission.

### Previous COPD Hospitalizations

Having had previous hospital admissions for COPD has been consistently associated with the risk of COPD admission, irrespective of the study design, population, and setting (12,14,20–22). It has been suggested that "frequent exacerbations" are a consistent feature within a patient, since correlation of exacerbation number from one year to the following was found in a panel study following more than 100 COPD patients for four years (28). In this study, the frequency of exacerbations—defined by symptoms—was related to the frequency of admissions during the same period of time (28). Whether the number of previous COPD admissions or exacerbations is a marker of severity of the disease, not totally explained by forced expiratory volume in one second ($FEV_1$), or is determinant of medical decisions is not known, but most likely both explanations could be true. Another explanation is that in the presence of strong correlation between many different risk factors from susceptibility to lifestyle and environment, autocorrelation of admissions may be consequence of autocorrelation of its determinants.

### Comorbidities

The presence of comorbidities (other chronic medical conditions that affect subjects with COPD) was related to a higher risk of COPD admission in a large primary care sample (19). However, in another primary case-based study and in several hospital-based follow-up studies, there was no association between the presence of or the number of comorbidities and the risk of COPD admission (12,14,18,20,21). It is likely that managing comorbidities as a score does not allow identification of the specific chronic diseases that could affect the risk of COPD exacerbation or admission. The history of ischemic heart disease independently increased the risk of COPD admission in a COPD sample from the general population (15), in agreement with a previous study relating cardiovascular disorders to admissions for chronic bronchitis (29). Although diabetes has been related to more severe exacerbations (30), the studies including diabetes as potential risk factor for admission have not yielded any independent association (15,20,21). The presence of comorbidities could also act by influencing the medical decision in case of exacerbation, partly because it affects quality of life even in mild COPD (31).

### C. Functional Status

### Lung Function

Although the influence of airflow limitation in the risk of COPD admission has been considered controversial (32), the current evidence suggests that it is a strong independent risk factor of this event. Lower $FEV_1$ was independently related to a higher risk of COPD admission in most of the mentioned studies, including different design, settings, and methods, irrespective of many other clinical and functional variables, such as symptoms, quality of life, or blood gas exchange (14,15,19–22). Other studies have reported no differences in the risk of COPD admission according to $FEV_1$ level (8,10,11,13,16–18). However, this lack of association could be the result of a small sample size and/or narrow variability in the lung function level, as already stated by the authors in their corresponding manuscripts. Actually, deterioration of lung function leads to a poor response to the increase of oxygen demand in case of exacerbation, which could relate to the risk of admission (33). Since there is the concern that $FEV_1$ does not completely reflect the respiratory functional status of moderate and severe COPD patients (1), further studies should incorporate complete, both static and dynamic, measures of lung function to better understand their independent role in explaining the risk of admission.

### Blood Gases Exchange and Hemodynamics

Gas exchange impairment (measured as hypoxemia or hypercapnia, at rest or during exercise) and pulmonary hemodynamic worsening (high pulmonary arterial pressure) have been independently associated with a higher risk of COPD hospital admission in several studies, including different designs, settings, and methods (8,10,17,18,20,21). Two studies did not find differences in blood gases between hospitalized and stable patients, but again this could have been the result of a small sample size, inappropriate design, or small variability (13,16). The fact that the described associations were independent of airflow obstruction (8,20,21) is interesting for the interpretation of results and for the consideration of these variables in further studies.

### Muscle Function

Respiratory (maximal inspiratory and expiratory pressures) and peripheral (quadriceps) muscle forces were associated with COPD admission in a case-control study of COPD patients with high use of health care resources compared with a group not admitted in the previous year (13). However, the retrospective nature of this study does not allow identifying whether the muscle weakness was previous or secondary to the admissions. Unfortunately, neither respiratory nor peripheral muscle function has been tested in longitudinal studies as potential risk factors for COPD admission. In favour of the association, one could argue that muscle weakness either relates to more severe disease (which was not the case in the mentioned study) or increases patients' complaints and then the possibility of being admitted to the hospital.

### Exercise Tolerance

Although the role of exercise tolerance in mortality of COPD patients has been tested in several studies, its effect on COPD admission is hardly known. Only four of the studies in Table 1 have tested it. The lack of association between walking distance and COPD admission in a case-control study could be the result of a small sample size, inappropriate design, or small variability (13). A second study found walking distance related to a higher risk of COPD readmission only in the univariate analysis (18). The remaining two studies found an independent association between walking distance and COPD admission in small samples of COPD patients after considering a wide range of potential confounders (16,17). It could be hypothesized that better tolerance to exercise allows for better tolerance to the exacerbation in terms of respiratory and cardiovascular response as well as in terms of patients complaints.

### D.  Lifestyle

### Smoking

It would be plausible that smoking status related to the risk of COPD admission. Quitting smoking, even after the age of 60 years, may reduce the lung function decline (34,35), while current smoking increases the risk for bacterial colonization in stable patients (36). Unfortunately, experimental studies about the effects of quitting smoking on COPD admission are not available, and data from observational studies do not support this hypothesis. Most of the studies previously mentioned have found no effect of smoking on the risk of COPD admission (10,11,14,18,19). More surprisingly, the EFRAM study found that current smoking was associated with a reduced risk of COPD admission (20). It has been discussed whether the benefits of quitting smoking can be compared between subjects with preclinical disease and patients with symptomatic disease, given that the latter most likely quit in response to their symptoms and disability, and they do not do well afterward (37). This could explain why studies of patients with well-established disease would have often not shown a reduction in mortality with smoking cessation (38,39).

### Physical Activity

The EFRAM cohort study first described an association between higher level of usual physical activity and a reduction in the risk of COPD admission (21). Results were highly consistent with those found in a longer follow-up of a large population-based COPD sample and in a small study of hospital-based COPD patients (15,16). In all of them, using different samples and different methods to assess physical activity and being from different environmental and climatic characteristics, the amount of activity needed to obtain a reduction in the admission risk was relatively small (walking or cycling 2 hr/wk or more). Previous studies that found an association between performance status (functional limitation) scores (10,22) and the physical (12) or activity (14) scales in the quality of life questionnaires, with COPD admission, support the described association. The potential mechanisms underlying this association include effects in cardiovascular function, muscle function, exercise capacity, and inflammation, all of them able to modulate the physiological response to an exacerbation.

### Alcohol Consumption

The potential role of high alcohol consumption as a risk factor for COPD admission was tested in few studies, but no statistically independent associations were found (15,20,21).

### Adherence to Medication

Adherence to medication was measured in the EFRAM study using different approaches, but none of them led to differences in the risk of COPD admission (20,21). However, it is interesting to note that an intervention study that reduced the risk of COPD admission (40) also improved treatment adherence and correctness with the inhaler maneuver (41), thus suggesting that better adherence led to a better effect of drugs with a subsequent lower risk of exacerbation.

## III. Conclusion

The present review shows consistent data supporting the fact that the main factors of hospital admission for a COPD exacerbation are those related to the severity of the disease, i.e., previous COPD admissions, lung function, blood gases, or exercise tolerance. Health-related quality of life has also been consistently associated with the risk of admission. Physical activity appears as a consistent modifiable factor that may reduce the risk of admission and therefore would require intervention. All these factors are likely to be both risk factors of the exacerbation through pathophysiological mechanisms and risk factors of the admission in the case that an exacerbation appears. The fact that most of them are strongly correlated has so far made difficult the identification of the independent contribution of each one to the risk of COPD admission. Further longitudinal studies including a large number of patients as well as a wide range of variability for most of these factors are still needed. Age and symptoms seem playing a role only when the range of severity is wide, as in the primary care or the population-based samples. The effects of BMI, comorbidities, or muscle function in the COPD admission cannot be interpreted, because of a small number of studies or inappropriate methodological approaches, and need further research. A better knowledge about risk factors of COPD admission is necessary both to prevent admissions by changing modifiable risk factors and to identify targets for a better management and evaluation of treatment.

## References

1. Celli BR, Macnee W, and committee members of the ATS/ERS Task force. Standards for the diagnosis and treatment of patients with COPD: a summary of the ATS/ERS position paper. Eur Respir J 2004; 23:932–946.
2. Pauwels R, Calverley P, Buist AS, et al. COPD exacerbations: the importance of a standard definition. Respir Med 2004; 98(2):99–107.
3. Seemungal TA, Donaldson GC, Bhowmik A, et al. Time course and recovery of exacerbations in patients with chronic obstructive pulmonary disease. Am J Respir Crit Care Med 2000; 161(5):1608–1613.
4. Burge S, Wedzicha JA. COPD exacerbations: definitions and classifications. Eur Respir J 2003; 21(suppl 41):46s–53s.
5. Kesley JL, Thompson WD, Evans AS. Biological and statistical concepts. In: Kesley JL, Thompson WD, Evans AS, eds. New York, NY: Oxford University Press, 1986:23–45.
6. Kleinbaum DG, Kupper LL, Morgenstern H. Confounding. In: Kleinbaum DG, Kupper LL, Morgenstern H, eds. Epidemiologic Research. Belmont, California: Lifetime Learning Publications, 1982:242–265.
7. Abramson JH. Formulating the objectives. In: Abramson JH, ed. Survey Methods in Community Medicine, 2nd ed. Edinburgh: Churchill Livingstone, 1979:22–28.
8. Braun SR, Dixon RM, Keim NL, et al. Predictive clinical value of nutritional assessment factors in COPD. Chest 1984; 85(3):353–357.
9. Chailleux E, Laaban JP, Veale D. Prognostic value of nutritional depletion in patients with COPD treated by long-term oxygen therapy: data from the ANTADIR observatory. Chest 2003; 123(5):1460–1466.
10. Ringbaek TJ, Viskum K, Lange P. BMI and oral glucocorticoids as predictors of prognosis in COPD patients on long-term oxygen therapy. Chron Respir Dis 2004; 1 (2):71–78.
11. Osman IM, Godden DJ, Friend JA, et al. Quality of life and hospital re-admission in patients with chronic obstructive pulmonary disease. Thorax 1997; 52(1):67–71.
12. Fan VS, Curtis JR, Tu SP, et al. Using quality of life to predict hospitalization and mortality in patients with obstructive lung diseases. Chest 2002; 122(2):429–436.
13. Decramer M, Gosselink R, Troosters T, et al. Muscle weakness is related to utilization of health care resources in COPD patients. Eur Respir J 1997; 10(2):417–423.
14. Gudmundsson G, Gislason T, Janson C, et al. Risk factors for rehospitalisation in COPD: role of health status, anxiety and depression. Eur Respir J 2005; 26(3):414–419.
15. Garcia-Aymerich J, Lange P, Benet M, et al. Regular physical activity reduces hospital admission and mortality in chronic obstructive pulmonary disease: a population based cohort study. Thorax 2006; 61(9):772–778.
16. Pitta F, Troosters T, Probst VS, et al. Physical activity and hospitalization for exacerbation of COPD. Chest 2006; 129(3):536–544.

17. Emtner MI, Arnardottir HR, Hallin R, et al. Walking distance is a predictor of exacerbations in patients with chronic obstructive pulmonary disease. Respir Med 2007; 101(5):1037–1040.
18. Kessler R, Faller M, Fourgaut G, et al. Predictive factors of hospitalization for acute exacerbation in a series of 64 patients with chronic obstructive pulmonary disease. Am J Respir Crit Care Med 1999; 159(1):158–164.
19. Miravitlles M, Guerrero T, Mayordomo C, et al. Factors associated with increased risk of exacerbation and hospital admission in a cohort of ambulatory COPD patients: a multiple logistic regression analysis. The EOLO Study Group. Respiration 2000; 67(5):495–501.
20. Garcia-Aymerich J, Monso E, Marrades RM, et al. Risk factors for hospitalization for a chronic obstructive pulmonary disease exacerbation. EFRAM study. Am J Respir Crit Care Med 2001; 164(6):1002–1007.
21. Garcia-Aymerich J, Farrero E, Felez MA, et al. Risk factors of readmission to hospital for a COPD exacerbation: a prospective study. Thorax 2003; 58(2):100–105.
22. Roberts CM, Lowe D, Bucknall CE, et al. Clinical audit indicators of outcome following admission to hospital with acute exacerbation of chronic obstructive pulmonary disease. Thorax 2002; 57(2):137–141.
23. Burrows B, Cline MG, Knudson RJ, et al. A descriptive analysis of the growth and decline of the FVC and FEV1. Chest 1983; 83(5):717–724.
24. Prescott E, Bjerg AM, Andersen PK, et al. Gender difference in smoking effects on lung function and risk of hospitalization for COPD: results from a Danish longitudinal population study. Eur Respir J 1997; 10(4):822–827.
25. Prescott E, Lange P, Vestbo J. Socioeconomic status, lung function and admission to hospital for COPD: results from the Copenhagen City Heart Study. Eur Respir J 1999; 13(5):1109–1114.
26. Prescott E, Vestbo J. Socioeconomic status and chronic obstructive pulmonary disease. Thorax 1999; 54(8):737–741.
27. Engelen MP, Schols AM, Baken WC, et al. Nutritional depletion in relation to respiratory and peripheral skeletal muscle function in out-patients with COPD. Eur Respir J 1994; 7(10):1793–1797.
28. Donaldson GC, Seemungal TA, Bhowmik A, et al. Relationship between exacerbation frequency and lung function decline in chronic obstructive pulmonary disease. Thorax 2002; 57(10): 847–852.
29. Ball P, Harris JM, Lowson D, et al. Acute infective exacerbations of chronic bronchitis. QJM 1995; 88(1):61–68.
30. Loukides S, Polyzogopoulos D. The effect of diabetes mellitus on the outcome of patients with chronic obstructive pulmonary disease exacerbated due to respiratory infections. Respiration 1996; 63(3):170–173.
31. Ferrer M, Alonso J, Morera J, et al. Chronic obstructive pulmonary disease stage and health-related quality of life. The Quality of Life of Chronic Obstructive Pulmonary Disease Study Group. Ann Intern Med 1997; 127(12):1072–1079.
32. Wouters EF. Management of severe COPD. Lancet 2004; 364(9437):883–895.
33. Barberà JA, Roca J, Ferrer A, et al. Mechanisms of worsening gas exchange during acute exacerbations of chronic obstructive pulmonary disease. Eur Respir J 1997; 10(6);1285–1291.
34. Fletcher C, Peto R. The natural history of chronic airflow obstruction. Br Med J 1977; 1(6077): 1645–1648.
35. Higgins MW, Enright PL, Kronmal RA, et al. Smoking and lung function in elderly men and women. The Cardiovascular Health Study. JAMA 1993; 269(21):2741–2748.
36. Monsó E, Rosell A, Bonet G, et al. Risk factors for lower airway bacterial colonization in chronic bronchitis. Eur Respir J 1999; 13(2):338–342.
37. Anthonisen NR. Smoking, lung function, and mortality. Thorax 2000; 55(9):729–730.
38. Burrows B, Earle RH. Prediction of survival in patients with chronic airway obstruction. Am Rev Respir Dis 1969; 99(6):865–871.

39. Anthonisen NR, Wright EC, Hodgkin JE. Prognosis in chronic obstructive pulmonary disease. Am Rev Respir Dis 1986; 133(1):14–20.

40. Casas A, Troosters T, Garcia-Aymerich J, et al. Integrated care prevents hospitalisations for exacerbations in COPD patients. Eur Respir J 2006; 28(1):123–130.

41. Garcia-Aymerich J, Hernandez C, Alonso A, et al. Effects of an integrated care intervention on risk factors of COPD readmission. Respir Med 2007; 101(7):1462–1469.

# 19

# Effect of Exacerbations on Disease Progression and Mortality

**JAMES J. P. GOLDRING and GAVIN C. DONALDSON**
Academic Department of Respiratory Medicine, Royal Free and
University College Medical School, London, U.K.

## I. Introduction

The rate of forced expiratory volume in one second ($FEV_1$) decline is a physiological measure of disease progression and is widely used as an outcome measure for clinical trials of chronic obstructive pulmonary disease (COPD) treatment because it is predictive of morbidity, mortality, quality of life, and hospitalization rates (1). Estimates of the decline in $FEV_1$ in nonsmoking men and women vary between 29.6 and 19.6 mL/yr (2,3). The rate of decline classically accelerates with age, but might appear to slow at the very upper end of the age range, as only those people with the slower rates of decline survive.

Smoking accelerates lung function decline, although only 10% to 15% of smokers experience a rate of decline in $FEV_1$ that is fast enough to result in the respiratory impairment and breathlessness that are the symptoms of COPD. The smokers most at risk are those who lose between 50 and 100 mL/yr. Why some COPD patients experience a faster $FEV_1$ decline than others remains elusive. The patients thought to decline fastest are those with either bronchial hyperreactivity or mucus hypersecretion and frequent chest infections. The former is called the "Dutch hypothesis," which suggests that some individuals develop an allergic response to cigarette smoke akin to hyperreactivity in asthma. Some of the evidence involves the finding of increased numbers of peripheral blood eosinophils in COPD patients (4). A number of large follow-up studies have shown an association between airway hyper-reactivity with early development of symptoms and accelerated lung function decline (5). However, these studies may be flawed because of lack of adjustment for baseline $FEV_1$ or retrospective assessment of hyperreactivity. The latter is the so-called British hypothesis, which suggests that mucus hypersecretion as a marker of airway infection leads to lung function decline. A general flaw in this hypothesis is that airway infections can occur without increase or any mucus production. The vast majority of COPD exacerbations are now known to be precipitated by either viral or bacterial infection and the ensuing host inflammatory response (6), and so, the British hypothesis is essentially making the link between exacerbations and lung function decline.

## II.  Studies That Have Investigated the Effect of Exacerbations on Disease Progression

The great London smog between 5 and 9 December, 1952, is still widely quoted as the stimulus for numerous studies into the effects of atmospheric pollutants. It is not however widely known that it also resulted in the establishment of a committee under the British Medical Research Council to fund research into chronic bronchitis. In 1960, this committee funded Fletcher and colleagues (7) to perform a prospective study of the effects of smoking, mucus hypersecretion, and respiratory tract infections on lung function in a group of London workingmen. At this time, the term "exacerbation" was not used in the same context as it is today. Consequently, for this study and subsequent studies thereafter, terms synonymous with lower respiratory tract illness (LRTI) could be interpreted as surrogates for exacerbation.

In the study, 792 postal and transport workers were followed up six monthly over a period of eight years. Sputum volume and spirometry were measured and a questionnaire was used to judge the frequency of LRTI in the preceding six months. Importantly, there was no correlation found between $FEV_1$ decline and either mucus hypersecretion or LRTI after adjusting for age, height, and baseline $FEV_1$. The adjustment for baseline $FEV_1$ was made because the authors noted that a low $FEV_1$ at study entry would in itself be associated with a steeper $FEV_1$ decline over time because it was related to the rate of change of $FEV_1$ prior to the study. It could be argued, however, that a correlation was not seen because the cohort comprised mainly young asymptomatic men with an impressive mean $FEV_1$ of 3.22 L. Additionally, exacerbations were retrospectively self-reported and were therefore likely to have been underreported.

Another prospective cohort study was performed by Howard (8) over a period of 11 years from 1956. In this study, 159 male industrial workers who were "healthy" volunteers completed symptom questionnaires and spirometry periodically. The men self-reported any "chest illness" that had necessitated time off work. In agreement with Fletcher et al. (7), neither mucus hypersecretion nor "chest illness" appeared to be related to $FEV_1$ decline. In contrast, however, there was also no difference in the rate of decline of $FEV_1$ between smokers and nonsmokers. A major confounder might have been high levels of atmospheric pollution in London at the time.

At a similar time, Bates analyzed data on 149 workingmen who were followed up with pulmonary function tests annually for 10 years (9). This time, the men had an established diagnosis of chronic bronchitis, although they had only very mild airflow obstruction, and it was perhaps for this reason that, overall, the $FEV_1$ decline did not differ significantly from the age expected decline. However, the group was not homogenous, and 31 of the men experienced deterioration in one or more of their pulmonary function tests greater than twice predicted. They were age matched to others who showed no such decline, and a paired analysis demonstrated that those with a more rapid lung function decline smoked more cigarettes and had more respiratory symptoms. However, the number of self-reported LRTI and more objectively, the number of days of sick leave was the same for both groups.

So, the earliest studies were restricted to occupational cohorts and appeared to show no association between $FEV_1$ decline and exacerbations. In an attempt to select a more representative population, Kanner et al. (10) recruited 84 patients with COPD through the media and local physicians and recorded interval spirometry over 2 to 10 years. They contacted their cohort weekly by telephone so as to minimize underreporting of exacerbations, which was a limitation of previous studies. They found a mean rate of change of $FEV_1$ of 69.2 mL/yr and demonstrated the following significant associations with $FEV_1$ decline: LRTI ($p < 0.001$), low $\alpha_1$-antitrypsin level, younger age at study entry, longer duration of smoking, greater bronchodilator reversibility, and higher socioeconomic class. These results though have to be interpreted with some caution as patients with coexistent asthma or bronchiectasis were not excluded and the population consisted predominantly of males and those with mild airflow obstruction.

The effect of LRTI and, in particular, its interaction with smoking was revisited more recently in 2001, with an analysis of the Lung Health Study (LHS) data (11). In the analysis, 5887 participants with a mean age of 49 years and a mean $FEV_1$ percentage predicted as 78% were followed up over five years with annual spirometry and symptom questionnaires. Participants were also asked annually to recall any visits that they made to physicians in the preceding year for management of an LRTI. They were categorized as sustained quitters, intermittent smokers, and continuous smokers. The average number of physician visits for LRTI per year for all categories was 0.24, and participants with chronic bronchitis had more than this. Sustained quitters had fewer LRTI and no effect of this was seen on $FEV_1$ decline. However, in both the continuous and intermittent smokers, the estimated effect of one LRTI per year was an additional 7 mL/yr to the average annual lung function decline. A potential source of bias in this study was that participants in the different smoking groups may have had differing health beliefs that might in turn have affected their decision to consult a physician.

The largest study to date of $FEV_1$ decline, COPD exacerbation, and mucus hypersecretion was performed by Vestbo and colleagues (12). They examined a subset of 9435 male and female subjects who were enrolled in the Copenhagen Heart Study and who had had spirometry performed at two visits, five years apart. Subjects with chronic mucus hypersecretion were identified through an MRC (British Medical Research Council) questionnaire and they were noted to have a lower baseline $FEV_1$. Subjects were further categorised by the intensity of their smoking habit and also by whether the mucus hypersecretion was persistent between the visit intervals or whether it had either appeared or disappeared. Combined nonsmokers, nonhypersecretors had an $FEV_1$ decline of 30.0 mL/yr in men and 25.4 mL/yr among women. As expected, smoking was associated with a faster decline in lung function. Mucus hypersecretion was statistically associated with an excess $FEV_1$ decline after adjustment for age, height, smoking status, and weight change, and this was more prominent in males and in those with persisting hypersecretion. So, for males whose mucus hypersecretion was present at both visits, there was an excess decline in $FEV_1$ of 22.8 mL/yr and in females, 12.6 mL/yr. The authors also repeated the whole analysis, taking into account the baseline $FEV_1$ so as to remove this as a potential confounder, but the association remained significant, although slightly weaker, at least among the men. Arguably, this is the only study to date that has demonstrated a positive tripartite relationship between exacerbation, $FEV_1$ decline, and mucus hypersecretion, a relationship previously described in this chapter as the British hypothesis.

Aware of the lack of serial lung function data for subjects with moderate-severe COPD, Donaldson et al. (13) investigated such a group over a four-year period. A strength of this study was that lung function and symptom counts were self-recorded each day and the cohort of 109 patients were instructed to contact the study team as soon as they recognized exacerbation symptoms. Additionally, they were seen three monthly so as not to miss "unreported" exacerbations. Subjects were recruited from National Health Service outpatient clinics. Median age was 68.1 years and $FEV_1$ 1 L and 74% were male. The median exacerbation rate was 2.92, with those experiencing less than this being categorised as "infrequent exacerbators" and those with more labeled as "frequent exacerbators." $FEV_1$ decline in the frequent exacerbators was significantly higher than in the infrequent exacerbators at 40.1 mL/yr versus 32.1 mL/yr. The percentage change in $FEV_1$ over the four years is shown in Figure 1. Although dyspnea and wheeze were significantly more likely in the frequent exacerbators, there were no differences between the groups with respect to age, body mass index, sex, lung function, arterial blood gases, and smoking habits.

A similar study, Makris et al. (14) looked at 102 COPD patients who had six-monthly spirometry over three years. Exacerbations were self-reported by patients who had been instructed to use a diary card to record any change in their respiratory symptoms. The patients' demographics were similar to the Donaldson et al. (13) study, apart from only 38% of the patients being treated with inhaled corticosteroids in contrast to the 92% reported by Donaldson. The median exacerbation rate was also very similar at 2.85/yr. Again, frequent exacerbators had a higher rate of decline in $FEV_1$ compared with patients with infrequent exacerbations. The highest rate of decline was seen in current smokers with frequent exacerbations. In contrast to Kanner (11), there was still a significantly higher $FEV_1$ decline in nonsmoking frequent exacerbators.

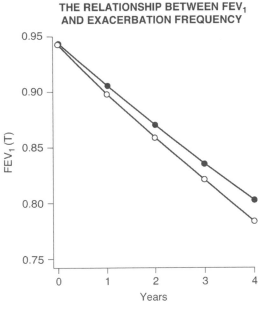

**Figure 1**   Absolute change in $FEV_1$ with standard errors over 4 years. (*Open circles*) Infrequent exacerbators. (*Closed circles*) Frequent exacerbators. *Source*: From Ref. 13.

## III. Studies That Have Investigated the Mechanisms Behind FEV$_1$ Decline in COPD Exacerbations

One of the earliest papers to ascribe a more rapid FEV$_1$ decline to increased airway inflammation was that by Stanescu et al. (15). Forty-six male ex-steelworkers who were a mixture of current smokers and ex-smokers were followed up over 15 years. The median age at entry was 49 years, and the FEV$_1$ percentage predicted was 86.4%. Pulmonary function tests and induced sputum were obtained at entry and again at 6, 13, and 15 years later. The average decline in FEV$_1$ was 19.4 mL/year. A significantly higher percentage of sputum neutrophils were found in those with airway obstruction and also those with mucus hypersecretion. Importantly, the rate of decline in FEV$_1$ was correlated with the percentage neutrophils.

Donaldson et al. (16) looked at the relationship between airway and systemic inflammation, but in an arguably more defined COPD population and with a larger panel of markers. In the study, 148 patients with COPD and median FEV$_1$ 0.98 were followed up for a median of 2.91 years with FEV$_1$ measurement taken at least three monthly. Sputum was collected for bacteria, neutrophil count, interleukin 6 (IL-6), IL-8 and blood was collected for fibrinogen. Both the sputum and blood inflammatory markers gradually increased with time and were higher still at exacerbation. The rise in IL-6 and fibrinogen was significantly faster in the frequent exacerbators. Furthermore, following adjustment for smoking, gender, and baseline FEV$_1$, higher inflammatory markers, with the exception of IL-8, and higher bacterial loads were associated with a significantly faster decline in FEV$_1$. Thus, this study provides a mechanism to link exacerbations to FEV$_1$ decline via the increased bacterial load and systemic and airway inflammation that occurs at exacerbation.

The relationship between bacterial load and FEV$_1$ decline had already been alluded to in an earlier study (17). Here 30 patients, again with moderate-severe COPD, were followed up over a year. The mean annual rate of decline in FEV$_1$ was 57.6 mL/yr. Sputum was obtained either by spontaneous expectoration or by induction at the beginning and at the end of the study. All sputum samples grew significant numbers of bacteria with a mean bacterial count of $10^{7.47}$ colony forming units mL$^{-1}$ suggesting lower airway bacterial colonization. Patients with an increasing airway bacterial load demonstrated a more severe decline in FEV$_1$ over the study period compared with those patients with stable or decreasing bacterial load. In addition, the 50% of patients whose airway bacteria species changed from the first sample to the second exhibited a significantly greater FEV$_1$ decline.

Viruses are also likely to play a role in promoting airway inflammation, which in turn accelerates FEV$_1$ decline (18). Over a two-year period, 241 stable state sputum samples from 74 patients with mild-to-moderate COPD were collected three monthly either by spontaneous expectoration or by sputum induction. Polymerase chain reaction (PCR) was used to detect respiratory syncytial virus (RSV). Sputum IL-6, IL-8, myeloperoxidase (MPO), and bacterial load were also measured. RSV was detected in 32.8% of samples. This rate was the approximately the same regardless of the time of year the sample was taken. Patients were divided into two groups on the basis of whether less than or equal to 50% of their sputum samples were RSV-PCR positive or more than 50% of their samples were RSV-PCR positive and were referred to as the "low RSV" and "high RSV" group, respectively. After accounting for differences in smoking status, bacterial load, exacerbation frequency, and baseline FEV$_1$ between the two groups, the FEV$_1$ decline for the high

RSV group was 114.7 mL/yr as compared with the low RSV group whose $FEV_1$ declined at a rate of 56.6 mL/yr ($p < 0.05$). Furthermore, detection of RSV was associated with higher levels of IL-6, IL-8, and MPO and also of bacterial load.

In summary, $FEV_1$ decline appears greatest in those COPD patients with greater airway inflammation as assessed by neutrophil count and sputum IL-6, which might be due to the presence of chronic infections with bacteria or RSV.

## IV.  Evidence from Other Diseases That Lung Function Decline is Related to Infection and Inflammation

If the hypothesis that inflammation arising from respiratory infections hastens lung function decline is correct, then a similar effect would be expected in patients with other respiratory diseases.

### A.  Asthma

A recent study of 93 asthmatic patients showed that those who experienced fewer (<0.1/yr) severe exacerbations, requiring either hospitalization or involving a drop in $FEV_1$ of 500 mL or 20%, had a smaller decline in $FEV_1$ of 14.6 mL/yr [95% confidence interval (CI) 1.9–27.3] compared with patients experiencing more frequent exacerbations, who had a decline of 31.5 mL/yr (95% CI 18.2–44.8). The difference between the groups was 16.9 mL/yr (95% CI 1.5–32.2; $p = 0.03$) (19).

### B.  Cystic Fibrosis

A common feature of cystic fibrosis is colonization of the lungs with *Pseudomonas aeruginosa*. There are various clinical stages in the infection, starting with first detection of *P. aeruginosa*, colonization, first mucoid detection, and chronic mucoid colonization. A comparison of the two years preceding transition with the subsequent two years were for the last two stages associated with a significant worsening in the annual rate of change in $FEV_1$. For transition to first mucoid PA detection, there was a mean annual change of 4.6% (percentage predicted) to −4.3% and for the transition to chronic mucoid PA colonization a change from 7.3% to −4.8% (20).

## V.  Effects of Exacerbation on Mortality

The inhospital mortality rate following an admission for an acute exacerbation of COPD (AECOPD) ranges from 2.5% (21) to 11% (22) depending on the population studied, and almost half of patients admitted for an AECOPD are dead within two years (22).

There are many determinants related to survival following an AECOPD such as patient age (22), hypoxia (22), hypercapnia (23), and comorbidity (24), and these factors largely reflect disease severity. However, until recently it has not been clear whether the exacerbation event per se is independently related to mortality. Soler-Cataluña and colleagues (25) investigated this specific question in a study of 302 all-male participants. In the first year, a record was kept of all exacerbations requiring inpatient or outpatient management, enabling classification of the cohort into frequent, infrequent, and non-exacerbators. In the five-year follow-up period, 116 deaths (38.2%) were recorded. The frequent and infrequent exacerbators had a significantly higher risk of death than the nonexacerbators, with hazard ratios of 4.13 and 2.00, respectively, and this was independent of age, comorbidity, body mass index, $FEV_1$, partial pressure of oxygen ($PaO_2$), partial pressure of carbon dioxide ($PaCO_2$), and use of long-term oxygen therapy. Thus, this study would appear to suggest that exacerbations themselves adversely affect prognosis.

Indirect evidence of the effect of exacerbation frequency on mortality was also seen in the much-debated TORCH (TOwards a Revolution in COPD Health) trial (26). This randomized controlled trial, the largest of its kind, set out to analyze the effects of pharmacological intervention, namely salmeterol and fluticasone propionate, on all-cause mortality in COPD patients over a period of three years. These medications, either on their own or in combination, significantly reduced the annual rate of exacerbations and when used in combination there was a nonsignificant ($p = 0.052$) but nevertheless remarkable 17.5% reduction in mortality.

## VI.  Summary

Over the last three decades, there has been increasing recognition of the importance of COPD exacerbations, their relationship to airway infection, and the host response and their contribution to important outcome measures such as lung function decline and mortality.

### References

1. Wise RA. The value of forced expiratory volume in 1 second decline in the assessment of chronic obstructive pulmonary disease progression. Am J Med 2006; 119:S4–S11.
2. Johannessen A, Lehmann S, Omenaas ER, et al. Post-bronchodilator spirometry reference values in adults and implications for disease management. Am J Respir Crit Care Med 2006; 173(12):1316–1325.
3. Roca J, Burgos F, Sunyer M, et al. References values for forced spirometry. Eur Respir J 1998; 11: 1354–1362.
4. Perng DW, Huang HY, Chen HM, et al. Characteristics of airway inflammation and bronchodilator reversibility in COPD: a potential guide to treatment. Chest 2004; 126(2):375–381.
5. Postma DS, Boezen HM. Rationale for the Dutch hypothesis. Allergy and airway hyperresponsiveness as genetic factors and their interaction with environment in the development of asthma and COPD. Chest 2004; 126(2 suppl):S96–S104.
6. Papi A, Bellettato CM, Braccioni F, et al. Infections and airway inflammation in chronic obstructive pulmonary disease severe exacerbations. Am J Respir Crit Care Med 2006; 173:1114–1121.
7. Fletcher C, Peto R, Tinker C, et al. The Natural History of Chronic Bronchitis and Emphysema. Oxford: Oxford University Press; 1976.
8. Howard P. A long-term follow-up of respiratory symptoms and ventilatory function in a group of working men. Br J Ind Med 1970; 27:326–333.
9. Bates DV. The fate of the chronic bronchitic: a report of the ten-year follow-up in the Canadian department of veteran's affairs coordinated study of chronic bronchitis. Am Rev of Respir Dis 1973; 108:1043–1065.
10. Kanner R, Renzettin A, Klauber M, et al. Variables associated with changes in spirometry in patients with obstructive lung diseases. Am J Med 1979; 67:44–50.

11. Kanner RE, Anthonisen NR, Connet JE. Lower respiratory illnesses promote $FEV_1$ decline in current smokers but not ex-smokers with mild chronic obstructive pulmonary disease. Am J Respir Crit Care Med 2001; 164:358–364.

12. Vestbo J, Prescott E, Lange P. Association of chronic mucus hypersecretion with $FEV_1$ decline and chronic obstructive pulmonary disease morbidity. Am J Respir Crit Care Med 1996; 143:1530–1535.

13. Donaldson GC, Seemungal TA, Bhowmik A, et al. Relationship between exacerbation frequency and lung function decline in chronic obstructive pulmonary disease. Thorax 2002; 57:847–852.

14. Makris D. Moschandreas J, Damianaski A, et al. Exacerbations and current lung function decline in COPD: New insights in current and ex-smokers. Resp Med 2007; 101:1305–1312.

15. Stanescu D, Sanna A, Veriter C, et al. Airways obstruction, chronic expectoration, and rapid decline of $FEV_1$ in smokers are associated with increased levels of sputum neutrophils. Thorax 1996; 51:267–271.

16. Donaldson GC, Seemungal TAR, Patel IS, et al. Airway and systemic inflammation and decline in lung function in chronic obstructive pulmonary disease. Chest 2005; 128:1995–2004.

17. Wilkinson TMA, Patel IS, Wilks M, et al. Airway bacterial load and $FEV_1$ decline in patients with chronic obstructive pulmonary disease. Am J Respir Crit Care Med 2003; 167:1090–1095.

18. Wilkinson TMA, Donaldson GC, Johnston SL, et al. Respiratory syncytial virus, airway inflammation and $FEV_1$ decline in patients with chronic obstructive pulmonary disease. Am J Respir Crit Care Med 2006; 173:871–876.

19. Bai TR, Vonk JM, Postma DS, et al. Severe exacerbations predict excess lung function decline in asthma. Eur Respir J 2007; 30(3):452–457.

20. Ballmann M, Rabsch P, von der Hardt H. Long-term follow up of changes in FEV1 and treatment intensity during Pseudomonas aeruginosa colonization in patients with cystic fibrosis. Thorax 1998; 53(9):732–737.

21. Patil SP, Krishnan JA, Lechtzin N, et al. In-hospital mortality following acute exacerbations of COPD. Arch Intern Med 2003; 163:1180–1186.

22. Connors AF, Dawson NV, Thomas C, et al. Outcomes following acute exacerbation of severe chronic obstructive pulmonary disease. Am J Respir Crit Care Med 1996; 154:959–967.

23. Groenewegen KH, Schols AMWJ, Wouters E. Mortality and mortality-related factors after hospitalization for acute exacerbation of COPD. Chest 2003; 124:459–467.

24. Incalzi RA, Fuso L, DeRosa M, et al. Co-morbidity contributes to predict mortality of patients with chronic obstructive pulmonary disease. Eur Respir J 1997; 10:2794–2800.

25. Soler-Cataluña JJ, Martinez-Garcia MA, Roman Sanchez P, et al. Severe acute exacerbations and mortality in patients with chronic obstructive pulmonary disease. Thorax 2005; 60:925–931.

26. Calverly PMA, Anderson JA, Celli BC, et al. Salmeterol and fluticasone propionate and survival in chronic obstructive pulmonary disease. N Engl J Med 2007; 356:775–789.

# 20
# Health Economic Consequences of COPD Exacerbations

**MARC MIRAVITLLES**
Department of Pneumology, Clinical Institute of Thorax (IDIBAPS), Hospital Clínic, Barcelona, Spain

## I. Introduction

Obstructive lung diseases, particularly chronic obstructive pulmonary disease (COPD), are one of the main causes of morbidity and mortality in developed countries. It is estimated that more than 15 million persons in the United States suffer from COPD and more than 12 million from chronic bronchitis (1). Furthermore, the number of individuals affected has grown over recent decades. The age-adjusted mortality rate from COPD doubled from 1970 to 2002 in the United States, whereas rates from stroke and heart disease decreased by 63% and 52%, respectively (2).

The prevalence of COPD in Spain is 9% in adults aged between 40 and 70 years, although only 22% are diagnosed (3). The situation in the future will not improve. A recent international survey showed that up to 11.8% of subjects aged between 20 and 44 years had GOLD (Global Initiative for Chronic Obstructive Lung Disease) stage 0 COPD, characterised by chronic respiratory symptoms and 3.6% had GOLD stages I to III COPD with impairment in lung function (4), which is remarkable, considering the young age of the participants.

Considering its high prevalence and the chronic and progressive course of COPD, it is easy to understand that this disease represents a high societal and economic burden. Exacerbations, particularly the most severe that require hospital admission, are the main cause of the high use of resources generated by these patients (5,6). A significant proportion of hospitalizations derive from failure of ambulatory treatment of exacerbations. Different studies consistently show a failure rate of ambulatory treatment of exacerbations that ranges from 15% to 26% (7,8). Relapse after initial treatment for acute exacerbation may lead to prolonged disability, impairment in health-related quality of life (HRQL), and increased costs (9).

## II. Costs of COPD

It is necessary to understand the high burden associated with the management of COPD before analyzing the impact of exacerbations. Studies of the costs of COPD have been performed in different countries using different methodology (1).

An example of the variation that can be observed in the calculation of costs is provided by the analysis of different studies in the same country, as in Spain. Using statistical and epidemiological data, one study reported costs figures of around €800 million annually in 1994 (10), including both direct and indirect costs. In a follow-up study performed in 1510 patients with ambulatory COPD followed over one year, the average direct annual cost per patient was of $1876 (for 2001) (11). With this data, it is possible to estimate from the focus of prevalence the approximate annual cost generated by COPD in Spain. Considering the estimated number of patients diagnosed with COPD (3) multiplied by the annual average, a total of $506.52 million annually in direct health care costs generated by COPD is obtained. It is interesting to compare the distribution of the costs obtained in both models. The hospital costs, mainly derived from exacerbations constituted between 36.3% and 43% of the total costs (10,11).

Other European studies have found higher costs. A prospective study in Italy on a cohort of 268 patients found a mean annual direct cost of €3040, and hospital admissions accounted for 40% of the total amount (12). Costs obtained in France were a mean of €2863 per patient per year with approximately 36% generated by hospitalizations. The costs derived from attention to the patients with COPD, not restricted to the cost of treating COPD accounted for 3.5% of the total medical expenditures (13). A population-based study in Denmark attributed a total cost of COPD for the whole country of €256 million, or 6% of the total annual cost of treating the population of 40 years or more, which represents a mean of €4436 per patient per year with COPD (14), very similar to the cost in France.

The economic impact of COPD in 1993 was estimated to be more than $15.5 billion in the United States, with $6.1 billion for hospitalization (1). In a study undertaken in the United States in a cohort of 413 patients with COPD, direct costs were found to range from $1681 for mild patients to $5037 for moderate and $10,812 for severe patients (15). These costs are higher than those observed in Spain and more similar to those observed in France, Denmark, and Italy, which may be due to a variety of factors among which the most important is the selection of patients from a population with COPD registered either in the hospital or the community. Other studies carried out regarding the cost of COPD in different countries are shown in Table 1.

All estimates indicate that the situation will not improve in the near future. The impact of aging and changes in smoking habits are responsible for an estimated increase of more than 60% of total life years lost and an increased loss of 75% of disability-adjusted life years from 1990 to 2020 in the Netherlands (16). New projections performed until 2025 provide similar results with an increase in prevalence and costs of COPD, despite the campaigns against tobacco smoking (17)

## III.  Economic Impact of Exacerbations

Exacerbations are a frequent event in the natural history of COPD. Patients included in clinical trials have a frequency of 0.8 to 2.5 exacerbations per year (18). The mortality of patients admitted to hospital with a COPD exacerbation is about 10% to 14% and the mortality of those admitted to an intensive care unit (ICU) for exacerbations may be as high as 24% (18).

A study performed in the United States on the basis of national statistics estimated that the total burden of exacerbations was $1592 million (for 1995) (5). Mean cost of an

**Table 1** Comparison of the Costs Published on COPD in Different Countries

| Reference | Country | Costs | Cost/patient/yr | Global cost/yr |
|---|---|---|---|---|
| Morera, 1992 (10) | Spain | Direct and indirect | €959 | Direct €319 M<br>Indirect €541 M |
| Sullivan, 2000 (40) | United States | Direct | $2300 | $1700 M |
| Hilleman, 2000 (15) | United States | Direct | Stage I = $1681<br>Stage II = $5037<br>Stage III=$10,812 | |
| Jacobson, 2000 (21) | Sweden | Direct and indirect | | Direct €109 M<br>Indirect €541 M |
| Wilson, 2000 (22) | United States | Direct | Emphysema $1341<br>Chronic Bronchitis $816 | $14,500 M |
| Rutten van Mölken, 2000 (41) | Netherlands | Direct | $876 | |
| Dal Negro, 2001 (42) | Italy | Direct | Stage I= €151<br>Stage II= €3001<br>Stage III= €3912 | |
| Jansson, 2002 (43) | Sweden | Direct and indirect | $1284 | $871 M |
| Miravitlles, 2003 (11) | Spain | Direct | Stage I= €1185<br>Stage II= €1640<br>Stage III= €2333 | €427 M |
| Masa, 2004 (20) | Spain | Direct | €909.5 | €238.8 M |
| Izquierdo, 2004 (29) | Spain | Direct | Stage I= €1657<br>Stage II= €2425<br>Stage III= €3303 | |
| Borg, 2004 (44) | Sweden | Direct and indirect | Direct costs<br>GOLD I= €92<br>GOLD II= €631<br>GOLD III= €2144<br>GOLD IV= €8678 | |
| Detournay, 2004 (13) | France | Direct | €2863 | €3500 M |
| Koleva, 2007 (12) | Italy | Direct | GOLD I= €1046<br>GOLD II= €2319<br>GOLD III= €3752<br>GOLD IV= €5033 | |
| Bilde, 2007 (14) | Denmark | Direct (COPD and non–COPD related) | €4436 | €256 M |

$ = costs in U.S. dollars
M = million
€ = costs in Euro
*Abbreviations*: COPD, chronic obstructive pulmonary disease; GOLD, Global Initiative for Chronic Obstructive Lung Disease.

exacerbation managed in outpatient clinic was $159, and interestingly, drug costs represented only 11.2% of the costs in inpatients and 15% in outpatients (5). The average cost of hospitalization for COPD in a cohort of severe patients in the Unites States was estimated to be $7100 (19). Some studies have determined that hospitalization costs represent between 40% and 65% of total direct costs generated by patients with COPD (11,12,20–22) and this percentage may be as high as 63% in severe patients (21). Since acute exacerbations are the main cause of hospitalization among COPD patients, it can be concluded that the economic burden of acute exacerbations is considerable. However, only a small proportion of exacerbations require hospitalization. A recent observational study performed in a cohort of COPD patients followed by primary care physicians observed that 22% were admitted during one year (23). In another prospective study performed in primary care, 16.5% of all exacerbations required hospital admission (8). The costs of exacerbations that require hospitalization increase dramatically compared with those that can be treated in an ambulatory setting. Another analysis derived from a clinical trial in patients with COPD demonstrated that 15% of exacerbations, that is, those requiring admission, generated 90% of the costs associated with exacerbations (24). In fact, a small group of COPD patients may generate most of the hospital visits and admissions. This highly demanding population usually has an older age, more severe indices of bronchial obstruction, and more hypoxemia at rest (25). In addition, a previous admission is a risk factor for higher use of health care resources and costs in the future (26). Previous hospitalization and frequent exacerbations are also significant and independent risk factors for failure in future exacerbations of COPD (27).

A Swedish study observed that exacerbations accounted for 35% to 45% of the total per capita health care costs for COPD (28). Another report observed that exacerbations generated a mean yearly cost of €415 in severe patients, €382 in moderate patients, and €228 in mild patients (29).

The mean total cost of an acute exacerbation of COPD was estimated to be $159 in a study on primary care in Spain, the main part being due to hospitalizations that represented 58% of the total cost, followed by the total drug acquisition cost of 32.2% (6). Interestingly, this was exactly the same estimate obtained by Niederman et al. (5) for the United States in 1995 using a different methodology. Using the unit costs in different Latin American countries and applying the same method of cost calculation, estimates of the cost of exacerbations may be obtained for these countries. A large variation exists, based mainly on the large differences in costs for health care resources. The highest cost was observed in Argentina, with an equivalent to $329 (of year 2000), and the lowest in Colombia, with $98 (30). A summary of studies reporting costs of exacerbations of COPD is presented in Table 2.

Another example of the high burden of exacerbations of COPD derives from the calculation of the excess cost generated by this patient population compared with a control population without the disease. This exercise was performed for England and Wales from 1994 to 1995 and the total excess cost of primary care associated with exacerbations was calculated at £35.7 million (31). The largest component of primary care costs was the excess cost of all prescription medicines, which totaled £27.8 million and the excess cost arising from inpatient hospital episodes included £8.3 million (31).

Failure implies a significant increase in costs of exacerbation. The cost of failure depends on disease severity in the study population. In a study on respiratory infections in one general practice, Davey et al (32) observed that repeated consultation due to failure

**Table 2** Comparison of the Costs of Exacerbations of COPD in Different Countries

| Study (ref.) | Country | Design | Setting | Cost/episode |
|---|---|---|---|---|
| Connors, 1996 (19) | United States | Observational study in 5 hospitals | Admitted patients with pCO₂>50 mm Hg | Median cost $7100 (IQ range $4100–$16,000) |
| Niederman, 1999 (5) | United States | Estimation from national statistics | Inpatients and outpatients with chronic bronchitis | Hospital cost (>65 yr) $5497. Ambulatory $159 |
| McGuire, 2001 (31) | United Kingdom | Prevalence-based, excess-cost-of-illness analysis based on national statistics | Primary care | Excess cost associated with AECB was £35.7 M/yr |
| Andersson, 2002 (28) | Sweden | Mail survey to 202 patients with COPD | Outpatients and inpatients | Mean cost SEK 3,163. Ranging from mild exacerbations SEK 120 to severe SEK 21,852 |
| Grassi, 2002 (45) | Italy | Randomised, open label clinical trial | Inpatients and outpatients | Moxifloxacin treated €1993 and ceftriaxone treated €2219 |
| Miravitlles, 2002 (6) | Spain | Observational study on 2414 patients | Outpatients in primary care | Exacerbation cost $159. Cost per failure $477.5 |
| Miravitlles, 2003 (30) | Latin America | Estimation from local statistics | Outpatients in primary care | Costs ranged from $98 in Colombia to $329 in Argentina. Failure accounted for 52% of costs |
| Borg, 2004 (44) | International | Computer simulation model | Outpatients and inpatients | Mild SEK 191, moderate SEK 2111, severe SEK 21,852 |
| Izquierdo, 2004 (29) | Spain | Observational study on 570 patients | Outpatients | Mild COPD €228/yr; moderate COPD €382/yr and severe COPD €415/yr |
| Llor, 2004 (46) | Spain | Observational study on 1456 patients | Outpatients in primary care | Mean cost €118.6 (95% CI 92.2–144.9) |
| Oostenbrink, 2004 (24) | Netherlands and Belgium | Randomised clinical trial with 519 patients | Outpatients | Mean cost €720. Ranging from €86 in mild to €4007 in severe exacerbations |

*Abbreviation:* SEK, Swedish krone.

incurred a maximum cost of £28.54, including indirect costs. It is of note that their population included patients of all ages with a great variety of respiratory infections, some of which were benign. This population of previously well patients with lower respiratory tract disease has demonstrated a very low rate of relapse. In contrast, patients with exacerbated COPD treated in the community present a failure rate ranging from 15% to 26% (7,8) and costs of failure represent from 40% to 65% of the total costs associated with treatment of ambulatory patients (11,12,20–22). As an example, from the total mean cost obtained of $159 in a large study in the community, $100.3 were derived from the cost of relapse. Ideally, if relapse in the global population were completely avoided, the mean cost of exacerbation would be reduced to only $58.7, or in the case that the relapse rate could be reduced by half, costs would be reduced to $107 (6). On the basis of these results, it can be speculated that a new treatment that is able to reduce failure rate, particularly in severe patients with high risk of hospitalization, may easily be a cost-effective strategy (33). Factors associated with high cost of exacerbations include severity indices of the baseline disease, of the exacerbation, and the antibiotic choice, such as use of long-term home oxygen, increased need of rescue bronchodilators, and the use of a less active antibiotic (33,34).

Other strategies that have been useful in reducing the costs associated with exacerbations include the implementation of measures aimed at reducing the length of stay in hospital for exacerbated patients. Supported discharge (35,36) and programs of home hospitalization using well-defined criteria to identify suitable patients in the early phase of clinical stability (37) have demonstrated to effectively reduce the length of stay and costs. Another area of interest is the implementation of self-management plans for patients with previous hospitalization for COPD. When a case manager is assigned to follow up 50 patients per year, the self-management intervention will be cost saving relative to usual care, with a cost-saving of $2149 per patient per year and a cost of $1326 per prevented hospitalization (38). This cost is clearly inferior to the cost of an admission for COPD. Finally, organizational aspects of the hospitals are crucial for the saving of important resources. A U.K. national audit in 234 hospitals showed that the length of stay was reduced in units with more respiratory consultants, better organization of care scores, an early discharge scheme, and local COPD management guidelines (39). Therefore reducing costs of exacerbations of COPD should be centered not only in reducing their frequency and severity, but also in improving the standards of care of hospitalized patients.

## IV.  Conclusions

The costs of management of acute exacerbations of COPD are high and are so particularly due to the high costs associated with relapse. Strategies to improve the outcome of ambulatory treatment of exacerbations may easily be cost-effective, especially in more severe patients who are at increased risk of hospital admission because of therapeutic failure.

Appropriate treatment of baseline disease and self-management plans have been successful in reducing the frequency of exacerbations. Strategies aimed at improving the standards of care of hospitalized patients have demonstrated to be cost saving.

Economic evaluation of the new treatments is increasingly recognized as an important part of the evaluation of new drugs, not only by the health care payers, but also by clinicians. Researchers must provide the data necessary for these analyses to be adequately performed.

## References

1. Chapman KR, Mannino DM, Soriano JB, et al. Epidemiology and costs of chronic obstructive pulmonary disease. Eur Respir J 2006; 27:188–207.
2. Jemal A, Ward E, Hao Y, et al. Trends in the leading causes of death in the United States, 1970–2002. JAMA 2005; 294:1255–1259.
3. Sobradillo V, Miravitlles M, Gabriel R, et al. Geographical variations in prevalence and under-diagnosis of COPD. Results of the IBERPOC multicentre epidemiological study. Chest 2000; 118:981–989.
4. De Marco R, Accordini S, Cerveri I, et al. An international survey of chronic obstructive pulmonary disease in young adults according to GOLD stages. Thorax 2004; 59:120–125.
5. Niederman MS, McCombs JS, Unger AN, et al. Treatment cost of acute exacerbations of chronic bronchitis. Clin Ther 1999; 21:576–591.
6. Miravitlles M, Murio C, Guerrero T, et al. Pharmacoeconomic evaluation of acute exacerbations of chronic bronchitis and COPD. Chest 2002; 121:1449–1455.
7. Adams SG, Melo J, Luther M, et al. Antibiotics are associated with lower relapse rates in outpatients with acute exacerbations of COPD. Chest 2000; 117:1345–1352.
8. Miravitlles M, Murio C, Guerrero T. Factors associated with relapse after ambulatory treatment of acute exacerbations of chronic bronchitis. A prospective multicenter study in the community. Eur Respir J 2001; 17:928–933.
9. Doll H, Miravitlles M. Quality of life in acute exacerbations of chronic bronchitis and chronic obstructive pulmonary disease: a review of the literature. Pharmacoeconomics 2005; 23:345–363.
10. Morera Prat J. Enfermedad pulmonar obstructiva crónica. Magnitud del problema. En: Enfermedad Pulmonar Obstructiva Crónica. Conceptos Generales. Vol. 1. Barcelona: MCR, 1992:57–65.
11. Miravitlles M, Murio C, Guerrero T, et al. Costs of chronic bronchitis and COPD. A one year follow-up study. Chest 2003; 123:784–791.
12. Koleva D, Motterlini N, Banfi P, et al. Healthcare costs of COPD in Italian referral centres: a prospective study. Respir Med 2007; 101: 2312–2320.
13. Detournay B, Pribil C, Fournier M, et al. The SCOPE study: health-care consumption related to patients with chronic obstructive pulmonary disease in France. Value Health 2004; 7:168–174.
14. Bilde L, Svenning AR, Dollerup J, et al. The cost of treating patients with COPD in Denmark: a population study of COPD patients compared with non-COPD controls. Respir Med 2007; 101:539–546.
15. Hilleman DE, Dewan N, Malesker M, et al. Pharmacoeconomic evaluation of COPD. Chest 2000; 118:1278–1285.
16. Feenstra TL, van Genugten MLL, Hoogenveen RT, et al. The impact of aging and smoking on the future burden of chronic obstructive pulmonary disease. Am J Respir Crit Care Med 2001; 164:590–596.
17. Hoogendoorn M, Rutten-van Mölken MPMH, Hoogenveen RT, et al. A dynamic population model of disease progression in COPD. Eur Respir J 2005; 26:223–233.
18. Donaldson GC, Wedzicha JA. COPD exacerbations. 1: epidemiology. Thorax 2006; 61:164–168.
19. Connors AF Jr., Dawson NV, Thomas C, et al. Outcomes following acute exacerbation of severe chronic obstructive pulmonary disease. Am J Respir Crit Care Med 1996; 154:959–967.
20. Masa JF, Sobradillo V, Villasante C, et al. Costs of chronic obstructive pulmonary disease in Spain: estimation from a population-based study. Arch Bronconeumol 2004; 40:72–79.
21. Jacobson L, Hertzman P, Löfdahl CG, et al. The economic impact of asthma and chronic obstructive pulmonary disease (COPD) in Sweden in 1980 and 1991. Respir Med 2000; 94:247–255.
22. Wilson L, Devine EB, So K. Direct medical costs of chronic obstructive pulmonary disease: chronic bronchitis and emphysema. Respir Med 2000; 94:204–213.
23. Miravitlles M, Mayordomo C, Artés M, et al. Treatment of chronic obstructive pulmonary disease and its exacerbations in general practice. Respir Med 1999; 93:173–179.

24. Oostenbrink JB, Rutten-van Mölken MPMH. Resource use and risk factors in high-cost exacerbations of COPD. Respir Med 2004; 98; 883–891.

25. Soler JJ, Sánches L, Latorre M, et al. The impact of COPD on hospital resources: the specific burden of COPD patients with high rates of hospitalization. Arch Bronconeumol 2001; 37:375–381.

26. Mapel DW, McMillan GP, Frost FJ, et al. Predicting the costs of managing patients with chronic obstructive pulmonary disease. Respir Med 2005; 99: 1325–1333.

27. Miravitlles M, Llor C, Naberan K, et al. Variables associated with recovery from acute exacerbations of chronic bronchitis and chronic obstructive pulmonary disease. Respir Med 2005; 99: 955–965.

28. Andersson F, Borg S, Jansson S-A, et al. The costs of exacerbations in chronic obstructive pulmonary disease (COPD). Respir Med 2002; 96: 700–708.

29. Izquierdo-Alonso JL, de Miguel-Díez J. Economic impact of pulmonary drugs on direct costs of stable chronic obstructive pulmonary disease. J COPD 2004; 1: 215–223.

30. Miravitlles M, Jardim JR, Zitto T, et al. Pharmacoeconomic study of antibiotic therapy for exacerbations of chronic bronchitis and chronic obstructive pulmonary disease in Latin America. Arch Bronconeumol 2003; 39: 549–553.

31. McGuire A, Irwin DE, Fenn P, et al. The excess cost of acute exacerbations of chronic bronchitis in patients aged 45 and older in England and Wales. Value in Health 2001; 4: 370–375.

32. Davey PG. Cost management in community-acquired lower respiratory tract infection. Am J Med 1995; 99(suppl 6B):20S–23S.

33. Simoens S, Decramer M, Laekeman G. Economic aspects of antimicrobial therapy of acute exacerbations of COPD. Respir Med 2007; 101:15–26.

34. Llor C, Naberan K, Cots JM, et al. Risk factors for increased cost of exacerbations of chronic bronchitis and chronic obstructive pulmonary disease. Arch Bronconeumol 2006; 42:175–182.

35. Skwarska E, Cohen G, Skwarski KM, et al. Randomised controlled trial of supported discharge in patients with exacerbations of chronic obstructive pulmonary disease. Thorax 2000; 55:907–912.

36. Sala E, Alegre L, Carrera M, et al. Supported discharge shortens hospital stay in patients hospitalized because of an exacerbation of COPD. Eur Respir J 2001; 17:1138–1142.

37. Hernandez C, Casas A, Escarrabill J, et al. Home hospitalisation of exacerbated chronic obstructive pulmonary disease patients. Eur Respir J 2003; 21:58–67.

38. Bourbeau J, Collet JP, Schwartzman K, et al. Economic benefits of self-management education in COPD. Chest 2006; 130:1704–1711.

39. Price LC, Lowe D, Hosker HSR, et al. UK national COPD audit 2003: impact of hospital resources and organisation of care on patient outcome following admission for acute COPD exacerbation. Thorax 2006; 61:837–842.

40. Sullivan SD, Ramsey SD, Lee TA. The economic burden of COPD. Chest 2000; 117 (suppl 2): 5S–9S.

41. Rutten van Mölken MPMH, Postma MJ, Joore MA, et al. Current and future medical costs of asthma and chronic obstructive pulmonary disease in the Netherlands. Respir Med 2000; 93:779–787.

42. Dal Negro R, Berto P, Tognella S, et al. Cost-of-illness of lung disease in the TriVeneto Region, Italy: the GOLD Study. Monaldi Arch Chest Dis 2002; 57:3–9.

43. Jansson SA, Andersson F, Borg S, et al. Costs of COPD in Sweden according to disease severity. Chest 2002; 122:1994–2002.

44. Borg S, Ericsson A, Wedzicha J, et al. A computer simulation model of the natural history and economic impact of chronic obstructive pulmonary disease. Value in Health 2004; 7:153–167.

45. Grassi C, Casali L, Curti E, et al. Efficacy and safety of short course (5-day) moxifloxacin vs 7-day ceftriaxone in the treatment of acute exacerbations of chronic bronchitis (AECB). J Chemother 2002; 14:597–608.

46. Llor C, Naberan K, Cots JM, et al. Economic evaluation of the antibiotic treatment of exacerbations of chronic bronchitis and COPD in primary care centers. Int J Clin Pract 2004; 58:937–944.

# 21

## Use of Bronchodilators and Mucolytics at COPD Exacerbations

**WIM JANSSENS and MARC DECRAMER**
Department of Respiratory Medicine, University of Leuven, Leuven, Belgium

## I. Introduction

Acute exacerbations of chronic obstructive pulmonary disease (AECOPD) are defined as events in the natural course of the disease characterised by a change in the patients baseline dyspnea, cough, and/or sputum that is beyond the normal day-to-day variations, is acute at onset, and may warrant a change in regular medication (1). Early recognition of exacerbations and prompt medical treatment improves patient's recovery, reduces risk of hospitalization, and is associated with a better health-related quality of life (2). Pharmacological treatment consists of an "ABC approach," an acronym for antibiotics, bronchodilators, and corticosteroids, which are the mainstay for treatment in exacerbations (3). Nonpharmacological approaches, namely oxygen therapy and ventilatory support, are also widely used, particularly in more severe presentations of the disease (4). In addition to these evidence-based medical treatments for AECOPD, other therapeutic options, such as mucus clearance strategies and respiratory stimulants have been proposed. Although these treatments have been the subject of different clinical studies during more than 30 years, solid evidence, if any, for a beneficial effect is still lacking (5). In general, these alternatives are no longer recommended in the current guidelines for treatment of AECOPD (1).

This chapter focuses on bronchodilators and mucolytics in the treatment of acute exacerbations. It will review the main concepts of their mechanism of action, their potential benefits and drawbacks, and their current role in the treatment of AECOPD according to evidence-based literature. The role of bronchodilators and mucolytics in the prevention of exacerbations is subject of another chapter and will not be addressed here.

## II. Bronchodilators

### A. Rationale

AECOPD are common events, resulting in an increased airflow obstruction and augmented air trapping with substantial deterioration of gas exchange and of pulmonary hemodynamics. Worsening hypoxemia is primarily produced by the consequent ventilation perfusion mismatch compounded by a decreased mixed venous $PO_2$ that results from increased oxygen consumption (6–8). Reduced airway diameter, with increased airway resistance and impaired expiratory flow, should improve as the exacerbation resolves, but changes in these measures during an AECOPD are relatively small and do not relate well to symptomatic response (9). Improvements in the operating lung volumes, such as an increase of inspiratory capacity (IC) and increase of forced vital capacity (FVC), however, are more important as an AECOPD recovers, and correlate well with the reduction in dyspnea (10).

At least in stable COPD, the use of a bronchodilator reduces end expiratory volume (EEV) and improves IC, which relates to lower symptom intensity and increased exercise capacity (11,12). Similarly, during AECOPD bronchodilators may not only improve the expiratory flow as assessed by an increase of forced expiratory volume in one second $FEV_1$ but may also reduce EEV and residual volume (RV), thereby allowing greater operational lung volumes. This may explain why the symptomatic relief of bronchodilators during an AECOPD is sometimes way above the effect a reversibility test on $FEV_1$ at that time would suggest (10,13). As the improvement of expiratory flow can also enhance the effectiveness of cough, bronchodilators might be also considered as cough clearance promoters (14).

Commonly used bronchodilators in COPD include β2-agonists, anticholinergics, and methylxanthines. Whereas long-acting β2-agonists and long-acting anticholinergics are routinely used in the maintenance treatment of COPD, short-acting bronchodilators are typically used for immediate relief and during exacerbations. The role of methylxanthines in the treatment of AECOPD is still unclear (Table 1).

### Short-Acting Bronchodilators

Short-acting inhaled β2-agonists (SABAs; salbutamol, albuterol, fenoterol, metaproterenol, terbutaline) and short-acting inhaled anticholinergic agents (ipatropium bromide, oxitropium bromide) remain the main treatment modality for AECOPD. SABAs selectively act on cellular β2-receptors, while anticholinergics are nonselective muscarinic antagonists. Inhalation of both agents results in the relaxation of airway smooth muscle cells with consequent bronchodilation.

**Table 1**  Bronchodilators in AECOPD

---

*Short-acting inhaled bronchodilators*
- improve symptoms, $FEV_1$, FVC, and IC
- no difference between β2-agonists and anticholinergics
- no additional benefit with combinations
- increasing dose and/or frequency of existing classes
- discrete side effects

*Methylxanthines*
- marginal improvement of $FEV_1$
- inconsistent benefit on symptoms
- numerous side effects

*Long-acting inhaled bronchodilators*
      no evidence in AECOPD

---

*Abbreviation*: AECOPD, acute exacerbations of chronic obstructive pulmonary disease.

Current guidelines recommend an increasing dose and frequency of SABAs during exacerbations with the association of an anticholinergic if a prompt response to the treatment does not occur (1,15–17). Several issues, however, deserve more attention.

In AECOPD, there is no evidence that the degree of bronchodilation achieved with a SABA is greater than that using ipratropium bromide (18). Specifically, the administration of a bronchodilator can increase $FEV_1$, FVC, and IC by 10% to 29% over a period of 60 to 120 minutes (10,19) When inhaled, the effects of SABAs begin within 5 minutes with maximum peaks at 30 minutes. Ipatropium starts to become effective within 15 minutes with a peak effect at 30 to 60 minutes. The effects of both classes of bronchodilators starts to decline after two to three hours and can last as long as four to six hours (20).

Unlike stable COPD where the simultaneous or concurrent administration of short-acting bronchodilators is more efficacious than either agent given alone (21), the combination of both classes during AECOPD does not provide additional benefit (18,22).

A systematic review of the route of delivery of short-acting bronchodilators found no significant difference in $FEV_1$ between the use of handheld metered-dose inhaler (MDI) with a good inhaler technique (with or without a spacer device) and nebulizers (23). In general, an MDI is recommended for low doses, whereas a nebulizer is more convenient for sicker patients admitted emergently and for patients with physical incapabilities (3,17).

Anticholinergics have little important side effects. Increasing doses of SABAs, in contrast, may augment the risk for cardiovascular events, especially in patients with cardiovascular morbidity due to tachycardia, potassium depletion, and increased oxygen consumption (24). In a large cohort study, however, no increased risk of acute myocardial infarction could be found when using SABAs (25). In addition, SABAs are known to worsen the ventilation perfusion inequality with transient decreases in $PaO_2$ in stable COPD (26), but this could not be confirmed in exacerbations (27). Taken together, SABAs may still be considered as the preferred bronchodilators in AECOPD with the addition of anticholinergics in the absence of a prompt response (28).

### Methylxanthines

Methylxanthines are nonspecific phosphodiesterase inhibitors that exert a direct bronchodilator effect through the relaxation of airway smooth muscle cells. Despite its bronchodilation, most studies comparing intravenous theophylline with placebo have only shown marginal and inconsistent benefits on symptoms and lung function variables. Side effects such as vomiting, nausea, and also tremor and palpitations occurred more frequently. Given the current evidence, methylxanthines can no longer be recommended in the treatment of AECOPD, and the consideration of using methylxanthines as rescue or second-line therapy is probably no longer valuable (1,19,29,30). The recent finding that low doses of theophyllines activate histone deacetylases (31)—enzymes that are involved in the switching off of activated inflammatory genes—may though be of interest in the chronic treatment of COPD and the prevention of exacerbations (32).

### Long-Acting Bronchodilators

Regular treatment with long-acting β2-agonists (salmeterol, formoterol) or long-acting anticholinergics (tiotropium) is more effective and convenient than treatment with short-acting bronchodilators. They improve health status, $FEV_1$, exercise capacity and reduce the rate of exacerbations (33–37). Many patients are therefore on long-acting bronchodilators or combination therapy with inhaled steroids for the moment they experience an exacerbation. For COPD, it is currently unclear if these long-acting bronchodilators need to be continued during the acute phase of an exacerbation together with the repetitive doses of short-acting bronchodilators (3). Studies evaluating the effect of short-acting bronchodilators in the acute setting did not address this issue, which might be important as both short-acting and long-acting agonists use the same receptor and receptor saturation may occur. Theoretically, immediate bronchodilation is not obtained with long-acting agonists, which might explain the preference for short-acting drugs. On the other hand, the maximal effect of formoterol occurs within one hour (38), and increasing the dose of formoterol (with budesonide) is an accepted approach for immediate relief treatment in asthma (39).

## III.  Mucolytics

### A.  Rationale

The airways of most COPD patients contain excessive amounts of mucus that is markedly increased above that in control subjects and relates to globlet hyperplasia, submucosal gland hypertrophy and disturbed mucociliary clearance (40,41). Airway luminal mucus is a complex dilute aqueous solution of lipids, proteins, and glycoconjugates. The long polymeric gel-forming glycoproteins or mucins that are produced in globlet cells or submucosal glands mainly determine the viscoelastic properties of the mucus (42). In COPD, a specific increase of the mucin MUC5B in the bronchiolar lumen has been described (43). AECOPD are associated with increased mucus production and with changes in color and tenacity of the mucus by inflammation and/or infection (44,45). The expectoration of such airway pus during AECOPD is an important mechanism to reduce the ongoing inflammation and to improve airway function (3,17,46). Many patients, however, complain of sputum retention in acute exacerbations, which is often caused by a combination of decreased airflow, muscle weakness, disturbed mucociliary clearance, and increased mucus viscosity. Mucoactive medications like expectorants, mucokinetics, and mucolytics, which tend to improve airway clearance, are therefore of potential benefit in acute exacerbations (42,47,48) (Table 2).

### Expectorants

Expectorants are medications that increase airway water and sputum volume presumably to improve the effectiveness of cough, and although numerous expectorants are widely available, none has proven effectiveness in COPD so far (14,49). As patients with an AECOPD often report more sputum, which is more difficult to expectorate, increasing the sputum volume in such circumstances may eventually lead to sputum impaction. Hyperosmolar agents like mannitol and hypertonic saline are probably of benefit in noncystic fibrosis bronchiectasis (50) but in COPD and certainly during acute exacerbations, they may even be harmful by the induction of further bronchoconstriction (51).

### Mucokinetic Agents

Mucokinetic agents can increase mucociliary clearance either by a direct stimulation of ciliary beat frequency or by unsticking highly adhesive secretions from the airway walls

**Table 2** Mucoactive Agents in AECOPD

---

*Expectorants*
- increase of sputum volume
- hypertonic saline/mannitol
  contraindicated in AECOPD (bronchoconstriction)

*Mucokinetic agents*
- bronchodilators—cough clearance promotor
- surfactant—mucociliary clearance promotor
  no evidence in AECOPD

*Mucolytic agents*
- decrease viscosity of sputum
- peptide mucolytics—only in cystic fibrosis
- classical mucolytics and *N*-acetylcysteine
  no effect on $FEV_1$
  inconsistent benefit on symptoms
  poor evidence in AECOPD

---

*Abbreviation*: AECOPD, acute exacerbations of chronic obstructive pulmonary disease.

thereby promoting ciliary movements (14). Although most bronchodilators stimulate cilia in vitro, their benefit in vivo is only marginal. As bronchodilators may also increase the expiratory flow, their mucokinetic effect is probably more related to the promotion of cough with consequent airway clearance (52,53). Surfactant is a promising medication, as it might decrease the tenacity of the mucus and thus increase the transportability of sputum (54). One trial demonstrated a beneficial effect of surfactant by aerosol in patients with stable COPD (55), but this has not been confirmed by others, and surfactants have never been tested for AECOPD.

### Mucolytic Drugs

Mucolytics are medications that degrade mucins to a lower viscosity with the aim to improve sputum evacuation by mucociliary clearance and cough. Classical mucolytics depolymerize the mucin glycoprotein polymers by hydrolyzing disulfide bonds that link mucin monomers together (14,48). Peptide mucolytics like DNAse and F-actin depolymerizing agents are specifically designed for cystic fibrosis and will not be discussed here (56).

There are several classical mucolytics commercially available [*N*-acetylcysteine (NAC), ambroxol, erdosteine, carbocysteine, iodinated glycerol], and many of these drugs are often prescribed in the treatment of COPD. No data convincingly demonstrate that any of these mucolytics consistently improve the ability to expectorate mucus (14), and if any clinical benefit was reported, its effect was only marginal. A recent meta-analysis on the effect of oral mucolytics in the chronic treatment of stable COPD (57), could only show a small reduction of acute exacerbations, an effect that may apply only to those patients not already receiving inhaled corticosteroids (58,59).

The best known mucolytic, NAC is of particular interest as it has also important antioxidative characteristics (60). In view of these properties, NAC has not only been the subject of several controlled trials in stable COPD, but some authors also investigated the effect of NAC during AECOPD that are typically accompanied by bursts of oxidative stress (61–63). To date, patients receiving NAC in conjunction with standard therapy for AECOPD had more reduced inflammatory markers, improved bacterial eradication, and better subjective outcomes when compared with placebo. However, no statistically significant difference in length of hospitalization and change of $FEV_1$ could be observed—a finding that might be explained by the low patient number and lack of statistical power. Alternatively, given the short half-life of NAC, it has been suggested that the doses to obtain a considerable antioxidative effect in vivo are beyond the current recommended dosage of 600 mg (58,60). At least, the benefit of a daily dose of 1800 mg NAC in the treatment of idiopathic lung fibrosis is consistent with this hypothesis (64).

In summary, the role of mucolytics in stable COPD and at acute exacerbations remains questionable. Given the absence of convincing evidence, guidelines cannot recommend their widespread use at present (1). However, certain individuals or subgroups of COPD patients might still benefit from the use of mucolytics (65) and applications with higher antioxidative doses of NAC may still have potential for the future.

## References

1. Rabe KF, Hurd S, Anzueto A, et al. Global strategy for the diagnosis, management, and prevention of chronic obstructive pulmonary disease: GOLD executive summary. Am J Respir Crit Care Med 2007; 176(6):532–555.
2. Wilkinson TM, Donaldson GC, Hurst JR, et al. Early therapy improves outcomes of exacerbations of chronic obstructive pulmonary disease. Am J Respir Crit Care Med 2004; 169(12): 1298–1303.
3. Rodriguez-Roisin R. COPD exacerbations .5: management. Thorax 2006; 61(6):535–544.
4. Jeffrey AA, Warren PM, Flenley DC. Acute hypercapnic respiratory failure in patients with chronic obstructive lung disease: risk factors and use of guidelines for management. Thorax 1992; 47(1):34–40.
5. McCrory DC, Brown C, Gelfand SE, et al. Management of acute exacerbations of COPD: a summary and appraisal of published evidence. Chest 2001; 119(4):1190–1209.
6. Barbera JA, Roca J, Ferrer A, et al. Mechanisms of worsening gas exchange during acute exacerbations of chronic obstructive pulmonary disease. Eur Respir J 1997; 10(6):1285–1291.
7. Kessler R, Faller M, Fourgaut G, et al. Predictive factors of hospitalization for acute exacerbation in a series of 64 patients with COPD. Am J Respir Crit Care Med 1999; 159(1):158–164.
8. Parker CM, Voduc N, Aaron SD, et al. Physiological changes during symptom recovery from moderate exacerbations of COPD. Eur Respir J 2005; 26(3):420–428.
9. Seemungal TA, Donaldson GC, Bhowmik A, et al. Time course and recovery of exacerbations in patients with COPD. Am J Respir Crit Care Med 2000; 161(5):1608–1613.
10. Stevenson NJ, Walker PP, Costello RW, et al. Lung mechanics and dyspnea during exacerbations of COPD. Am J Respir Crit Care Med 2005; 172(12):1510–1516.
11. Newton MF, O'Donnell DE, Forkert L. Response of lung volumes to inhaled salbutamol in a large population of patients with severe hyperinflation. Chest 2002; 121(4):1042–1050.
12. O'Donnell DE, Lam M, Webb KA. Spirometric correlates of improvement in exercise performance after anticholinergic therapy in COPD. Am J Respir Crit Care Med 1999; 160(2):542–549.
13. Hay JG, Stone P, Carter J, et al. Bronchodilator reversibility, exercise performance and breathlessness in stable chronic obstructive pulmonary disease. Eur Respir J 1992; 5(6):659–664.
14. Rubin BK. Mucolytics, expectorants, and mucokinetic medications. Respir Care 2007; 52(7):859–865.
15. Celli BR, Macnee W. Standards for the diagnosis and treatment of patients with COPD: a summary of the ATS/ERS position paper. Eur Respir J 2004; 23(6):932–946.

16. Halpin D. NICE guidance for COPD. Thorax 2004; 59(3):181–182.
17. Willaert W, Daenen M, Bomans P, et al. What is the optimal treatment strategy for chronic obstructive pulmonary disease exacerbations? Eur Respir J 2002; 19(5):928–935.
18. McCrory DC, Brown CD. Anti-cholinergic bronchodilators versus beta2-sympathomimetic agents for acute exacerbations of COPD. Cochrane Database Syst Rev 2002;(4):CD003900.
19. Stoller JK. Clinical practice. Acute exacerbations of COPD. N Engl J Med 2002; 346(13):988–994.
20. Rennard SI. Treatment of stable COPD. Lancet 2004; 364(9436):791–802.
21. Routine nebulized ipratropium and albuterol together are better than either alone in COPD. The COMBIVENT Inhalation Solution Study Group. Chest 1997; 112(6):1514–1521.
22. Patrick DM, Dales RE, Stark RM, et al. Severe exacerbations of COPD and asthma. Incremental benefit of adding ipratropium to usual therapy. Chest 1990; 98(2):295–297.
23. Turner MO, Patel A, Ginsburg S, et al. Bronchodilator delivery in acute airflow obstruction. A meta-analysis. Arch Intern Med 1997; 157(15):1736–1744.
24. Salpeter SR, Ormiston TM, Salpeter EE. Cardiovascular effects of beta-agonists in patients with asthma and COPD: a meta-analysis. Chest 2004; 125(6):2309–2321.
25. Suissa S, Assimes T, Ernst P. Inhaled short acting beta agonist use in COPD and the risk of acute myocardial infarction. Thorax 2003; 58(1):43–46.
26. Khoukaz G, Gross NJ. Effects of salmeterol on arterial blood gases in patients with stable COPD. Comparison with albuterol and ipratropium. Am J Respir Crit Care Med 1999; 160(3):1028–1030.
27. Polverino E, Gomez FP, Manrique H, et al. Gas exchange response to short-acting beta2-agonists in COPD severe exacerbations. Am J Respir Crit Care Med 2007; 176(4):350–355.
28. Joos GF. Are beta2-agonists safe in patients with acute exacerbations of COPD? Am J Respir Crit Care Med 2007; 176(4):322–323.
29. Barr RG, Rowe BH, Camargo CA Jr. Methylxanthines for exacerbations of chronic obstructive pulmonary disease: meta-analysis of randomised trials. BMJ 2003; 327(7416):643.
30. Duffy N, Walker P, Diamantea F, et al. Intravenous aminophylline in patients admitted to hospital with non-acidotic exacerbations of chronic obstructive pulmonary disease: a prospective randomised controlled trial. Thorax 2005; 60(9):713–717.
31. Cosio BG, Tsaprouni L, Ito K, et al. Theophylline restores histone deacetylase activity and steroid responses in COPD macrophages. J Exp Med 2004; 200(5):689–695.
32. Barnes PJ. Theophylline for COPD. Thorax 2006; 61(9):742–744.
33. Calverley PM, Anderson JA, Celli B, et al. Salmeterol and fluticasone propionate and survival in chronic obstructive pulmonary disease. N Engl J Med 2007; 356(8):775–789.
34. Mahler DA, Donohue JF, Barbee RA, et al. Efficacy of salmeterol xinafoate in the treatment of COPD. Chest 1999; 115(4):957–965.
35. Mahler DA. The effect of inhaled beta2-agonists on clinical outcomes in chronic obstructive pulmonary disease. J Allergy Clin Immunol 2002; 110(6 Suppl):S298–S303.
36. Niewoehner DE, Rice K, Cote C, et al. Prevention of exacerbations of COPD with tiotropium, a once-daily inhaled anticholinergic bronchodilator: a randomized trial. Ann Intern Med 2005; 143(5): 317–326.
37. Vincken W, Van Noord JA, Greefhorst AP, et al. Improved health outcomes in patients with COPD during 1 yr's treatment with tiotropium. Eur Respir J 2002; 19(2):209–216.
38. Seberova E, Andersson A. Oxis (formoterol given by Turbuhaler) showed as rapid an onset of action as salbutamol given by a pMDI. Respir Med 2000; 94(6):607–611.
39. Rabe KF, Pizzichini E, Stallberg B, et al. Budesonide/formoterol in a single inhaler for maintenance and relief in mild-to-moderate asthma: a randomized, double-blind trial. Chest 2006; 129(2): 246–256.
40. Hogg JC. Pathophysiology of airflow limitation in COPD. Lancet 2004; 364(9435):709–721.
41. Maestrelli P, Saetta M, Mapp CE, et al. Remodeling in response to infection and injury. Airway inflammation and hypersecretion of mucus in smoking subjects with chronic obstructive pulmonary disease. Am J Respir Crit Care Med 2001; 164(10 pt 2):S76–S80.

42. Houtmeyers E, Gosselink R, Gayan-Ramirez G, et al. Regulation of mucociliary clearance in health and disease. Eur Respir J 1999; 13(5):1177–1188.
43. Caramori G, Di GC, Carlstedt I, et al. Mucin expression in peripheral airways of patients with chronic obstructive pulmonary disease. Histopathology 2004; 45(5):477–484.
44. Anthonisen NR. Bacteria and exacerbations of COPD. N Engl J Med 2002; 347(7):526–527.
45. Burge S, Wedzicha JA. COPD exacerbations: definitions and classifications. Eur Respir J Suppl 2003; 41:46S–53S.
46. Vestbo J, Prescott E, Lange P. Association of mucus hypersecretion with FEV1 decline and COPD morbidity. Copenhagen City Heart Study Group. Am J Respir Crit Care Med 1996; 153(5): 1530–1535.
47. Henke MO, Shah SA, Rubin BK. The role of airway secretions in COPD—clinical applications. COPD 2005; 2(3):377–390.
48. Rogers DF, Barnes PJ. Treatment of airway mucus hypersecretion. Ann Med 2006; 38(2):116–125.
49. Houtmeyers E, Gosselink R, Gayan-Ramirez G, et al. Effects of drugs on mucus clearance. Eur Respir J 1999; 14(2):452–467.
50. Wills P, Greenstone M. Inhaled hyperosmolar agents for bronchiectasis. Cochrane Database Syst Rev 2006;(2):CD002996.
51. Taube C, Holz O, Mucke M, et al. Airway response to inhaled hypertonic saline in patients with moderate to severe COPD. Am J Respir Crit Care Med 2001; 164(10 pt 1):1810–1815.
52. Hasani A, Pavia D, Agnew JE, et al. Regional lung clearance during cough and forced expiration technique (FET): effects of flow and viscoelasticity. Thorax 1994; 49(6):557–561.
53. Hasani A, Toms N, Agnew JE, et al. Mucociliary clearance in COPD can be increased by both a D2/beta2 and a standard beta2 agonists. Respir Med 2005; 99(2):145–151.
54. Albers GM, Tomkiewicz RP, May MK, et al. Ring distraction technique for measuring surface tension of sputum: relationship to sputum clearability. JAP 1996; 81(6):2690–2695.
55. Anzueto A, Jubran A, Ohar JA, et al. Effects of aerosolized surfactant in patients with stable chronic bronchitis: a prospective randomized controlled trial. JAMA 1997; 278(17):1426–1431.
56. Henke MO, Ratjen F. Mucolytics in cystic fibrosis. Paediatr Respir Rev 2007; 8(1):24–29.
57. Poole PJ, Black PN. Mucolytic agents for chronic bronchitis or chronic obstructive pulmonary disease. Cochrane Database Syst Rev 2006; 3:CD001287.
58. Decramer M, Rutten-van MM, Dekhuijzen PN, et al. Effects of N-acetylcysteine on outcomes in COPD (BRONCUS): a randomised placebo-controlled trial. Lancet 2005; 365(9470):1552–1560.
59. Sutherland ER, Crapo JD, Bowler RP. N-acetylcysteine and exacerbations of chronic obstructive pulmonary disease. COPD 2006; 3(4):195–202.
60. Dekhuijzen PN. Antioxidant properties of N-acetylcysteine: their relevance in relation to chronic obstructive pulmonary disease. Eur Respir J 2004; 23(4):629–636.
61. Black PN, Morgan-Day A, McMillan TE, et al. Randomised, controlled trial of N-acetylcysteine for treatment of acute exacerbations of COPD. BMC Pulm Med 2004; 4:13.
62. Reichenberger F, Tamm M. N-acetylcystein in the therapy of chronic bronchitis. Pneumologie 2002; 56(12):793–797.
63. Zuin R, Palamidese A, Negrin R, et al. High-dose N-acetylcysteine in patients with exacerbations of COPD. Clin Drug Investig 2005; 25(6):401–408.
64. Demedts M, Behr J, Buhl R, et al. High-dose acetylcysteine in idiopathic pulmonary fibrosis. N Engl J Med 2005; 353(21):2229–2242.
65. Petty TL. The National Mucolytic Study. Results of a randomized, double-blind, placebo-controlled study of iodinated glycerol in chronic obstructive bronchitis. Chest 1990; 97(1):75–83.

# 22
## Corticosteroids in the Management of Acute Exacerbations

**DENNIS E. NIEWOEHNER and KATHRYN RICE**
Pulmonary Section, Minneapolis Veterans Affairs Medical Center, Department of Medicine, University of Minnesota, Minneapolis, Minnesota, U.S.A.

## I.  Introduction

Exacerbations of chronic obstructive pulmonary disease (COPD) have a major adverse impact on health status and place a serious burden on health care systems, particularly when they entail a visit to an emergency department or hospital admission (1). In 2000, COPD was responsible for 1.5 million emergency department visits and 726,000 hospitalizations in the United States (2). A hospital admission for COPD in the United States incurs average costs in excess of $16,000, so that hospitalization accounts for a large proportion of the total medical costs of caring for this disease (3,4). Because severe exacerbations are common, treatments that shorten their duration to even a small extent may provide substantial human and financial benefits in absolute terms.

Administering systemic corticosteroids to patients with severe COPD exacerbations has been fairly widespread for several decades, but only in recent years has a sound scientific basis been established for this practice. Authoritative guidelines now strongly recommend systemic corticosteroids as a standard component of care for severe COPD exacerbations (5–8). It appears that this recommendation is widely followed. A recent retrospective cohort study of 69,820 admissions for COPD exacerbations at 360 hospitals encompassing all regions in the United States reported that 85% had received systemic corticosteroids (9). The rationale for the use of systemic corticosteroids in this clinical setting will be reviewed.

## II.  Evidence for Clinical Efficacy

Albert and his colleagues published the first randomized, double-blind, placebo-controlled trial designed to evaluate the efficacy of systemic corticosteroids for COPD exacerbations (10). Forty-four patients hospitalized for COPD randomly received either intravenous methylprednisolone, 0.5 mg/kg every six hours, or placebo for three days. All patients received other usual components of care. The forced expiratory volume in 1 second ($FEV_1$), but not the forced vital capacity or arterial blood gases, improved at a significantly faster rate in those patients who received methylprednisolone. Most corticosteroid-induced improvement in the postbronchodilator $FEV_1$ was evident within the first 36 hours, with an average increase over placebo of approximately 75 mL. The observation period stopped after three days and the investigators made no attempt to evaluate clinical efficacy outcomes.

Two earlier trials evaluated short-term effects of systemic corticosteroids on COPD exacerbations in an emergency department setting. Emerman and his associates administered a single 100-mg dose of IV methylprednisolone or placebo to 96 patients (11). Over a subsequent five-hour observation period, there were no treatment-related differences in spirometry, nor were there any differences in hospitalizations or unscheduled emergency department visits over the ensuing 48 hours. Bullard and his colleagues administered hydrocortisone, 100 mg IV every four hours, or placebo to 113 patients who presented to an emergency facility (12). They also observed no effect of systemic corticosteroids on short-term spirometric changes or on subsequent hospitalization, intubation, or mortality rates.

The duration of therapy in the aforementioned trials may have been insufficient to detect benefit. Thompson and associates enrolled 27 patients with exacerbations, also in an outpatient setting, but administered a longer, nine-day tapering course of prednisone or placebo (13). They reported that prednisone had a relatively large effect on the $FEV_1$, amounting to a treatment difference of nearly 200 mL at 3 days and approximately 400 mL at 10 days. Additionally, prednisone-treated patients exhibited improved arterial blood gases, reported less dyspnea, and experienced fewer treatment failures. However, these very positive results must be viewed in the context of a small study having been conducted at a single site.

A study group, Systemic Corticosteroids in Chronic Obstructive Pulmonary Disease Exacerbations (SCCOPE), supported by the Veterans Affairs Cooperative Studies Program designed and executed a trial to evaluate the effects of systemic corticosteroids on clinical outcomes in patients with severe COPD exacerbations (14). SCCOPE randomized 271 hospitalized patients at 25 study centers into one of the three treatment arms. The two active treatment arms received intravenous methylprednisolone, 125 mg every six hours, for three days, followed by a tapering course of prednisone over eight weeks in one arm and two weeks in the second arm. The third arm received placebo throughout. All subjects received other standard measures of care, such as oxygen, inhaled bronchodilators, and antibiotics. The primary outcome was a composite definition of treatment failure that included all cause mortality, intubation and mechanical ventilation, hospital readmission for COPD, or the need to intensify pharmacological treatment, such as with open-label prednisone.

At study days 30 and 90, systemic corticosteroids, compared with placebo, statistically significantly reduced the absolute treatment failure rate by 10% and 11%, respectively ($p < 0.05$ for both comparisons) (Fig. 1). Patients receiving active treatment, compared with placebo, experienced a faster improvement in the $FEV_1$ by about 100 mL over the first three days of treatment, and they were discharged from the hospital one to two days sooner. None of the primary and secondary efficacy outcomes significantly differed between the two- and eight-week treatment arms.

In a concurrent smaller, single-site trial, Davies and associates obtained results similar to those of SCCOPE (15). Those investigators randomized 56 patients who were admitted to the hospital for COPD exacerbations to oral prednisolone, 30 mg, once daily for two weeks, or placebo. The postbronchodilator $FEV_1$ was the primary outcome; on average it improved faster in the patients who received prednisolone, as compared with placebo. This improvement amounted to about 60 mL/day over the five-day interval since enrollment, an increase somewhat larger than that seen with systemic corticosteroids in SCCOPE.

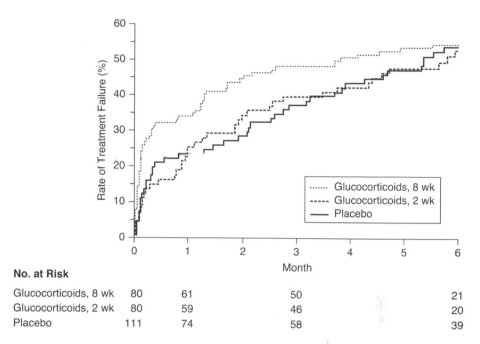

| No. at Risk | | | | |
|---|---|---|---|---|
| Glucocorticoids, 8 wk | 80 | 61 | 50 | 21 |
| Glucocorticoids, 2 wk | 80 | 59 | 46 | 20 |
| Placebo | 111 | 74 | 58 | 39 |

**Figure 1**  First treatment failure according to treatment assignment in COPD patients hospitalized for exacerbation and enrolled in the SCCOPE trial. Compared with the placebo arm, treatment failure rates in the combined active treatment arms are significantly ($p < 0.05$) decreased at one month and at three months, but not at six months. *Source*: From Ref. 14.

As was observed in SCCOPE, patients receiving active treatment were able to leave the hospital a couple of days sooner than the patients who received placebo.

A Canadian trials group evaluated the benefits of systemic corticosteroid therapy for COPD exacerbations in patients who sought emergency department care (16). They randomized 147 patients at 10 study sites to either placebo or 40 mg prednisone daily for 10 days. The primary outcome was the relapse rate at 30 days, defined as an unscheduled visit to a physician's office or return to the emergency department because of worsening dyspnea. The relapse rate was significantly lower in the patients who received prednisone (27% vs. 43%, $p = 0.04$) (Fig. 2). Additionally, the $FEV_1$ improved more rapidly in the prednisone-treated patients (difference over placebo of 140 mL by study day 10), as did dyspnea.

## III.  Dose, Duration, and Route of Administration

As described above, strong evidence now exists that systemic steroids improve clinical outcomes in the management of acute COPD exacerbations (13–16). The design of these trials varied widely in terms of daily corticosteroid dosage (30–600 mg in prednisone equivalents) and treatment duration (10–56 days). In some trials, study drug was administered orally and in others it was given intravenously. Hence, practical questions remain as

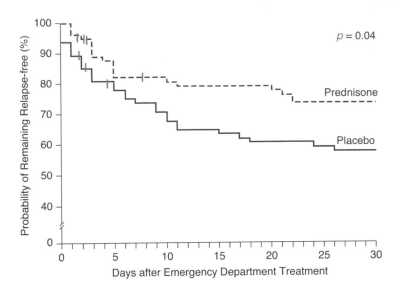

**Figure 2**  Kaplan–Meier estimates of the probability of remaining relapse free at 30 days in prednisone and placebo groups. Compared with placebo, the likelihood was significantly reduced
($p < 0.05$) in those patients who received prednisone. *Source:* From Ref. 16.

to how to best maximize treatment benefit while minimizing systemic corticosteroid
exposure and its attendant adverse effects.

The SCCOPE trial clearly demonstrated that most exacerbating patients need no
more than two weeks of systemic corticosteroid treatment, as no added clinical benefit was
detected in patients given an eight-week course of treatment (14). Results from another trial
suggested that 10 days of treatment might be sufficient, though no direct comparisons were
made to a 14-day treatment regimen (16). Sayiner and colleagues compared a three-day
treatment regimen with a 10-day regimen in 36 patients hospitalized for a COPD exacerbation (17). Subjects in both treatment arms received methylprednisolone, 0.5 mg/kg
intravenously every six hours for three days. At this point, treatment with tapering doses of
methylprednisolone was given to one study arm and placebo to the other arm for an
additional seven days. After 10 days, the $FEV_1$ had improved by an average of 236 mL over
baseline in the 10-day active treatment arm compared with only 68 mL in the three-day
active treatment arm ($p = 0.02$). Favorable improvements in arterial blood gases were also
evident with longer treatment. Though not adequately powered to show differences in
clinical outcomes, this trial suggests that three days of systemic corticosteroid treatment is
inadequate for severe COPD exacerbations. Hence, available evidence suggests that the
optimal duration of therapy lies between 10 and 14 days for most patients.

While many hospitalized patients receive intravenous corticosteroids during the early
phases of treatment for exacerbations, orally administered prednisone and prednisolone are
known to have good bioavailability, raising the question as to whether the more expensive
and less convenient intravenous therapy is needed (18). The question of oral versus
intravenous corticosteroid therapy was recently addressed in a large Dutch trial (19). These

investigators randomized 210 patients hospitalized for COPD exacerbations to receive either 60 mg prednisolone daily by intravenous infusion or the same daily dose given orally, each for five days. Both treatment arms then received open-label, oral prednisolone, starting at 30 mg and tapered daily in 5 mg decrements. In terms of the primary outcome, there were fewer treatment failures at 90 days in the oral therapy arm as compared with the intravenous arm (56.3% vs. 61.7%, respectively). Formal statistical analysis confirmed noninferiority of oral corticosteroid therapy at the prespecified confidence level. Additionally, improvements in spirometry and health-related quality of life were comparable in the two treatment arms over the first week of the study.

While the conclusion of equivalence in this particular trial is likely correct, the conclusion may not be generalizable because of a design issue (19). Of the patients enrolled in the trial, 77% had already taken systemic corticosteroids immediately prior to the hospitalization during which they were enrolled. This raises the distinct possibility that carryover effects could have obscured treatment differences during the trial. It was for this reason that previous placebo-controlled trials excluded patients who had taken a systemic corticosteroid during the previous 30 days (14–16).

Inhaled corticosteroids are widely used for stable obstructive lung diseases in preference to systemic corticosteroids because the inhalational route improves airway function while minimizing adverse systemic effects. Two small trials compared nebulized budesonide with prednisolone in patients hospitalized for COPD exacerbations and reported no statistically significant treatment-related differences in spirometry after five days in one study and after 10 days in the other (20,21). Maltais and associates executed a three-arm trial comparing oral prednisolone (30 mg twice daily for 3 days, followed by 40-mg daily for 7 days) versus budesonide (2 mg by nebulization every 6 hours for 72 hours, followed by 2000 μg by inhalation daily for 7 days) versus placebo in 199 nonacidotic patients hospitalized for COPD (22). The postbronchodilator $FEV_1$ at study day 3 was the primary outcome, and values were statistically significantly better in both active treatment arms compared with placebo. The mean improvement in the $FEV_1$ was 60 mL greater in the oral prednisolone arm as compared with the budesonide arm, but that difference was not statistically significant. Secondary outcomes also showed benefits for both corticosteroid arms over placebo but with prednisolone-treated patients tending to show larger improvements than those patients receiving inhaled budesonide. A second trial enrolled a comparable patient population with a similar three-arm design (oral prednisolone, inhaled budesonide, and placebo) and showed that spirometry and arterial blood gases improve in response to inhaled budesonide (23). However, neither of these trials was designed to adequately show clinical superiority of inhaled budesonide over placebo or clinical equivalence of inhaled budesonide with oral prednisolone. Hence, inhaled budesonide cannot be recommended as a proven therapy or as an adequate substitute for systemic corticosteroids when treating severe COPD exacerbations.

## IV.  Adverse Effects of Short-Term Systemic Corticosteroids

Short-term administration of systemic corticosteroids causes substantial glucose intolerance, even in subjects not previously known to have diabetes mellitus (24). Thus, it is no surprise that COPD patients receiving systemic corticosteroids for an exacerbation commonly exhibit hyperglycemia. Albert and associates reported that patients treated with high doses of methylprednisolone (2 mg/kg/24 hours) for three days had a mean glucose level that was 25 mg/dL greater than the mean value in controls (10). The highest value in a corticosteroid-treated patient was 265 mg/dL without mention being made of any specific treatment. Davies and associates reported transient glycosuria in six of their 29 corticosteroid-treated subjects, but again made no mention of the need for treatment (15). The SCCOPE investigators listed hyperglycemia as a complication only if it required a new treatment or change in existing treatment (14). Such events occurred in only 3.6% of the placebo patients but were identified in 18.8% of patients receiving systemic corticosteroids. Because of chance, a substantial imbalance occurred in the allocation of subjects with known diabetes (4.5% in placebo v. 14.4% in active treatment), and this might partly account for the higher rate of hyperglycemic treatment in patients receiving active study drug. The overall clinical importance of corticosteroid-related hyperglycemia in this setting is difficult to judge. Physicians should monitor patients for hyperglycemia, and some patients will require specific treatment. Hyperglycemia is generally transient and published trials have made no mention of associated serious or fatal events, though that possibility clearly exists if the condition goes unrecognized.

Systemic corticosteroids are potent immunosuppressive agents that place patients at some increased dose- and duration-dependent risk for infectious complications (25). The absolute risk for a serious infection secondary to a 10 to 14 day prednisone course commonly used to treat an exacerbation is unknown but probably quite small. The SCCOPE investigators found no statistically significant excess of secondary infections in patients who received systemic corticosteroids (14). However, there were more cases of pneumonia requiring rehospitalization among patients who received eight weeks of systemic cortico-steroids (11%), as compared with patients who received two weeks of corticosteroids (1%) or placebo (4%). No mention has been made of infectious complications in other trials that have evaluated systemic corticosteroids for COPD exacerbations. There are numerous case reports of serious pneumonia due to bacteria, fungi, and viruses, but nearly all infections occurred only after extended periods of systemic corticosteroid therapy and frequently with high doses (26–28).

Acute psychosis and a number of milder neuropsychiatric disorders are also well-recognized complications of systemic corticosteroids. A meta-analyses of randomized, placebo-controlled trials confirmed that corticosteroid therapy given for a variety of conditions was associated with a significant increase in the number of acute psychoses, but the absolute increase in risk was calculated to be only 0.2% overall (29). Milder disorders appear to be more common. Aaron and associates reported that 48% of patients receiving prednisone complained of insomnia compared with only 21% in the placebo arm (16). They also noted trends toward more depression and anxiety in subjects who received prednisone.

Systemic corticosteroids may cause an acute or chronic myopathy in patients treated for obstructive lung disease and it is important that physicians be aware of this potentially serious complication (30–32). Myopathies are not uncommon in an acute-care setting, but the contribution of corticosteroids is difficult to determine with certainty (33). Because of multiple confounding factors, inferences about causality must rely on statistical associations (30,32). Indeed, it is possible that interactions with other acute illness factors might increase susceptibility to corticosteroid-induced myopathy. Limited information indicates that a brief course of systemic corticosteroids in an outpatient setting does not seriously affect muscle function. Detailed physiological studies failed to detect any evidence of muscle dysfunction among 25 stable COPD patients who were given oral prednisolone, 30 mg daily, for two weeks (34).

Many health care workers view systemic corticosteroids as a risk factor for upper gastrointestinal bleeding, but this perception may be subject to confounding. A large systematic review of numerous trials found no association between gastrointestinal bleeding and systemic corticosteroid administration, once adjustment was made for concomitant nonsteroidal anti-inflammatory drug use (35).

Even relatively short courses of systemic corticosteroids are known to cause measurable reductions in trabecular bone density, but these effects are small and their long-term clinical significance is not known (36). Chronic systemic corticosteroid therapy poses a far greater risk of osteoporotic fractures (37). Similarly, other well-known complications of corticosteroids, such as cataract formation, skin bruisability, and adrenal insufficiency, are usually seen only with long-term corticosteroid use (38).

## V. Mechanisms of Response to Corticosteroids in COPD Exacerbations

While systemic corticosteroids have been found clinically effective for treating COPD exacerbations, little is known of the specific mechanisms. Worsening airflow obstruction and air trapping are held to be central pathophysiological features of severe exacerbations, being largely responsible for the clinical features of worsening dyspnea and, in some instances, respiratory failure. It is presumed that some combination of mucus accumulation inside airways, smooth muscle contraction, and edema formation within bronchial walls causes narrowing of airway lumens with a consequent increase in airflow resistance and possibly complete airway closure of some instances. As detailed pathological studies of the bronchial tree during exacerbations are lacking, these considerations remain somewhat conjectural. A close linkage does exist between decreases in airflow obstruction and positive clinical outcomes during exacerbations, suggesting that improved airway function is the key to clinical recovery (39).

Increased bronchial inflammation, as evidenced by purulent sputum, is a hallmark of many COPD exacerbations. Studies of sputum, bronchial biopsies, and exhaled breath condensate during exacerbations have shown increased numbers of several inflammatory cell types, of cytokines, and of products of oxidative stress (40–43). The corticosteroid related anti-inflammatory activities of greatest clinical importance remain to be identified, and this failure is due in no small part to the ubiquity of the cortisol receptor and complexity of transduction pathways among various lung cells (44,45). Corticosteroids might also improve lung function via mechanisms not generally considered to be anti-inflammatory. For example, corticosteroids might simply increase the sensitivity of airway smooth muscle to inhaled or endogenous adrenergic agents by increasing transcription of the $\beta$-adrenergic receptor (46).

A question of potential clinical importance is whether subpopulations of prednisone "responders" and "nonresponders" might exist. Mendella and associates reported that stable COPD patients exhibited a clear bimodal response to two weeks of oral methylprednisolone; compared with placebo, the $FEV_1$ increased by a mean of 54% in 8 of 46 subjects who were given methylprednisolone (47). In contrast, average $FEV_1$ change in the remaining 38 subjects did not differ significantly between placebo and active drug. In other similarly designed trials, investigators were unable to identify such a distinct subgroup of systemic corticosteroid "responders" (48–50). Additionally, secondary analysis of data from the SCCOPE trial failed to identify a discrete subset of responders (39). Several studies have reported that the presence of sputum eosinophilia or levels of exhaled nitric oxide have value in predicting the magnitude of $FEV_1$ increases following short-term treatment of stable COPD patients with inhaled corticosteroids or systemic corticosteroids (51–53). These measurements have not been assessed during COPD exacerbations, and it remains unknown as to whether they might have any clinical predictive value.

## VI.  Summary

A brief course of systemic corticosteroids decreases treatment failure by an absolute rate of about 10% in patients who are hospitalized for COPD exacerbations. In addition, systemic corticosteroids improve lung function and shorten the length of hospital stay by one or two days. Prednisone confers similar benefits when COPD exacerbations are treated in an emergency department setting, as it reduces the absolute relapse rate by about 15%. The optimal duration of therapy appears to be between 10 and 14 days. The optimal dose is not known, though clinical improvement has been observed with daily doses as low as 30 to 40 mg of prednisone or its equivalent. Tapering of doses is probably unnecessary. Adverse effects of systemic corticosteroids appear to be acceptably low when given for periods of no more than 14 days. Transient hyperglycemia that usually requires no specific treatment is relatively common, and rare instances of secondary infection, myopathy, and psychosis should be anticipated. Better airway function is probably the main factor in improving clinical outcomes. Cellular targets and the molecular mechanisms of corticosteroid therapy in this clinical setting remain unknown. It is also not known whether some patients with COPD exacerbations are more responsive to systemic corticosteroids than others.

## References

1. Spencer S, Jones PW. Time course of recovery of health status following an infective exacerbation of chronic bronchitis. Thorax 2003; 58:589–593.
2. Mannino DM, Homa DM, Akinbami LJ, et al. Chronic obstructive pulmonary disease surveillance – United States, 1971-2000. MMWR 2002; 51:1–16.
3. HCUP Nationwide Inpatient Sample (NIS). Agency for Healthcare Research and Quality. Available at: http://hcupnet.ahrq.gov/HCUPnet.jsp. Accessed October 10, 2007.
4. Strassels SA, Smith DH, Sullivan SD, et al. The costs of treating COPD in the United States. Chest 2001; 119:344–352.
5. Bach PB, Brown C, Gelfand SE, et al. Management of acute exacerbations of chronic obstructive pulmonary disease: a summary and appraisal of published evidence. American College of Physicians–American Society of Internal Medicine; American College of Chest Physicians. Ann Intern Med 2001; 134:600–620.
6. Global Initiative for Chronic Obstructive Lung Disease. Global strategy for the diagnosis, management and prevention of COPD. 2006. Available at: http://www.goldcopd.org.
7. O'Donnell DE, Aaron S, Bourbeau J, et al. Canadian Thoracic Society recommendations for management of chronic obstructive pulmonary disease—2003. Can Respir J 2003; 10(suppl A):11A–65A.
8. National Collaborating Centre for Chronic Conditions. Chronic obstructive pulmonary disease. National clinical guideline on management of chronic obstructive pulmonary disease in adults in primary and secondary care. Thorax 2004; 59(suppl 1):1–232.

9. Lindenauer PK, Pekow P, Gao S, et al. Quality of care for patients hospitalized for acute exacerbations of chronic obstructive pulmonary disease. Ann Intern Med 2006; 144:894–903.

10. Albert RK, Martin TR, Lewis SW. Controlled clinical trial of methylprednisolone in patients with chronic bronchitis and acute respiratory insufficiency. Ann Intern Med 1980; 92:753–758.

11. Emerman CL, Connors AF, Lukens TW, et al. A randomized controlled trial of methylprednisolone in the emergency treatment of acute exacerbations of COPD. Chest 1989; 95:563–567.

12. Bullard MJ, Liaw SJ, Tsai YH, Min HP. Early corticosteroid use in acute exacerbations of chronic airflow obstruction. Am J Emerg Med 1996; 14:139–143.

13. Thompson WH, Nielson CP, Carvalho P, et al. Controlled trial of oral prednisone in outpatients with acute COPD exacerbation. Am J Respir Crit Care Med 1996; 154:407–412.

14. Niewoehner DE, Erbland ML, Deupree RH, et al. Effect of systemic glucocorticoids on exacerbations of chronic obstructive pulmonary disease. N Engl J Med 1999; 340:1941–1947.

15. Davies L, Angus RM, Calverley PMA. Oral corticosteroids in patients admitted to hospital with exacerbations of chronic obstructive pulmonary disease: a prospective randomised controlled trial. Lancet 1999; 354:456–460.

16. Aaron SD, Vendemheen KL, Hebert P, et al. Outpatient oral prednisone after emergency treatment of chronic obstructive pulmonary disease. N Engl J Med 2003; 348:2618–2625.

17. Sayiner A, Aytemur ZA, Cirit M, et al. Systemic glucocorticoids in severe exacerbations of COPD. Chest 2001; 119:726–730.

18. Ferry JJ, Horvath AM, Bekersky I, et al. Relative and absolute bioavailability of prednisone and prednisolone after separate oral and intravenous doses. J Clin Pharmacol 1988; 28:81–87.

19. de Jong YP, Uil SM, Grotjohan HP, et al. Oral or IV prednisolone in the treatment study of COPD exacerbations: a randomized, controlled, double-blind study. Chest 2007; 132:1741–1747.

20. Morice AH, Morris D, Lawson-Matthew P. A comparison of nebulized budesonide with oral prednisolone in the treatment of exacerbations of obstructive pulmonary disease. Clin Pharmacol Ther 1996; 60:675–678.

21. Mirici A, Meral M, Akgun M. Comparison of the efficacy of nebulised budesonide with parenteral corticosteroids in the treatment of acute exacerbations of chronic obstructive pulmonary disease. Clin Drug Invest 2003; 23:55–62.

22. Maltais F, Ostivelli J, Bourbeau J, et al. Comparison of nebulized budesonide and oral prednisolone with placebo in the treatment of acute exacerbations of chronic obstructive pulmonary disease. Am J Respir Crit Care Med 2002; 165:698–703.

23. Gunen H, Hacievliyagil SS, Yetkin O, et al. The role of nebulised budesonide in the treatment of exacerbations of COPD. Eur Respir J 2007; 29:660–667.

24. Pagano G, Bruno A, Cavallo-Perin P, et al. Glucose intolerance after short-term administration of corticosteroids in healthy subjects. Prednisone, deflazacort, and betamethasone. Arch Intern Med 1989;149:1098–1101.

25. Stuck AE, Minder CE, Frey FJ. Risk of infectious complications in patients taking glucocorticoids. Rev Inf Dis 1989; 11:954–963.

26. Weist PM, Flanigan T, Salata RA, et al. Serious infectious complications of corticosteroid therapy for COPD. Chest 1989; 95:1180–1184.

27. Rodrigues J, Niederman MS, Fein AM, et al. Nonresolving pneumonia in steroid-treated patients with obstructive lung disease. Am J Med 1992; 93:29–34.

28. Palmer LB, Greenberg HE, Schiff MJ. Corticosteroid treatment as a risk factor for invasive aspergillosis in patients with lung disease. Thorax 1991; 46:15–20.

29. Conn H, Poynard T. Corticosteroids and peptic ulcer: meta-analysis of adverse events during steroid therapy. J Intern Med 1994; 236:619–632.

30. Decramer M, Lacquet LM, Fagard R, Rogiers P. Corticosteroids contribute to muscle weakness in chronic airflow obstruction. Am J Respir Crit Care Med 1994; 150:11–16.

31. Hanson P, Dive A, Brucher JM, et al. Acute corticosteroids myopathy in intensive care medicine. Muscle Nerve 1997; 20:1371–1380.

32. Amaya-Villar R, Garnacho-Montero J, Garcia-Garmend JL, et al. Steroid-induced myopathy in patients intubated due to exacerbation of chronic obstructive pulmonary disease. Intensive Care Med 2005; 31:157–161.
33. Laghi F, Tobin MJ. Disorders of the respiratory muscles. Am J Respir Crit Care Med 2003; 168:10–48.
34. Hopkinson NS, Man WD–C, Dayer MJ, et al. Acute effect of oral steroids on muscle function in chronic obstructive pulmonary disease. Eur Respir J 2004; 24:137–142.
35. Conn HO, Blitzer BL. Nonassociation of adrenocorticosteroid therapy and peptic ulcer. N Engl J Med 1976; 294:473–479.
36. Laan RFJM, van Riel PLCM, van de Putte LBA, et al. Low-dose prednisone induces rapid reversible axial bone loss in patients with rheumatoid arthritis; a randomized, controlled study. Ann Intern Med 1993; 119:963–968.
37. McEvoy CE, Ensrud KE, Bender E, et al. Association between corticosteroid use and vertebral fractures in older men with chronic obstructive lung disease. Am J Respir Crit Care Med 1998; 157:704–709.
38. McEvoy CE, Niewoehner DE. Adverse effects of corticosteroid therapy for chronic obstructive pulmonary disease. A critical review. Chest 1997; 111:732–743.
39. Niewoehner DE, Collins D, Erbland ML. Relation of $FEV_1$ to clinical outcomes during exacerbations of chronic obstructive pulmonary disease. Am J Respir Crit Care Med 2000; 161:1201–1205.
40. Saetta M, Di Stefano A, Maestrelli P, et al. Airway eosinophilia in chronic bronchitis during exacerbations. Am J Respir Crit Care Med 1994; 150:1646–1652.
41. Bhowmik A, Seemungal TAR, Sapsford RJ, et al. Relation of sputum inflammatory markers to symptoms and lung function changes in COPD exacerbations. Thorax 2000; 55:114–120.
42. Biernacki WA, Kharitonov SA, Barnes PJ. Increased leukotriene B4 and 8-isoprostane in exhaled breath condensate of patients with exacerbations of COPD. Thorax 2003; 58:294–298.
43. Papi A, Bellettato CM, Braccioni F, et al. Infections and airway inflammation in chronic obstructive pulmonary disease severe exacerbations. Am J Respir Crit Care Med 2006; 173:1114–1121.
44. Barnes PJ. Anti-inflammatory actions of glucocorticoids: molecular mechanisms. Clin Sci 1998; 94:557–572.
45. Adcock IM, Ito K. Glucocorticoid pathways in chronic obstructive pulmonary disease therapy. Proc Am Thorac Soc 2005; 2:313–319.
46. Mak JCW, Nishikawa Barnes PJ. Glucocorticosteroids increase $B_2$-adrenergic receptor transcription in human lung. Am J Physiol 1995; 268:L41–L46.
47. Mendella LA, Manfreda J, Warren PW, et al. Steroid response in stable chronic obstructive pulmonary disease. Ann Int Med 1982; 96:17–21.
48. Shim S, Stover DE, Williams MH Jr. Response to corticosteroids in chronic bronchitis. J Allergy Clin Immunol 1978; 62:363–367.
49. Blair GP, Light RW. Treatment of chronic obstructive pulmonary disease with corticosteroids: comparison of daily vs alternate-day therapy. Chest 1984; 86:524–528.
50. Eliasson O, Hoffman J, Trueb D, et al. Corticosteroids in COPD: a clinical trial and reassessment of the literature. Chest 1986; 89:484–490.
51. Brightling CE, Monteiro W, Ward R, et al. Sputum eosinophilia and short term response to prednisolone in chronic obstructive pulmonary disease: a randomised trial. Lancet 2000; 356:1480–1485.
52. Brightling C, McKenna S, Hargadon B, et al. Sputum eosinophilia and the short term response to inhaled mometasone in chronic obstructive pulmonary disease. Thorax 2005; 60:193–198.
53. Zietkowski Z, Kucharewicz I, Bodzenta-Lukaszyk A. The influence of inhaled corticosteroids on exhaled nitric oxide in stable chronic obstructive pulmonary disease. Respir Med 2005; 99:816–824.

# 23
# Antibiotic Therapy at COPD Exacerbations

**ROBERT WILSON and MITZI NISBET**
Royal Brompton Hospital, London, U.K.

## I. Introduction

Antibiotics are widely prescribed empirically for clinically diagnosed respiratory tract infections accounting for three-quarters of such community prescriptions. Tonsillopharyngitis is the most frequent indication followed by bronchitis, and most of the latter are prescribed to adult patients who are experiencing an exacerbation of chronic lung disease (1). An analysis of acute exacerbations of chronic obstructive pulmonary disease (COPD) in the United States illustrates the size of the problem (2). Using 1994 data to make their calculations, the survey estimated that there were 280,000 hospital admissions and 10 million outpatient visits primarily due to COPD. The majority of patients in both groups were 65 years or older, and older patients had a longer hospital stay. Most patients were given an antibiotic, so the volume prescribed for this indication was enormous. The average cost of a doctor's office visit was estimate to be $74, whereas the average cost of a hospital admission was $5516. Antibiotics accounted for only a small proportion of the hospital costs. Therefore any effective therapy that reduces the need for hospitalization will be highly cost effective because of the large difference in the cost of care in the two settings.

Antibiotics are often given either to speed up recovery in an illness, which might be expected to resolve in any case when the host defences overcome the infection, or in a defensive manner to avoid the risk of infection causing deterioration in a more compromised patient. This might either be deterioration in the established lung disease or in a comorbid condition. In recent years both these practices have been questioned, because of concerns about the size of benefit against a background of rising antibiotic resistance among common respiratory pathogens (3). Penicillin and macrolide antibiotic resistance in *Streptococcus pneumoniae* and β-lactamase production by nontypeable *Haemophilus influenzae* and *Moraxella catarrhalis* have become relatively common, although most studies have shown considerable geographical variation. Broadly speaking, the volume of antibiotics that are used in a community is reflected in the amount of antibiotic resistance in a particular class. Pediatric antibiotic consumption is also a factor, because children spread resistant strains among themselves by direct contact during play in day care and school and also pass strains on to family members. Probably use of antibiotics in animal husbandry and agriculture has contributed as well.

Although a link has been established between in vitro antibacterial resistance and clinical treatment failure in patients with community acquired pneumonia (4), there is virtually no evidence to date in acute exacerbations of COPD. However, at the most severe end of the spectrum of acute exacerbations, patients with COPD requiring admission to the ICU for mechanical ventilation had increased mortality if they were given inappropriate antibiotic treatment of their infection, which was judged when antibiotic sensitivities were known (5), and it seems likely that adverse outcomes would also occur as a consequence of antibiotic resistance in less severe cases.

COPD is a heterogeneous condition both in terms of severity and in that it encompasses several pathologies (airflow obstruction, chronic bronchitis, bronchiolitis, and emphysema), which usually coexist. Mucus hypersecretion, the hallmark of chronic bronchitis, is particularly associated with bacterial infection and identifies a subgroup of young adults at risk of developing COPD independently of smoking habits (6). Bacteria have marked affinity for mucus, and mucociliary clearance is impaired in COPD (3). Bacteria inhaled or aspirated from the nasopharynx may use stationery mucus as the first step when they infect the mucosa. Mucus hypersecretion is associated with COPD mortality from an infectious cause (7). Purulent sputum during an exacerbation has been shown in several studies to be a good predictor of the presence of bacterial infection (8–10). An informative study was performed by Soler and colleagues (11) who bronchoscoped patients admitted with an exacerbation of COPD to directly investigate the presence or absence of bacterial airway infection. Purulent sputum, $FEV_1$ less than 50% of predicted, four or more exacerbations in the last year, and previous hospitalizations due to COPD were associated with the presence of pathogenic bacteria $10^2$ colony forming units/mL or more, which is accepted as a significant level.

## II. Meta-Analysis of Placebo-Controlled Antibiotic Trials in COPD

Although there is evidence that higher exacerbation frequency leads to more rapid progression of COPD (12), as well as worse quality of life for patients (13,14), only one of four older prospective studies showed that more frequent episodes of infection caused a more rapid decline in lung function (15). A meta-analysis of nine placebo controlled trials published in 1995 concluded that there was a small but significant benefit from antibiotic treatment of acute exacerbations of COPD in terms of overall recovery and change in peak flow (16). There have also been nine prospective, placebo-controlled, randomized trials to investigate whether continuous antibiotic treatment reduces the frequency of exacerbations (15). Five trials showed no reduction in frequency of exacerbations, whereas four did show a significant reduction versus placebo. Two of the five trials that showed no benefit did show significantly less time lost from work in the antibiotic group, which suggests that exacerbations occurring while taking continuous antibiotics were shorter and less severe, although the overall frequency was unchanged. Patients most likely to benefit from continuous antibiotic treatment were those suffering frequent exacerbations, which were classified as four or more per year.

In the study of Anthonisen et al. (17), which was the largest study in the above meta-analysis (16), 173 patients with COPD were followed for 3.5 years during which time they had 362 exacerbations. Antibiotics or placebo were given in a randomized, double-blind, crossover fashion. Three levels of severity of exacerbation were defined: the most severe (type 1) comprised worsening dyspnea with increased sputum volume and purulence, type 2 was only two of these symptoms, and type 3 was any one of the symptoms with evidence of fever and/or an upper respiratory tract infection. Three antibiotics were used: amoxicillin, trimethoprim/sulfamethoxazole, and doxycycline, the choice being made by the physician. There was a significant benefit for antibiotics, which was largely accounted for by type 1 exacerbations, whereas there was no significant difference between antibiotic and placebo in patients with type 3 exacerbations. However, even with type 1 exacerbations, 43% of patients recovered in the placebo group within 21 days, emphasizing that most bacterial infection–provoked exacerbations of COPD are mucosal infections, which will be cleared without antibiotic treatment by the host defences. Another consideration is the benefit to the patients' quality of life, and future disease control, by shortening the time of infection with antibiotics. In patients with multiple exacerbations, the duration of antibiotic-treated exacerbations averaged 2.2 days less than those treated with placebo ($p = 0.02$). However, when all patients were considered and treatment failures were eliminated from the analysis, the benefit of antibiotics on speed of recovery was only 0.9 days (NS). Peak flow returned to baseline in both groups during the study period, but the rate of increase was faster in antibiotic-treated exacerbations.

A study by Allegra et al. (18) was not included in the Saint meta-analysis (16). Amoxicillin/clavulanate acid was compared with placebo and showed a clear overall superiority for the antibiotic-treated group. The analysis also showed that patients with more severe impairment of $FEV_1$ and with a history of more frequent exacerbations derived the greatest benefit.

A Cochrane review (19) was completed recently, and was compromised by the small number of trials considered adequate. A significant benefit for antibiotics versus placebo was found for mortality (relative risk ratio = 0.23), but this result was heavily influenced by a single study (ofloxacin vs. placebo) in patients with very severe exacerbations requiring ventilator support (20). The need for antibiotics to be given to all patients in this setting is now proven. Antibiotics also influenced treatment failure (relative risk ratio = 0.47), and the number of patients needed to treat to avoid a failure was three. Antibiotics influenced resolution of sputum purulence but did not influence recovery of peak flow nor gas exchange.

## III.  Bacterial Infection Causing Exacerbations of COPD

There are several possible causes of an exacerbation of COPD. These include air pollution, allergic responses, and patients forgetting to take their medication. However, evidence of an infectious cause was found in 78% of patients hospitalized because of an exacerbation. Thirty percent had bacterial infection, 23% viral, and 25% viral and bacterial coinfection (21). In this study, infectious exacerbations had longer hospitalizations and greater impairment of lung function. These data indicate that infection is the major driver of COPD exacerbations that are severe and that management needs to be focused on preventing and treating infection and its consequences.

Isolation of bacteria from about half of exacerbations has been the finding in many different studies (3). The most frequent species isolated are nontypeable *H. influenzae*, *S. pneumoniae*, and *M. catarrhalis*. These species colonize the nasopharynx of healthy individuals and can therefore be picked up during expectoration of sputum and might not therefore represent true lower airway infection. A number of bronchoscopy studies have been performed to examine the lower airways directly. Monso et al. (22) studied one group of patients with COPD in a stable phase and another group during an exacerbation. They found 25% of stable patients colonized with *H. influenzae* and *S. pneumoniae*. The number of positive cultures increased to 50% at times of exacerbation, and importantly concentrations of the same species of bacteria were much higher during exacerbations. Similarly, hospitalized patients with COPD sputum yielding a bacterial growth of $10^7$ colony forming units/mL were significantly more frequent at exacerbation as compared with convalescence when the patient had recovered (21).

However, the host-bacterial interaction is likely to be much more complex than simple bacterial numbers determining the level of neutrophilic inflammatory response, because this difference in numbers between stable state and exacerbation has not been found in all studies (23). Sethi and colleagues (24) studied a cohort of patients with COPD, seeing them at monthly intervals, with extra visits arranged for exacerbations. Samples (sputum and blood) were taken at each visit, allowing longitudinal bacteriological (including molecular techniques to "fingerprint" strains of bacteria) and immunological investigations to be performed. They showed that 33% of clinic visits associated with acquisition of a new strain were accompanied by an exacerbation, as compared with 15.4% of visits, without a new strain being found. One hypothesis to explain this observation would be that the new strain, not being recognized by the immune system, can multiply and invade the mucosa, thereby stimulating local and systemic inflammatory responses, which cause the symptoms of an exacerbation. Such invasion of the mucosa by *H. influenzae* has been shown in biopsy studies (25). Sethi and colleagues went on to show that when a new strain was associated with an exacerbation, a specific systemic antibody response occurred that gave positive results in bactericidal assay (26). This finding adds weight to the argument that the bacteria are having a causative role in the exacerbation by participating in the generation of a host response intended to eliminate them. The bacterial species involved might also be important in determining the outcome of a host-bacteria encounter, in that Murphy and colleagues (27) found that *H. influenzae* was often carried by patients for long periods, whereas *M. catarrhalis* was eliminated quickly, even in the absence of antibiotic treatment. Therefore exacerbations provoked by *H. influenzae* are more likely to be followed by persistent infection.

Lower airway bacterial colonization in stable COPD probably represents a balance in which impaired host defences are able to limit the numbers of bacteria, but not eradicate them. This is a dynamic process, so that strains may be carried for variable periods of time before being lost and replaced by others (28). After acquisition of the new strain, if an exacerbation does not occur, development of an adaptive immune response may limit proliferation of the pathogen, or regulatory mechanisms could dampen the inflammation, despite the pathogen persisting. Three studies, one using sputum and two lavage have shown that bacterial colonization by potential pathogens when the patients' condition is stable is associated with chronic inflammation (29–31). In one study colonization was also associated with higher concentrations of fibrinogen in plasma and poorer health status (31), which suggests a systemic as well as local inflammatory response. Whether bacterial colonization is driving these results or whether bacteria are passengers taking advantage of the local environment in the airway created by inflammation with another cause is uncertain. However, the following studies infer an active role for bacteria. White et al. (32) showed that resolution of bronchial inflammation following antibiotic treatment of an exacerbation is dependent on bacterial eradication. Antibody responses to bacteria following an exacerbation are of greater intensity, although they do also occur with bacterial colonization in the stable state (33). Finally, "pulsed" antibiotic treatment given to patients at regular intervals during stable COPD significantly reduces exacerbation frequency, particularly for a group of patients who produce purulent sputum when stable (34).

## IV. Aims of Antibiotic Therapy at Acute Exacerbations of COPD

Cigarette smoking is the major cause of COPD. Bacterial infection is an important cause of acute exacerbations, and bacterial colonization probably plays some part in stimulating chronic airway inflammation when the patient's condition is stable. There are therefore several points in these acute and chronic cycles where antibiotic treatment will influence the level of inflammation, and hence the severity of symptoms, which are illustrated in Figure 1. Antibiotic treatment of acute exacerbations is almost always empiric, in that the results of sputum culture and antibiotic sensitivities, even when it is performed, are delayed for 48 hours. The aim is to rapidly sterilize the airway leading to a resolution of the inflammatory response. The success or failure of treatment will depend on many factors:

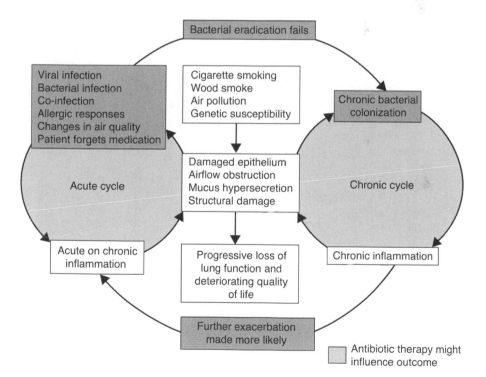

**Figure 1** Pathogenesis of exacerbations of COPD. Points at which antibiotic treatment will influence acute and chronic inflammation (*shaded boxes*).

the extent of infection and virulence of the strain, sensitivity of the strain to the antibiotic chosen, potency of the antibiotic, pharmacokinetics of the antibiotic, whether bacterial infection is the only factor provoking the exacerbation, the severity of the patients' lung disease and therefore the efficacy of their local host defences, and comorbid illness, e.g., heart failure or poorly controlled diabetes. Failure to eradicate the bacterial infection will lead into the chronic cycle and make relapse of the same infection, or a future exacerbation more likely. However some patients acquire bacterial strains that lead to colonization, and this does not necessarily cause an exacerbation. The reason for this is not known, but innate immunity, the severity of the airways disease, and current smoking habit have all been shown to influence whether colonization is present or not (29,35–37).

In one study (38) comparing the quinolone antibiotic moxifloxacin with the macrolide antibiotic clarithromycin, there was superior bacteriological eradication in patients treated with the quinolone (77% compared to 62%) due to persistence of *H. influenzae* in the clarithromycin-treated patients. However, the primary endpoint of the study, which was whether the patient had recovered sufficiently shortly after the course of antibiotic not to require more antibiotic treatment, showed no difference between moxifloxacin and clarithromycin (89% compared to 88% recovery). An analysis of paired sputum samples in the study showed that the explanation for this result was that many patients with persistent *H. influenzae*, who had been treated with clarithromycin, recovered as judged by the criteria used in this trial. Two further studies have suggested that persistent bacterial infection after antibiotic treatment might lead to incomplete recovery and a shorter time until the next exacerbation (39,40).

Further studies are needed to clarify the importance of bacterial eradication after antibiotic therapy at COPD exacerbation and its relationship to recovery and the level of chronic airway inflammation. The studies need to incorporate careful bacteriology and more sensitive measures of patient responses to treatment. Patient-reported outcome (PRO) measures may well prove useful in this regard, and studies need to be longer than the standard design to capture the consequences of bacterial persistence when it occurs (41,42). Another consideration is the speed of action of an antibiotic in killing bacteria, which will differ for bactericidal versus bacteriostatic antibiotics. One study has suggested that this antibiotic property influences the rate of recovery (43), but how early the antibiotic is given after the onset of exacerbation, and therefore the time the infection has to become established, could be more important.

Goals for antibiotic treatment of exacerbations are set out in Table 1, and many of these are generic for all treatments. This is an important consideration, since an antibiotic is only one aspect of management, which should be aimed at reducing airway inflammation as quickly and completely as possible.

**Table 1**  Aims of Antibiotic Therapy at COPD Exacerbations

| Clinical | Biological |
| --- | --- |
| Quick resolution of symptoms | Bacterial eradication |
| Return to baseline health status | Resolution of airway inflammation |
| Avoid relapse | Resolution of systemic inflammation |
| Long exacerbation-free interval | Return of lung function to baseline |
| Maintain health-related quality of life | Avoid disease progression |
| No side effects of treatment | Avoid antibiotic resistance development |

## V. Current Guidelines for Antibiotic Treatment at COPD Exacerbations

Guidelines for this indication have been produced by many national/international societies and national health agencies. They are intended to promote selection of antibiotics to minimize the risk of treatment failure, while containing the development and spread of antibacterial resistance. Therefore equal emphasis is placed on which patients suffering an exacerbation need not be given an antibiotic. Most guidelines attempt to be evidence based. However, they are constrained in this regard because few antibiotics have been tested against a placebo treatment group, and the active comparator-controlled clinical trials are only powered to show equivalence, not superiority, of one antibiotic over another (3).

Broadly speaking, three guideline approaches have been taken (44–53), although the differences are more to do with emphasis rather than any difference of opinion. In the first, "Scandinavian" view COPD is seen as an inflammatory disorder in which for the most part bacteria are passengers taking advantage of a favorable environment in the airway during an exacerbation. First-line treatment is with systemic corticosteroids and in most cases the host defences alone will clear the bacteria. Clinical features and investigations are used to determine the severity of the exacerbation (20) and those patients needing an antibiotic (47). The second approach taken by the majority of guidelines is based on the study by Anthonisen et al. (17) described earlier. Type 3 patients (1 cardinal symptom) should not be given an antibiotic, whereas types 1 and 2 should. Some guidelines place greater emphasis on sputum purulence because of the evidence that this is a signal of bacterial infection, e.g., type 2 patients (2 cardinal symptoms) without sputum purulence do not need an antibiotic. The third "Canadian" approach (48) is to define characteristics that define patients at risk of greater morbidity and mortality. This is a rational approach, since these patients have more severe disease and thus more frequent exacerbations. Therefore, they have received more antibiotics in the past and as a consequence are at more risk of carrying resistant strains. They also have less respiratory reserve if antibiotic failure leads to clinical deterioration (3,44,45). Unfortunately, the use of patient stratification by clinical criteria as a basis for selecting an antibiotic has only been incorporated into very few clinical studies to date.

Martinez et al. (46) divided patients on the basis of $FEV_1$, the number of exacerbations in the last year, comorbidity, and sputum production. They showed that regardless of therapy, the group with the more severe disease, which they termed "complicated," demonstrated lower clinical and microbiological success than uncomplicated patients without those features. Uncomplicated patients were randomized to receive either short-course levofloxacin or azithromycin and complicated patients standard-course levofloxacin or amoxicillin/clavulanate. However, there were no differences in outcome within each group so the benefits or otherwise of the stratification for guiding antibiotic treatment remained unproven.

Choice of antibiotic is usually argued on a number of factors, including suspected etiology, clinical features, and local patterns of antibacterial resistance. A number of studies have shown that the bacteria most commonly isolated vary with the severity of airflow obstruction. *H. influenzae* is the most common isolate overall. In patients with mild airflow obstruction *S. pneumoniae* and other gram-positive cocci are more frequently isolated, whereas *Pseudomonas aeruginosa* and other gram-negative bacilli account for a significant number of isolates in patients with severe airflow obstruction but are very rare in mild cases (49–51). The GOLD guidelines (52) use need for hospitalization to choose between older agents, including amoxicillin for the outpatient setting or amoxicillin/clavulanate, which protects amoxicillin against β-lactamases produced by *H. influenzae* and *M. catarrhalis*. This approach also draws attention to two other factors: cost and tolerability, since amoxicillin/clavulanate is more costly and less well tolerated because of side effects (gastrointestinal) from clavulanate.

French guidelines (53) are interesting in that they refer to pharmacokinetics of antibiotics and their ability to penetrate bronchial tissue and mucus (quinolones, macrolides, ketolides better, betalactams worse) and propensity of the antibiotic to induce resistance. These are potentially very important factors but there is no evidence that they should influence choice of antibiotic in COPD. Development of antibiotic resistance in a community is best achieved by not prescribing antibiotics to otherwise well patients with an exacerbation of mild COPD; nor to Anthonisen types 2 (without purulent sputum) and 3 patients; using short courses of treatment; using correct dosages; and antibiotic diversity. A general principle should be not to use the same antibiotic on every occasion and to try to vary the antibiotic class when managing patients with frequent exacerbations. Although the benefits of cycling antibiotics are unproven in terms of overall resistance development (54), in an individual patient a recent antibiotic course makes a resistant strain more likely (3).

Most guidelines have an alternative recommendation if first-line treatment fails. However, in these circumstances one should first question the diagnosis of a bacterial exacerbation of COPD and ask whether the relapse or failure could be due to another condition such as asthma or heart failure. Investigations, e.g., sputum culture or chest radiograph, should be considered. Usually the second-line antibiotics are those that are active against strains resistant to first-line older agents (trimethoprim-sulphamethoxazole, amoxicillin, tetracycline, trimethoprim, macrolides). These would include betalactam/betalactamase inhibitors (e.g., amoxicillin/clavulanate), ketolides (e.g., azithromycin, telithromycin), quinolones (e.g., moxifloxacin, levofloxacin), and second or third generation cephalosporins. Ciprofloxacin or high-dose levofloxacin are the only oral antibiotics active against *P. aeruginosa*.

## VI.  Patient Characteristics Which Might Influence Choice of Antibiotic

The MOSAIC study (40) was a large, multicenter, double-blind trial in which patients enrolled were middle aged or older, had a heavy-smoking history, a history of frequent exacerbations, significant comorbidity, and, in many cases, severe COPD. They were randomized to receive the quinolone antibiotic moxifloxacin (400 mg once daily for 5 days) or one of the older agents, amoxicillin, cefuroxime, or clarithromycin (standard dosages for 7 days), as selected by the enrolling doctor. Patients were assessed in a stable phase to measure their health status so that following treatment of an exacerbation judgement could be made about their full or partial recovery. When patients had an Anthonisen type 1 exacerbation, they were randomized to one of the treatment groups. In terms of symptomatic improvement shortly after the end of treatment, which was the primary endpoint, the two groups were equivalent. However, moxifloxacin resulted in superior bacteriological eradication and possibly, as a result of this, a better clinical cure rate as assessed by a return to baseline health status. Moxifloxacin was associated with fewer requirements for additional antibiotics (7.6% in the moxifloxacin arm compared with 14.1% in the comparator arm $p = 0.006$) in the weeks following the exacerbation (fewer cases of rapid relapse), and an extended time to the next exacerbation (14 days $p = 0.03$) so that the superiority of moxifloxacin over comparator was significant for five months after the initial exacerbation.

Not all studies have shown a longer exacerbation-free interval in patients treated with a quinolone antibiotic as opposed to a macrolide. The study by Lode et al. (55) compared levofloxacin with clarithromycin. Levofloxacin was associated with a higher bacteriological eradication rate but a similar exacerbation-free interval to clarithromycin. A reason for the difference in outcome compared with the MOSAIC study could be the characteristics of the patients enrolled. Approximately 75% of patients recruited for the Lode et al. study only had moderate airflow obstruction and would therefore be less prone to frequent exacerbations, also nonsmokers and patients having type 2 exacerbations were enrolled.

The MOSAIC study database was interrogated to identify those patient characteristics that influence short (failure to return to baseline health status after acute treatment) and long-term (time to next exacerbation) outcomes of an exacerbation (56). Frequent exacerbations ($\geq 4$ in the past year), low $FEV_1$ ($<50\%$ predicted), randomization to comparator antibiotic (cefuroxime, amoxicillin, clarithromycin), and wheeze during the acute episode were risk factors for both adverse outcomes; whereas comorbid cardiopulmonary disease was a risk factor for clinical failure and older age ($>65$ years) was a risk factor for shorter time to next exacerbation. The superiority of moxifloxacin with respect to rapid relapse was largely accounted for by patients with frequent exacerbations and 65 years or older (53). These findings of the post hoc analysis of the MOSAIC study are similar to other published studies (57), and describe a more vulnerable patient in whom choice of antibiotic might be more important. Other risk factors for poor outcome that have been described include low body mass index, current smoking habit, alcohol consumption, and duration of chronic bronchitis. Not all of the characteristics are amenable to antibiotic treatment. For example a wheezy patient will not do well, even if the bacterial infection is eradicated, unless that aspect of their management is dealt with.

Patel and colleagues (35) used high-resolution computed tomography in a well-characterized group of stable patients with moderate to severe COPD to determine the prevalence of bronchiectasis and emphysema and their relationship to exacerbations, bacterial colonization of the airway in stable state, and airway inflammation. There was no relationship between the degree of emphysema and bacterial colonization or the nature of exacerbations. Bronchiectasis, which was present in half of patients, was associated with bacterial colonization, high levels of airway inflammation, and long exacerbations.

Taking all the above into consideration, we have constructed the algorithm shown in Figure 2. Patients at risk for poor clinical outcome fit within group B of the GOLD guidelines (52) and might be considered for hospital admission. Amoxicillin/clavulanate or a respiratory quinolone would be an appropriate choice of antibiotic; whereas older agents such as amoxicillin and doxycycline are an appropriate choice for low-risk patients. Patients at risk of *P. aeruginosa* should be given an active quinolone such as ciprofloxacin, although care must be taken in patients sick enough to require hospital admission to provide adequate gram-positive cover with a second antibiotic, e.g., benzyl penicillin.

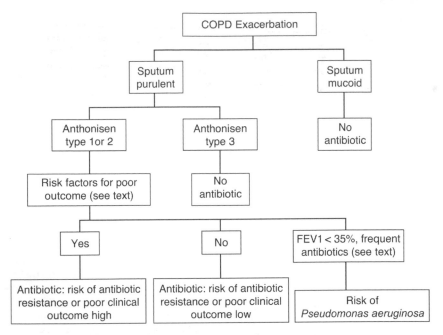

**Figure 2**  An algorithm showing which patients with an acute exacerbation of COPD should receive antibiotic therapy and clinical features influencing choice of antibiotic.

## VII.  Other Issues

### A.  *Pseudomonas aeruginosa*

Patients with severe airflow obstruction (FEV$_1$ <35% predicted), previous frequent antibiotic consumption, recent hospital admission, chronic corticosteroid use, and presence of bronchiectasis are at risk of infection with the gram-negative bacillus *Pseudomonas aeruginosa* (49–51). Patients can become chronically infected and may produce larger volumes of purulent sputum than is usual in COPD on a daily basis. Management is problematic because resistance to ciprofloxacin commonly occurs with repeated use. Parenteral antibiotics may be required, although an alternative is long courses of azithromycin, which have been used successfully in bronchiectasis (58).

## VIII.  Length of Antibiotic Course and Dosage

There is very little information available about the length of antibiotic course that should be prescribed, and 7 to 10 day courses have traditionally been used. New antibiotics have sought a five-day licence on the grounds of greater potency and/or better pharmacokinetics. Some of the registration trials for these antibiotics have compared short versus longer courses of the same new antibiotic or a short course of the new antibiotic versus a longer course of the older agent. The results have shown equivalence, but these trials exclude sicker patients who are more likely to fail and the conclusion that shorter courses can be used in all cases must be made with caution. Shorter courses of antibiotics have several advantages. They will improve patient compliance, reduce total antibiotic consumption and therefore the risk of resistance development, and likely reduce side effects and cost.

Similarly, there are few studies that have addressed dosage in different patient groups. The recommended dosage of amoxicillin/clavulanate and levofloxacin has been increased in some countries to counter rising resistance levels. Broadly speaking, higher dosage leads to more side effects. However, in patients with more damaged lungs, who harbor higher levels of bacterial infection and in whom the risk of resistance development is greater, an increase in dosage might be a more successful strategy rather than increasing the length of the treatment course.

## IX. Biomarkers

A rapid, specific test to identify bacterial lower respiratory tract infections would provide a major improvement in the management plan outlined in Figure 2. C-reactive protein has been found to be unsatisfactory in terms of both sensitivity and specificity (59). Procalcitonin, a small protein, which is increased neither by inflammation that is autoimmune nor by sole viral infection, has produced more encouraging results (60,61). In one study, procalcitonin-guided decision making led to a reduction in antibiotics prescribed to patients admitted with acute exacerbations of COPD without adverse outcomes (62). More studies are required, particularly in centers not used to this approach, because physician judgement plays a big part in current studies when patients have intermediate values. Furthermore, a placebo-controlled study is needed in patients with low values to determine whether any benefit is derived from antibiotic therapy in this group. Development of a rapid diagnostic kit would also mean that the test could be used in the community (63).

## X. Atypical Bacterial Infections

*Mycoplasma pneumoniae* and *Chlamydia pneumoniae* are intracellular bacteria that share some of the characteristics of viruses. There is considerable disagreement in the literature about their importance in acute exacerbations of COPD (64,65). This is because of the various methods used to diagnose infection and the different criteria used for serological tests. Chronic infection by *C. pneumoniae* seems to be quite common in COPD, the significance of which is uncertain (66). If only studies with rigorous methodology are included *M. pneumoniae* is a rare cause of COPD exacerbation, and *C. pneumoniae* is uncommon.

## XI. Viral and Bacterial Coinfection

Rhinovirus, respiratory syncytial virus, and influenza have been associated with exacerbations (21,67). Coinfection by virus and bacteria does seem to increase the severity of the exacerbation (21,68,69) with more symptoms, larger fall in $FEV_1$, higher bacterial loads, more systemic inflammation, longer hospital stay, and slower outpatient recovery. Sputum eosinophilia is associated with viral infections, and it is likely that the inflammatory

**Table 2** Proposed Endpoints for Future Antibiotic Trials in COPD Exacerbations

Patient-reported outcome measures
Speed of recovery
Return to baseline lung function/symptom score
Clinical failure to include rapid relapse in a given time period, e.g., 6 wk following exacerbation
Induced sputum or new biomarkers to assess bacteriological eradication/resolution of inflammation

processes are different when there is coinfection (21), and there is evidence that bacterial infection in turn increases rhinovirus binding to cells and virus-induced chemokine responses (70). Exploration of these interactions should provide new opportunities for therapeutic intervention.

## XII. Future Research

There is an urgent need for more studies to inform appropriate antibiotic therapy at COPD exacerbations. Key questions that remain unanswered are the consequences (if any) of not prescribing antibiotics to COPD patients who do have bacterial infection but relative intact host defences; the importance of antibiotic resistance; should antibiotic prescription be modified in patients who have risk factors for poor outcome; and the effect of bacterial persistence after an exacerbation and lower airway bacterial colonization in the stable state on exacerbation frequency. In the past, most antibiotic studies have been conducted as part of registration trials for new antibiotics. These equivalence studies have provided no help in answering these questions (71).

Patient selection and trial design will both be important, and the studies must be sufficiently powered to either show superiority of one comparator over another, or have a placebo arm. New endpoints should replace the present definition of antibiotic failure, which is requirement for further antibiotic therapy because this has not differentiated between antibiotics despite significant differences in bacteriological outcome (38–40). Table 2 lists possible new endpoints. The MOSAIC study enrolled a homogeneous population of patients with significant COPD and stratified at randomization for the use of corticosteroids, which were anticipated to lessen the difference between comparator antibiotic therapy by reducing airway inflammation independent of bacterial eradication or persistence. Further analysis (42) showed that between group differences could still be confounded by underlying factors related to medical history (e.g., comorbid cardiopulmonary disease), the severity of the disease (e.g., $FEV_1$), and the use of concomitant medication (e.g., long-acting bronchodilators). The analysis suggests that future clinical trials of antibiotic therapy at COPD exacerbation should systematically take these factors into account either a priori (at randomization) or a posteriori (statistical analysis) to increase the sensitivity of the studies to detect differences between antibiotic regimens.

## References

1. Carbon C, Bax RP. Regulating the use of antibiotics in the community. BMJ 1998; 317:663–665.
2. Niederman MS, McCombs JS, Unger AN, et al. Treatment cost of acute exacerbations of chronic bronchitis. Clin Ther 1999; 21:576–591.

3. Wilson R. Bacteria, antibiotics and COPD. Eur Respir J 2001; 17:995–1007.
4. Rzeszutek M, Wierzbowski A, Hoban DJ, et al. A review of clinical failures associated with macrolide-resistant *Streptococcus pneumoniae*. Int J Antimicrob Agents 2004; 24:95–104.
5. Nseir S, Di Pompeo C, Cavestri B, et al. Multiple-drug-resistant bacteria in patients with severe acute exacerbation of chronic obstructive pulmonary disease: prevalence, risk factors and outcome. Crit Care Med 2006; 12:2959–2966.
6. de Marco R, Accordini S, Cerven I, et al. Incidence of chronic obstructive pulmonary disease in a cohort of young adults according to the presence of chronic cough and phlegm. Am J Resp Crit Care Med 2007; 175:32–39.
7. Prescott E, Lange P, Vestbo J, Chronic mucus hypersecretion in COPD and death from pulmonary infection. Eur Resp J 1995; 8:1333–1338.
8. Hill AT, Campbell EJ, Hill SL, et al. Association between airway bacterial load and markers of airways inflammation in patients with stable chronic bronchitis. Am J Med 2000; 108:288–295.
9. Stockley RA, O'Brien C, Pye A, et al. Relationship of sputum color to nature and outpatients management of acute exacerbations of COPD. Chest 2000; 117:1638–1645.
10. Allegra L, Bias F, Diano PL, et al. Sputum color as a marker of acute bacterial exacerbations of chronic obstructive pulmonary disease. Respir Med 2005; 99:742–747.
11. Soler N, Agusti C, Angrill J, et al. Bronchoscopic validation of the significance of sputum purulence in severe exacerbations of chronic obstructive pulmonary disease. Thorax 2007; 62:29–35.
12. Donaldson GC, Seemungal TAR, Bhowmik A, et al. Relationship between exacerbation frequency and lung function decline in chronic obstructive pulmonary disease. Thorax 2002; 57:847–852.
13. Seemungal TAR, Donaldson GC, Paul EA, et al. Effect of exacerbation on quality of life in patients with chronic obstructive pulmonary disease. Am J Respir Crit Care Med 1998; 157:1418–1422.
14. Spencer S, Calverley PMA, Sherwood Burge PS, et al. Health status deterioration in patients with chronic obstructive pulmonary disease. Am J Respir Crit Care Med 2001; 163:122–128.
15. Murphy TF, Sethi S. Bacterial infection in chronic obstructive pulmonary disease. Am Rev Respir Dis 1992; 146:1067–1083.
16. Saint SK, Bent S, Vittinghoff E, et al. Antibiotics in chronic obstructive pulmonary disease exacerbations: a meta-analysis. JAMA 1995; 273:957–960.
17. Anthonisen NR, Marfreda J, Warren CPW, et al. Antibiotic therapy in exacerbations of chronic obstructive pulmonary disease. Ann Intern Med 1987; 106:196–204.
18. Allegra F, Blasi F, de Bernardi B, et al. Antibiotic treatment and baseline severity of disease in acute exacerbations of chronic bronchitis: a re-evaluation of previously published data of a placebo-controlled randomized study. Pulm Pharmacol Ther 2001; 14:149–155.
19. Ram FSF, Rodriquez-Roisin R, Granados-Navarrete A. Antibiotics for exacerbations of chronic obstructive pulmonary disease. Cochrane Database Syst Rev 2006; 2:CD004403.
20. Nouira S, Marghli S, Belghith M, et al. Once daily oral ofloxacin in chronic obstructive pulmonary disease exacerbations requiring mechanical ventilation: a randomised placebo – controlled trial. Lancet 2001; 358:2020–2025.
21. Papi A, Bellettato CM, Braccioni F, et al. Infections and airway inflammation in chronic obstructive pulmonary disease severe exacerbations. Am J Respir Crit Care Med 2006; 173:1114–1121.
22. Monso E, Rosell AI, Boret G, et al. Risk factors of lower airway bacterial colonization in chronic bronchitis. Eur Respir J 1999; 13:338–342.
23. Sethi S, Sethi R, Eschberger K, et al. Airway bacterial concentrations and exacerbations of chronic obstructive pulmonary disease. Am J Respir Crit Care Med 2007; 176:356–361.
24. Sethi S, Evans N, Grant BJB, et al. New strains of bacteria and exacerbations of chronic obstructive pulmonary disease. N Engl J Med 2002; 347:465–471.
25. Bandi V, Apicella MA, Mason E, et al. Nontypeable *Haemophilus influenzae* in the lower respiratory tract of patients with chronic bronchitis. Am J Respir Crit Care Med 2001; 164:2114–2119.

26. Sethi S, Wrona C, Grant BJB, et al. Strain specific immune response to nontypeable *Haemophilus influenzae* in chronic obstructive pulmonary disease. Am J Respir Crit Care Med 2004; 169:448–453.

27. Murphy TF, Brauer AL, Grant BJB, et al. *Moraxella catarrhalis* in chronic obstructive pulmonary disease: burden of disease and immune response. Am J Respir Crit Care Med 2005; 172:195–199.

28. Murphy TF. *Haemophilus influenzae* in chronic bronchitis. Semin Respir Infect 2000; 15:41–51.

29. Soler N, Ewig S, Torres A, et al. Airway inflammation and bronchial microbial patterns in patients with stable chronic obstructive disease. Eur Respir J 1999; 14:1015–1022.

30. Sethi S, Maloney J, Grove L, et al. Airway inflammation and bronchial bacterial colonization in chronic obstructive pulmonary disease. Am J Respir Crit Care Med 2006; 173:991–998.

31. Banerjee D, Khair OA, Honeybourne D. Impact of sputum bacteria on airway inflammation and health status in clinical stable COPD. Eur Respir J 2004; 23:685–691.

32. White AJ, Gompertz S, Bayley DL, et al. Resolution of bronchial inflammation is related to bacterial eradication following treatment of exacerbations of chronic bronchitis. Thorax 2003; 58:680–685.

33. Wilson R. Bacteria and airway inflammation in chronic obstructive pulmonary disease. Am J Respir Crit Care Med 2005; 172:147–148.

34. Sethi S. Pulse moxifloxacin usage and its long-term impact on the reduction of subsequent exacerbations. Presented at: the European Respiratory Society, Stockholm 2007.

35. Patel IS, Seemungal TA, Wilks M, et al. Relationship between bacterial colonization and the frequency, character and severity of COPD exacerbations. Thorax 2002; 57:759–764.

36. Berenson CS, Wrona CT, Grove LJ, et al. Impaired alveolar macrophage response to *Haemophilus* antigens in chronic obstructive pulmonary disease. Am J Respir Crit Care Med 2006; 174:31–40.

37. Berenson CS, Garlipp MA, Grove LJ, et al. Impaired phagocytosis of nontypeable *Haemophilus influenzae* by human alveolar macrophages in chronic obstructive pulmonary disease. J Infect Dis 2006; 194:1375–1384.

38. Wilson R, Kubin R, Ballin I, et al. Five day moxifloxacin therapy compared with seven day clarithromycin therapy for the treatment of acute exacerbations of chronic bronchitis. J Antimicrob Chemother 1999; 44:501–530.

39. Wilson R, Schentagg JJ, Ball P, et al. A comparison of gemifloxacin and clarithromycin in acute exacerbations of chronic bronchitis and long-term clinical outcomes. Clin Ther 2002; 24:639–652.

40. Wilson R, Allegra L, Huchon G, et al. Short-term and long-term outcomes of moxifloxacin compard to standard antibiotic treatment in acute exacerbations of chronic bronchitis. Chest 2004; 125:953–964.

41. Van Parys BA, Sethi S, Lode H, et al. Patient reported outcome (PRO) measure in AECOPD. Preliminary findings: observational clinical study. ICAAC 2007; presentation L-1156.

42. Wilson R. Treatment of COPD exacerbations: antibiotics. Eur Respir Rev 2005; 14:32–38.

43. Miravitlles M, Ferrer M, Pont A, et al. Characteristics of a population of COPD patients identified from a population-based study. Focus on previous diagnosis and never smokers. Respir Med 2005; 99:985–995.

44. Blasi F, Ewig S, Torres A, et al. A review of guidelines for antibacterial use in acute exacerbations of chronic bronchitis. Pulm Pharmacol Ther 2006; 19:361–369 (epub 2005, Nov 10).

45. Rodriguez-Roisin R. COPD exacerbations – 5: Management. Thorax 2006; 61:535–544.

46. Martinez FJ, Grossman RF, Zadeikis N, et al. Patient stratification in the management of acute bacterial exacerbation of chronic bronchitis: the role of levofloxacin 750 mg. Eur Respir J 2005; 25:1001–1010.

47. Sachs APE, Koeter GH, Groenier KH, et al. Changes in symptoms, peak expiratory flow, and sputum flora during treatment with antibiotics of exacerbations in patients with chronic obstructive pulmonary disease in general practice. Thorax 1995; 50:758–763.

48. Balter MS, La Forge J, Low DE, et al. Canadian guidelines for the management of acute exacerbations of chronic bronchitis. Can Respir J 2003; 10(suppl B):3B–32B.

49. Eller J, Ede A, Schaberg T, et al. Infective exacerbations of chronic bronchitis: relation between bacteriologic aetiology and lung function. Chest 1998; 113:1542–1548.
50. Miravitlles M, Espinosa C, Fernando-Laso E, et al. Relationship between bacterial flora in sputum and functional impairment in patients with acute exacerbations of COPD. Chest 1999; 116:40–46.
51. Soler N, Torres A, Ewig S, et al. Bronchial microbial patterns in severe exacerbations of chronic obstructive pulmonary disease requiring mechanical ventilation. Am J Respir Crit Care Med 1998; 157:1498–1505.
52. Global Initiative for Chronic Obstructive Pulmonary Disease. Global strategy for the diagnosis, management and prevention of chronic obstructive pulmonary disease. Executive summary 2005. Available at www.goldcopd.com.
53. Societé de Pneumologie de Langue Francaise. Guidelines for the clinical management of COPD. Exacerbations/acute respiratory failure: antibiotherapy. Rev Mal Respir 2003; 20:565–568.
54. Brown EM, Nathwani D. Antibiotic cycling or rotation: a systematic review of the evidence of efficacy. J Antimicrob Chemother 2005; 55:6–9.
55. Lode H, Eller J, Linnhoff A, et al. Levofloxacin versus clarithromycin in chronic obstructive pulmonary disease exacerbation: focus on exacerbation-free interval. Eur Respir J 2004; 24: 947–953.
56. Wilson R, Jones P, Schaberg T, et al. Antibiotic treatment and factors influencing short and long term outcomes of acute exacerbations of chronic bronchitis. Thorax 2006; 61:337–342.
57. Wilson R. Outcome predictors in bronchitis. Chest 1995; 108:535–575.
58. Davies G, Wilson R. Prophylactic antibiotic treatment of bronchiectasis with azithromycin. Thorax 2004; 59:539–540.
59. van der Meer V, Neven AK, van den Broek PJ, et al. Diagnositic value of C-reactive protein in infections of the lower respiratory tract: systematic review. BMJ 2005; 331:26–31.
60. Christ-Crain M, Jaccord Stolz D, Bingisser R. Effect of procalcitonin-guided treatment on antibiotic use and outcome in lower respiratory tract infections: cluster-randomised, single-blinded intervention trial. Lancet 2004; 363:600–607.
61. Martinez FJ, Curtis JL. Procalcitonin-guided antibiotic therapy in COPD exacerbations: closer but not quite there. Chest 2007; 131:1–2.
62. Stolz D, Christ-Crain M, Bingisser R, et al. Antibiotic treatment of exacerbations of COPD: a randomised controlled trial comparing procalcitonin-guidance with standard therapy. Chest 2007; 131:9–19.
63. Galetto-Lacour A, Zamora SA, Gervaix A. Bedside procalcitonin and c-reactive protein tests in children with fever without localizing signs of infection seen in a referral centre. Paediatrics 2003; 112:1054–1060.
64. White AJ, Gompertz S, Stockley RA. Chronic obstructive pulmonary disease 6: The aetiology of exacerbations of chronic obstructive pulmonary disease. Thorax 2003; 58:680–685.
65. Anzueto A, Sethi S, Martinez FJ. Exacerbations of chronic obstructive pulmonary disease. Proc Am Thorac Soc 2007; 4:554–564.
66. Blasi F, Damato S, Cosentini R, et al. Chlamydia pneumoniae and chronic bronchitis: association with severity and bacterial clearance following treatment. Thorax 2002; 57: 672–676.
67. Wedzicha JA. Role of viruses in exacerbations of chronic obstructive pulmonary disease. Proc Am Thorac Soc 2004; 1:115–120.
68. Seemungal T, Harper-Owen R, Bhowmik A, et al. Detection of rhinovirus in induced sputum at exacerbations of chronic obstructive pulmonary disease. Eur Respir J 2000; 16:677–683.
69. Wilkinson TMA, Hurst JR, Perera WR, et al. Effects of interactions between lower airway bacterialand rhinoviral infection in exacerbations of COPD. Chest 2006; 129:317–324.
70. Sajjan US, Jia Y, Newcomb DC, et al. *Haemophilus influenzae* potentiates airway epithelial cell responses to rhinovirus by increasing ICAM-1 and TLR3 expression. FASEB J 2006; 20:212–213.
71. Miravitlles M, Torres A. No more equivalence trials for exacerbations of COPD, please. Chest 2004; 125:811–813.

# 24

## Noninvasive Ventilatory Support in Acute Exacerbations of COPD

**STANLEY D. W. MILLER and MARK W. ELLIOTT**
Department of Respiratory Medicine, St. James's University Hospital, Leeds, U.K.

## I. Introduction

Patients with acute exacerbations of chronic obstructive pulmonary disease (COPD) form the largest single group of those treated successfully using noninvasive ventilation (NIV) (1). The respiratory muscle pump in patients with severe COPD is often functioning close to the point at which it can no longer maintain effective ventilation due to hyperinflation, airways obstruction, and intrinsic positive end-expiratory pressure (PEEP). During an acute exacerbation, the load on the respiratory muscle pump becomes excessive and effective ventilation can no longer be maintained, worsening hypoxia, hypercapnia, and most importantly acidosis. Worsening acidosis causes further impairment of respiratory muscle function, which in turn has a deleterious effect on pH and arterial blood gas tensions. The use of NIV aims to break this vicious circle.

## II. NIV in Acute COPD

Even short periods of NIV are usually sufficient to break the vicious circle produced by acidosis, while other therapies take effect upon the precipitating cause. It is striking that in some studies NIV was administered for only a relatively short period (2,3) (mean 7.6 hours and 6 hours daily, respectively) or at very modest levels for a longer period (4). In a large multicenter randomized controlled trial of NIV in the United Kingdom (5), "treatment failure," a surrogate for the need for intubation defined by a priori criteria, was reduced from 27% to 15% by NIV and in-hospital mortality was reduced from 20% to 10%. The early introduction of NIV (pH < 7.35 on admission to the ward) resulted in a better outcome than providing no ventilatory support for acidotic patients outside the ICU. A prospective randomized controlled trial of NIV versus immediate endotracheal intubation and invasive mechanical ventilation (IMV), in sicker patients with an exacerbation of COPD [acute exacerbations of chronic obstructive pulmonary disease (AECOPD)] and a mean pH of 7.2, showed that NIV was no worse than IMV (6). In those who could be managed successfully with NIV, there was an advantage not only in the short term but also in the year after hospital discharge in terms of a reduction in the need for hospital admission and de novo long-term oxygen therapy. The intubation rate of 52% in the NIV group in the study was higher than in other randomized controlled trials, which is not surprising given that these were a sicker group of patients. However, it does reinforce the view that NIV is best instituted early (7). In all but the sickest patients with an exacerbation of COPD, there is little to be lost, and much to be gained, by a trial of NIV.

## III.  NIV vs. IMV

The most important advantage of NIV when compared with IMV in the treatment of AECOPD relates to the reduction in nosocomial infections, in particular, ventilator-associated pneumonia (VAP). VAP is consistently associated with increased length of ventilation, increased stay in the ICU and hospital, increased costs, and a worse outcome. The impairment of local defences to infection secondary to intubation, aspiration of contaminated secretions pooled above the endotracheal cuff, supine position, nasogastric tube insertion, enteral feeding, reintubation, tracheotomy, failure to maintain adequate inflation pressure of the endotracheal cuff, excessive frequency of ventilator tube changes, and gastric alkalization all increase the risk of VAP with IMV (8). NIV has been shown consistently to reduce the incidence of nosocomial infections, particularly VAP, when compared with IMV (9–12). Relating specifically to COPD, NIV has been shown to result in lower rates of nosocomial infections, lower rates of VAP, lower use of antibiotics for treating these infections, lower length of ICU and hospital stays, and lower mortality compared with IMV and is independently linked with a reduced risk of death (3,13,14). The reduction in complications, particularly infections, makes NIV preferable to invasive ventilation if deemed clinically appropriate.

## IV.  Indications for NIV in AECOPD

Ideally, NIV should be instituted when the pH is less than 7.35 and the respiratory rate is more than 23 breaths/min and after optimized medical treatment has been evaluated (5). In most patients, therefore, NIV should not be started until an hour or two has elapsed. The arterial blood gas tensions should be measured, and if the pH is less than 7.35 and the patient is hypercapnic, NIV should be initiated (15) (Table 1). It should be noted that approximately 20% of patients with COPD who are acidotic at the time of arrival in the emergency room will correct their pH completely into the normal range with standard medical therapy alone including, most importantly, properly controlled oxygen therapy (16). This can apply to patients with very severe acidosis. In addition, in the pH range 7.30–7.35, 80% of patients will get better without NIV, but only 10 patients need to receive NIV to avoid one intubation (5). Once the pH is less than 7.30, however, the outcome without NIV is much

**Table 1**   Indications for NIV in Acute COPD

| |
| --- |
| pH < 7.35 |
| Hypercapnia |
| Respiratory rate >23 breaths/min |

All above after optimized medical treatment has been evaluated (5)

worse, and these patients should be encouraged very strongly to use NIV. There is no lower limit of pH contraindicating the use of NIV, but the more severe the acidosis, the greater the chance that NIV will not be successful (17). One group has even used NIV successfully in very sick comatose patients (18). We would suggest starting with an inspiratory positive airway pressure (IPAP) of 10 cm $H_2O$ and an expiratory positive airway pressure (EPAP) of 5 cm $H_2O$ and then increase the IPAP depending upon response over the following hour or so to 15 to 20 cm $H_2O$. If necessary, patients can be persuaded to tolerate high pressures, though once the IPAP gets above 20 cm $H_2O$, there may be a marked increase in leak (19). It is advisable to have some EPAP to counterbalance intrinsic PEEP, reduce carbon dioxide rebreathing, and in some cases stabilize the upper airway during sleep.

## V.  Where Should NIV be Given?

For the purposes of this discussion, the following definitions are used.

ICU: A high ratio of staff to patients and facilities for invasive ventilation and monitoring.

Intermediate respiratory ICU or high-dependency unit (HDU): Continuous monitoring of vital signs in a specified clinical area with a staffing ratio between an ICU and a general ward.

General ward: Patients with a variety of medical conditions and degrees of severity cared for in the same area with variable nursing levels that are not as intensive as HDU/ICU.

There have been no direct comparisons between these three locations regarding the outcome from NIV, but there is ample other evidence to help decide where NIV should be given. When NIV was studied in the ICU (3,4,20,21), the most striking finding was a reduction in the need for subsequent endotracheal intubation and mechanical ventilation (3). In this setting, NIV reduces the need for intubation (3,4), improves survival, reduces the length of both ICU and hospital stays (3), and markedly reduces complications (3,9–14). However, many patients find their experience of ICU to be unpleasant (22). Factors including the likelihood of NIV failure, whether subsequent intubation is appropriate, the presence of any comorbidities or other system failure, and the severity of respiratory failure in a particular patient will help determine the appropriateness of ICU care. If NIV is only to be provided in an ICU setting, the number of patients needing ICU care will increase, causing obvious pressures on bed availability for IMV. Although NIV has been shown to be cost effective in the ICU setting (23), if it can be performed outside the ICU, there are greater savings to be made (24,25). There have been a number of prospective randomized controlled studies of NIV outside the ICU either on general wards or in accident and emergency departments (2,5,26–30). NIV was instituted at a higher pH than that reported in the ICU studies, and most studies failed to show any significant advantage of NIV when analyzed on an intention-to-treat basis. However, in one study (2), a significant survival benefit was seen when those unable to tolerate NIV were excluded. NIV is an option on general wards (5), but the outcome if the pH is less than 7.3 is not as good as that seen for patients in a higher-dependency setting. However, for reasons of training, throughput, quality of service, and skill retention, NIV is best performed in a single location in an intermediate respiratory unit (16). A dedicated intermediate care unit with particular expertise in NIV may provide the best environment, both in terms of outcome and cost effectiveness (31). Staff training and experience is more important than location, and adequate numbers of staff skilled in NIV must be available 24 hours per day (31). These units are not widely available throughout Europe (32), but data from the United States suggest that they are cost effective (33). As NIV in the more severely ill patient may require as much input as IMV (34), there should be one nurse responsible for no more than three or four patients. In the less severely affected patient, NIV can be successfully delivered with a lower level of staffing (5).

## VI.  Contraindications

There are no absolute contraindications to NIV, although quite a few have been suggested (35,36). These include coma or confusion, inability to protect the airway, severe acidosis at presentation, significant comorbidity, vomiting, bowel obstruction, upper gastrointestinal bleeding, uncontrolled arrhythmia, hemodynamic instability, radiological evidence of consolidation, and orofacial abnormalities that interfere with the mask-face interface. In part, these contraindications have been determined by the fact that they were exclusion criteria for controlled trials. It is therefore more correct to state that NIV is not proven in these circumstances rather than that it is contraindicated. Decisions regarding these contraindications should be made on a case-by-case basis. If IMV has been deemed inappropriate and NIV has been determined as the ceiling of treatment, the potential contraindications listed above fail to become a barrier to the use of NIV. Under these circumstances, there is nothing to be lost by a trial of NIV, but any worsening of the relevant clinical condition, such as bowel obstruction or hemodynamic instability, should be closely watched for.

## VII.  Choice of Ventilator Type

Ventilators used for NIV in exacerbations of COPD are either volume or pressure targeted. In stable patients, little difference in gas exchange is seen between these ventilator types (37,38). Volume-targeted ventilators have been shown to produce more complete off-loading of the respiratory muscles, but this is at the expense of comfort (39). Pressure-targeted ventilators have much better leak compensating abilities than volume-targeted ventilators, but even this can vary depending on the device used (40). In terms of outcome, there is no difference between volume-targeted or pressure-targeted machines, but pressure-targeted machines are generally tolerated better (41). In addition, these pressure-cycled machines are usually cheaper. Several alternative modes and strategies of NIV have been explored. Proportional assist ventilation (PAV) has been shown to improve gas exchange and dyspnea in stable COPD (42). It has also been shown to decrease patient effort, work of breathing, and neuromuscular drive in patients with COPD being weaned off mechanical ventilation (43,44). PEEP added during NIV has beneficial effects, off-loading the respiratory muscles, by counterbalancing intrinsic PEEP (45) and lavaging carbon dioxide from the mask (46). Both mask continuous positive airway pressure (CPAP) (47–49) and negative pressure ventilation (NPV) (50–52) have been shown to have beneficial effects in exacerbations of COPD, but these modes lack the same wealth of evidence that noninvasive positive pressure ventilation (NIPPV) enjoys. In addition, the degree of unloading with CPAP is less than with NIPPV in stable patients (37).

## VIII. Interfaces

The development of various interfaces has made the delivery of effective ventilation to patients without intubation possible. A good interface is crucial to the success of NIV. Essentially, there are four different types of factory-made interfaces: Full face masks (enclose mouth and nose), nasal masks, nasal pillows or plugs (insert directly into the nostrils), and mouthpieces. The use of an appropriate-sized mask is vital, and equal attention should be directed toward the choice of the correct size of headgear. Other interfaces include the helmet and semicustomized masks, consisting of a prefabricated frame into which a quick-drying filler is injected and the mask moulded to the patient's face. In acute NIV, facial masks are most widely used (63%) followed by nasal masks (31%) and nasal pillows (6%). This is in contrast to chronic NIV use where nasal masks predominate (73%) (53). A full face mask is a definite advantage in a patient who is mouth-breathing, a common occurrence in acute COPD. This type of mask results in better quality of ventilation, in terms of improved minute ventilation and blood gases (54,55). The improvement in arterial blood gas tensions appears to be slower in studies using nasal masks compared with face masks (56). The nasal mask has a role in the post-acute situation, however, by switching from the full face mask to encourage prolonged compliance with NIV (57). The use of the helmet has been described in both hypoxemic acute respiratory failure (58) and in acute exacerbations of COPD (59). When compared with the full face mask, the helmet has been shown to be less efficient in reducing inspiratory effort and worsens patient-ventilator synchrony (59). As both helmet and facial mask are equally tolerated and patient comfort is comparable, the helmet may prove to be an alternative for patients who do not tolerate the mask or serve as an additional tool to prevent skin breakdown when NIV is applied for prolonged periods of time.

The three main challenges when choosing an interface for a particular patient are to (*i*) minimize any leak, (*ii*) maximize patient comfort, and (*iii*) reduce dead space to a minimum. Leak, which results from a poor fit between the mask and the skin or through the open mouth, reduces alveolar ventilation and synchrony between the patient and the machine and may also compromise the quality of sleep (60). It should be monitored, but however good the interface, some leak is inevitable. An interface that is comfortable and does not cause side effects such as nasal bridge sores, eye irritation, or dryness is best. With most face masks, continuous flow throughout expiration reduces the total dynamic dead space to close to the physiological dead space (61). Once the PEEP or EPAP is reduced below 4 to 6 cm $H_2O$, $CO_2$ rebreathing is markedly increased in the absence of a non-rebreathing valve (46). The position of the exhalation port within a mask is important and affects the dynamic dead space with ports over the nasal bridge being best followed by ports elsewhere in the mask and then those at the junction of mask and ventilator circuit (61). Interestingly, there is a poor relationship between the static volume of a mask and dynamic dead space (61), which may explain why the helmet, with a large static dead space, can be used effectively. Masks that do not have optimally positioned ports may still maintain a small dynamic dead space by benefiting from a small amount of unintentional leak around the nasal bridge (62).

## IX. Monitoring the Patient on NIV

Monitoring serves two roles: to warn of impending problems and to facilitate optimization of ventilator settings. Although the evaluation of patient-ventilator asynchrony is difficult without visualization of flow and pressure waveforms (63), it should be remembered that

**Table 2**  Monitoring During NIV

---

***Essential***
Regular clinical observation by experienced staff
Continuous pulse oximetry
Arterial blood gases after 1–4 hr NIV and after 1 hr of any change in ventilator settings or $FiO_2$
Respiratory rate

***Desirable***
Electrocardiogram
More detailed physiological information such as leak, expired $V_T$, and measure of ventilator-patient
   asynchrony

---

*Abbreviations*: NIV, noninvasive ventilation; $FiO_2$: inspiratory oxygen fraction; $V_T$: tidal volume.

high-technology monitoring is never a substitute for good clinical observation (64). The oxygen saturation should be maintained at around 92% (65) to avoid hypoxia. A higher $SaO_2$ target is not necessary as these patients will be well acclimatized to hypoxia, and a high $FiO_2$ may worsen hypercapnia by altering the dead space-to-$V_T$ ratio (66). Arterial blood gases should be checked at baseline and after one to four hours as the change in arterial blood gas tensions predicts a successful outcome (see "Predictors of Success and Outcome"). In addition, arterial blood gas tensions should be checked within one hour of any change in ventilator settings or $FiO_2$. The recording of the respiratory rate may be useful in determining the likely outcome with NIV (see "Predictors of Success and Outcome"). The monitoring required during NIV is summarized in Table 2.

## X.  Predictors of Success and Outcome

Data available at the time NIV is initiated and after a short period can predict the likelihood of success or failure with a reasonable degree of precision. Patients with high APACHE II (Acute Physiology and Chronic Health Evaluation II) scores or pneumonia or those who are underweight or have a greater level of neurological deterioration are more likely to fail on NIV (35,36). A reduction in respiratory rate with NIV has been shown in a number of studies, with larger falls generally being associated with a successful outcome (3,36,67), though this is not always seen (68). The change in arterial blood gas tensions, particularly pH, after a short period of NIV predicts a successful outcome (2,3,35,36,56,67). An improvement in pH and/or carbon dioxide tension in arterial blood at 30 minutes (69), one hour (67), or after a longer period (36,67) predicts successful NIV. After four hours of therapy, improvement in acidosis and/or a fall in respiratory rate is associated with success (70). Although NIV results in lower rates of nosocomial infections compared with IMV, colonization with nonfermenting gram-negative bacilli, mainly *Pseudomonas aeruginosa*, is strongly associated with NIV failure in exacerbations of COPD (71). The tolerance of NIV also predicts subsequent outcome. Patients with an inability to minimize the amount of mask leak or an inability to coordinate with NIV are less likely to improve with NIV (36), and there should be a low threshold for IMV. In addition, NIV is more likely to fail if there is reduced compliance with ventilation (35). NIV is less likely to be successful if there are

**Table 3**    Predictors of Likely Success and Failure in NIV

**Predictors of success**

Large reduction in respiratory rate (3,36,67)

Improvement in pH and/or carbon dioxide tension at 30 min (69), 1 hr (67), or after a longer period (36,67)

Improvement in acidosis and/or a fall in respiratory rate after 4 hr of therapy (70)

**Predictors of failure**

*Patient factors*

High APACHE II scores (35,36)

Low BMI (35)

Low level of consciousness (35,36)

Pneumonia (35)

Colonization with nonfermenting gram-negative bacilli (*Pseudomonas aeruginosa*) (71)

Excessive secretions (36)

Poor premorbid condition (72,73)

Low pH prior to starting NIV (35)

Late failure after initially successful NIV (72)

*Technical factors*

Inability to minimize leak (36)

Inability to coordinate with NIV (36)

Reduced compliance with ventilation (35)

*Abbreviations*: NIV, noninvasive ventilation; APACHE II, Acute Physiology and Chronic Health Evaluation II; BMI, body mass index.

associated complications or if the patient's premorbid condition is poor (72,73). Late failure after initially successful NIV is a bad prognostic factor, with over half the patients dying even with IMV (72). The predictors of success and failure of NIV in COPD are summarized in Table 3.

Although there have been a number of studies to ascertain predictors of outcome for patients with COPD requiring NIV (17,35,36,69,70,74,75), these studies have a number of limitations. Most have recruited small numbers of patients from a small number of centers and have been retrospective, and important variables that have been shown to be predictive in other studies may not have been included. Furthermore, the outcome variable is usually survival to hospital discharge. There is little data about longer-term outcome, postdischarge health status, or the longer-term outcome of patients who fail an initial trial of NIV and either receive no further treatment or receive IMV. The clinician needs to make two decisions: first, the likelihood of success of a particular technique in the short term [most patients who fail with NIV do so in the first 12–24 hours (3)], and second, the effect of an intervention upon longer-term outcome. It is possible that ready recourse to IMV results in better short-term results but worse long-term survival than NIV, and there is some evidence to support this theory (76). There is therefore a need for a prospective study of predictors of outcome for patients receiving NIV in a wide variety of different centers. It is important that the predictors be those that are readily available at the time when decisions need to be made. At the time of writing, the European Predictors of Outcome from Ventilation (EPOV) study coordinated from Leeds, United Kingdom, was recruiting patients to determine more robust predictors of outcome.

## XI. Conclusion

NIV is now very well established as the primary intervention for patients with ventilatory failure due to an acute exacerbation of COPD. There are a few absolute contraindications to its use, and the advantages are such that it should be offered to most patients requiring ventilatory support. It should be initiated when the pH remains less than 7.35 after a period of time has elapsed to see if patients will improve anyway with standard medical therapy and controlled oxygen. There are no data on which to base recommendations of how long NIV should be continued, but in most cases it can be stopped after 48 to 72 hours.

## References

1. Lightowler JV, Wedzicha JA, Elliott MW, et al. Non-invasive positive pressure ventilation to treat respiratory failure resulting from exacerbations of chronic obstructive pulmonary disease: cochrane systematic review and meta-analysis. BMJ 2003; 326:185–189.
2. Bott J, Carroll M, Conway J, et al. Randomised controlled trial of nasal ventilation in acute ventilatory failure due to chronic obstructive airways disease. Lancet 1993; 341:1555–1557.
3. Brochard L, Mancebo J, Wysocki M, et al. Noninvasive ventilation for acute exacerbations of chronic obstructive pulmonary disease. N Engl J Med 1995; 333(13):817–822.
4. Kramer N, Meyer T, Meharg J, et al. Randomized, prospective trial of noninvasive positive pressure ventilation in acute respiratory failure. Am J Respir Crit Care Med 1995; 151:1799–806.
5. Plant P, Owen J, Elliott M. Early use of non-invasive ventilation for acute exacerbations of chronic obstructive pulmonary disease on general respiratory wards: a multicentre randomised controlled trial. Lancet 2000; 355:1931–1935.
6. Conti G, Antonelli M, Navalesi P, et al. Noninvasive vs. conventional mechanical ventilation in patients with chronic obstructive pulmonary disease after failure of medical treatment in the ward: a randomized trial. Intensive Care Med 2002; 28(12):1701–1707.
7. Evans TW. International consensus conferences in intensive care medicine: non-invasive positive pressure ventilation in acute respiratory failure. Intensive Care Med 2001; 27(1):166–178.
8. Kollef M. The prevention of ventilator-associated pneumonia. N Engl J Med 1999; 340:627–634.
9. Antonelli M, Conti G, Rocco M. A comparison of noninvasive positive-pressure ventilation and conventional mechanical ventilation in patients with acute respiratory failure. N Engl J Med 1998; 339:429–435.
10. Carlucci A, Richard J, Wysocki M, et al. Noninvasive versus conventional mechanical ventilation. An epidemiologic survey. Am J Respir Crit Care Med 2001; 163:874–880.
11. Guerin C, Girard R, Chemorin C, et al. Facial mask noninvasive mechanical ventilation reduces the incidence of nosocomial pneumonia. A prospective epidemiological survey from a single ICU. Intensive Care Med 1997; 23:1024–1032.
12. Nourdine K, Combes P, Carton M, et al. Does noninvasive ventilation reduce the ICU nosocomial infection risk? A prospective clinical survey. Intensive Care Med 1999; 25:567–573.
13. Girou E, Brun-Buisson C, Taille S, et al. Secular trends in nosocomial infections and mortality associated with noninvasive ventilation in patients with exacerbation of COPD and pulmonary oedema. JAMA 2003; 290:2985–2991.
14. Girou E, Schortgen F, Delclaux C, et al. Association of noninvasive ventilation with nosocomial infections and survival in critically ill patients. JAMA 2000; 284:2361–2367.
15. British Thoracic Society Standards of Care Committee. Non-invasive ventilation in acute respiratory failure. Thorax 2002; 57(3):192–211.
16. Plant PK, Owen JL, Elliott MW. One year period prevalence study of respiratory acidosis in acute-exacerbations of COPD: implications for the provision of non-invasive ventilation and oxygen administration. Thorax 2000; 55(7):550–554.

17. Confalonieri M, Garuti G, Cattaruzza MS, et al. A chart of failure risk for noninvasive ventilation in patients with COPD exacerbation. Eur Respir J 2005; 25(2):348–355.
18. Diaz GG, Alcaraz AC, Talavera JCP, et al. Noninvasive positive-pressure ventilation to treat hypercapnic coma secondary to respiratory failure. Chest 2005; 127(3):952–960.
19. Tuggey JM, Elliott MW. Titration of non-invasive positive pressure ventilation in chronic respiratory failure. Respir Med 2006; 100(7):1262–1269.
20. Celikel T, Sungur M, Ceyhan B, et al. Comparison of noninvasive positive pressure ventilation with standard medical therapy in hypercapnic acute respiratory failure. Chest 1998; 114(6):1636–1642.
21. Martin TJ, Hovis JD, Costantino JP, et al. A randomized, prospective evaluation of noninvasive ventilation for acute respiratory failure. Am J Respir Crit Care Med 2000; 161(3):807–813.
22. Easton C, MacKenzie F. Sensory-perceptual alterations: delirium in the intensive care unit. Heart Lung 1988; 17:229–237.
23. Keenan S, Gregor J, Sibbald W, et al. Noninvasive positive pressure ventilation in the setting of severe, acute exacerbations of chronic obstructive pulmonary disease: more effective and less expensive. Crit Care Med 2000; 28:2094–2102.
24. Plant PK, Owen JL, Parrott S, et al. Cost effectiveness of ward based non-invasive ventilation for acute exacerbations of chronic obstructive pulmonary disease: economic analysis of randomised controlled trial. BMJ 2003; 326:956–961.
25. Carlucci A, Delmastro M, Rubini F, et al. Changes in the practice of non-invasive ventilation in treating COPD patients over 8 years. Intensive Care Med 2003; 29:419–425.
26. Angus R, Ahmed A, Fenwick L, et al. Comparison of the acute effects on gas exchange of nasal ventilation and doxapram in exacerbations of chronic obstructive pulmonary disease. Thorax 1996; 51:1048–1050.
27. Avdeev SN, Tret'iakov AV, Grigor'iants RA, et al. Study of the use of noninvasive ventilation of the lungs in acute respiratory insufficiency due exacerbation of chronic obstructive pulmonary disease. Anesteziol Reanimatol 1998; 3(3):45–51.
28. Barbe F, Togores B, Rubi M, et al. Noninvasive ventilatory support does not facilitate recovery from acute respiratory failure in chronic obstructive pulmonary disease. Eur Resp J 1996; 9:1240–1245.
29. Bardi G, Pierotello R, Desideri M, et al. Nasal ventilation in COPD exacerbations:early and late results of a prospective, controlled study. Eur Resp J 2000; 15:98–104.
30. Wood K, Lewis L, Von Harz B, et al. The use of noninvasive positive pressure ventilation in the Emergency Department. Chest 1998; 113:1339–1346.
31. Elliott MW, Confalonieri M, Nava S. Where to perform noninvasive ventilation? Eur Resp J 2002; 19(6):1159–1166.
32. Nava S, Confalonieri M, Rampulla C. Intermediate respiratory intensive care units in Europe: a European perspective. Thorax 1998; 53:798–802.
33. Elpern E, Silver M, Rosen R, et al. The noninvasive respiratory care unit. Patterns of use and financial implications. Chest 1991; 99:205–208.
34. Nava S, Evangelisti I, Rampulla C, et al. Human and financial costs of noninvasive mechanical ventilation in patients affected by COPD and acute respiratory failure. Chest 1997; 111:1631–1638.
35. Ambrosino N, Foglio K, Rubini F, et al. Non-invasive mechanical ventilation in acute respiratory failure due to chronic obstructive pulmonary disease: correlates for success. Thorax 1995; 50(7):755–757.
36. Soo Hoo GW, Santiago S, Williams AJ. Nasal mechanical ventilation for hypercapnic respiratory failure in chronic obstructive pulmonary disease: determinants of success and failure. Crit Care Med 1994; 22(8):1253–1261.
37. Elliott MW, Aquilina R, Green M, et al. A comparison of different modes of noninvasive ventilatory support: effects on ventilation and inspiratory muscle effort. Anaesthesia 1994; 49(4): 279–283.
38. Meecham Jones DJ, Wedzicha JA. Comparison of pressure and volume preset nasal ventilator systems in stable chronic respiratory failure. Eur Respir J 1993; 6(7):1060–1064.

39. Girault C, Richard JC, Chevron V, et al. Comparative physiologic effects of noninvasive assist-control and pressure support ventilation in acute hypercapnic respiratory failure. Chest 1997; 111 (6):1639–1648.
40. Mehta S, McCool FD, Hill NS. Leak compensation in positive pressure ventilators: a lung model study. Eur Respir J 2001; 17(2):259–267.
41. Vitacca M, Rubini F, Foglio K, et al. Non-invasive modalities of positive pressure ventilation improve the outcome of acute exacerbations in COPD patients. Intensive Care Med 1993; 19(8): 450–455.
42. Ambrosino N, Vitacca M, Polese G, et al. Short-term effects of nasal proportional assist ventilation in patients with chronic hypercapnic respiratory insufficiency. Eur Respir J 1997; 10(12): 2829–2834.
43. Appendini L, Purro A, Gudjonsdottir M, et al. Physiologic response of ventilator-dependent patients with chronic obstructive pulmonary disease to proportional assist ventilation and continuous positive airway pressure. Am J Respir Crit Care Med 1999; 159(5):1510–1517.
44. Wrigge H, Golisch W, Zinserling J, et al. Proportional assist versus pressure support ventilation: effects on breathing pattern and respiratory work of patients with chronic obstructive pulmonary disease. Intensive Care Med 1999; 25(8):790–798.
45. Appendini L, Patessio A, Zanaboni S, et al. Physiologic effects of positive end-expiratory pressure and mask pressure support during exacerbations of chronic obstructive pulmonary disease. Am J Respir Crit Care Med 1994; 149(5):1069–1076.
46. Ferguson GT, Gilmartin M. $CO_2$ rebreathing during BiPAP ventilatory assistance. Am J Respir Crit Care Med 1995; 151(4):1126–1135.
47. de Lucas P, Tarancon C, Puente L, et al. Nasal continuous positive airway pressure in patients with COPD in acute respiratory failure. A study of the immediate effects. Chest 1993; 104(6): 1694–1697.
48. Miro AM, Shivaram U, Hertig I. Continuous positive airway pressure in COPD patients in acute hypercapnic respiratory failure. Chest 1993; 103(1):266–268.
49. Potgieter PD, Rosenthal E, Benatar SR. Immediate and long-term survival in patients admitted to a respiratory ICU. Crit Care Med 1985; 13(10):798–802.
50. Corrado A, Bruscoli G, Messori A, et al. Iron lung treatment of subjects with COPD in acute respiratory failure. Evaluation of short- and long-term prognosis. Chest 1992; 101(3):692–696.
51. Corrado A, Confalonieri M, Marchese S, et al. Iron lung vs mask ventilation in the treatment of acute on chronic respiratory failure in COPD patients : a multicenter study. Chest 2002; 121(1): 189–195.
52. Corrado A, De Paola E, Gorini M, et al. Intermittent negative pressure ventilation in the treatment of hypoxic hypercapnic coma in chronic respiratory insufficiency. Thorax 1996; 51(11): 1077–1082.
53. Schonhofer B, Sortor-Leger S. Equipment needs for noninvasive mechanical ventilation. Eur Respir J 2002; 20(4):1029–1036.
54. Navalesi P, Fanfulla F, Frigerio P, et al. Physiologic evaluation of noninvasive mechanical ventilation delivered with three types of masks in patients with chronic hypercapnic respiratory failure. Crit Care Med 2000; 28(6):1785–1790.
55. Brochard L. What is really important to make noninvasive ventilation work. Crit Care Med 2000; 28(6):2139–2140.
56. Meduri GU, Turner RE, Abou-Shala N, et al. Noninvasive positive pressure ventilation via face mask. First-line intervention in patients with acute hypercapnic and hypoxemic respiratory failure. Chest 1996; 109(1):179–193.
57. Elliott MW. The interface: crucial for successful noninvasive ventilation. Eur Respir J 2004; 23(1):7–8.
58. Antonelli M, Conti G, Pelosi P, et al. New treatment of acute hypoxemic respiratory failure: noninvasive pressure support ventilation delivered by helmet—a pilot controlled trial. Crit Care Med 2002; 30(3):602–608.

59. Navalesi P, Costa R, Ceriana P, et al. Non-invasive ventilation in chronic obstructive pulmonary disease patients: helmet versus facial mask. Intensive Care Med 2007; 33(1):74–81.
60. Teschler H, Stampa J, Ragette R, et al. Effect of mouth leak on effectiveness of nasal bilevel ventilatory assistance and sleep architecture. Eur Respir J 1999; 14(6):1251–1257.
61. Saatci E, Miller DM, Stell IM, et al. Dynamic dead space in face masks used with noninvasive ventilators: a lung model study. Eur Respir J 2004; 23(1):129–135.
62. Hill NS, Carlisle C, Kramer NR. Effect of a nonrebreathing exhalation valve on long-term asal ventilation using a bilevel device. Chest 2002; 122(1):84–91.
63. Kacmarek R. NIPPV: patient-ventilator synchrony, the difference between success and failure? Intensive Care Med 1999; 25:645–647.
64. Tobin M. Respiratory monitoring. JAMA 1990; 264:244–251.
65. Jubran A, Tobin M. Reliability of pulse oximetry in titrating supplemental oxygen therapy in ventilator-dependent patients. Chest 1990; 97:1420–1425.
66. Stradling J. Hypercapnia during oxygen therapy in airways obstruction: a reappraisal. Thorax 1986; 41:897–902.
67. Meduri GU, Abou-Shala N, Fox R, et al. Noninvasive face mask mechanical ventilation in patients with acute hypercapneic respiratory failure. Chest 1991; 100:445–454.
68. Anton A, Guell R, Gomez J, et al. Predicting the result of noninvasive ventilation in severe acute exacerbations of patients with chronic airflow limitation. Chest 2000; 117:828–833.
69. Poponick JM, Renston JP, Bennett RP, et al. Use of a ventilatory support system (BiPAP) for acute respiratory failure in the emergency department. Chest 1999; 116(1):166–171.
70. Plant PK, Owen JL, Elliott MW. Non-invasive ventilation in acute exacerbations of chronic obstructive pulmonary disease: long term survival and predictors of in-hospital outcome. Thorax 2001; 56(9):708–712.
71. Ferrer M, Ioanas M, Arancibia F, et al. Microbial airway colonization is associated with non-invasive ventilation failure in COPD exacerbation. Crit Care Med 2005; 33:2003–2009.
72. Moretti M, Cilione C, Tampieri A, et al. Incidence and causes of non-invasive mechanical ventilation ventilation failure after initial success. Thorax 2000; 55:819–825.
73. Scala R, Bartolucci C, Naldi M, et al. Co-morbidity and acute decompensations of COPD requiring non-invasive positive-pressure ventilation. Intensive Care Med 2004; 30:1747–1754.
74. Lightowler JV, Elliott MW. Predicting the outcome from NIV for acute exacerbations of COPD. Thorax 2000; 55(10):815–816.
75. Putinati S, Ballerin L, Piattella M, et al. Is it possible to predict the success of non-invasive positive pressure ventilation in acute respiratory failure due to COPD? Respir Med 2000; 94 (10):997–1001.
76. Confalonieri M, Parigi P, Scartabellati A, et al. Noninvasive mechanical ventilation improves the immediate and long-term outcome of COPD patients with acute respiratory failure. Eur Respir J 1996; 9(3):422–430.

# 25

## Invasive Mechanical Ventilation and Weaning at COPD Exacerbation

**ANTONIO ANZUETO**

Division of Pulmonary and Critical Care Medicine at the South Texas Veterans Health Care System, Audie L Murphy Division and the University of Texas Health Science Center at San Antonio, San Antonio, Texas, U.S.A.

**ANDRÉS ESTEBAN and FERNANDO FRUTOS-VIVAR**

Intensive Care Unit, Hospital Universitario de Getafe, Madrid, Spain

## I. Introduction

Chronic obstructive pulmonary disease (COPD) affects large number of patients and is associated with significant morbidity, disability, and mortality (1,2). COPD is complicated by frequent and recurrent acute exacerbations, which are known to be associated with enormous health care expenditures and high morbidity (1–3). Exacerbations of COPD results in over 110,000 deaths and over 500,000 hospitalizations per year, with over $18 billion spent in direct costs annually (4,5). In addition to the financial burden required to care for these patients, other "costs," including days missed, need to be considered. In this review, we will address the indications and use of invasive mechanical ventilation and weaning modalities in patients with COPD exacerbation and acute respiratory failure.

## II. Impact of Exacerbations on Mortality

Acute exacerbation of COPD is associated with significant morbidity and mortality. Hospital mortality of patients admitted for a hypercarbic COPD exacerbation is approximately 10%, and the long-term outcome is poor (6). Mortality reaches 40% in one year in those needing mechanical support, and all-cause mortality is even higher (up to 49%) three years after hospitalization for a COPD exacerbation (6–10). These studies identified the risk factors associated with mortality in these patients. The Study to Understand Prognosis and Preferences for Outcomes and Rates of Treatment (SUPPORT) (6) enrolled 1016 patients who had severe acute exacerbation of COPD at hospital admissions due to respiratory infections, including pneumonia (48%), congestive heart failure (26%), worsening respiratory failure due to lung cancer (3.3%), pulmonary emboli (1.4%), and pneumothorax (1%). This study reported an in-hospital mortality rate of 11% in patients with acute

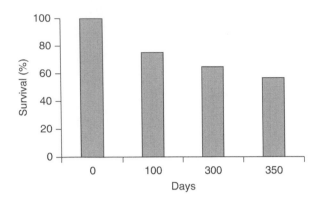

**Figure 1** Survival associated with severe exacerbation of COPD. *Abbreviation*: COPD, chronic obstructive pulmonary disease. *Source*: From Ref. 6.

hypercapnic respiratory failure. The 180-day mortality rate was 33%, and the two-year mortality rate was 49% (Fig. 1). Significant predictors of mortality include acute physiology and chronic health evaluation (APACHE III) score, body mass index, age, functional status two weeks prior to admission, lower ratio of $PO_2$ to $FiO_2$ (hypoxemia), congestive heart failure, serum albumen level, cor pulmonale, lower activities of daily living scores, and lower scores on the Duke Activity Status Index. This study also reported the long-term impact of an acute exacerbation, only 25% of patients were both alive and able to report a good, very good, or excellent quality of life six months after discharge.

Health care resource utilization including emergency room visit and hospital admission for acute exacerbation of COPD has been recognized as an important indicator of a patient's poor prognosis. None of these studies have specifically examined the prognostic influence of acute exacerbation by itself. Soler-Cataluna et al. (10) were the first to report that severe exacerbations of COPD have an independent negative prognostic impact with mortality increasing with the frequency of severe exacerbations and those requiring hospitalization. Multivariate techniques were used to analyze the prognostic influence of acute exacerbation of COPD that required hospitalization and included patient age, smoking status, body mass index, comorbidity, long-term oxygen therapy, spirometry parameters, and arterial blood gases (both hypoxemia and hypercarbia). The study was performed in a prospective cohort of 304 men with COPD followed for up to five years. Only older age [hazard ratio (HR) 5.28, 95% CI, 1.75–15.93], arterial carbon dioxide tension ($PaCO_2$) (HR 1.07, 95% CI, 1.02–1.12), and acute exacerbations of COPD were found to be independent indicators of poor prognosis. A total of 116 deaths (38.2%) were recorded; 78 (25.7%) were due to respiratory causes and 38 (12.5%) died of cardiovascular disease, 7 (2.3%) cerebrovascular disease of different causes, 11 (3.6%) from cancer. Patients with frequent exacerbations had the highest mortality rate ($p < 0.001$) with a risk of death 4.3 times greater (95% CI, 2.62–7.02) than for patients requiring no hospital management. Eighty-nine patients (29.3) were admitted to hospital at least once during the study period. Mortality in this group after 12, 24, 36, 48, and 60 months were 11.6%, 25.9%, 40.2%, 46.6%, and 55.2%, respectively (Fig. 2). Therefore, exacerbations are significant factors associated with increased mortality in COPD.

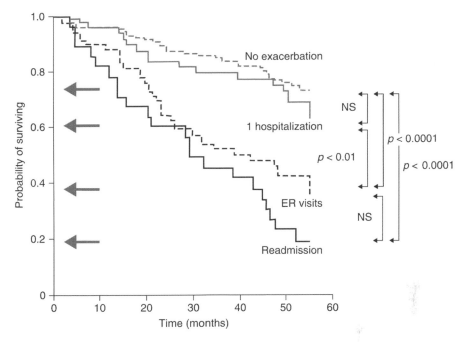

**Figure 2** Probability of survival in relation to the frequency of exacerbations and resource utilization (emergency room visit, hospital admission). *Source*: From Ref. 10.

Patients with COPD exacerbation and acute respiratory failure will require admission to intensive care units (ICUs) and ventilator support. This decision is mainly based on the clinician perception of patients' outcome and futility of care. In general, physicians will have a "pessimistic" prognosis in these patients. Windman et al. carried out a multicenter observational cohort study including 832 patients aged 45 and older admitted to ICUs because of COPD exacerbation (11). On admission, the physicians were to estimate the patient's probability of survival at 180 days after admission. Clinicians predicted that 49% patients will survive 180 days, but the actual survival rate was 62%. Furthermore, for patients with the poorest prognosis, clinicians predicted a survival rate of 10%, whereas the actual rate was 40%. Although we have discussed that COPD exacerbation can be associated with poor outcome, in this review we will demonstrate that invasive mechanical ventilation in these patients results in a better outcome as compared with other causes of acute respiratory failure.

## III. Physiological Impairment in Acute Respiratory Failure in Patients with COPD Exacerbation

Worsening ventilation/perfusion relationships in exacerbations of COPD are multifactorial and relate to airway inflammation and edema, mucus hypersecretion, and bronchoconstriction, which affect ventilation and hypoxic vasoconstriction of pulmonary arterioles, which reduces perfusion (12). Alveolar hypoventilation and respiratory muscle fatigue also

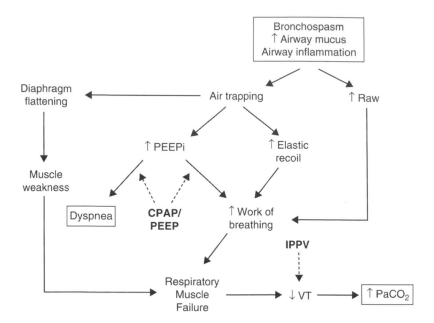

**Figure 3** Pathophysiology of NPPV in patients with COPD exacerbation. *Abbreviations*: NPPV, noninvasive positive pressure ventilation; COPD, chronic obstructive pulmonary disease; Raw, airway resistance; PEEPi, intrinsic positive end-expiratory pressure; CPAP, continuous positive airway pressure; IPPV, intermittent positive pressure ventilation; VT, tidal volume. *Source*: From Ref. 1, 2.

contribute to hypoxemia, hypercapnia, and respiratory acidosis, leading to severe respiratory failure and death. Hypoxia and respiratory acidosis produce pulmonary vasoconstriction imposing an additional load on the right ventricle (1,2). Morphologically, there are widespread airway obstruction due to mucus gland enlargement, mucus plugs, bronchial wall thickening, acute/chronic inflammation that will result in airway narrowing, obliteration, and obstruction. Patients may also show different patterns of ventilation/perfusion distribution due to different dispersions of blood flow, or ventilation, or both (13). These patients also have significant shunt and increased dead space. The physiological effect of ventilator support is to improve ventilation/perfusion relationship and rest fatigued respiratory muscles.

In these patients, arterial blood gases improve because of an increase in alveolar ventilation without significant modifications in the lung ventilation/perfusion mismatching and gas exchange. Application of continuous positive airway pressure (CPAP) during pressure support ventilation (PSV) and positive end-expiratory pressure (PEEP) provide a greater reduction of the work of breathing than either alone, because CPAP and PEEP counterbalances the intrinsic PEEP or auto-PEEP (1,2) (Fig. 3).

## IV. Respiratory Failure and Supplemental Oxygen

Respiratory failure during COPD exacerbation can be manifested with hypoxemia and/or hypercarbia. The differential diagnosis should consider other conditions that can precipitate acute respiratory failure in these patients, such as acute infectious process (community-acquired pneumonia), congested heart failure, pulmonary embolism, or spontaneous pneumothorax (14).

Severe exacerbations are accompanied by a significant worsening of pulmonary gas exchange (due mostly to increased ventilation/perfusion inequality) and respiratory muscle fatigue (12). Supplemental oxygen is considered a cornerstone of treatment in patients that are hypoxic during an acute exacerbation of COPD (15). Among the multiple potential benefits are reduction of pulmonary vasoconstriction, decrease in right heart strain and possible ischemia, and improvement of cardiac output and oxygen delivery to the central nervous system and other vital organs (16). Administration of 100% oxygen can result in rapid nitrogen washout of alveolar units, even in patients with poorly ventilated areas with low or very low ventilation/perfusion mismatch. The deterioration of the ventilation/ perfusion relationship will result in a significant increase in $PaCO_2$. These effect can be influence by the Haldane effect (17). Several investigators have also shown that in patients with COPD exacerbation airway resistance is decreased while breathing higher inspired oxygen fraction ($FiO_2$) (18). Thus, this bronchodilatation increases the volume of the conducting airways, and as a consequence, there is an increase in dead space. A systematic review found that the administration of supplemental oxygen therapy was associated with an increase in arterial oxygen pressure ($PaO_2$), although most patients did not require subsequent mechanical ventilation (16). Patients with combined baseline hypercarbia and more severe hypoxemia experienced the highest risk of requiring mechanical ventilation following the administration of supplemental oxygen (16). In general, oxygen should be administered for patients with a COPD exacerbation under close monitoring, with a goal of oxygen saturations of 90% to 92% ($PaO_2$ 60 mm Hg–65 mm Hg) (3). It is important to consider the oxygen delivery system. Patients with COPD exacerbation that have hypoxemia with or without hypercarbia should not receive high-flow oxygen using a nasal cannula. Instead, supplemental oxygen should be titrated using a Venturi mask.

## A. Indications for Mechanical Ventilation

The institution of mechanical ventilation should be considered when, despite "optimal" medical therapy and oxygen administration, one of the following conditions occur: (*i*) there is persistent respiratory failure with tachypnea, evident use of accessory respiratory muscles, and abdominal paradox; (*ii*) refractory hypoxemia; and/or (*iii*) moderate-to-severe acidosis (pH < 7.36) and hypercapnia ($PaCO_2$) more than 6 to 8 kPa (45–60 mm Hg) (1,2,19). Figure 4 illustrates a suggested "flowchart" for the indications of invasive mechanical ventilation and noninvasive positive pressure ventilation (NPPV) in patients with COPD exacerbation and acute respiratory failure (1,2). Factors associated with success of NPPV include appropriate selection of patients (i.e., younger age, ability to cooperate, lower acuity of illness), experienced team of caregivers, and availability of resources (monitoring).

## B. Modes of Mechanical Ventilation

According to the results of the largest prospective international study in mechanically ventilated patients, 10% of critically ill patients received mechanical ventilation for COPD exacerbation (19). Mechanical ventilation is delivered using different interfaces between patient and ventilator: (*i*) through an endotracheal tube bypassing the upper airway, i.e., conventional or invasive mechanical ventilation or (*ii*) via nasal or face mask,

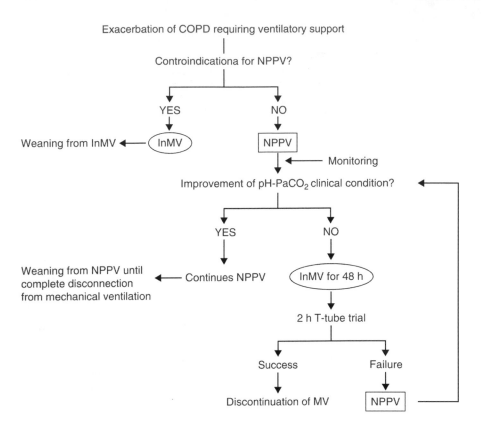

**Figure 4** Algorithm for the use of NPPV. *Abbreviation*: NPPV, noninvasive positive pressure ventilation. *Source*: From Ref. 1,2.

"noninvasive" mechanical ventilation, using different modalities. The latter include CPAP, bi-level ventilation using CPAP and PSV. In this review, we will refer to noninvasive ventilation as NPPV. Table 1 summarizes the contraindications for NPPV. Mechanical ventilation is a form of life support until the underlying cause that precipitates the acute respiratory failure is reversed with medical therapy, other therapies including the use of corticosteroids, bronchodilators, antibiotics, etc., are discussed in another chapter (1–3).

## C. Invasive Mechanical Ventilation

Invasive mechanical ventilation should not be the first mode to support patients with acute respiratory failure due to COPD exacerbation. However, in the multicenter study by Brochard et al. (20), only 29% of patients admitted to the ICU were eligible for NPPV. Thus, invasive mechanical ventilation is used in patients with a contraindication or who have failed NPPV (1,2) (Table 2). The use of NPPV in COPD exacerbation is discussed in another chapter.

**Table 1** Contraindications for Noninvasive Ventilator Support in COPD Exacerbation

- s/p respiratory arrest
- cardiovascular instability (hypotension, arrhythmias, myocardial infarction)
- impaired mental status, somnolence, inability to cooperate
- copious and/or viscous secretions with high aspiration risk
- recent facial or gastro-oesophageal surgery
- craniofacial trauma and/or fixed nasopharyngeal abnormality
- burns
- extreme obesity

*Abbreviation*: s/p, status post.
*Source*: From Refs. 1–3.

**Table 2** Indications for Endotracheal Intubation in Patients with NPPV

- NPPV failure (worsening of arterial blood gases and/or pH in 1–2 hr or lack of improvement in arterial blood gases and/or pH after 4 hr)
- severe acidosis (pH < 7.25) and hypercapnia [$PaCO_2$ > 8 kPa (60 mm Hg)]
- life-threatening hypoxemia [arterial oxygen tension/inspiratory oxygen fraction < 26.6 kPa (200 mm Hg)]
- tachypnea >35 breaths·$min^{-1}$
- Other complications include metabolic abnormalities, sepsis, pneumonia, pulmonary embolism, barotraumas, and massive pleural effusion.

*Abbreviations*: NPPV, noninvasive positive pressure ventilation; $PaCO_2$, arterial carbon dioxide tension.
*Source*: From Refs. 1–3.

Patients with worsening respiratory/metabolic acidosis and/or refractory hypoxemia should be considered for invasive mechanical ventilation (19). The International Mechanical Ventilation Study completed in 1998 included 5183 consecutive eligible patients from 20 countries, demonstrating that 10% patients that received mechanical ventilation was due to COPD exacerbation (21). From this cohort, we reported a retrospective analysis of COPD patients that required invasive mechanical ventilation (22). In this report we studied 522 patients, mean age 67 (SD ± 10); mean SAPS (simplified acute physiology score) II 41 (SD ± 15); and 65% males. The prior functional activity of these patients was as follow: normal in 10%, exercise-induced dyspnea in 49%, dyspnea at rest in 31%. Twenty-nine percent patients were on home oxygen, and 4% received some form of ventilator support at home. At the beginning of mechanical ventilation, 78% patients had respiratory acidosis; mean $PaCO_2$ was 79 (SD ± 19), and $PaO_2/FiO_2$ was 187 (SD ± 84). ICU and hospital mortality were 22% and 30%, respectively. Variables associated with mortality were cardiovascular dysfunction, renal failure, and duration of ventilator support for more than 18 days. Median durations were mechanical ventilation 4 days (P25: 2, P76: 6), ICU stay 8 days (P25: 5, P76: 13), and hospital stay 17 days (P25: 10, P76: 27).

We recently conducted a second international observational study of mechanically ventilated patients, using methodology similar to the original study (21,23). The objectives of the second study were to (*i*) describe current mechanical ventilation practices, (*ii*) compare current results with those of the 1998 cohort study, and (*iii*) judge the concordance of practice change (or lack thereof) with interval reports of randomized trials. We reported in 2004 that the proportion of patients with COPD exacerbation that received invasive mechanical ventilation decreased to 5%, and NPPV increased from 17% to 44% (23). In these studies, the use of mechanical ventilation, including ventilator parameters (mode, tidal volume, positive pressure at the end of expiration, etc.), and complications were similar as compared with other condition that required mechanical ventilation (21,23). When we compared COPD patients with patients with other conditions such as acute respiratory distress syndrome (ARDS), there were differences in the duration of ventilator support and ICU and hospital length of stay. The duration of ventilator support in patients with COPD exacerbation was mean (SD) 5.1 (5.3) and median (IQR) 4 (2–6) days; duration of weaning was mean (SD) 4.7 (7.8) and median (IQR) 2 (1–5) days; while in patients with ARDS, the duration of ventilator support was mean (SD) 8.8 (8.5) and median (IQR) 6 (3–11) days; duration of weaning was mean (SD) 5 (5.6) and median (IQR) 3 (1–6) days ($p < 0.001$). The length of ICU stay in COPD patients was mean (SD) 11.2 (10.6) and median (IQR) 8 (5–13) days; and length of hospital stay was mean (SD) 21.2 (17.7) and median (IQR) 17 (10–27) days; while in patients with ARDS, the length of ICU stay was mean (SD) 14.3 (17.7) and median (IQR) 9 (5–20) days; and length of hospital stay was mean (SD) 24.5 (24.8) and median (IQR) 19 (9–31) days ($p < 0.01$). These variables were similar in patients with other causes of acute respiratory failure (community-acquired pneumonia, or congestive heart failure, etc.) (21). Ely et al. (24) reported that duration of mechanical ventilation of patients with COPD was similar to that of the other ventilated patients (5.5 vs. 5 days) and their data are similar to that of the international study.

In the International Mechanical Ventilation Study, the ICU mortality of the whole cohort was 31% (95% CI, 29–32%) and 28% in COPD patients (21,22). Figure 5 shows that the overall mortality in COPD patients was lower compared with other causes of acute respiratory failure. Furthermore, univariate and multivariate analysis of factors associated with ICU mortality receiving mechanical ventilation due to COPD exacerbation was not a factor associated with increased mortality (16). These data are similar to two retrospective studies involving more than 150 patients with COPD exacerbation and mechanical ventilation that reported hospital mortality of 32% and 28% (19,20).

Several studies have evaluated the risk factors associated with mortality in COPD exacerbation that require mechanical ventilation. These factors include basal dyspnea (25); spirometry parameters (forced expiratory volume) (26), or development of multiple organ failure (27,28). In the study by Esteban et al. and Frutos et al. (21,22), development of renal and/or cardiac complications as well as the duration of mechanical ventilation were independent factors associated with increased mortality. Nseir et al. in a prospective, observational case study reported that in COPD patients that required intubation, ventilator-associated pneumonia (VAP) was associated with increased mortality and longer duration of mechanical ventilation and ICU stay (29). The clinician should be aware of these conditions and, when possible, avoid renal toxic medications and start weaning trials as soon as possible.

Thus, invasive mechanical ventilation in COPD patients with an acute exacerbation has better clinical course and lower duration of mechanical ventilation, weaning, and ICU and hospital length of stay when compared with patients ventilated due to other conditions. Therefore, clinicians should not hesitate to utilize invasive ventilator support in COPD patients with contraindications for NPPV or those who failed NPPV.

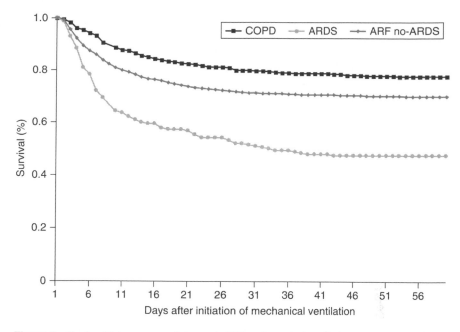

**Figure 5** Kaplan-Meier curves of the probability of survival over time on mechanical ventilation based on underlying conditions. *Source*: From Ref. 21.

## V. Weaning

Weaning and liberation from mechanical ventilation should be initiated as soon as possible to reduce the duration of ventilator support (21,30). Clinical studies have identified the 'readiness to wean' criteria: improvement in the cause of respiratory failure, $PaO_2/FiO_2$ more than 200 mm Hg, PEEP less than or equal to 5 cm of water, and stable cardiovascular function with no vasoactive drugs (31). Evidence-based guidelines recommend a trail of spontaneous breathing to determine, in any given patient, whether mechanical ventilation can be successfully discontinued (30). Routine screening of the patient's ability to breathe spontaneously has been shown to be the most important approach for speeding extubation. Investigators have shown that the implementation of a weaning protocol based on daily screening of weaning parameters shortened weaning time (31,32). These studies have demonstrated that between 60% and 80% of patients can be extubated when they first meet these criteria. With this approach, the length of time needed for mechanical ventilation was shortened to an average of four days; the mean stay in the ICU also decreased from 20 to 16 days. In the recent publication of the International Mechanical Ventilation Study group, the majority (77%) of patients were successfully extubated after this first trial and did not need any additional weaning (22–24). In patients who failed their first trial, there was an increase in the use of gradual reductions in pressure support and a moderate decrease in the use of daily spontaneous breathing trials as weaning methods. This study also reported a marked reduction in the use of synchronized intermittent mandatory ventilation (SIMV) as a weaning modality. The reduction in the use of SIMV is because this method has been shown to result in worse outcome (31,32).

Clinical studies reported the use of NPPV as the first line of ventilator support in patients with COPD exacerbation (20,33,34). NPPV has been used in these patients after failed extubation (35). Furthermore, investigators have proposed to extubate COPD patients that do not meet conventional weaning criteria to NPPV. Nava et al. (36) studied 50 COPD patients who needed mechanical ventilation due to hypercapnic failure (pH 7.18, $PaCO_2$ 94). Patients were then randomized to receive invasive PSV via an endotracheal tube or to be extubated and received noninvasive PSV via a face mask. Both groups received similar pharmacological therapy. The main results of the study were, that at 60 days, 88% of patients ventilated with NPPV were successfully weaned as compared with 68% of patients ventilated invasively (Fig. 6). The mean duration of mechanical ventilation was 17 days for the invasive ventilation group and 10 days for the NPPV group, this difference was not significant. There were significant survival rates at 60 days, 92% for NPPV group versus 72% invasive group. These investigators also reported a significant decrease of complications, none of the patients randomized to the NPPV developed VAP. The authors attributed the excessive mortality in the invasive group to this complication. Although the 60-day mortality was significant, other parameters were different but not significant. At this time, we cannot recommend that patients intubated because of COPD exacerbation that do not meet standard weaning criteria be extubated and placed on NPPV.

Other investigators have shown that NPPV will be useful in extubation failure in COPD patients. Hilbert et al. (37) studied the efficacy of NPPV in 30 COPD patients with

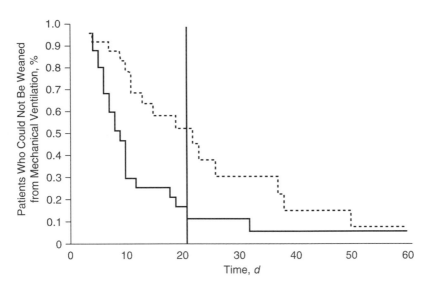

**Figure 6**   Kaplan-Meier curves for patients who could not be weaned from mechanical ventilation in the group of NPPV or invasive ventilator support. The probability of weaning failure was lower in the NPPV group. The vertical line represents day 21, considered by the investigators as the threshold between weanable and unweanable patients. *Abbreviation*: NPPV, noninvasive positive pressure ventilation. *Source*: From Ref. 33.

postextubation hypercapnic respiratory insufficiency compared with 30 historically matched control patients who were treated conventionally. Patients were included in the study if within 72 hours after extubation, they presented with respiratory distress, defined as the combination of a respiratory frequency of more than 25 breath/min, an increase in $PaCO_2$ more than 20% compared with the postextubation value, and a pH < 7.35. The use of NPPV reduced the need for endotracheal intubation, 20% versus 67%, with associated shorter duration of mechanical ventilation, 6 versus 11 days, and the length of ICU stay, 8 versus 14 days. It is important to point out that the hospital mortality was not different, 7% versus 20%, this could be due to the small sample size. The better outcome of NPPV was associated with lower incidence of complications that are related to prolonged endotracheal intubation, such as VAP and the need for tracheostomy.

Girault et al. reported the use of NPPV in patients with acute-on-chronic respiratory failure (not all with COPD), failing one single weaning attempt, and variable period of conventional mechanical ventilation (38). NPPV resulted in a mild reduction of the duration of endotracheal ventilation among patients randomized to early extubation but no improvement in other outcomes. Jiang et al. (39) reported patients who had NPPV applied directly after being weaned and extubated in the conventional manner from mechanical ventilation. All the randomized patients followed planned or self-extubation to either NPPV or usual treatment and found no benefit from NPPV. This study included a very high number of patient who self-extubated (40%). More recently, Ferrer et al. (40) reported a prospective, randomized, controlled study in 43 mechanically ventilated patients who failed a weaning trail for three consecutive days. This study has a mixed patient population, but 77% of patients had chronic lung disease (mainly COPD exacerbation). Patients were randomly extubated, receiving NPPV or remained intubated, following a conventional weaning approach of daily weaning attempts. The investigators showed that the NPPV group had shorted duration of invasive ventilation (9.5 ± 8.3 vs. 20 ± 13 days, $p = 0.003$) (Fig. 7), ICU (14.1 ± 9.2 vs. 25 ± 12.5, $p = 0.002$) and hospital stays (27.8 ± 14.6 vs. 40.8 ± 21.4, $p = 0.026$). The patients assigned to the NPPV also had lower complications, decreased incidence of VAP and septic shock, and less need for tracheostomy. The main limitation of this study is that the control group had a much higher morbidity (50% developed VAP; 27% required reintubation; 50% had tracheostomy) and mortality (34%) as compared with other studies.

We reported data in a heterogeneous group of patients (mainly non-COPD) where NPPV was used after failing extubation. In these patients, NPPV was not effective in averting the need for reintubation, did not improve survival, and may in fact be harmful (41). A post hoc analysis of COPD patients did not show any benefit of NPPV in postextubation failure.

Thus, the literature supports that in COPD exacerbation, weaning should be used using standard criteria. Furthermore, there is a limited role for NPPV in patients that do not meet these criteria or failed extubation.

## VI. Conclusion

COPD exacerbations represent an important event in the natural history of this disease and are associated with significant morbidity and mortality. Though substantial progress has been made in the understanding of the etiology of exacerbations in COPD, much still needs

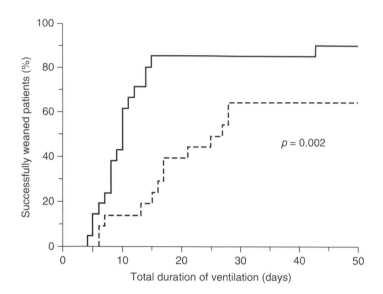

**Figure 7** Kaplan-Meier curves for patients successfully weaned from mechanical ventilation. The probability of weaning success was significantly higher for patients from NPPV group (solid lined) than in the conventional weaning group (dashed line) (log-rank test). *Abbreviation*: NPPV, non-invasive positive pressure ventilation. *Source*: From Ref. 39.

to be learned. Invasive and noninvasive mechanical ventilation should be considered in patients with associated acute respiratory failure. Current data suggest that clinicians are not able to predict patients' outcome and have a pessimistic view when using forms of ventilator support in these patients (11). In this chapter, we demonstrated that mechanical ventilation should be considered in patients with acute respiratory failure due to COPD exacerbation. Furthermore, patients' outcome is better as compared with other conditions when these therapeutic modalities are used. Liberation from mechanical ventilation can be achieved in most patients using current weaning criteria. NPPV can be used during the weaning process by early removal of endotracheal tube or in cases that failed extubation. There is a need for careful selection of patients until clinical trails are complete and probe the benefit of routine use of this technique.

## References

1. Celli BR, MacNee W. Standards for the diagnosis and treatment of patients with COPD: a summary of the ATS/ERS position paper. Eur Respir J 2004; 23:932–946.
2. Rabe K, Hurd S, Anzueto A, et al. Global initiative for chronic obstructive lung disease. Global strategy for the diagnosis, management, and prevention of chronic obstructive pulmonary disease. GOLD Executive Summary. Am J Respir Crit Care Med 2007; 176:532–555.
3. Stoller, J. Acute exacerbations of chronic obstructive pulmonary disease. N Engl J Med 2002; 346:988–994.
4. Statistical Abstract of the United States 1997. U.S. Department of Commerce, , Bureau of the Census, . Washington, DC. U.S. Department of Commerce, 1997.

5. Healthcare Cost and Utilization Project. 1997 Nationwide Inpatient Sample. Agency for Healthcare Research and Policy. Available at: www.ahcpr.gov/data/hcup/hcupnet.htm.
6. Connors AF Jr., Dawson NV, Thomas C, et al. Outcomes following acute exacerbation of severe chronic obstructive lung disease. The SUPPORT investigators (Study to Understand Prognoses and Preferences for Outcomes and Risks of Treatments). Am J Respir Crit Care Med 1996; 154(4 pt 1): 959–967.
7. Almagro P, Calbo E, Ochoa de Echaguen A, et al. Mortality after hospitalization for COPD. Chest 2002; 121:1441–1448.
8. Groenewegen KH, Schols AMWJ, Wauters E. Mortality and mortality-related factors after hospitalization for acute exacerbation of COPD. Chest 2003; 124:459–467.
9. Fuso L, Incalzi RA, Pistelli R, et al. Predicting mortality of patients hospitalized for acute exacerbated chronic obstructive pulmonary disease. Am J Med 1995; 98:272–277.
10. Soler-Cataluna JJ, Martinez-Garcia MA, Roman Sanchez P, et al. Severe acute exacerbations and mortality in patients with chronic obstructive pulmonary disease. Thorax 2005; 60:925–931.
11. Wildman MJ, Sanderson C, Groves J, et al. Implications of prognostic pessimism in patients with chronic obstructive pulmonary disease (COPD) or asthma admitted to intensive care in the UK with in the COPD and asthma outcome study (CAOS): multicenter observational cohort study. BMJ 2007; 335:1132. [Epub 2007 Nov 1].
12. Gunen H, Hacievliyagil SS, Kosar F, et al. Factors affecting survival of hospitalised patients with COPD. Eur Respir J 2005; 26(2):234–241.
13. Rodriguez-Roisin R. Ventilation-perfusion relationships. In: Pinsky MR, Dhainaut JFA, ed. Pathophysiologic Foundations of Critical Care. Baltimore: Williams & Wilkins, 1993:389–413.
14. Barbera JA, Roca J, Ferrer A, et al. Mechanisms of worsening gas exchange during acute exacerbations of chronic obstructive pulmonary disease. Eur Respir J 1997; 10(6):1285–1291.
15. Carrera M, Sala E, Cosio BG, et al. Hospital treatment of chronic obstructive pulmonary disease exacerbation: an evidence-based review. Arch Bronchoneumol 2005; 41:220–229.
16. McCrory DC, Brown C, Gelfand SE, et al. Management of acute exacerbations of COPD: a summary and appraisal of published evidence. Chest 2001; 119:1190–1209.
17. Aubier M, Murciano D, Milic-Emili J, et al. Effect of the administration of O2 on ventilation and blood gases in patients with chronic obstructive pulmonary disease during acute respiratory failure. Am Rev Respir Dis 1980; 122:747–754.
18. Libby DM, Briscoe WA, King TKC. Relief of hypoxia-related bronchoconstriction by breathing 30 percent of oxygen. Am Rev Respir Dis 1981; 123:171–175.
19. Vitacca M, Clini E, Porta R, et al. Acute exacerbations in patients with COPD: predictors of need for mechanical ventilation. Eur Respir J 1996; 9:1487–1493.
20. Brochard L, Mancebo J, Wysocki M, et al. Noninvasive ventilation for acute exacerbation of chronic obstructive pulmonary disease. N Engl J Med 1995; 333:817–822.
21. Esteban A, Anzueto A, Frutos F, et al. Characteristics and outcomes in adult patients receiving mechanical ventilation: a 28-day international study. JAMA 2000; 287:345–355.
22. Frutos-Vivar F, Esteban A, Anzueto A, et al. Pronostico de los enfermos con enfermedad pulmonary obstructive cronica reagudizada que precisan ventilacion mecanica. Med Intensiva 2006; 30:52–61.
23. Esteban A, Ferguson N, Frutos F, et al. Evolution of mechanical ventilation in response to clinical research. Am J Respir Critic Care Med 2008; 177:170–177.
24. Ely EW, Baker AM, Evans Gw, et al. The distribution of cost of care in mechanically ventilated patients with chronic obstructive pulmonary disease. Crit Care Med 2000; 28:408–413.
25. Seneff MG, Wagner DP, Wagner RP, et al. Hospital and 1-year survival of patients admitted to intensive care units with acute exacerbation of chronic obstructive pulmonary disease. JAMA 1995; 274:1852–1857.
26. Nevis ML, Epstein SK. Predictor of outcome for patients with COPD that requiring invasive mechanical ventilation. Chest 2001; 119:1840–1849.

27. Lázaro A, López-Mesa J, Aragón C, et al. Evolución a corto y largo plazo de 100 enfermos con EPOC tratados con ventilación mecánica. Med Intensiva 1990; 14:245–248.
28. Añón JM, García de Lorenzo A, Zarazaga A, et al. Mechanical ventilation of patients on long-term oxygen therapy with acute exacerbations of chronic obstructive pulmonary disease: prognosis and cost-utility analysis. Intensive Care Med 1999; 25:452–457.
29. Nseir S, De Pompeo CD, Soubier S, et al. Impact of ventilator-associated pneumonia on outcome in patients with COPD. Chest 2005; 128:1650–1656.
30. MacIntyre NR, Cook DJ, Ely EW Jr., et al. Evidence-based guidelines for weaning and discontinuing ventilatory support: a collective task force facilitated by the American College of Chest Physicians, American College for Respiratory Care, and the American College of Critical Care Medicine. Chest 2001; 120(suppl):375S–399S.
31. Esteban A, Alia I, Gordo F, et al. Extubation outcome after spontaneous breathing trials with T-tube or pressure support ventilation. Am J Respir Crit Care Med 1997; 156:459–465.
32. Ely EW, Baker AM, Dunagan DP, et al. Effect on the duration of mechanical ventilation of identifying patients capable of breathing spontaneous. N Engl J Med 1996; 335:1864–1869.
33. Celikel T, Sungur M, Ceyhan B, et al. Comparison of non-invasive positive pressure ventilation with standard medical therapy in hypercarbic acute respiratory failure. Chest 1998; 114:1636–1642.
34. Plant PK, Owen JL, Elliott MW. Early use of non-invasive ventilation for acute exacerbations of chronic obstructive pulmonary disease on general respiratory wards: a multicentre randomised controlled trial. Lancet 2000; 355(9219):1931–1935.
35. International Consensus conferences in Intensive Care Medicine: Non-invasive positive pressure ventilation in acute respiratory failure. Am J Respir Crit Care Med 2001; 163:283–291.
36. Nava S, Ambrosino N, Clini E, et al. Noninvasive mechanical ventilation in the weaning of patients with respiratory failure die to chronic obstructive pulmonary disease. A randomized controlled trial. Ann Intern Med 1998; 128:721–728.
37. Hilbert G, Gruson D, Portel L, et al. Noninvasive pressure support ventilation in COPD patients with postextubation hypercapnic respiratory insufficiency. Eur Respir J 1998; 11:1349–1353.
38. Girault C, Daudenthun I, Chevron V, et al Noninvasive ventilation as a systematic extubation and weaning technique in acute-on-chronic respiratory failure: a prospective, randomized controlled study. Am J Respir Crit Care Med 1999; 160:86–92.
39. Jiang JS, Kao SI, Wang SN. Effect of early application of biphasic positive airway pressure on the outcome of extubation in ventilator weaning. Respirology 1999; 4161–4165.
40. Ferrer M, Esquinas A, Arancibia F, et al. Noninvasive ventilation during persistent weaning failure. A randomized controlled trial. Am J Respir Med Crit Care Med 2003; 168:70–76.
41. Esteban A, Frutos-Vivar F, Ferguson ND, et al. Noninvasive positive-pressure ventilation for respiratory failure after extubation. N Engl J Med 2004; 350:2452–2460.

# 26
## Oxygen Therapy and Exacerbations

**A. G. DAVISON**
Southend University Hospital, Prittlewell Chase, Westcliff-on-Sea, Essex, U.K.

**RONAN O'DRISCOLL**
Respiratory Medicine, Salford Royal University Hospital, Salford, Great Manchester, U.K.

**LUKE HOWARD**
Hammersmith Hospital, Imperial College Healthcare NHS Trust and National Heart and Lung Institute, Imperial College London, London, U.K.

## I. Introduction

Oxygen therapy is generally considered as beneficial and, at worst, harmless. In most conditions, there has, until recently, been little good evidence that this statement is incorrect, and as a consequence, oxygen is often given liberally to avoid hypoxemia, which may be fatal. Chronic obstructive pulmonary disease (COPD) is one of the few conditions in which this does not hold true, and there is in fact good evidence that oxygen can be harmful. This chapter will review the key pathophysiological derangements relevant to oxygen administration before discussing how best to approach the issue of how to deliver and monitor oxygen therapy during acute exacerbations of COPD (AECOPD).

## II. Blood Gas Pathophysiology in AECOPD

The major pathological features in COPD that result in abnormal arterial blood gas physiology are ventilation-perfusion ($V_A/Q$) mismatch and the inability to increase effective alveolar ventilation. The building block of the lung is the alveolar-capillary unit; here, efficient gas exchange ensures equilibration of oxygen and carbon dioxide across the alveolar-capillary membrane so that there is no alveolar-end capillary gradient. A healthy lung will consist largely of normal alveolar-capillary units. Because of gravitational effects on blood flow distribution, not all alveolar-capillary units will have matched ventilation to perfusion, but this effect is small, producing a small alveolar-arterial gradient.

In COPD with significant emphysema, alveolar destruction will lead to areas of very high $V_A/Q$ ratio, increasing dead space ventilation and thus decreasing effective alveolar ventilation. Areas of airflow obstruction produce areas of low $V_A/Q$ ratio, and blood leaving these units will have relatively low oxygen and high carbon dioxide content. This will be partially compensated by mixing with blood from high $V_A/Q$ ratio units, but by definition, these units contribute less flow and, therefore, mixed pulmonary venous blood will be dominated by low $V_A/Q$ ratio units for a given amount of ventilation.

One physiological "solution" to this problem is hypoxic pulmonary vasoconstriction (HPV) (1), whereby alveolar hypoxia, present in low $V_A/Q$ ratio units, will produce pulmonary arteriolar vasoconstriction and, in the longer-term, remodeling, thus diverting blood flow to better-ventilated alveolar-capillary units. The other solution is increased overall ventilation, although with the increased dead space in COPD, much of this will be wasted in high $V_A/Q$ ratio areas. As the shape of the hemoglobin oxygen dissociation curve is sigmoid and oxygen is poorly soluble in plasma, increases in alveolar $PO_2$ and therefore end-capillary $PO_2$ in well-ventilated areas will not significantly increase oxygen content of pulmonary venous blood leaving these areas as a result of increased ventilation.

In the physiological range, carbon dioxide carriage in the blood (largely as bicarbonate) has a linear relationship with $PCO_2$, and therefore, any decrease in $PCO_2$ from high $V_A/Q$ ratio areas can counterbalance the higher carbon dioxide content of blood leaving alveolar-capillary units with low $V_A/Q$ characteristics. The overall effect of these two fundamental differences in oxygen and carbon dioxide carriage is that increases in ventilation in COPD can normalize $PaCO_2$, but not $PaO_2$. Type 2 respiratory failure, therefore, only develops when the respiratory system is incapable of increasing ventilation because of prohibitive airflow obstruction and respiratory muscle fatigue.

During an AECOPD, both $V_A/Q$ mismatch and respiratory mechanics will worsen. Consequently, hypoxia will worsen and, as described above, increased ventilation will only partially correct this; therefore, additional oxygen therapy will be required to elevate alveolar $PO_2$ in low $V_A/Q$ ratio areas. The mechanical effects of an exacerbation will decrease the capacity of the respiratory system to augment overall ventilation to maintain effective alveolar ventilation in the face of increased dead space ventilation, and this may lead to hypercapnic respiratory failure, unless respiratory support is given. Furthermore, during an AECOPD, both oxygen consumption and carbon dioxide production will rise, thus placing further demand upon gas exchange requirements.

Although increasing oxygen will increase alveolar $PO_2$ in low $V_A/Q$ ratio areas, it will further worsen $V_A/Q$ mismatch by releasing HPV in these areas. As they remain low-ventilation areas, but with higher flow, pulmonary venous $PCO_2$ will rise further. Although the inability of the respiratory system to increase ventilation is the reason for failure to clear carbon dioxide, the effect of worsening $V_A/Q$ mismatch is the principal reason behind the deterioration with oxygen therapy. It has previously been felt, and indeed is still widely erroneously taught today, that loss of hypoxic ventilatory drive is responsible for the rise in $PaCO_2$ seen in susceptible patients with COPD on receiving oxygen therapy (2). Two empirical observations suggest in fact that worsening $V_A/Q$ mismatch is responsible and not loss of hypoxic drive (3–8), although it still remains a matter of debate (9,10). The first observation is that overall ventilation does not change significantly when oxygen is given during exacerbations, despite seeing a rise in $PaCO_2$, and the second, and perhaps more convincing, observation is that $PaCO_2$ continues to rise with increasing $PaO_2$ above 13 kPa, although carotid sinus discharge will have become largely attenuated above 13 kPa.

Additional physiological disturbances contribute to worsened hypercapnia with oxygen therapy during AECOPD. These include decreased buffering capacity of carbon dioxide by oxyhemoglobin compared with deoxyhemoglobin (known as the Haldane Effect). Levels of inspired oxygen greater than 30% to 50% can produce absorption atelectasis, leading to a shunt, an extreme form of $V_A/Q$ mismatch.

## III. Critical Hypoxemia in Normal Subjects

It is difficult to estimate a precise level of hypoxemia that is dangerous to normal subjects because the physiological effects will vary considerably depending on the degree and the speed of onset of hypoxemia and on several characteristics of the subject such as age, illness, and acclimatization. Tolerance of hypoxemia is increased by acclimatization and decreased by advancing age of the subject. An acclimatized climber may climb Mount Everest (8848 m) without oxygen despite an estimated $PaO_2$ of only 28 mm Hg (3.7 kPa) at the summit and oxygen saturation below 70% (11,12). However, acute exposure to the same altitude causes dramatic symptoms. Twenty-five volunteers who removed their oxygen masks in an unpressurized airplane at 8500 m made errors in simple tasks and developed tremor within 50 to 178 seconds (13). This was followed by a period of confusion or apathy, and the subjects suffered imminent unconsciousness at 100 to 210 seconds and recovered when their oxygen mask was replaced. The mean blood oxygen saturation was 64% at the time when the subjects started to make errors, and no errors were made while the oxygen saturation was above 84%. The mean oxygen saturation was 56% at the time when unconsciousness was imminent (range 40–73%). The work of Yoneda et al. has shown that the time of useful consciousness in hypoxic conditions is diminished in subjects older than 40 years (14).

Millions of people live at altitudes above 3500 m with oxygen saturation of about 88% at rest, and healthy people have no symptoms due to hypoxemia during commercial air travel, although the oxygen saturation may fall to an average minimum value of 89% (range 80–93%) (15). However, it is known that sudden exposure to altitudes above 4000 m for a few hours or days can cause mountain sickness, high altitude cerebral edema, or high altitude pulmonary edema (16). Graduated exposure to hypoxemia in a decompression chamber (down to saturation 52%) was associated with periodic breathing, apneas, and disturbed sleep quality (17). Medium-term and long-term hypoxemia at high altitude causes physiological derangements, including pulmonary hypertension. Hypoxic hepatitis has been reported in patients with chronic respiratory failure associated with oxygen levels below or 34 mm Hg (4.5kPa) (18).

In summary, it would appear that young adults can tolerate acute hypoxemia with saturation down to about 85% without any clinical symptoms and much lower levels with gradual acclimatization, although there may be adverse long-term physiological consequences.

## IV. Levels of Hypoxemia Found in AECOPD

Refsum examined levels of consciousness compared with measured levels of $PaO_2$ in AECOPD (Tables 1 and 2) (19). The lowest level of $PaO_2$ that can exist and produce no adverse effects is not known. Campbell used mental clarity as his index of tissue oxygenation rather than any particular value in the arterial blood and concluded that the physiological effects are gradual, although the damaging effects are sudden (2). He considered that there was little evidence of damage with a $PaO_2$ of 40 mm Hg (5.3 kPa) (or a saturation of 70%) and above. Hutchinson et al. concluded that a $PaO_2$ of 50 mm Hg (6.7 kPa) will prevent immediate death from hypoxemia but congestive heart failure may

**Table 1** Lowest Levels of PaO$_2$ and Highest Levels of PaCO$_2$ When Breathing Air Found in Studies of Exacerbations of COPD

| Study | Number of patients | Lowest level of PaO$_2$ | | Highest level of PaCO$_2$ | |
|---|---|---|---|---|---|
| | | mm Hg | kPa | mmHg | kPa |
| Refsum 1963 (19) | 129 | 20–22 | 2.7–2.9 | 88 | 11.7 |
| Hutchinson et al. 1964 (20) | 8 | 23 | 3.1 | 100 | 13.3 |
| McNicol et al. 1965 (41) | 81 | 19 | 2.5 | 88 | 11.7 |
| King et al. 1973 (34) | 40 | 24 | 3.2 | 95 | 12.7 |
| Warren et al. 1980 (26) | 108 | 19 | 2.5 | 97 | 12.9 |

Refs. are shown in parenthesis.

**Table 2** Blood Gas Measurements and Levels of Consciousness in Acute Exacerbations of COPD

| | n | Mean pH | Mean PaCO$_2$ | | Mean PaO$_2$ | |
|---|---|---|---|---|---|---|
| | | | mm Hg | kPa | mm Hg | kPa |
| Conscious | 114 | 7.34 | 68 | 9.1 | 38.8 | 5.2 |
| Semiconscious | 8 | 7.26 | 84 | 11.2 | 25.9 | 3.5 |
| Unconscious | 7 | 7.25 | 84 | 11.2 | 25.3 | 3.4 |

develop and proposed that the aim of oxygen therapy should be to provide a PaO$_2$ of at least this level (20), as did Mithoefer et al. (21). Smith et al. described the management of 34 patients, with the aim to improve oxygen saturations to 70% to 75% [approximately PaO$_2$ of 50 mm Hg (6.7 kPa)], without a concomitant dangerous increase in the severity of respiratory acidosis (22). Jeffrey et al. aimed to increase the PaO$_2$ without causing a fall in pH below 7.26 (23).

Levels of PaO$_2$ down to 19 to 24 mm Hg (2.5–3.2 kPa) have been recorded in exacerbations of COPD. Patients with higher levels could have died before reaching hospital. On the other hand, many studies have found that mortality in hospital after an AECOPD is not correlated with the level of hypoxemia on admission (23–26). The evidence and general consensus is that if the PaO$_2$ is above 50 mm Hg (6.7 kPa), death will not occur from hypoxemia. This is equivalent to an oxygen saturation of about 75% (Evidence 3).

## V. Hypercapnia

The most critical consequence of hypercapnia is arguably narcosis. Westlake et al. concluded that semiconsciousness or coma occurred if the PaCO$_2$ was 120 mm Hg with a pH below 7.1 and mental clarity was maintained if the PaCO$_2$ was below 80 mm Hg or the pH was greater than 7.3 (27). Sieker and Hickam came to similar conclusions and with similar values [PaCO$_2$ of 130 mm Hg (17.3 kPa) and pH < 7.14 for semiconsciousness or coma and PaCO$_2$ < 90 mm Hg (12 kPa) and pH > 7.25 for mental clarity] (28) (Evidence 3).

A number of studies on patients with AECOPD have emphasized that the mortality increases as the pH falls below 7.25 or 7.26 (20,23,26–28). Jeffrey found that death occurred in 27% when the pH fell to 7.26 or below compared with 7% when it remained above 7.26 (23). Plant et al. showed that acidosis on admission was the only variable on multivariate analysis, which was associated with subsequent admission to intensive care (29), and there was a significantly greater chance of being intubated if the pH was below 7.3. This study differed from the other studies quoted, in that patients had been treated with uncontrolled oxygen (Evidence 3).

## VI. Effect of Continuous High Concentrations of Oxygen in AECOPD

High concentrations of oxygen in COPD exacerbations may (but not universally) produce worsening hypercapnic respiratory failure, leading to drowsiness, coma, and death. Westlake et al. described a series of patients with exacerbations of COPD who had been treated with 40% to 50% inspired oxygen and developed severe symptomatic hypercapnia, resulting in death, coma, semicoma, or drowsiness (27) (Evidence 3).

Campbell reported three scenarios from his clinical experience concerning the effects of uncontrolled oxygen (2): (*i*) In 10% of patients, the clinical state and PaCO$_2$ either improves or does not change. (*ii*) Sixty percent of patients become or remain drowsy. The PaCO$_2$ slowly rises in 12 hours by up to 20 mm Hg (2.7 kPa) and then stabilizes. (*iii*) Thirty percent of patients rapidly become unconscious, cough becomes ineffective, and the PaCO$_2$ rises at a rate of 30 mm Hg (4 kPa) or more per hour. The absence of a rise in PaCO$_2$ in oxygen therapy is not necessarily indicative of a good prognosis, however, as 5 of 18 patients in another study with this response died in hospital (26).

## VII. Effect of Intermittent Oxygen Therapy or Stopping Oxygen in AECOPD

In the 1950s, intermittent oxygen therapy was recommended as a means of improving PaO$_2$ while avoiding progressive respiratory acidosis (30); however, this is dangerous and can lead to rebound hypoxemia. When the concentration of inspired oxygen is changed, PAO$_2$ and thus PaO$_2$ will change within one to two minutes, but changes in PACO$_2$ and PaCO$_2$ will take 10 to 20 minutes because of the body's capacity to store oxygen (31). Consequently, if oxygen therapy has led to an increase in PaCO$_2$, and therefore, PACO$_2$, then, according to the alveolar gas equation, on cessation, rebound alveolar hypoxia, and hypoxemia will develop. This was confirmed clinically by Massaro et al. in 1962 (32) (Evidence 3).

## VIII. High-Flow Low-Concentration Oxygen Using a 24–28% Venturi Mask

Smith et al. described 27 patients with an AECOPD who were treated with controlled oxygen (22 received 24%; 3 received 28%, and 2 received 24% and then 28%) (22). The mean oxygen saturation rose from 61% to 82%, and the mean PaCO$_2$ changed from 64 to

61 mm Hg (8.5–8.1 kPa). Rises of 3 mm Hg (0.4 kPa) or more in the $PaCO_2$ were observed in 16 patients. In two of these, there was a dangerous fall in pH to below 7.25, and treatment was modified. One patient on 24% oxygen required ventilation, the arterial saturation increased from 56% to 76% at four hours, the $PaCO_2$ increased from 72 to 74 mm Hg, and the pH fell from 7.27 to 7.24. The other improved when the 28% oxygen was reduced to 24%, but at four hours the oxygen saturation had increased from 55% to 77%, the $PaCO_2$ had increased from 69 to 82 mm Hg, and the pH had fallen from 7.31 to 7.24. On 24% oxygen, 70% of the patients had an oxygen saturation that was 88% or below and 60% had an oxygen saturation of 85% or below.

Warrell et al., in 1970, described seven patients treated initially with 24% and then 28% oxygen (33). The mean increases in $PaO_2$ were 11 and 21 mm Hg (1.5–2.8 kPa) and, in $PaCO_2$, 4 and 8 mm Hg (0.53–1.1 kPa), respectively. In two of the five patients, the $PaCO_2$ increased markedly and was associated with decreased levels of consciousness. Both these patients required ventilation.

King et al. reported 40 patients admitted to a pulmonary intensive care unit with an AECOPD (34). All were treated with 24% oxygen. Blood gases were remeasured at 30–60 minutes. Mean $PaO_2$ increased from 40.4 to 57.3 mm Hg (5.2–7.6 kPa) and oxygen saturation increased from 69% to 83.9%. There was no significant change in $PaCO_2$ (mean 63 mm Hg) (8.3 kPa) or pH (mean 7.35). There was no significant correlation between the initial $PaO_2$ and the change in $PaO_2$. No patient developed carbon dioxide narcosis.

Mithoefer et al. reported that 70% of patients admitted to hospital treated with 24% oxygen achieved a $PaO_2$ of less than 50 mm Hg (6.6 kPa) (21). The authors regarded this as less than adequate. The change in $PaO_2$ produced by 24%, 28%, and 35% oxygen masks was unpredictable.

DeGaute et al. gave 28% oxygen for one hour to 35 patients who had exacerbations of COPD (35). The mean $PaO_2$ increased from 45 (6 kPa) to 68 mm Hg (9.1 kPa) and the $PaCO_2$ increased from 59 (7.9 kPa) to 63 mm Hg (8.4 kPa).

## IX. Use of Nasal Cannulae (Prongs) to Provide Controlled Oxygen

It has been shown that there is variability of oxygen delivery using nasal cannulae (36). Nasal cannulae using oxygen flow chart rates of 1 to 4 L/min produce approximately the same change in oxygen saturation as Venturi masks of 24% to 40%. Augusti et al. compared oxygen arterial saturation ($SaO_2$), in AECOPD in a randomized crossover study, produced by Venturi masks and nasal cannulae (37). $SaO_2$ was less than 90% for 3.7 ± 3.8 hours in 24 hours using Venturi masks and for 5.4 ± 5.9 hours in 24 hours using nasal prongs ($p < 0.05$) (Evidence 2).

## X. Recent Studies on AECOPD

There have been a number of recent studies of admissions to hospital with AECOPD. One major difference in practice is that more recently ambulances have been equipped with oxygen. High-concentration masks are often the only ones available. Plant et al. published a prospective prevalence study of 983 patients admitted to a hospital for one year (29).

Eleven required immediate intubation, 20% of the remaining had a respiratory acidosis [(pH < 7.35 and $PaCO_2$ > 45 mm Hg (6 kPa)], an oxygen tension of 75 mm Hg (10 kPa) being associated with acidosis in the most hypercapnic patients. The authors were only able to show an association between acidosis and oxygen tension rather than a causative relationship because patients had received oxygen in ambulances and accident and emergency (A&E) departments before blood gas analysis. The authors concluded that the $PaO_2$ should be maintained at 54.8 to 75 mm Hg (7.3–10 kPa). Oxygen saturations were not measured in this study, and they estimated that these correlated to oxygen saturations of 85% to 92%; however, they probably correlated with the range 88–93%.

Denniston et al. found that if the initial management in ambulances or the A&E department included oxygen therapy with an $FiO_2$ above 0.28, the hospital mortality (14%) was significantly greater than if an $FiO_2$ of 0.28 or below was used (2%) (38). An $FiO_2$ of greater than 0.28 was used in 80% of patients in ambulances and 39% of accident and emergency cases. There was also poor recognition of COPD by the patients (35%) and by the ambulance crew (32%). Patients recognized as having COPD received a lower $FiO_2$. Durrington et al. showed that 40% of admissions had initially received oxygen therapy in the ambulances on $FiO_2$ of greater than 0.28 (39). Following a change of protocol, this was reduced to 25%. Patients receiving a high $FiO_2$ were significantly more acidotic and had a higher $PaCO_2$ and higher $PaO_2$ than patients receiving a lower $FiO_2$ and also had significantly more complicated admissions (40.8% compared with 25.2%).

## XI.  Oxygen Alert Cards and 24 or 28% Venturi Masks for COPD Patients Who have had an Episode of Hypercapnic Respiratory Failure

These patients should be issued with an oxygen alert card and 24% or 28% Venturi masks. The recommended oxygen saturation will usually be 88% to 92%. If the patient has developed retention at a lower oxygen saturation, then a lower-target saturation of 85% to 88% can be recommended. Patients are instructed to show the card to the ambulance staff and the A&E department staff so that high concentrations of oxygen are avoided. This scheme has been shown to be successful (40). Ambulance control should also be informed which patients are issued with a card.

## References

1.  Cutaia M, Rounds S. Hypoxic pulmonary vasoconstriction. Physiologic significance, mechanism, and clinical relevance. Chest 1990; 97(3):706–718.
2.  Campbell EJ. The J. Burns Amberson Lecture. The management of acute respiratory failure in chronic bronchitis and emphysema. Am Rev Respir Dis 1967; 96(4):626–639.
3.  Aubier M, Murciano D, Milic-Emili J, et al. Effects of the administration of O2 on ventilation and blood gases in patients with chronic obstructive pulmonary disease during acute respiratory failure. Am Rev Respir Dis 1980; 122(5):747–754.
4.  Berry RB, Mahutte CK, Kirsch JL, et al. Does the hypoxic ventilatory response predict the oxygen-induced falls in ventilation in COPD? Chest 1993; 103(3):820–824.

5.  Castaing Y, Manier G, Guenard H. Effect of 26% oxygen breathing on ventilation and perfusion distribution in patients with cold. Bull Eur Physiopathol Respir 1985; 21(1):17–23.

6.  Dick CR, Liu Z, Sassoon CS, et al. O2-induced change in ventilation and ventilatory drive in COPD. Am J Respir Crit Care Med 1997; 155(2):609–614.

7.  Erbland ML, Ebert RV, Snow SL. Interaction of hypoxia and hypercapnia on respiratory drive in patients with COPD. Chest 1990; 97(6):1289–1294.

8.  Pain MC, Read DJ, Read J. Changes of arterial carbon-dioxide tension in patients with chronic lung disease breathing oxygen. Austr Ann Med 1965; 14(3):195–204.

9.  Feller-Kopman D, Schwartzstein R. The role of hypoventilation and ventilation-perfusion redistribution in oxygen-induced hypercapnia during acute exacerbations of chronic obstructive pulmonary disease. Am J Respir Crit Care Med 2001; 163(7):1755.

10. Robinson TD, Freiberg DB, Regnis JA, et al. The role of hypoventilation and ventilation-perfusion redistribution in oxygen-induced hypercapnia during acute exacerbations of chronic obstructive pulmonary disease. Am J Respir Crit Care Med 2000; 161(5):1524–1529.

11. Peacock AJ, Jones PL. Gas exchange at extreme altitude: results from the British 40th Anniversary Everest Expedition. Eur Respir J 1997; 10(7):1439–1444.

12. West JB, Hackett PH, Maret KH, et al. Pulmonary gas exchange on the summit of Mount Everest. J Appl Physiol 1983; 55(3):678–687.

13. Hoffman C, Clark R, Brown E. Blood oxygen saturations and duration of consciousness in anoxia at high altitudes. Am J Physiol 1946; 145:685–692.

14. Yoneda I, Tomoda M, Tokumaru O, et al. Time of useful consciousness determination in aircrew members with reference to prior altitude chamber experience and age. Aviat Space Environ Med 2000; 71(1):72–76.

15. Cottrell JJ, Lebovitz BL, Fennell RG, et al. Inflight arterial saturation: continuous monitoring by pulse oximetry. Aviat Space Environ Med 1995; 66(2):126–130.

16. Duplain H, Sartori C, Scherrer U. High-altitude related illness. Rev Med Suisse 2007; 3(120): 1766–1769.

17. Anholm JD, Powles AC, Downey R III, et al. Operation Everest II: arterial oxygen saturation and sleep at extreme simulated altitude. Am Rev Respir Dis 1992; 145(4 pt 1):817–826.

18. Henrion J, Minette P, Colin L, et al. Hypoxic hepatitis caused by acute exacerbation of chronic respiratory failure: a case-controlled, hemodynamic study of 17 consecutive cases. Hepatology 1999; 29(2):427–433.

19. Refsum HE. Relationship between state of consciousness and arterial hypoxaemia and hypercapnia in patients with pulmonary insufficiency, breathing air. Clin Sci 1963; 25:361–367.

20. Hutchison DC, Flenley DC, Donald KW. Controlled oxygen therapy in respiratory failure. Br Med J 1964; 2(5418):1159–1166.

21. Mithoefer JC, Karetzky MS, Mead GD. Oxygen therapy in respiratory failure. N Engl J Med 1967; 277(18):947–949.

22. Smith JP, Stone RW, Muschenheim C. Acute respiratory failure in chronic lung disease. Observations on controlled oxygen therapy. Am Rev Respir Dis 1968; 97(5):791–803.

23. Jeffrey AA, Warren PM, Flenley DC. Acute hypercapnic respiratory failure in patients with chronic obstructive lung disease: risk factors and use of guidelines for management. Thorax 1992; 47(1):34–40.

24. Asmundsson T, Kilburn KH. Survival of acute respiratory failure. A study of 239 episodes. Ann Intern Med 1969; 70(3):471–485.

25. Bone RC, Pierce AK, Johnson RL Jr. Controlled oxygen administration in acute respiratory failure in chronic obstructive pulmonary disease: a reappraisal. Am J Med 1978; 65(6):896–902.

26. Warren PM, Flenley DC, Millar JS, et al. Respiratory failure revisited: acute exacerbations of chronic bronchitis between 1961-68 and 1970-76. Lancet 1980; 1(8166):467–470.

27. Westlake EK, Simpson T, Kaye M. Carbon dioxide narcosis in emphysema. Q J Med 1955; 24(94):155–173.

28. Sieker HO, Hickam JB. Carbon dioxide intoxication: the clinical syndrome, its etiology and management with particular reference to the use of mechanical respirators. Medicine (Baltimore) 1956; 35(4):389–423.

29. Plant PK, Owen JL, Elliott MW. One year period prevalence study of respiratory acidosis in acute exacerbations of COPD: implications for the provision of non-invasive ventilation and oxygen administration. Thorax 2000; 55(7):550–554.

30. Cohn JE, Carroll DG, Riley RL. Respiratory acidosis in patients with emphysema. Am J Med 1954; 17(4):447–463.

31. Campbell EJ. Respiratory failure: the relation between oxygen concentrations of inspired air and arterial blood. Lancet 1960; 2:10–11.

32. Massaro DJ, Katz S, Luchsinger PC. Effect of various modes of oxygen administration on the arterial gas values in patients with respiratory acidosis. Br Med J 1962; 2(5305):627–629.

33. Warrell DA, Edwards RH, Godfrey S, et al. Effect of controlled oxygen therapy on arterial blood gases in acute respiratory failure. Br Med J 1970; 1(5707):452–455.

34. King TK, Ali N, Briscoe WA. Treatment of hypoxia with 24 percent oxygen. A new approach to the interpretation of data collected in a pulmonary intensive care unit. Am Rev Respir Dis 1973; 108(1):19–29.

35. DeGaute JP, Domenighetti G, Naeije R, et al. Oxygen delivery in acute exacerbation of chronic obstructive pulmonary disease. Effects of controlled oxygen therapy. Am Rev Respir Dis 1981; 124(1):26–30.

36. Bazuaye EA, Stone TN, Corris PA, et al. Variability of inspired oxygen concentration with nasal cannulas. Thorax 1992; 47(8):609–611.

37. Agusti AG, Carrera M, Barbe F, et al. Oxygen therapy during exacerbations of chronic obstructive pulmonary disease. Eur Respir J 1999; 14(4):934–939.

38. Denniston AK, O'Brien C, Stableforth D. The use of oxygen in acute exacerbations of chronic obstructive pulmonary disease: a prospective audit of pre-hospital and hospital emergency management. Clin Med 2002; 2(5):449–451.

39. Durrington HJ, Flubacher M, Ramsay CF, et al. Initial oxygen management in patients with an exacerbation of chronic obstructive pulmonary disease. QJM 2005; 98(7):499–504.

40. Gooptu B, Ward L, Ansari SO, et al. Oxygen alert cards and controlled oxygen: preventing emergency admissions at risk of hypercapnic acidosis receiving high inspired oxygen concentrations in ambulances and A&E departments. Emerg Med J 2006; 23(8):636–638.

41. McNicol MW, Campbell EJ. Severity of Respiratory Failure. Arterial Blood-Gases in Untreated Patients. Lancet 1965; 1:336–338.

# 27

# End-of-Life Issues and COPD Exacerbations

**ANITA K. SIMONDS**
Academic Department of Sleep & Breathing, Royal Brompton Hospital, London, U.K.

## I. Mortality and Morbidity of Severe Acute Exacerbations

Prospective study has shown that severe exacerbations of chronic obstructive pulmonary disease (COPD) requiring hospital management are independently associated with all-cause mortality and the patients at highest risk of dying are those presenting with more than three exacerbations, especially if these required inpatient care. Connors and colleagues (1) reported an in-hospital mortality rate of 11% in patients with acute hypercapnic respiratory failure, with subsequent mortality of 43% and 49% at one and two years, respectively. Seneff et al. (2) found an inpatient mortality of 24%, with this figure increasing to 59% at one year. In a more recent study (3) of patients receiving noninvasive ventilation (NIV) for an acute hypercapnic exacerbation, 73% survived the admission, but by one year after discharge, 80% had been readmitted, 63% had experienced another life-threatening event, and almost 50% had died. Survivors spent a median of 12% of the following year in hospital. A low body mass score predicted early readmission or death, and early death was more frequent in highly dyspneic patients [medical research council (MRC) score, $p < 0.001$]. Budweiser et al. (4) have also shown that nutritional status, base excess, and extent of hyperinflation (as index of physiological severity) are reliable predictors of mortality in keeping with the previously established body mass, obstruction, dyspnea, and exercise capacity (BODE) index.

These studies confirm that acute severe exacerbations are associated with high morbidity and mortality, and those who experience them recurrently despite optimum therapy are coming to the end of their life. In the huge amount of attention directed toward the acute exacerbation, this simple fact needs to be acknowledged and addressed. It is also increasingly recognized that not only is there a very significant symptom burden associated with the exacerbation, the overall symptom burden for those with steady-state disease is substantial and often poorly managed. Acute exacerbations are also associated with a reduction in health-related quality of life (5) and may precipitate depression and anxiety. Furthermore, even though the mortality following an acute severe exacerbation is high, many patients are not involved in advance decision-making, and so important decisions on intubation and the resuscitation status of the patient end up being made in crisis situations.

This is particularly important as, though prognostic indices are helpful on a population basis, for the individual patient it is not always clear which exacerbation is likely to be the last.

## II.  Symptom Burden

The Support study, which described the last year of life in patients admitted to the hospital in the United States between 1989 and 1994, was one of the first to highlight the high level of symptoms in patients with COPD. Less is known about patients in the community, and to address this lacuna, Elkington et al. (6) have recently examined symptoms, day-to-day functioning, contact with health carers and social services, and place of death in over 200 patients with COPD who died at an average age of 77 years in London, United Kingdom. Ninety-eight percent of this cohort were breathless all of the time or some of the time in their last year of life, 96% experienced fatigue or weakness, low mood occurred in 77%, and pain in 70%. Breathlessness was relieved by treatment in only 57%. More starkly, low mood was effectively treated in only 8% and 82% received no treatment for low mood. Over 40% of patients were housebound or left the house less than once a month. Sixty-three percent were aware they might die, but according to relatives, over a third did not know they were dying. This despite the fact that almost 50% had been admitted to the hospital in the past year, although a third saw their general practitioner (GP) less than once every three months or never.

This is reinforced by an earlier study in which Gore et al. (7) showed that 90% of COPD patients experienced anxiety of depression compared to 42% of patients with non-small cell lung cancer, and unlike the lung cancer patients, none of the COPD patients had access to palliative or supportive care services.

This work exposes a mass of missed opportunities to communicate at primary and secondary care levels. As a result, COPD patients suffer unnecessarily, and those who are not aware they are dying are denied the chance to participate in decision making or sort their affairs, say good-bye to family members, and achieve closure.

### A.  Supportive Care

To rationalize care of these individuals, particularly those with chronic disorders, the concept of supportive care has been developed. This embraces palliative medicine and end-of-life care but emphasizes the broader nature of patient and family care (Table 1).

### B.  Dissection of Symptom Burden

A change in symptoms or failure to respond to previous effective therapy should always provoke a clinical assessment to ascertain as fully as possible the cause and whether new problems or comorbidities have arisen. Measurement of pulmonary function, a chest X ray and echocardiogram, respectively, will help identify the need for intensification in airway

**Table 1**  Supportive Care

- Involves patients in decision making about their treatment
- Provides information about the condition, treatments, social support
- Deals with side effects of treatment and comorbidities
- Promotes access to social support
- Provides rehabilitation after treatment
- Provides emotional and spiritual support to the individual and family

maintenance therapy or demonstrate the development of a complicating problem such as lung cancer with pleural effusion or bronchial obstruction, cardiac failure, or thromboembolism.

## C. Depression and Anxiety

Evidence from multiple studies supports the importance of depression and anxiety in contributing to a poor quality of life and as a determinant of admissions. Yohannes et al. (8) using a simple screening score in COPD patients [mean forced expiratory volume in one second (FEV₁), 0.89l, aged 60–89 years] attending a university teaching hospital in the United Kingdom found 425 of patients were clinically depressed. The prevalence of anxiety was 37% in depressed patients, but only 5% in nondepressed patients. Thirty percent of patients were mildly depressed and a disturbing 68% were moderately depressed; few were on treatment for depression. In a cohort of COPD patients on long-term oxygen therapy (LTOT) in Quebec, Canada, Lacasse et al. (9) found that 57% [confidence interval (CI), 47–66] of individuals demonstrated depressive symptoms and 18% were severely depressed. Of those who met criteria for depression, only 6% were taking an antidepressant medication. In a Nordic study (10) using the Hospital Anxiety and Depression scale and St. George's respiratory questionnaire, anxiety occurred more often in females than males (47% vs. 34%, $p = 0.009$) and current smokers had a higher rate of both depression (43% vs. 23%) and anxiety (54% vs. 37%) than ex-smokers ($p < 0.01$). Crucially, depression influences the outcome of hospitalization from exacerbations and may affect readmission rates. In a prospective study, Ng et al. (11) examined the impact of depression on mortality, hospital stay, and readmissions. Forty-four percent of COPD patients were depressed on admission, and multivariate analysis showed that during follow-up over the subsequent year the presence of depression was associated with higher mortality (hazard ratio = 1.93; 95% CI, 1.04–3.58), longer hospital stay, a higher likelihood of persistent smoking at six months (odds ratio = 2.3; 95% CI, 1.17–4.52), and worse levels of symptoms, activities, and total score of the St. George's Respiratory Questionnaire, even when controlling for severity of COPD, comorbidities, and socioeconomic variables. In a further prospective study, Gudmundsson et al. (12) found that risk of rehospitalization in the year following an index exacerbation was significantly increased in COPD patients with anxiety (hazard ratio = 1.76; 95% CI, 1.16–2.68). The effects of depression and anxiety on preferences for mechanical ventilation and resuscitation are considered below.

Serotonin reuptake inhibitors may be particularly helpful in depression, panic, and anxiety. However, cognitive therapy and an exploration of fears should be considered as vital counterparts.

## D. Oxygen Therapy

Many patients with end-stage COPD will be on LTOT as determined by guidelines, and the evidence base for this in hypoxemic patients is well established. Short-burst oxygen therapy is often prescribed by GPs for management of dyspnea in end-stage COPD patients, but ideal prescription rates and evidence of efficacy are limited. It is important that relevant outcome measures are selected when assessing the value of an intervention for symptom palliation. Many studies of short-burst oxygen therapy have used exercise tests as a primary outcome measure, e.g., six-minute walk or shuttle walk. While this may be relevant to some COPD patients, for end-stage patients, a decrease in simple breathlessness score may be far more important than walking a longer distance.

Booth et al. (13) have systematically reviewed studies assessing the use of oxygen for palliation of breathlessness. There have been no large randomized controlled trials. Five studies have examined the effects of oxygen therapy at rest on visual analog score (VAS) of dyspnea. One study showed a reduction in breathlessness and another showed similar improvements with air at 4 L/min compared with $O_2$ at 4 L/min, with no significant difference between the cylinders. When comparing the effects of oxygen before, during, and after exercise on VAS scores, the authors found no benefit from preoxygenation, but the majority of studies showed less breathlessness on oxygen at an equivalent level of exercise compared with air. In some cases, oxygen may speed recovery of breathlessness after exercise, but this is not universally seen.

### E. Opiates

Use of opiates in COPD has been explored over many years with conflicting results. As a consequence, there are differing views from consensus reports, although, as with oxygen therapy, there have been few large randomized trials. In a recent Cochrane analysis, the authors identified 18 studies of which half involved oral or parenteral opiates and the other half nebulized opioids. A significant improvement in breathlessness was seen in patients receiving oral and parenteral opiates, whereas no reduction in breathlessness was found in patients receiving nebulized drug. The Cochrane analysis included patients with end-stage cancer as well as COPD, but carrying out a subgroup analysis with COPD patients alone did not change the overall message from the study.

As benefit with oral or parenteral opiates is seen, there is the additional need to balance reduction in dyspnea against side effects such as constipation and oversedation and harmful consequences such as ventilatory decompensation. Abernethy et al. (14) carried out a randomized double-blind placebo-controlled crossover trial of sustained release morphine 20 mg in 48 COPD patients (although severity of disease was not well defined) in an outpatient setting. Docusate and senna were also provided. The primary outcome measure was dyspnea measured on VAS. In the 38 patients who completed the trial (3 withdrawals due to morphine side effects), there was a significant reduction in refractory dyspnea, and sleep quality improved, although constipation was worse in the morphine period, despite laxatives. This was a short-term four-day study, and therefore it is not possible to determine whether further cumulative effects would follow. There is therefore still a crucial need to further investigate the role of opiates and opiate analogs for symptom control in COPD.

### F. Noninvasive Ventilation

NIV is a well-established therapy in acute exacerbations of COPD and has been shown to halve mortality and reduce ICU admissions (15). Interestingly, even the earliest studies of NIV in acute COPD showed it reduced dyspnea more rapidly than standard therapy (16), and therefore the role of NIV in palliating symptoms has been explored.

It is clear too that NIV is used in a substantial group of patients where it is the ceiling of ventilatory care, i.e., in Do Not Intubate Patients (17). In a survey (18) of end-of-life care in European respiratory high-dependency units, NIV was a ceiling of ventilatory care in 31% of admissions (Fig. 1). For any patient receiving NIV as a palliative strategy, clear goals should be set at the start of therapy. As well as reducing dyspnea, NIV may be used to control $PaCO_2$ and associated hypercapnic symptoms in patients requiring opiate or

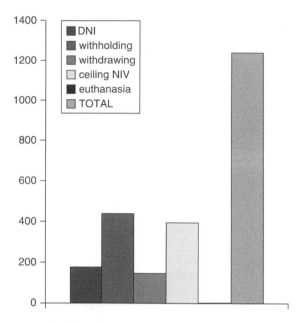

ERS Task Force from ref 18

**Figure 1** End-of-life decisions in European respiratory high-dependency-units: NIV as ceiling of ventilatory care. *Abbreviation*: NIV, noninvasive ventilation.

sedative therapy or to buy time to allow patient and family to explore options and take part in decisions. If these goals are not being met (and dyspnea should be resolved within hours), then NIV can be discontinued and therapy redirected to other means.

## G. Practical Measures

Pulmonary rehabilitation is effective at reducing breathlessness and improving quality of life, but in one study of patients who were housebound due to breathlessness, no improvement was seen (19). Rather than dismissing exercise or pulmonary rehabilitation in this end-stage group, additional tactics may be required, especially to address depression and social isolation. Despite physical limitations, most COPD patients have a strong desire to participate and be engaged in activities, and the importance of social interaction as well as improving functional performance should not be forgotten. Scooters, wheelchairs, and stairlifts are not a "defeat," but enable many to maintain some autonomy, get out of the home, and join in family events. Ambulatory oxygen systems, which are easily portable, should be provided so that patients are not limited by their oxygen supply.

## H. Decision Making About Invasive Mechanical Ventilation

There has been renewed interest in this important area with the recognition of the centrality of autonomy in decision making, while at the same time acknowledging that individuals cannot request futile interventions. Curtis et al. (20) examined patient's views on the type of end-of-life care they would like to receive and found differences between preferences in those with cancer, AIDS, and COPD. On the whole, COPD patients wanted further education in the areas of diagnosis and disease progress, treatment, prognosis, what dying might be like, and advance care planning.

As indicated above, the presence of depression and anxiety may have a major influence on the choices patients make. In the Support study of seriously ill hospitalized patients, preference for Do Not Resuscitate status was strongly correlated with depression, and a reduction in depression score at two-month follow-up was associated with a fivefold increase in the likelihood of the patient changing their preference to want cardiopulmonary resuscitation. Stapleton et al. (21) examined the effects of depressive symptoms and health-related quality of life on preferences for life-sustaining therapies in COPD patients receiving LTOT (median age 67 years, median $FEV_1$, 26.3% predicted). Depression was associated with a wish to forego resuscitation (50% of depressed patients vs. 23% of patients without depression), although there was no relationship with the wish to receive mechanical ventilation or not. Importantly, health-related quality of life scores were *not* *r*elated to either resuscitation or mechanical ventilation preferences. The latter point is crucial as health care professionals often assume that these choices will be closely correlated with patient-reported quality of life—and therein may lie the genesis of an important mismatch between patient and physician expectations.

In a Canadian study (22) of pulmonologists, it was found that doctor/patient discussion about mechanical ventilation tended to take place at an advanced stage in the condition. About 43% of pulmonologists felt they would discuss mechanical ventilation with 40% or less of their COPD patients before an exacerbation requiring ventilatory support. Most felt that the decision was collaborative between patient and physician, although a significant proportion of physicians reported modifying the information presented to patients in an attempt to influence ("frame") their decision. In fact, "shared" decision-making is often viewed quite differently by health care professional and patients or their family. Health care professionals tend to underestimate patients' need for information and overestimate their understanding and awareness of their prognosis and end-of-life issues (23). This clearly indicates a need to repeatedly review the patients' understanding, treatment preferences, and care options.

It is worth noting too that patients are capable of balancing quite complex information and possible outcomes, providing it is presented appropriately. Fried et al. (24) have examined treatment preferences regarding life-sustaining interventions in a range of patients with limited life expectancy due to cancer, congestive cardiac failure, or COPD. Individuals of average age, approximately 73 years, were asked whether they would wish to receive a given treatment if the outcome was certain, or if there were differing likelihoods of an adverse outcome. Crucially, participants were able to balance the outcome against the burden of treatment (e.g., length of hospital stay, invasiveness of procedure). For example, a low-burden treatment that returned the individual to previous functioning level would be accepted by nearly all participants (98.7%), but 11.2% would not accept this option if the treatment had a high burden. Conversely, if the likely outcome was survival but with severe functional or cognitive impairment, 74.4% and 88.8% would not want to receive low- and high-burden treatment, respectively. There was no difference between choices between the diagnostic groups, although there was a trend for COPD and cancer patients to refuse high-burden therapy. This work demonstrates that patients can compute varying outcomes and that impact on functional and cognitive outcomes play a greater part in preferences than survival itself. This should help inform discussion with patients. Clearly, they also need to know the probable consequences of *nonintervention* to make a valid decision to undergo or forego a treatment.

## I. Improving Communication

Opportunities to discuss treatment preferences arise during pulmonary rehabilitation sessions (although in group meetings general topics rather than specific management plans are easier to address) and outpatient consultations. For example, Heffner et al. (25) carried out a two-site prospective evaluation of advance directive education during a pulmonary rehabilitation course to assess the effects on completion of (*i*) living wills, (*ii*) durable powers of attorney (i.e., identifying a proxy decision maker), (*iii*) patient-physician discussion about end-of-life issues (*iv*) decisions about life support, and (*v*) patient impression that their physician understood their end-of-life preferences. The group that received education on these topics was subsequently significantly more likely to discuss these issues and complete advance directives and felt more assured that their physicians understood their preferences. It has been demonstrated that COPD patients in particular want further information on their disease, its likely course, and treatments from their doctors, but may not necessarily raise these topics without prompting. The way the topics are broached is also important. Most individuals welcome discussion, but this is usefully directed to the symptom control approach through the remainder of the patient's life, rather than an exclusive focus on their death. Striking a realistic and kindly balance between maintaining hope and a pragmatic expectation of deterioration is part of the clinical judgment health care workers should exercise and adapt with the individual.

The barriers to effective communication about resuscitation status and mechanical ventilation have been explored by Knauft et al. (26), who found that only 32% of patients had taken part in such discussion with their physician. Frequently cited barriers for the patient were "I'd rather concentrate on staying alive" and "I'm not sure what doctor will be taking care of me." Physicians ranked the most important barriers as "There was too little time during our appointment to discuss everything we should" or "I worry that discussing end-of-life care will take away his/her hope" and "The patient is not ready to talk about the care they would like to receive if and when she/he is sick."

There are echoes of these findings in a London-based GP survey (27), assessing whether the GPs entered into discussion about prognosis and end-of-life care with COPD patients. While the majority recognized the importance of these discussions in primary care, only a minority (42%) reported they often or always discussed prognosis. In those who rarely or never had these discussions, the majority felt ill prepared to discuss the subject and 64% found it hard to initiate discussions. This is a particularly revealing finding as there is evidence that patients would like the medical team to raise this topic, so it is easy to see how decision-making gets deferred or missed till it is too late.

On a positive note, Knauft et al. (26) found a number of facilitators that made effective communication more likely. These included the patient's experience of friends or family who had died, the fact that the patient trusted their physician, and the feeling that their physician was good for caring for lung disease and that he/she viewed them as a person rather than focusing purely on the lung condition.

### J.   Advance Care Plans

A further method of enhancing understanding between patient and health care team are advance care plans or directives. When formulated and recorded by a competent individual, these enable that person to give direction to health care providers about the treatments they would like to receive and how these decisions might change if they were, for example, incapacitated by senility or coma. In most jurisdictions, individuals can appoint proxy decision makers if they lose the capacity to make decisions. Only around 30% of the U.S. residents make advance directives, and in other countries, this is considerably lower. Advance plans are particularly valuable in chronic conditions but may work less well in other circumstances, and this may be a particular problem in ICU admissions. Instructions may be too vague to be of use or too medically specific to be applied in common situations. Advance directives tend to focus on the right to refuse treatment with little emphasis on the underlying goals or values of the patient. Once completed, they are often not reviewed even when health declines. These directives are based on patient autonomy, but in some cultures, decisions are family or religion based. There are concerns from some disability groups that directives deal predominantly with treatment refusal, where some groups would like to emphasize their continued wish for treatment. Having said that, advance directives can and usually do work well for individuals with advanced lung disease.

### K.   Management of Comorbidities

Supportive care of patients with end-stage COPD should take into account the fact that most are likely to have other conditions, such as peripheral vascular disease, ischemic heart disease, osteoarthritis, or disorders exacerbated by therapy such as osteoporosis. These will have a cumulative effect on health-related quality of life, and the treatment of comorbidities needs to be carefully factored into comprehensive care plans, bearing in mind the risks of polypharmacy, the likelihood of benefit (e.g., what exactly is the risk/benefit of a cholesterol-lowering statin in a COPD patient in the last few months of life?), and the psychological consequences of stopping therapy (28).

### L.   Support for Carers

Carers for end-stage COPD patients are often elderly partners who are not in good health themselves. Any care plan should embrace their needs. It is vital to recognize that while many patients prefer to die at home, unless the carer is supported, plans in this respect are likely to disintegrate, to the distress of all concerned. Comprehensive care pathways, e.g., Liverpool Care Pathway, acknowledge this role and provide support to the carer after the patient's death.

## III.   Conclusions

The previous miserablist approach to end-stage COPD is now disappearing, but much still needs to be done to improve supportive care and facilitate the patient and families' full understanding of COPD and central role in decision making. While respiratory medicine has much to learn from palliative and supportive care services, it is unlikely that palliative medicine and hospice resources can cater for all end-stage COPD patients. It is therefore incumbent on respiratory teams to embrace fully this vital role. Raising of public awareness is also important as there are still misperceptions in the general population on end-of-life issues. In a study of outpatient attendees, Silverira and colleagues (29) found that almost 70% understood concepts of refusal of treatment, 46% correctly understood withdrawal of therapy, but 62% did not distinguish between assisted suicide and euathanasia. Perhaps, not surprisingly, the awareness of concepts was positively associated with college degree, personal experience of illness or death of a loved one, acting as a proxy for health care decisions, or having written an advance directive. Integration of these concepts into school and college courses and a wider public debate should help further understanding.

## References

1. Connors AF, Dawson NV, Thomas C, et al. Outcomes following acute exacerbations of severe chronic obstructive lung disease. Am J Respir Crit Care Med 1996; 154:959–967.
2. Seneff MG, Wagner DP, Wagner RP, et al. Hospital and 1-year survival of patients admitted to intensive care units with acute exacerbation of chronic obstructive pulmonary disease. JAMA 1995; 274:1852–1857.
3. Chu CM, Chan VL, Lin AWN, et al. Readmission rates and life threatening events in COPD survivors treated with non-invasive ventilation for acute hypercapnic respiratory failure. Thorax 2004; 59:1020–1025.
4. Budweiser S, Jorres RA, Riedl T, et al. Predictors of survival in COPD patients with chronic hypercapnic respiratory failure receiving noninvasive home ventilation. Chest 2007; 131: 1650–1658.
5. Seemungal TAR, Donaldson GC, Paul EA, et al. Effect of exacerbations on quality of life in patients with chronic obstructive pulmonary disease. Am J Respir Crit Care Med 1998; 157:1418–1422.
6. Elkington H, White P, Addington-Hall J, et al. The healthcare needs of chronic obstructive pulmonary disease patients in the last year of life. Palliat Med 2005; 19:485–491.
7. Gore JM, Brophy CJ, Greenstone MA. How well do we care for patients with end stage chronic obstructive pulmonary disease (COPD)? A comparison of palliative care and quality of life in COPD and lung cancer. Thorax 2000; 55:1000–1006.
8. Yohannes AM, Baldwin RC, Connolly MJ. Depression and anxiety in elderly outpatients with chronic obstructive pulmonary disease: prevalence, and validation of the BASDEC screening questionnaire. Int J Geriatr Psychiatry 2000; 15:1090–1096.
9. Lacasse Y, Rousseau L, Maltais F. Prevalence of depressive symptoms and depression in patients with severe oxygen-dependent chronic obstructive pulmonary disease. J Cardiopulm Rehabil 2001; 21:80–86.
10. Gudmundsson G, Gislason T, Janson C, et al. Depression, anxiety and health status after hospitalisation for COPD: a multicentre study in the Nordic countries. Respir Med 2006; 100: 87–93.
11. Ng TPNM, Tan WC, Cao Z, et al. Depressive symptoms and chronic obstructive pulmonary disease: effect on mortality, hospital readmission, syptom burden, functional status, and quality of life. Arch Intern Med 2007; 167:60–67.
12. Gudmundsson G, Gislason T, Janson C, et al. Risk factors for rehospitalisation in COPD: role of health status, anxiety and depression. Eur Respir J 2005; 26:414–419.
13. Booth S, Anderson H, Swannick M, et al. The use of oxygen in the palliation of breathlessness. A report of the expert working group of the scientific committee of the association of palliative medicine. Respir Med 2004; 98:66–77.
14. Abernethy AP, Currow DC, Frith P, et al. Randomised, double blind, placebo controlled crossover trial of sustained release morphine for the management of refractory dyspnoea. BMJ 2003; 327(7414):523–528.

15. Lightowler J, Wedzicha JA, Elliott MW, et al. Non-invasive positive pressure ventilation to treat respiratory failure resulting from exacerbations of chronic obstructive pulmonary disease: cochrane systematic review and meta-analysis. BMJ 2003; 326:185.

16. Bott J, Carroll MP, Conway JH, et al. Randomised controlled trial of nasal ventilation in acute ventilatory failure due to chronic obstructive airways disease. Lancet 1993; 341:1555–1557.

17. Levy M, Tanios MA, Nelson D, et al. Outcomes of patients with do-not-intubate orders treated with noninvasive ventilation. Crit Care Med 2004; 32:2002–2007.

18. Nava S, Sturani C, Hartl S, et al. End of life decision-making in respiratory intermediate care units: A European survey. Eur Respir J 2007; 30:156–164.

19. Wedzicha JA, Bestall JC, Garrod R, et al. Randomizes controlled trial of pulmonary rehabilitation in severe chronic obstructive pulmonary disease patients, stratified with the MRC dyspnoea scale. Eur Respir J 1998; 12:363–369.

20. Curtis JR, Wenrich MD, Carline JD, et al. Patients' perspectives on physician skill in end-of-life care. Differences between patients with COPD, cancer and AIDS. Chest 2002; 122:356–362.

21. Stapleton RD, Nielsen EL, Engelber' RA, et al. Association of depression and life-sustaining treatment preferences in patients with COPD. Chest 2005; 127:328–334.

22. McNeely PD, Hebert PC, Dales RE, et al. Deciding about mechanical ventilation in endstage chronic obstructive pulmonary disease: how respirologists perceive their role. Can Med Assoc J 1997; 156:177–183.

23. Hancock K, Clayton JM, Parker SM, et al. Discrepant perceptions about end-of-life communication: a systemtic review. J Pain Symptom Manage 2007; 34:190–200.

24. Fried TR, Bradley EH, Towle VR, et al. Understanding the treatment preferences of seriously ill patients. N Engl J Med 2002; 346:1061–1066.

25. Heffner JE, Fahy B, Hilling L, et al. Outcomes of advance directive education of pulmonary of pulmonary rehabilitation patients. Am J Respir Crit Care Med 1997; 155:1055–1059.

26. Knauft E, Nielsen EL, Engelberg RA, et al. Barriers and facilitators to end-of life-care communication for patients with COPD. Chest 2005; 127:2188–2196.

27. Elkington H, White P, Higgs R, et al. GPs views of discussions of prognosis in severe COPD. Fam Pract 2001; 18:440–444.

28. Stevenson J, Abernethy AP, Miller C, et al. Managing comorbidities in patients at the end of life. BMJ 2004; 329:909–912.

29. Silveira MJ, DiPiero A, Gerrity MS, et al. Patients' knowledge of options at the end of life: ignorance in the face of death. JAMA 2000; 284:2483–2488.

# 28
# Novel Models of Care for COPD Exacerbations

**MARTYN R. PARTRIDGE**
Department of Respiratory Medicine, NHLI Division, Imperial College London and Honorary Consultant Respiratory Physician, Imperial College Healthcare NHS Trust, London, U.K.

## I. Introduction

Over the last few decades, the burden of ill health in westernised countries has moved from a burden of acute illness to a burden of long-term disease such as diabetes, hypertension, asthma, and chronic obstructive pulmonary disease (COPD). Services for those with long-term diseases need to be structured differently from those appropriate for short-lived acute, usually infectious illness, and long-term medical conditions need more attention being paid to

- good communication,
- partnerships of care,
- giving control, where possible, to the patient,
- group support, and
- convenient follow-up.

Many long-term conditions such as COPD are, however, punctuated with more acute episodes of worsening (exacerbations), and how we handle such episodes from an organizational point of view requires thought and evaluation. Key features are likely to be as follows:

- Patient recognition of the worsening of their condition
- Patient appreciation of the significance of certain features of worsening (e.g., swelling of the ankles, or purulence of sputum)
- Easy access to appropriate healthcare for information and advice
- Patient self-treatment where appropriate
- Healthcare that is conveniently located, safely configured, and empathic to the wishes of the patient
- Healthcare that is cost effective

Traditionally the first step of treatment for an exacerbation or worsening of a condition such as COPD would be either self-treatment or the patient consulting with a general practitioner, a family physician, or a specialist based in the community. Treatment would be instituted, but if response was suboptimal, or the severity was of a degree that merited it, hospitalization would be the next step. Often the patient bypasses these first steps by directly attending an emergency department or by calling an ambulance. It is important to note that in this disease, perhaps especially, the decision to admit a patient to the hospital with an exacerbation of COPD is often influenced not only by the severity of the respiratory condition but by other factors such as social support, appropriateness of home accommodation, presence of depression (or other comorbidity), and sometimes the wishes of other family members.

More recently alternative models of care have been introduced in many parts of the world and these organizational changes are often referred to by different terms but would include systems described as

- nurse-led care,
- hospital-at-home schemes,
- admission avoidance schemes,
- cooperation schemes,
- case management,
- self-management,
- integrated care, and
- early (or assisted) discharge schemes.

This chapter is concerned with describing for the reader what may be involved in these different patterns of care and in teasing out interventions for which there is some evidence of benefit. Didactic concluding statements are particularly difficult in this field, and the reasons for that need to be outlined so that greater clarity can be applied to evaluation in future randomized controlled trials. The reasons for conflicting results are shared with other areas but some are specific to COPD. Reasons for confusion include the following:

- Too few trials
- Poorly described or poorly defined interventions so that it is difficult for others to emulate the study
- Small proportion of eligible patients being willing to enter trials such that general extrapolability of results is compromised (1)
- Inappropriate outcomes
- Lack of appreciation of the impact of comorbidity
- Lack of room for improvement in some parameters. The potential magnitude for improvement of some outcomes in COPD is going to be much less than it is for other more reversible diseases, meaning that trials often need to involve large numbers of patients if a clear answer is to be achieved.
- Study design that has often involved either a single intervention that may not be powerful enough by itself to alter outcomes, or complex interventions so that it is difficult to know the beneficial components.

In reality, when discussing optimal methods of organizing care for those with COPD, it is likely that there will be a synergism between several interventions, and it is possible that significant impacts will only be achieved when two, three, or more interventions out of a possible list of six, seven, or eight are applied in any one case.

In any study, it is essential to carefully describe the patient population and to describe what one is trying to avoid. In this chapter, the emphasis will be upon description and evaluation of techniques that have been used to reduce the need for those with an exacerbation of COPD to be admitted to the hospital. This emphasis is dictated by the health economic importance of avoiding admission, but is clearly also justified from studies of patients that have shown that dependency and hospitalization are feared and disliked much more in this condition than the symptoms of breathlessness, cough, or fatigue (2).

## II. Alternative Methods of Care That Have Been Described and Studied

It is thus both the patient's wish and that of healthcare providers to minimize the number of patients with COPD who need to be admitted to the hospital [54% of the total economic cost of COPD is from hospitalization (3)]. The following care delivery methods by which this may be undertaken have been reported.

### A. Admission Avoidance Schemes

Admission avoidance schemes have been described and evaluated in a number of studies. If the full impact of such a scheme is to be evaluated, it is essential that the patient population be clearly described, and it is always easier to demonstrate a reduction in admission rates if one was previously admitting patients, who in other localities might not have been admitted. Furthermore, one has to determine the likely *overall* benefits of different types of intervention. While admission avoidance might be attractive, it is likely to be suitable only for a minority of patients and *early (assisted) discharge schemes* may produce a greater overall benefit for the system (i.e., there may be a greater advantage in reducing the average duration of stay by one to two days for every patient admitted with a exacerbation of COPD rather than avoiding the admission altogether of only 5–25% of patients). An example of a randomized controlled trial in this area is that of Skwarska and colleagues (4), where suitable patients were randomized to either traditional hospital admission or home support, where they were visited by a nurse every few days until they recovered and they were then discharged. The majority of patients could not be randomized because the admission was regarded as obligatory, and it is likely from this study that, at most, approximately only a quarter of patients could be considered for this sort of scheme. Those supported at home were followed up for a slightly longer time before being deemed fit for discharge than those who had been admitted to the hospital, but the latter group were slightly more likely to have a further admission during a short period of follow-up. Patient satisfaction was good and the total health service costs for those who were supported at home were half that of those who were admitted to the hospital.

### B. Early Discharge Schemes

Early discharge schemes are likely to be suitable for a larger number of patients than admission avoidance schemes. More studies have been undertaken of such services and in more countries and such schemes are said to be available in over 40% of U.K. acute hospital trusts (5). Early discharge schemes are more likely to have been established in larger hospitals with higher number of COPD admissions, a speciality respiratory ward, and with a pulmonary rehabilitation service and availability of respiratory nurses. Proof of concept studies in Australia (6), Spain (7) and the United Kingdom (8) have demonstrated that such schemes that involve discharge from hospital after two or three days, with follow-up by a nurse at home, can significantly reduce overall hospital length of stay and do so safely with low rates of readmission. Some of these studies did however have rather short follow-up periods. Randomized controlled trials such as that by Cotton and colleagues (9), albeit involving relatively small numbers of patients, were able to show that such early discharge schemes could halve hospital inpatient stays with no excess of mortality and with subsequent readmission rates that are similar to those who had traditional inpatient care. In this study, patients were excluded if they were not resident in the locality, were homeless, were unable to give informed consent, or did not have access to a telephone. Those with significant medical comorbidity and those with life-threatening respiratory failure (acidosis) were similarly excluded. Over a 14-month period, 412 emergency admissions were evaluated, with 38 being excluded on the grounds of homelessness, inability to consent, or no access to a telephone, but the largest group (209 patients) was excluded because of significant medical comorbidity or severity and 37 patients declined to take part in the study. Eighty-one patients were randomized, and 36 underwent early supported discharge. Support needed in the home included loan of nebulizers, prescription of oxygen, and a respiratory nurse's visit to the patients on the first day after discharge and then according to the nurse's professional discretion. The median duration of nurse follow-up was 24 days and the median number of nurse visits was 11.

### C.  Hospital-at-Home Schemes

Hospital-at-home schemes include various methods of providing more intensive healthcare for patients within their own homes, and both admission avoidance and early discharge schemes as described above have clearly had to use what is in effect a hospital-at-home scheme. Such schemes have involved supervision by primary care physicians, daily or alternate day nurse visits, with additional interventions from pharmacists, physiotherapists, and occupational therapists, telephone support and more intensive schemes whereby patients are escorted to their homes from the emergency department and visited twice daily for a minimum of three subsequent days by a specialist nurse, with nighttime cover being available from generic district nurses. A scheme such as that described by Davies (10) showed similar hospital readmission rates among patients treated by the hospital-at-home team and those who had been managed in the traditional way, and no difference in mortality, nor in this study in subsequent quality of life. A systematic review of randomized control trials in this area by Ram and colleagues (11) included seven randomized controlled trials. Out of 2786 patients who presented with acute exacerbations and were evaluated in these trials, 26.7% were suitable for study entry with comorbidity being the commonest reason for exclusion. A subsequent guideline on hospital at home in chronic obstructive pulmonary disease (12) made recommendations as to which type of patient should *not* be offered hospital-at-home schemes and these are listed in Table 1.

In the published series the availability of hospital-at-home services has varied, with some working usual working hours on Monday to Fridays and some working seven days a week. The longer the service is available the more patients may be able to avail themselves of it, but the cost implications may alter. Lines of medical responsibility need to be clearly outlined with such schemes and most have involved respiratory nurse specialists but in some, non specialist district nurses have been involved and in a smaller number respiratory

**Table 1**  Patients Thought to be Unsuitable for Hospital at Home (12)

- Those with impaired level of consciousness
- Those with acute confusion
- Those with respiratory acidosis (pH < 7.35)
- Those with acute changes on a chest radiograph
- Those in whom comorbidity necessitates hospitalization
- Those with insufficient social support or lack of access to a telephone or long distance from hospital
- Those with apparently new onset hypoxemia (SpO2 ≤ 90%)
- Those for whom oxygen cannot be provided at home

physiotherapists. The second UK national COPD audit (13) confirmed that hospitals that had access to early discharge schemes had a shorter median length of stay for their COPD patients than did hospitals without access to such a scheme, and whilst all schemes showed that they were suitable for only a minority of patients, none suggested any resultant risk to patients. Whilst the health economic studies are limited they are likely to result in significant cost savings.

## D. Self-Treatment of an Exacerbation

One of the advantages of self-management education of those with COPD (see chap. 32) is the ability of the patient to recognize a worsening of their own condition and to institute by themselves changes in routine therapy or the starting of new therapies. The evidence of benefit from such self-treatment is slightly confusing in the literature, but it should be borne in mind that in the parallel field of asthma, one of the key features of self-management education has been the receipt by the patient of written personal asthma action plans. In many of the studies of COPD, patients were not issued with written action plans and indeed in the seven studies evaluated in the first Cochrane systematic review of this field (14), only two of the studies involved the patient receiving a written action plan, and in one of those, it was an *asthma* action plan that was given, which did not, for example, include self-institution by the patient of antibiotic therapy. A subsequent review (15) has shown that the use of action plans in COPD increases both the recognition by the patient of a severe exacerbation and increases their use of antibiotics and oral steroids. It did not, however, at the time of that review demonstrate any benefit in terms of change in healthcare utilization, quality of life, or symptom scores, but there were only three studies included in the systematic review. A subsequent study of integrated care in those with COPD over a two-year period by Sridhar and colleagues (16), which involved multiple interventions, did show that within a randomized controlled trial those who had been given a written COPD action plan and reserve supplies of antibiotics and steroids were much more likely to be the initiators of such treatment than a control group where the treatment for exacerbations was instituted by the primary care physician. As a result there was a very significant reduction in the need for unscheduled contact with the primary care physician in the intervention group compared with that in the control group: for every one patient receiving the intervention, there was

1.79 less unscheduled contacts with the GP, with potentially great economic savings and the likelihood of prompter treatment of exacerbations.

If self-treatment is to be advocated, we should recall that much information given to a patient is soon forgotten and reinforcement of spoken messages by the use of written action plans is usually recommended (Fig. 1). These may contain lifestyle advice and advice about usual treatment but specifically include advice for patients about when to start a course of antibiotics and, where appropriate, a course of steroid tablets. However, we should be aware that 10% to 15% of our patients may be unable to use health-related information leaflets and consideration should be given to the use of pictorial advice to patients as shown in one COPD action plan under trial in Figure 2.

These three systems of care described above, hospital-at-home, assisted discharge, and admission avoidance, along with patient self-treatment are all concerned with methods of care accessed by the patient at a time when they are experiencing a worsening of their condition. However, other types of care offered at other times also need description and

**Department of Respiratory Medicine**
**Charing Cross Hospital**

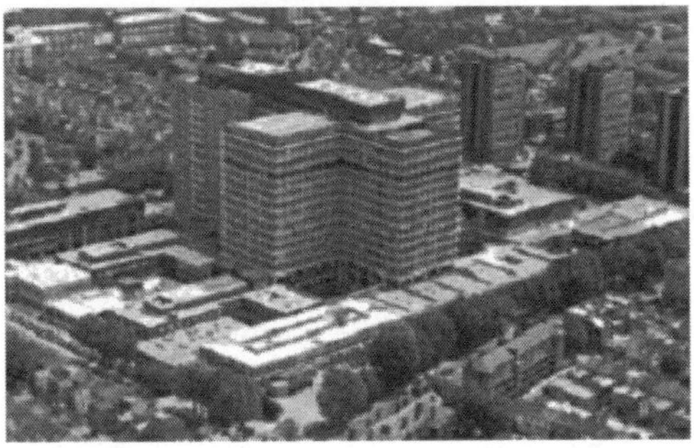

C.O.P.D. Self-management Card

Name: .............................................................

Hospital No.: ...................................................

Chest Consultant: .............................................

Respiratory Health Worker: ...................................

General Practitioner: ...........................................

**Figure 1** Fifty percent of all that we say to a patient is likely to be forgotten within 5 minutes of the consultation ending. Self-management advice that has been given orally needs reinforcement by leaflets that can be taken away by the patient. Such leaflets should contain lifestyle advice, advice about usual treatments and advice as to when to start additional therapies such as antibiotics and steroid tablets and when to seek medical attention.

**Charing Cross Hospital Copd Action Plan**

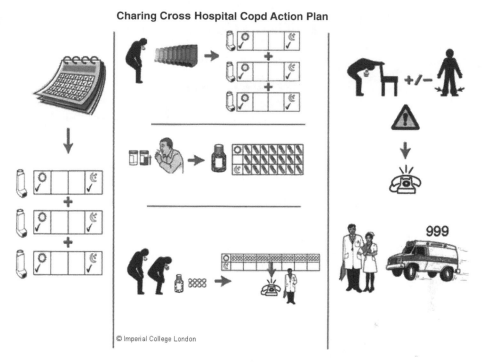

© Imperial College London

**Figure 2** A significant number of patients with COPD may be unable to use written health-related information. Pictures may represent a more usable method of giving information to both the literate and those with impaired literacy. The illustration shown here is a pictorial treatment plan currently being evaluated in the United Kingdom.

evaluation to determine whether they are beneficial to patients and result in a reduction in need for emergency health care. Such processes are described below.

### Disease Registers

Patients with COPD need regular review to reassess severity, assess lung function, ensure optimization of treatment, assess nutritional status, and to revise self-management education. Review frequency will be adjusted according to severity, but any form of recall involves knowledge of patients with such a diagnosis and disease registers are therefore recommended and a key feature of a successful chronic care model (17).

### Case Management and Regular Respiratory Nurse Support

Twenty to thirty years ago, care for patients with lung disease was provided either by primary care physicians or by specialists working in the community or within hospitals, with patients with severe disease being admitted to the hospital. In many countries there was very little in the way of integrated care by healthcare professionals or by teams working in *both* hospitals and within the community. One exception might have been tuberculosis nurses and health care workers and as tuberculosis declined in prevalence in many areas the tuberculosis health care workers took on additional respiratory duties in an increasing number of cases of chronic respiratory disease (18). More recently still such respiratory health workers have had their role evaluated in a number of studies of integrated care or nurse assisted community care of patients with COPD. One of the first studies was that of Cockroft et al. (19) in which 75 patients were randomized so that 42 were visited by a respiratory health worker and 33 were allocated to a controlled group. The patients were mainly suffering from chronic obstructive pulmonary disease and had had at least two previous hospital admissions. The patients were visited in their homes at approximately monthly intervals for education and support and encouraged to recognize signs of deterioration and take appropriate action. The study showed that visits were much appreciated by the patients but the quality of life as measured did not alter and whilst there was a beneficial effect upon survival, the duration of stay in hospital for respiratory reasons was longer in those who had been visited by the respiratory health worker than in the control group. A more recent study (20) showed rather similar results in that patients with COPD who were randomized to nurse-assisted management had no better quality of life results than the control group and no specifically beneficial effect in terms of need for unscheduled health care. Similarly, an Australian study of those with COPD offered a coordinated intervention led by GPs and supported by nurses showed no improvement in quality of life or reduction in admission rates in that continent (21).

The problem with all of these studies is that they often involved patients with differing severity of disease who have been offered interventions of varying intensities in a disease that we know is not dramatically responsive to therapies. Prompt identification and treatment of exacerbations may however be beneficial and a recent North American review (17) of interventions for COPD has shown that a possible beneficial effect can be made upon need for unscheduled care, when patients received at least two components from a list of chronic care model interventions that included

- advanced access to a knowledgeable health care provider (24 hr/day, 7 days a week),
- optimal care based on evidence-based guidelines,
- use of databases and registries and thus regular review, and
- self-management education.

### E.  Group Support

Group support is one aspect that has not been studied in this field. Many patients with COPD feel stigmatized and sense their own downhill course and often express feelings of hopelessness (22). Their exertional breathlessness contributes to social isolation; and yet, many who have run pulmonary rehabilitation programmes have experienced the tremendous fillip that patients experience from realizing that they are not alone. Indeed, after pulmonary rehabilitation programmes patients often exchange contact details to maintain contact with those they had spent the last four to six weeks; and in some countries either systematic follow-up has been offered or voluntary groups such as those run by the British Lung Foundation (23) have provided ongoing social support and an opportunity for reinforcement of the messages of pulmonary rehabilitation and the ongoing giving of information. Such group support has not been formally evaluated.

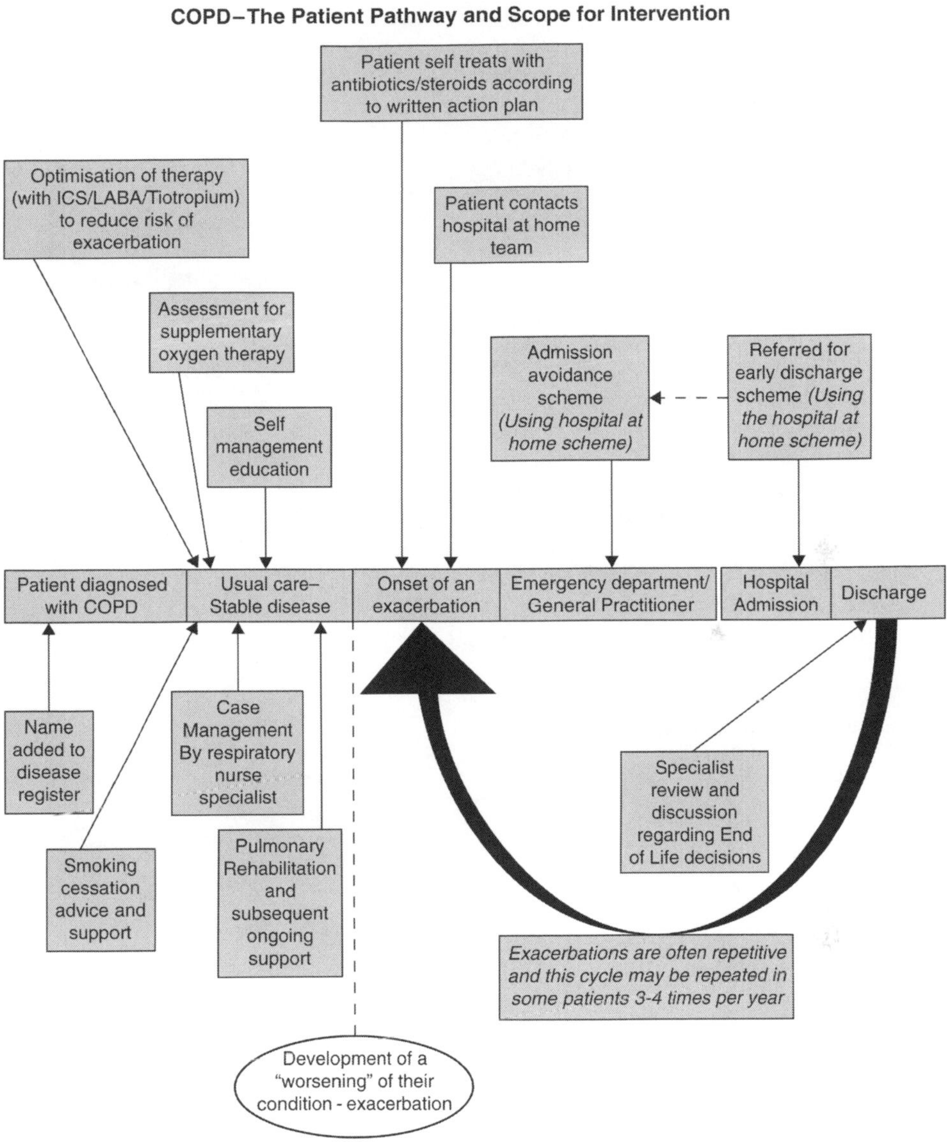

**COPD–The Patient Pathway and Scope for Intervention**

Patient self treats with antibiotics/steroids according to written action plan

Optimisation of therapy (with ICS/LABA/Tiotropium) to reduce risk of exacerbation

Patient contacts hospital at home team

Assessment for supplementary oxygen therapy

Admission avoidance scheme *(Using hospital at home scheme)*

Referred for early discharge scheme *(Using the hospital at home scheme)*

Self management education

| Patient diagnosed with COPD | Usual care– Stable disease | Onset of an exacerbation | Emergency department/ General Practitioner | Hospital Admission | Discharge |

Name added to disease register

Case Management By respiratory nurse specialist

Specialist review and discussion regarding End of Life decisions

Smoking cessation advice and support

Pulmonary Rehabilitation and subsequent ongoing support

*Exacerbations are often repetitive and this cycle may be repeated in some patients 3-4 times per year*

Development of a "worsening" of their condition - exacerbation

**Figure 3** Apart from pharmacological interventions, there are a number of other interventions shown here that may be of value to those with COPD. Some interventions such as self-treatment, admission avoidance schemes, and supported discharge schemes may reduce the burden of exacerbations to both individual and healthcare systems.

## III.  Conclusion

The patient pathway and scope for intervention in COPD is summarized in Figure 3. Many of the interventions that we may be able to offer to patients with COPD have not been fully evaluated, and there is still some ongoing confusion with regard to optimal interventions. However, there is much more to the good care of those with COPD than the writing of the prescription, and as the late Trevor Clay wrote in an editorial in *Thorax* (24),
"There is no cure, no magic, but there is always something that can be done."
In other chapters of this book, the benefits of self-management education, pulmonary rehabilitation, and the optimal use of oxygen have been described. Exacerbations are greatly feared by patients and hospitalization is disliked by them, and these are costly to the health service. More study is required over longer periods of time on the benefits of different organizational changes, but at this point in time, it seems reasonable to conclude that issuing a personal, written action plan to patients with COPD can lead to prompter therapy and a reduction in need for primary unscheduled healthcare. Optimization of therapy according to guidelines and review of patients by the maintenance of their names on a disease register is important. Rapid patient access, at time of need (but not routinely), to COPD-competent health professionals is beneficial, and if exacerbations occur, self-treatment is possible and a minority, but significant minority of those deemed to need hospitalization, can instead be cared for at home either by avoiding admission all together or by shortening admission using an early discharge scheme. Such an intervention is likely to be safe and cost effective.

### Acknowledgement

Dr. Nicola Roberts assistance with the development of the pictorial action plan (figure 2) is much appreciated.

### References

1.   Taylor R, Dawson S, Roberts N, et al. Why do patients decline to take part in a research project involving pulmonary rehabilitation? Respir Med 2007; 101(9):1942–1946.
2.   Haughney J, Partridge MR, Vogelmeier C, et al. Exacerbations of COPD: quantifying the patient's perspective using discrete choice modelling. Eur Respir J 2005; 26(4):623–629.
3.   Britton M. The burden of COPD in the U.K.: results from the Confronting COPD survey. Respir Med 2003; 97(suppl C):S71–S79.
4.   Skwarska E, Cohen G, Skwarski KM, et al. Randomized controlled trial of supported discharge in patients with exacerbations of chronic obstructive pulmonary disease. Thorax 2000; 55(11): 907–912.
5.   Quantrill SJ, Lowe D, Hosker HS, et al. Survey of early discharge schemes from the 2003 UK National COPD Audit. Respir Med 2007; 101(5):1026–1031.
6.   Murphy NM, Byrne CC, O'Neill SJ, et al. An outreach programme for patients with an exacerbation of chronic obstructive pulmonary disease. Ir Med J 2003; 96(5):137–140.
7.   Pascual-Pape T, Badia JR, Marrades RM, et al. (Results of a preventive program and assisted hospital discharge for COPD exacerbation. A feasibility study). Med Clin (Barc) 2003; 120(11): 408–411.

8. Mair FS, Wilkinson M, Bonnar SA, et al. The role of telecare in the management of exacerbations of chronic obstructive pulmonary disease in the home. J Telemed Telecare 1999; 5(suppl 1): S66–S67.

9. Cotton MM, Bucknall CE, Dagg KD, et al. Early discharge for patients with exacerbations of chronic obstructive pulmonary disease: a randomized controlled trial. Thorax 2000; 55(11):902–906.

10. Davies L, Wilkinson M, Bonner S, et al. "Hospital at home" versus hospital care in patients with exacerbations of chronic obstructive pulmonary disease: prospective randomised controlled trial. BMJ 2000; 321(7271):1265–1268.

11. Ram FS, Wedzicha JA, Wright J, et al. Hospital at home for patients with acute exacerbations of chronic obstructive pulmonary disease: systematic review of evidence. BMJ 2004; 329(7461):315.

12. British Thoracic Society. Intermediate care: Hospital-at-Home in chronic obstructive pulmonary disease: British Thoracic Society guideline. Thorax 2007; 62(3):200–210.

13. Roberts CM, Barnes S, Lowe D, et al. Evidence for a link between mortality in acute COPD and hospital type and resources. Thorax 2003; 58(11):947–949.

14. Monninkhof E, van der Valk P, van der Palen J, et al. Self-management education for patients with chronic obstructive pulmonary disease: a systematic review. Thorax 2003; 58(5):394–398.

15. Turnock A, Walters E, Walters J, et al. Action plans for chronic obstructive pulmonary disease. The Cochrane Database Syst Rev 2005; 4:CD005074.

16. Sridhar M, Taylor R, Dawson S, et al. A Nurse-Led intermediate care package in patients who have been hospitalised with an acute exacerbation of chronic obstructive pulmonary disease. Thorax 2007.

17. Adams SG, Smith PK, Allan PF, et al. Systematic review of the chronic care model in chronic obstructive pulmonary disease prevention and management. Arch Intern Med 2007; 167(6): 551–561.

18. Royal College of Physicians. Disabling chest disease: prevention and care. A report of the Royal College of Physicians by the College Committee on Thoracic Medicine. J R Coll Physicians Lond 1981; 15(2):69–87.

19. Cockcroft A, Bagnall P, Heslop A, et al. Controlled trial of respiratory health worker visiting patients with chronic respiratory disability. BMJ 1987; 294:225–228.

20. Coultas D, Frederick J, Barnett B, et al. A randomized trial of two types of nurse-assisted home care for patients with COPD. Chest 2005; 128(4):2017–2024.

21. Smith BJ, McElroy HJ, Ruffin RE, et al. The effectiveness of coordinated care for people with chronic respiratory disease. Med J Aust 2002; 177(9):481–485.

22. Oliver SM. Living with failing lungs: the doctor-patient relationship. Fam Pract 2001; 18 (4):430–439.

23. British Lung Foundation. About Breath Easy. Availabe at: http://www.lunguk.org/supporting-you/breathe-easy/aboutbreatheeasy.htm. (Accessed November 26, 2007).

24. Clay T. Pulmonary rehabilitation in chronic respiratory insufficiency. 9. How to keep the customer satisfied. Thorax 1994; 49(3):279–280.

# 29

# Physiotherapy at Exacerbation of COPD

**RACHEL GARROD**
Faculty of Health and Social Care Sciences, St. George's, University of London and Kingston University, Tooting, U.K.

**CHRISTINE MIKELSONS**
Physiotherapy Department, Royal Free Hospital, London, U.K.

## I.  Introduction

This chapter will consider the various physiotherapy techniques that may be used with a patient during an exacerbation of chronic obstructions of pulmonary disease (COPD). Two core tenets should be understood by the therapist: central to each successful intervention is an understanding of the evidence underlying treatment and, equally, an empathy with each patient in translating theory into practice.

## II.  Positioning

COPD is associated with hyperinflation of the lungs; because of this, the inspiratory muscles are in a permanently shortened position, leading to reduced efficiency and altered mechanics of breathing. This inefficiency contributes to the dyspnea perceived by patients with COPD and is likely to be exaggerated at exacerbation. Forward lean sitting (FLS) may be advocated in order to reduce work of breathing associated with hyperinflation. In this position, patients rest their forearms on a table or such surface, allowing forward movement of abdominal contents and fixation of the shoulder girdle, which in turn facilitates accessory respiratory muscle activity and increases thoracic cage volume. Studies evaluating FLS have shown improvements in lung volume (1) and relief of dyspnea while in a stable condition (2) and during the first five days of an exacerbation (3). In addition, for patients with severe airflow limitation, maximal inspiratory pressure is enhanced in the FLS position when performed during exacerbation (3). The FLS position may provide patients with sufficient relief to enable them to rest and hence help attenuate fatigue. A COPD exacerbation is frequently associated with pneumonia and unilateral consolidation. In this situation, maximizing the ventilation/perfusion ratio is an important aim of positioning. By utilizing gravitational effects on perfusion, the lateral decubitis position with the affected lung placed uppermost, may markedly improve gas exchange (4,5). Simple techniques such as effective positioning can have significant benefits for patients and may provide a window of opportunity for other therapies to take effect.

## III.  Breathing Techniques

Dyspnea in COPD is a major symptom, and at time of an exacerbation, dyspnea is markedly increased; indeed this is one of the defining characteristics of an exacerbation (6). Breathing techniques, encompassing a wide range of treatments such as diaphragmatic breathing (DB), breathing control, pursed lips breathing, and paced breathing, may be taught during exacerbation to help relieve breathlessness and aid relaxation. DB is probably most contentious. Using mainly abdominal motion and minimal upper thoracic motion, the patient is encouraged to inhale maximally. Anecdotally, it is thought that this movement reduces the work of breathing and improves ventilation perfusion matching. However, investigation of this technique in patients with severe COPD recovering from exacerbation has shown that while DB does improve blood gases, tidal volume, and respiratory rate compared with natural breathing, this is at the expense higher work of breathing and worsening dyspnea (7). The study by Vitacca et al. (7) confirms earlier work in severe stable COPD (8). Thus DB is unlikely to be particularly helpful during an acute exacerbation; the use of breathing control however may be more suitable for these patients. Breathing control is defined as "normal tidal breathing using the lower chest with relaxation of the upper chest and shoulders; it is performed at normal tidal volume, at a natural rate and expiration should not be forced" (9). The use of breathing control in conjunction with positioning such as FLS may facilitate greater relaxation. Where anxiety contributes to breathlessness breathing control facilitates slower deeper breathing, which in turn stimulates the parasympathetic nervous system, leading to a slower heart rate. However, it has been argued that in COPD patients, heart rate variability due to vagal stimuli is altered (10). At present we know little about the effects of breathing control on dyspnea during exacerbation and randomized trials are required that measure physiological and clinically relevant outcomes. Slow, deep breathing has positive effects on tidal volume and arterial blood gases, but during an exacerbation, imposing this breathing pattern on a patient may predispose to earlier diaphragmatic fatigue (11). Variability in responses and additional problems such as anxiety, fear and hyperventilation mean that treatment is required on an individual basis, with careful monitoring throughout. The technique of pursed lips breathing (PLB) may provide symptomatic benefit when work of breathing is increased. During PLB patients inhale through the nose and exhale actively through pursed lips, this maneuver helps to prevent airway collapse. In one randomized controlled trial, the effect of using PLB during activity was compared with natural breathing during activity. Outcomes measured were respiratory rate, dyspnea, time to recovery, and distance walked (12). PLB significantly reduced time to recovery and respiratory rate but had little effect on the other outcomes. However, there is significant variation amongst patients as to whether PLB provides relief of dyspnea or not. It is likely that it is most effective for patients who have low elastic recoil pressures (13). During an exacerbation, increased hyperinflation may mean that PLB is more likely to be beneficial. A trial of the technique is warranted. Ultimately, the aim of breathing techniques in COPD is to relieve dyspnea, reduce the work of breathing, to aid relaxation and rest. Clinical examination and objective measures will identify positions and techniques of benefit to the patient. Possibly, PLB is most suitable for patients with severe COPD and hyperinflation, whereas controlled breathing suitable for those with mild-to-moderate COPD; how things differ during exacerbation is unknown. Often patients are well aware of what helps them and may simply need support to achieve this.

## IV. Early Pulmonary Rehabilitation

During acute exacerbation and hospitalization for COPD performance of weight bearing activities are at a minimum, and the amount of walking a patient takes is strongly correlated with quadriceps muscle strength (14). Quadriceps weakness and low levels of physical activity are important predictors of hospital readmission (15) and utilization of health resources (16). Maintenance of physical fitness and peripheral muscle strength is therefore of primary importance during exacerbation and hospitalization. A simple inpatient rehabilitation program provided within eight days of an exacerbation has shown promising results (17). In this study, COPD patients were randomized to five daily-supervised walking sessions or usual care for 11 days. Improvements in walking distance were significantly greater in the active group compared with the control. However, not all health care providers have facilities for inpatient rehabilitation and outpatient programs may be more applicable. One such community program delivered within 10 days of discharge from hospital has demonstrated significant improvements in exercise tolerance and quality of life for patients with COPD (18). Importantly emergency visits were significantly reduced as a result of the early intervention and although only a trend, hospital admissions were down. What was striking about this study however, was the evidence that if no early intervention is provided after discharge, exercise tolerance further deteriorates. This downward spiral can only contribute to additional risk of hospitalization, muscle weakness, and mortality (19). This community delivered rehabilitation program was not unusual in the intensity, duration, and frequency of training delivered. Both rehabilitation programmes were well tolerated by patients and the research supports the premise that rehabilitative physiotherapy should be an essential component of follow-up for COPD patients after exacerbation.

## V. Early Rehabilitation of Intubated Patients with COPD

When the severity of the exacerbation is sufficient to warrant mechanical ventilation, other strategies may be employed to maximize physical function. Early mobilization remains the treatment of choice, although where impaired airway clearance problems contribute to morbidity, these should be treated as described below. In a comprehensive publication from Stiller and Phillips (20), guidelines are presented, outlining safety aspects to consider in the mobilization of critically ill patients. Physiotherapists need to make assessment of respiratory and cardiac reserve before deciding on the level of activity suitable for the patient. Where patients are stable, providing therapy that focuses on aerobic and muscular fitness appears to have beneficial effects. In one recent study, COPD patients who required mechanical ventilation for more than 14 days were randomized to usual care (without physiotherapy) or usual care plus a six-week program of strength training aimed at the upper and lower limbs, abdominal breathing exercises, and functional activities that included mobilization as able (21). There were impressive improvements in functional independence in the physiotherapy group compared with control, these were evident at three weeks and further increased by six weeks. Almost half of the control patients were able to mobilize with assistance by the end of the program, with a mean walking distance of 43 m. None in the control group were walking and functional status had deteriorated in these patients. While this study points the way forward for additional therapies in critical care, a comparison of mobilization therapy with or without additional limb training is warranted. Care must be taken when implementing these programmes with consideration of acute inflammatory responses. In healthy subjects, exercise is associated with increased inflammatory mediators; however, with longer-term training this acute response is attenuated (22). Early data have indicated that physical training in COPD may be associated with heightened cytokine response, in particular, TNF-α (tumor necrosis factor-alpha) (23); but more recent data refute this (24), and it may be hypothesized that rehabilitation itself provides anti-inflammatory benefits (25). Certainly strength training appears encouraging: one evaluation of transcutaneous electrical stimulation (TENS) applied in conjunction with active limb exercises resulted in greater muscle strength change compared with active exercise alone (26). These patients were severely acutely unwell; however, not only were no adverse events reported but patients in the TENS group were also able to perform independent transfer from bed to chair more quickly than the exercise-only control group. These data concerning rehabilitation for critically ill COPD patients support the need for greater physiotherapy input at the acute stage of COPD.

## VI.  Airway Clearance Therapies

Airway clearance may be impaired in some, but not all, patients with acute exacerbations of COPD, and in these patients airway clearance therapies may include chest physiotherapy (CP) [defined as percussion, postural drainage (PD) and vibration], active cycle of breathing techniques (ACBT), forced expiration technique (FET), autogenic drainage (AD), or devices delivering positive expiratory pressure, discussed in more detail below. A review of the literature concerning the use of these techniques identifies the difficulties in drawing conclusions about effectiveness because of lack of research, weaknesses in methodology, and differences in the international usage of the terminology. This calls for greater research in evaluating treatment techniques and clearer descriptions in the international literature of what is meant by the terminology used.

The efficacy of CP, other than in the cystic fibrosis (CF) group, has not been well studied, and guidelines suggest there is insufficient evidence to recommend its use other than in patients with CF (27). ACBT involves the use of repetitions of five to six thoracic expansion exercises, interspersed with breathing control followed by FET, and can be successfully performed independently by the patient in modified PD positions or sitting (28). AD consists of controlled expiratory airflow during tidal breathing to move secretions from the peripheral to the central airways, in three phases called "unstick," "collecting" and "evacuating" (29,30). Evidence supports the use of ACBT and AD in aiding sputum clearance in COPD and demonstrates their equal effectiveness in terms of improvements in lung function (31). While these techniques have shown both statistical and clinical improvements in pulmonary function, arterial blood gases, exercise tolerance, and dyspnea scores, some differences have been noted between the techniques: those using AD have demonstrated greater improvement in PEFR and $PaCO_2$ and those using ACBT, in $SaO_2$ (32). It remains unclear whether there is a significant clinical difference between the uses of the two techniques. FET has been shown to be effective in sputum clearance in COPD (33), with FET and PD being more effective than cough alone (34), but FET with PD was not found to be more effective than PD with cough (35). Key points in deciding which treatment techniques to use are an accurate assessment of the patient, identification of sputum clearance as a clear goal of treatment, concordance of the patient with the intervention, ease of performance of the technique, and the requirement of help from an assistant. Regimes for airway clearance regarding frequency and length of treatments will depend on the clinical presentation of each patient and treatments should be modified according to their condition.

A variety of devices delivering positive expiratory pressure are available to aid sputum clearance and include the PEP mask (Astra Meditec Ltd., Glouscester, U.K.) Flutter® (Scandipharm Intl., Powys, U.K.) Cornet (Pari Respiratory Equipment, Midlothian, Virginia, U.S.) or Acapella™ (Smiths Medical, Kent, U.K.). In addition, some of these devices also incorporate an oscillatory element, providing expiratory vibration (e.g., Flutter, Cornet, Acapella), which aids sputum movement into larger airways. These devices have been shown to be as effective when compared with conventional CP (PD, percussion, chest shaking, huffing, and directed coughing) with no clear difference in benefit between the devices demonstrated (31,36,37). While much of the evidence relates to the use of PEP devices in CF, Bellone and colleagues (36) found significant improvements in sputum removal in a small group of COPD patients using the Flutter during an acute exacerbation compared with PD during the first hour after treatment. Patients' preference may be a key feature in deciding on the use of such devices, where convenience in performing sputum clearance may be of prime importance (31).

The use of intermittent positive pressure breathing (IPPB) was shown in early studies to increase tidal volume in acute respiratory failure (38) and decrease the work of breathing (39). Its use has largely been replaced by the advent of more sophisticated noninvasive ventilators, the use of which is well supported in the literature in the treatment of acute exacerbations of COPD (40). Nevertheless, the use of IPPB may be of benefit in selected patients with exacerbations of COPD, who have retained secretions that they are unable to clear independently because of fatigue or increased work of breathing (41). An alternative, such as the mechanical insufflator/exsufflator, which applies high pressures (20–30 $H_2O$) followed by rapid reversal of pressure (–30—40 $H_2O$), is thought to be useful for patients with sputum retention as a result of neuromuscular disease but is not recommended for use in COPD. In a study comparing manually assisted cough with manually assisted cough and mechanical insufflation/exsufflation in patients with COPD, it was found that both produced detrimental falls in peak expiratory flow rate (42).

Other techniques such as intrapulmonary percussive ventilation (delivery of pneumatic, oscillating pressures via a jet venture) and high frequency chest wall oscillation (an inflatable jacket attached by hoses to a airflow generator producing pressures of $50cmH_2O$ of 5–25 Hz) have been investigated for use in CF patients and have not been extensively tested in the COPD group to date.

The evidence relating to inspiratory muscle training (IMT) demonstrates improvements in inspiratory muscle weakness, dyspnea, exercise tolerance, quality of life in patients with COPD (43,44). In addition, IMT may have a role in airway clearance in patients with an exacerbation of COPD and sputum retention, as Chatham et al. found that the use of resistive inspiratory maneuvers increased sputum production in patients with CF when compared with the use of ACBT (45).

The various physiotherapy techniques that can be used in an exacerbation of COPD have been described. In translating theory into practice, care should be taken to individualize therapy in a spirit of concordance, ensuring that the patient lies at the center of care.

## References

1. Barach AL. Chronic obstructive lung disease: postural relief of dyspnoea. Arch Phys Med Rehabil 1974; 55(11):494–504.
2. Sharp JT, Druz WS, Moisan T, et al. Postural relief of dyspnoea in severe chronic obstructive pulmonary disease. Am Rev Respir Dis 1980;122:201–211.
3. O'Neill S, McCarthy DS. Postural relief of dyspnoea in severe chronic airflow limitation: relationship to respiratory muscle strength. Thorax 1983; 38(8):595–600.
4. Dreyfuss D, Djedaini K, Lanore J, et al. A comparative study of the effects of almitrine bis-mesylate and lateral position during unilateral bacterial pneumonia with severe hypoxemia. Am Rev Respir Dis 1992; 146(2):295–299.
5. Remolina CK. Positional hypoxemia in unilateral lung disease. N Engl J Med 1981; 304(9): 523–525.
6. Global Initiative for Chronic Obstructive Lung Disease (GOLD). Global Strategy for the Diagnosis, Management and Prevention of COPD, 2006. National Institutes of Health, National Heart, Lung, and Blood Institute. Available at: http://www.goldcopd.org.
7. Vitacca M, Clini E, Bianchi L, et al. Acute effects of deep diaphragmatic breathing in COPD patients with chronic respiratory insufficiency. Eur Respir J 1998; 11(2):408–415.
8. Gosselink RA, Wagenaar RC, Rijswijk H, et al. Diaphragmatic breathing reduces efficiency of breathing in patients with chronic obstructive pulmonary disease. Am J Respir Crit Care Med 1995; 151(4):1136–1142.
9. Pryor JA, Webber BA. Physiotherapy techniques. In: Pryor JA, Prasad A, eds. Physiotherapy for Respiratory and Cardiac Problems. 3rd ed. Edinburgh, U.K.: Churchill Livingstone, 2002:182.
10. Volterrani M, Scalvini S, Mazzuero G, et al. Decreased heart rate variability in patients with chronic obstructive pulmonary disease. Chest 1994; 106(5):1432–1437.
11. Bellemare F, Grassino A. Force reserve of the diaphragm in patients with chronic obstructive pulmonary disease. J Appl Physiol 1983; 55(1 pt 1):8–15.
12. Garrod R, Dallimore K, Cook J, et al. An evaluation of the acute impact of pursed lips breathing on walking distance in nonspontaneous pursed lips breathing chronic obstructive pulmonary disease patients. Chron Respir Dis 2005; 2(2):67–72.
13. Ingram RH, Schilder DP. Effect of pursed lips expiration on the pulmonary pressure-flow relationship in obstructive lung disease. Am Rev Respir Dis 1967; 96(3): 381–388.
14. Pitta F, Troosters T, Probst VS, et al. Physical activity and hospitalization for exacerbation of COPD. Chest 2006; 129(3):536–544.
15. Garcia-Aymerich J, Farrero E, Felez MA, et al. Risk factors of readmission to hospital for a COPD exacerbation: a prospective study. Thorax 2003; 58(2):100–105.
16. Decramer M, Gosselink R, Troosters T, et al. Muscle weakness is related to utilization of health care resources in COPD patients. Eur Respir J 1997; 10(2):417–423.
17. Kirsten DK, Taube C, Lehnigk B, et al. Exercise training improves recovery in patients with COPD after an acute exacerbation. Respir Med 1998; 92(10):1191–1198.
18. Man WD, Polkey MI, Donaldson N, et al. Community pulmonary rehabilitation after hospital-isation for acute exacerbations of chronic obstructive pulmonary disease: randomised controlled study. BMJ 2004; 329(7476):1209.
19. Swallow EB, Reyes D, Hopkinson NS, et al. Quadriceps strength predicts mortality in patients with moderate to severe chronic obstructive pulmonary disease. Thorax 2007; 62(2):115–120.
20. Stiller K, Phillips A. Safety aspects of mobilising acutely ill inpatients. Physiother Theory Pract 2003; 19(4):239–257.
21. Chiang LL, Wang LY, Wu CP, et al. Effects of physical training on functional status in patients with prolonged mechanical ventilation. Phys Ther 2006; 86(9):1271–1281.
22. Petersen AM, Pedersen BK. The anti-inflammatory effect of exercise. J Appl Physiol 2005; 98(4):1154–1162.
23. Rabinovich RA, Figueras M, Ardite E, et al. Increased tumour necrosis factor-alpha plasma levels during moderate-intensity exercise in COPD patients. Eur Respir J 2003; 21(5):789–794.

24. Canavan J, Garrod R, Marshall J, et al. Measurement of the acute inflammatory response to walking exercise in COPD: effects of pulmonary rehabilitation. Int J Chron Obstruct Pulmon Dis 2007; 2(3):347–353.
25. Garrod R, Ansley P, Canavan J, et al. Exercise and the inflammatory response in chronic obstructive pulmonary disease (COPD)-Does training confer anti-inflammatory properties in COPD? Med Hypotheses 2007; 68(2):291–298.
26. Zanotti E, Felicetti G, Maini M, et al. Peripheral muscle strength training in bed-bound patients with COPD receiving mechanical ventilation: effect of electrical stimulation. Chest 2003; 124(1): 292–296.
27. McCool FD, Rosen MJ. Non-pharmacologic airway clearance therapies: ACCP evidence-based clinical practice guideline. Chest 2006; 129:S250–S259.
28. Webber BA. The active cycle of breathing exercises. Cystic Fibrosis News. August/September 1990:10–11.
29. Chevaillier J. Autogenic drainage. In: Lawson D, ed. Cystic Fibrosis: Horizons. London: Churchill Livingstone, 1984:65–78.
30. Miller S, Hall DO, Clayton CB, et al. Chest physiotherapy in cystic fibrosis: a comparative study of autogenic drainage and the active cycle of breathing techniques with postural drainage. Thorax 1995; 50:165–169.
31. Hess DR. The evidence for secretion clearance techniques. Cardiopulmon Phys Ther 2002; 13:7–22.
32. Savci S, Ince DI, Arikan H. A comparison of autogenic drainage and the active cycle of breathing techniques in patients with chronic obstructive pulmonary diseases. J Cardiopulm Rehabil 2000; 20:37–43.
33. van der Schans CP, Goldstein RS, Bach JR. Airway secretion management and oxygen therapy. Phys Med Rehabil Clin N Am 1996; 7:277–298.
34. Clarke SW. Management of mucus hypersecretion. Eur J Respir Dis Suppl 1987; 153:136–144.
35. Van Hengstrum M, Festen J, Beurskens C, et al. The effect of positive expiratory pressure versus forced expiration technique on tracheobronhial clearance in chronic bronchitis. Scand J Gastroenterol Suppl 1988; 143:114–118.
36. Bellone A, Lascioli R, Raschi S, et al. Chest physical therapy in patients with acute exacerbation of chronic bronchitis: effectiveness of three methods. Arch Phys Med Rehabil 2000; 81:558–560.
37. Main E, Prasad A, van der Schans. Conventional chest physiotherapy compared to other airway clearance techniques for cystic fibrosis. Cochrane Database Syst Rev 2005; CD002011.
38. Sukumalchantra Y, Park SS, Williams MH. The effect of intermittent positive pressure breathing in acute ventilatory failure. Am Rev Respir Dis 1965; 92:885–893.
39. Ayres SM, Kozam RL, Lukas DS. The effects of intermittent positive pressure breathing on intrathoracic pressure, pulmonary mechanics and work of breathing. Am Rev Respir Dis 1963; 87:370–379.
40. Ram FSF, Lightowler JV, Wedzicha JA. Non-invasive ventilation for treatment of respiratory failure due to exacerbations of chronic pulmonary disease. Cochrane Database Syst Rev 2003; (1):CD004104 [Update in Cochrane Database Syst Rev 2004; 3:CD004104].Issue
41. Pavia D, Webber B, Agnew JE, et al. The role of intermittent positive pressure breathing (IPPB) in bronchial toilet. Eur Respir J 1998; (1 suppl 2):250S.
42. Sivasothy P, Brown L, Smith IE, et al. Effect of manually assisted cough and mechanical insufflation on cough flow of normal subjects, patients with chronic obstructive pulmonary disease (COPD) and patients with respiratory muscle weakness. Thorax 2001; 56:438–444.
43. Beckerman M, Magadle R, Weiner M, et al. The effects of 1 year of specific inspiratory muscle training in patients with COPD. Chest 2005; 128:3177–3182.
44. Sanchez-Riera H, Montemayor RT, Ortega RF, et al. Inspiratory muscle training in patients with COPD: effect on dyspnoea, exercise performance, and quality of life. Chest 2001; 120:748–756.
45. Chatham K, Ionescu AA, Nixon LS, et al. A short- term comparison of two methods of sputum expectoration in cystic fibrosis. Eur Respir J 2004; 23:435–439.

# 30
## COPD Exacerbation and Pulmonary Rehabilitation

**WILLIAM D-C. MAN and MICHAEL I. POLKEY**
Respiratory Muscle Laboratory, Royal Brompton Hospital, London, U.K.

## I. Introduction

There has been growing realization that chronic obstructive pulmonary disease (COPD) severity and prognosis are determined only partially by lung function impairment; indeed once forced expiratory volume ($FEV_1$) is less than 50% predicted, it yields no prognostic value (1). This may explain the limited benefits of pulmonary pharmacological therapies and the rapidly expanding interest in therapies designed to treat the systemic consequences of COPD. Despite initial skepticism that COPD patients (with their pulmonary impairment) could achieve exercise levels necessary to produce a true physiological training effect (2), pulmonary rehabilitation (PR) has emerged as arguably the most effective non-pharmacological intervention in improving exercise capacity and health status in COPD patients, supported by a number of randomized-controlled trials and meta-analyses (3). However, the health-economic consequences of PR and its effects on acute exacerbation rate are less well established. Furthermore, most data have been obtained in stable chronic patients (free from recent exacerbation), and only in recent times have investigators begun studying the role of PR in the multidisciplinary management of the COPD patient with acute exacerbation.

## II. PR in the Prevention of Acute Exacerbations

PR is a multidisciplinary program of care for patients with chronic respiratory impairment that is designed to maximize each patient's physical and social performance, reduce symptoms, and restore autonomy. In general, PR consists of individually tailored exercise training and multidisciplinary education sessions that focus on psychosocial and lifestyle issues, with a particular emphasis on self-management. Many randomized controlled trials (and meta-analyses) have demonstrated clinically and statistically significant improvements in exercise capacity and health-related quality of life in COPD patients following PR (3–5). Although exacerbations and subsequent hospital admission comprise a significant proportion of healthcare costs in COPD (6), previous randomized controlled PR studies have generally not focused on exacerbation rate as a primary outcome. Consequently, data on healthcare resource usage and health economics, although present, are relatively sparse.

However, this bias may change in the future, as there is a growing realization that reduced usual physical activity is a major risk factor for hospital readmission (7). Furthermore, there is some evidence that exacerbation rate may influence decline in $FEV_1$ (8), and if PR indeed reduces exacerbation frequency, there is the intriguing prospect that PR could influence disease progression.

Several studies have suggested a reduction in exacerbation rate, hospitalization, and hospital days following PR when applied to stable patients. Guell and colleagues demonstrated that compared with a control group, a year-long PR program for stable patients significantly reduced exacerbation frequency from 6.9 to 3.7 exacerbations per patient over a 24-month period. However, the study was inadequately powered to show a statistically significant reduction in hospitalizations (9). In a randomized controlled trial of home PR in elderly housebound COPD patients, there was no reduction in the number of hospital admissions due to exacerbation, but there was a significant reduction in average length of stay (5.9 vs. 9.3 days) (10). Hui and Hewitt demonstrated a reduction in both number of hospital admissions for COPD exacerbations and mean length of stay in the 12 months following the completion a PR program, compared with the 12 months preceding the rehabilitation (11). Similarly, Stewart and colleagues showed a reduction in hospital days following PR (12), whilst Young and colleagues demonstrated a reduction in hospital admissions and courses of oral corticosteroids (13). These latter three studies reflect the findings of the original descriptions of PR (14,15), but like them, were uncontrolled studies. In a well-conducted randomized controlled study of outpatient PR, Griffiths and colleagues demonstrated fewer days spent in hospital and reduced frequency of admissions, but no reduction in number of patients needing to be admitted (4). Interestingly, this study also showed an increased number of consultations at primary care premises, but a reduced number of home visits by primary care physicians in the intervention group compared with the controls. The authors interpreted this as a more efficient use of primary care, which reflected either increased fitness of the intervention group or a change in behavior and attitude to their illness.

Not all studies have demonstrated similar reductions in hospitalizations. A Swedish randomized controlled study of a 12-month outpatient exercise program showed no reduction in hospital days despite improvement in exercise capacity (16). Interestingly, this study is one of the few in the PR literature that does not show improvements in health-related quality of life. Ries and colleagues also demonstrated significant improvements in exercise capacity, but no changes in health-related quality of life or hospital days (17), suggesting a link between these latter outcome measures, but not between exercise capacity and exacerbation rate. Presumably, improved self-management skills and better knowledge of the disease are responsible. This is supported by a recent randomized controlled trial that showed an outpatient program, consisting predominantly of self-management with an assigned case manager could reduce hospital admissions by 39.8% and unscheduled emergency department visits by 41% (18).

## III.   PR in the Treatment of Acute Exacerbations

Most of the data in the PR literature is based on stable patients with COPD who have been free from exacerbation for a defined period of time, usually several weeks. This is principally due to concerns that immediately following an exacerbation, COPD patients are unable to achieve or sustain sufficiently high exercise levels to produce a true physiological training effect. Furthermore, it is well recognized that a catabolic state exists during an exacerbation (19), and it is unknown whether the increased activity levels associated with PR could aggravate this process, or perhaps overtax already fatiguing muscles. Despite these concerns, investigators have recently studied the role of PR at the time of or shortly after an acute exacerbation with promising results.

There are several hypothetical reasons why PR may be useful at the time of an exacerbation. Exercise capacity is severely compromised, and activity levels are markedly reduced during and shortly after an exacerbation. This has been confirmed objectively by using activity monitors (20), as well as by self-reported diaries (21). This latter study also demonstrated that patients with frequent exacerbations were more likely to be house bound, and hence particularly likely to benefit from PR (21). The decline in activity levels associated with an exacerbation also contributes to significant skeletal muscle dysfunction, particularly of locomotor muscles such as the quadriceps (20). Although stable patients with COPD are well known to have quadriceps weakness (22), Spruit and colleagues demonstrated a further decline in quadriceps peak torque between days 3 and 8 of a hospital admission for an acute COPD exacerbation (23). Quadriceps strength showed only partial recovery by three months. Aside from the physical ramifications, patients also describe psychological distress and substantial decline in health-related quality of life associated with an exacerbation (24,25).

Given the proven benefits of PR in improving exercise capacity, activity level, skeletal muscle function, and health-related quality of life in the stable patient, it is surprising that investigators have only recently commenced studying systematically the effects of PR after acute exacerbation. With concerns about exercising patients recovering from an acute severe illness, early reports have focused on supervised in-patient rehabilitation. In a retrospective analysis, Make and colleagues demonstrated the feasibility of rehabilitating ventilator-dependent patients to functional independence (26), although the timing of rehabilitation was long after the initial illness that necessitated intubation and ventilation. Foster et al. showed that hypercapnic COPD patients benefited from an inpatient rehabilitation program with improvements in exercise capacity, lung function, and arterial blood gases (27). However, this study was neither randomized nor controlled. In a randomized controlled study of COPD patients admitted to a respiratory intensive care unit, a four-step inpatient rehabilitation program of increasing intensity, started within three to five days after admission, led to improvements in six-minute walking distance and breathlessness as measured by visual analogue scores (28). Similarly, Kirsten and colleagues demonstrated that a 10-day inpatient rehabilitation program (consisting of endurance walking exercise), commenced within four to seven days after admission, significantly improved exercise capacity and breathlessness (29). However, the follow-up period was limited only to the end of the rehabilitation program (i.e. day 11). The same group of investigators followed their initial in-patient rehabilitation program with firstly a six-month and then an 18-month largely unsupervised home-based training period following hospital discharge (30,31). Although exercise capacity at the end of the follow-up periods remained significantly better than at baseline, almost all the improvement occurred during the initial 10-day in-patient rehabilitation.

Inpatient rehabilitation is unfortunately not a viable option in many healthcare systems, where inpatient costs make up the majority of COPD expenditure and current ethos is to discharge safely to the community as soon as possible. With this in mind, Murphy and colleagues investigated the benefits of supervised home-exercise training as an extension to a hospital-at-home care program (32). Although there were only 12 training sessions in all, the investigators demonstrated an impressive 106-metre improvement in incremental shuttle walk in the intervention group, as well as improvements in health-related quality of life, as measured by the St. George's Respiratory Questionnaire and EuroQol-5D (32). However, between-group statistical comparisons were not documented.

Outpatient-based programs are a pragmatic solution to providing sufficient PR for the large number of COPD patients recovering from exacerbations. In a pilot study, Man and colleagues randomized 42 hospitalized patients to either usual medical care or community PR (at a choice of three locations in southeast London) within 10 days of hospital discharge (33). The program was similar at all three locations, run by the same multidisciplinary team and consisted of two supervised sessions per week for eight weeks, as well as an individualized home exercise program. At three months, they demonstrated clinically and statistically significant improvements in shuttle walk test, St. George's Respiratory Questionnaire Total Score, all four domains of the Chromic Respiratory Disease Questionnaire and the mental component score of the Short Form-36 (33) in the intervention group compared with controls. Secondary outcomes analysis also showed a significantly reduced number of unscheduled "Accident & Emergency" visits, and a 30% reduction in hospital admissions, although the trial was underpowered to demonstrate a statistical significance in this regard. Another trial of outpatient respiratory rehabilitation (lasting 6 months), which has been published in abstract form, showed similar improvements in exercise capacity, but also demonstrated reduced mortality in the intervention group at four years following rehabilitation (34). This corroborates the observation that adverse events have not been reported with PR shortly after an exacerbation (30,33), suggesting that exercise training is safe in this vulnerable group of patients.

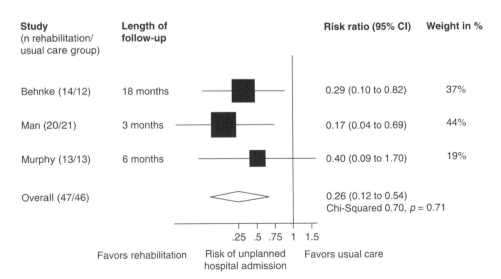

**Figure 1**  Effects of respiratory rehabilitation on unplanned hospital readmissions. Boxes with 95% confidence intervals represent point estimates for the risk ratio. *Source*: From Ref. 35.

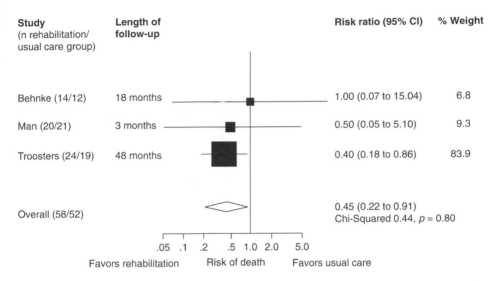

**Figure 2** Effects of respiratory rehabilitation on mortality. Boxes with 95% confidence intervals represent point estimates for the risk ratio. *Source*: From Ref. 35.

The existing research on PR in the acute exacerbation setting is promising, but most of the studies have consisted of small numbers of patients, and have been underpowered to look at health resource usage. Recently, Puhan and colleagues conducted a systematic review of existing clinical trials studying respiratory rehabilitation in COPD patients, following acute exacerbations (35). As well as showing the expected improvements in exercise capacity and health-related quality of life, this meta-analysis also demonstrated significantly reduced hospital readmissions and mortality (Figs. 1 and 2), suggesting that future larger trials should show a reduction in health costs.

## IV. Summary

Although PR is undoubtedly an effective intervention in COPD, data from well-conducted randomized controlled studies supporting its effects in reducing acute exacerbations in stable disease remain sparse and debatable. However, recent evidence suggests that PR that shortly follows an acute exacerbation is highly beneficial and should be considered an integral part of the multidisciplinary management of the postexacerbation recovery period.

### References

1. Swallow EB, Reyes D, Hopkinson NS, et al. Quadriceps strength predicts mortality in patients with moderate to severe chronic obstructive pulmonary disease. Thorax 2007; 62(2):115–120.
2. Belman MJ, Kendregan BA. Exercise training fails to increase skeletal muscle enzymes in patients with chronic obstructive pulmonary disease. Am Rev Respir Dis 1981; 123(3):256–261.

3. Lacasse Y, Brosseau L, Milne S, et al. Pulmonary rehabilitation for chronic obstructive pulmonary disease. Cochrane Database Syst Rev 2002; (3):CD003793.

4. Griffiths TL, Burr ML, Campbell IA, et al. Results at 1 year of outpatient multidisciplinary pulmonary rehabilitation: a randomised controlled trial. Lancet 2000; 355(9201):362–368.

5. Lacasse Y, Wong E, Guyatt GH, et al. Meta-analysis of respiratory rehabilitation in chronic obstructive pulmonary disease. Lancet 1996; 348(9035):1115–1119.

6. Britton M. The burden of COPD in the U.K.: results from the confronting COPD survey. Respir Med 2003; 97(suppl C):S71–S79.

7. Garcia-Aymerich J, Farrero E, Felez MA, et al. Risk factors of readmission to hospital for a COPD exacerbation: a prospective study. Thorax 2003; 58(2):100–105.

8. Donaldson GC, Seemungal TA, Bhowmik A, et al. Relationship between exacerbation frequency and lung function decline in chronic obstructive pulmonary disease. Thorax 2002; 57(10): 847–852.

9. Guell R, Casan P, Belda J, et al. Long-term effects of outpatient rehabilitation of COPD: A randomized trial. Chest 2000; 117(4):976–983.

10. Boxall AM, Barclay L, Sayers A, et al. Managing chronic obstructive pulmonary disease in the community. A randomized controlled trial of home-based pulmonary rehabilitation for elderly housebound patients. J Cardiopulm Rehabil 2005; 25(6):378–385.

11. Hui KP, Hewitt AB. A simple pulmonary rehabilitation program improves health outcomes and reduces hospital utilization in patients with COPD. Chest 2003; 124(1):94–97.

12. Stewart DG, Drake DF, Robertson C, et al. Benefits of an inpatient pulmonary rehabilitation program: a prospective analysis. Arch Phys Med Rehabil 2001; 82(3):347–352.

13. Young P, Dewse M, Fergusson W, et al. Improvements in outcomes for chronic obstructive pulmonary disease (COPD) attributable to a hospital-based respiratory rehabilitation programme. Aust N Z J Med 1999; 29(1):59–65.

14. Petty TL, Nett LM, Finigan MM, et al. A comprehensive care program for chronic airway obstruction. Methods and preliminary evaluation of symptomatic and functional improvement. Ann Intern Med 1969; 70(6):1109–1120.

15. Lertzman MM, Cherniack RM. Rehabilitation of patients with chronic obstructive pulmonary disease. Am Rev Respir Dis 1976; 114(6):1145–1165.

16. Engstrom CP, Persson LO, Larsson S, et al. Long-term effects of a pulmonary rehabilitation programme in outpatients with chronic obstructive pulmonary disease: a randomized controlled study. Scand J Rehabil Med 1999; 31(4):207–213.

17. Ries AL, Kaplan RM, Limberg TM, et al. Effects of pulmonary rehabilitation on physiologic and psychosocial outcomes in patients with chronic obstructive pulmonary disease. Ann Intern Med 1995; 122(11):823–832.

18. Bourbeau J, Julien M, Maltais F, et al. Reduction of hospital utilization in patients with chronic obstructive pulmonary disease: a disease-specific self-management intervention. Arch Intern Med 2003; 163(5):585–591.

19. Vermeeren MA, Schols AM, Wouters EF. Effects of an acute exacerbation on nutritional and metabolic profile of patients with COPD. Eur Respir J 1997; 10(10):2264–2269.

20. Pitta F, Troosters T, Probst VS, et al. Physical activity and hospitalization for exacerbation of COPD. Chest 2006; 129(3):536–544.

21. Donaldson GC, Wilkinson TM, Hurst JR, et al. Exacerbations and time spent outdoors in chronic obstructive pulmonary disease. Am J Respir Crit Care Med 2005; 171(5):446–452.

22. Man WD, Soliman MG, Nikoletou D, et al. Non-volitional assessment of skeletal muscle strength in patients with chronic obstructive pulmonary disease. Thorax 2003; 58(8):665–669.

23. Spruit MA, Gosselink R, Troosters T, et al. Muscle force during an acute exacerbation in hospitalised patients with COPD and its relationship with CXCL8 and IGF-I. Thorax 2003; 58(9): 752–756.

24. Kessler R, Stahl E, Vogelmeier C, et al. Patient understanding, detection, and experience of COPD exacerbations: an observational, interview-based study. Chest 2006; 130(1):133–142.
25. Schmier JK, Halpern MT, Higashi MK, et al. The quality of life impact of acute exacerbations of chronic bronchitis (AECB): a literature review. Qual Life Res 2005; 14(2):329–347.
26. Make B, Gilmartin M, Brody JS, et al. Rehabilitation of ventilator-dependent subjects with lung diseases. The concept and initial experience. Chest 1984; 86(3):358–365.
27. Foster S, Lopez D, Thomas HM, 3rd. Pulmonary rehabilitation in COPD patients with elevated PCO2. Am Rev Respir Dis 1988; 138(6):1519–1523.
28. Nava S. Rehabilitation of patients admitted to a respiratory intensive care unit. Arch Phys Med Rehabil 1998; 79(7):849–854.
29. Kirsten DK, Taube C, Lehnigk B, et al. Exercise training improves recovery in patients with COPD after an acute exacerbation. Respir Med 1998; 92(10):1191–1198.
30. Behnke M, Taube C, Kirsten D, et al. Home-based exercise is capable of preserving hospital-based improvements in severe chronic obstructive pulmonary disease. Respir Med 2000; 94(12): 1184–1191.
31. Behnke M, Jorres RA, Kirsten D, et al. Clinical benefits of a combined hospital and home-based exercise programme over 18 months in patients with severe COPD. Monaldi Arch Chest Dis 2003; 59(1):44–51.
32. Murphy N, Bell C, Costello RW. Extending a home from hospital care programme for COPD exacerbations to include pulmonary rehabilitation. Respir Med 2005; 99(10):1297–1302.
33. Man WD, Polkey MI, Donaldson N, et al. Community pulmonary rehabilitation after hospitalisation for acute exacerbations of chronic obstructive pulmonary disease: randomised controlled study. BMJ 2004; 329(7476):1209.
34. Troosters T, Gosselink R, De Paepe K. Pulmonary rehabilitation improves survival in COPD patients with a recent severe acute exacerbation. Am J Respir Crit Care Med 2002; 165:A16.
35. Puhan MA, Scharplatz M, Troosters T, et al. Respiratory rehabilitation after acute exacerbation of COPD may reduce risk for readmission and mortality: a systematic review. Respir Res 2005; 6:54.

# 31
## Pharmacological Prevention of COPD Exacerbations

**BIANCA BEGHÉ, FABRIZIO LUPPI, and LEONARDO M. FABBRI**
Section of Respiratory Diseases, Department of Oncology, Haematology and Respiratory Diseases,
University Hospital of Modena, University of Modena and Reggio Emilia, Modena, Italy

## I.  Introduction

Exacerbations of chronic obstructive pulmonary disease (COPD) are characterized by changes in the patient's baseline dyspnea, cough, and/or sputum that are beyond normal day-to-day variations, that are acute in onset, and that may warrant a change in regular medication (1). The frequency and severity of exacerbations increase with disease severity and are associated with poorer quality of life and health outcomes, with a greater burden on health care (2), accelerated decline of lung function (3), and increased risk of death. For all these reasons, exacerbations are a major target of prevention and treatment in patients with COPD (1).

While exacerbations are increasingly used as primary outcome or secondary pre-specified outcome in clinical trials in COPD, major limitations of the studies on COPD exacerbations are that the definition is based on symptoms and not on objective measurements. Furthermore, the definition varies between studies, and often comorbidities are not adequately taken into account. Worsening of daily respiratory symptoms, particularly dyspnea, could be associated with respiratory events such as pneumonia, or nonrespiratory events such as heart failure, thromboembolism, and renal failure, among others (4).

Long-acting bronchodilators alone or in combination with inhaled glucocorticosteroids are the most effective treatment for reducing the number and severity of COPD exacerbations—even though caution is required in interpreting the results of some trials. Suissa and coworkers, in their recent papers on methodological issues (5–7), suggest that the results of major, randomized controlled clinical trials that evaluate the effect of treatment on COPD exacerbations might be biased by the facts that many patients enrolled in the studies are already receiving inhaled therapy before randomization and that the results could be influenced by withdrawal from the ongoing effective therapy. Another bias might be that patients included in the trials are often not followed after discontinuation of treatment; considering the different rates of withdrawal between treatments and the different causes of withdrawal, this may severely affect the interpretation of the data (7). Statistical methods are also critical. A statistical approach that does not weigh the length of the follow-up (unweighted approach), and for the within- and between-subject variability of exacerbations, may lead to false-positive results. In particular, this bias applies to all but two trials (8,9) examining the effect of inhaled glucocorticosteroids on exacerbations, causing the authors of those studies to conclude that the positive effect of inhaled gluco-corticosteroids on exacerbations is not supported by solid evidence. With these limitations, however, randomized controlled trials are and will remain the fundamental tools for evaluating the benefit of COPD treatment, and the data collected so far, although with the potential biases, are the only evidence available to support treatment recommendations (7).

In this chapter, we review the various classes of medications commonly used in treating COPD. We focus on the most effective medications for preventing exacerbations, such as inhaled long-acting bronchodilators alone or in combination with inhaled gluco-corticosteroids. Also, considering their importance in the management of COPD, we briefly discuss the effects of smoking cessation and vaccinations on COPD exacerbations. We do not discuss the effects of treatment of exacerbations on subsequent exacerbations—obviously an important clinical aspect. In fact, short-term therapy with oral glucocorticosteroids after hospitalization for a COPD exacerbation reduces the likelihood of readmission for another exacerbation (10).

## II.  Smoking Cessation

Smoking cessation is the single most effective intervention for reducing the progression and mortality of COPD (11). Smoking cessation may also reduce use of health resources, whether related or unrelated to management of acute exacerbations (12,13). However, no randomized clinical trial has been performed to assess the effect of smoking cessation (induced with educational intervention and/or pharmacological support) on COPD exacerbations. While studies are urgently required in this important area, all guidelines strongly recommend cessation to smokers in general and to smokers with COPD in particular (1,14,15).

## III.  Vaccines

Influenza vaccination reduces morbidity, hospitalization, and mortality in the general population, particularly in the elderly (16). However, a recent meta-analysis (17) was unable to confirm the role of influenza vaccination in preventing COPD exacerbations.

Although proper randomized clinical trials are still lacking, the U.S. Centers for Disease Control and Prevention (CDC) (18) recommends vaccination against *Streptococcus pneumoniae* for all elderly people and for younger people at high risk for pneumonia. Pneumococcal vaccination may or may not protect against pneumonia or death, but it does significantly decrease the risk of invasive pneumococcal disease (19).

Despite a "level A" recommendation by the CDC, the use of pneumococcal poly-saccharide vaccination in patients with COPD is supported by limited data (20). Alfageme et al. (21) evaluated the clinical efficacy of the 23 serotype pneumococcal polysaccharide vaccine in COPD patients. They reported that the vaccine was efficacious in preventing community-acquired pneumonia in patients with COPD younger than 65 years and in those with severe airflow obstruction, even though no difference in mortality was observed between the groups studied. However, while pneumococcal vaccination may reduce the incidence of community-acquired pneumonia in COPD patients (21), its role in the prevention of COPD exacerbations remains to be established (17,22,23).

A recent systematic review on of OM-85 BV, an immunomodulatory agent derived from eight bacteria and used for prevention of exacerbations in persons with chronic lung disease, identified three useful trials conducted in patients with COPD and found that OM-85 BV had a small (though not statistically significant) effect in preventing COPD exacerbations (24). The authors concluded that the available evidence did not clearly demonstrate clinical benefit. Recently, Soler et al. (25) investigated the effect of OM-85 on acute exacerbations in patients with COPD. Although the study was relatively small, it showed a surprising 29% decrease in exacerbations in patients with mild disease and confirmed and extended the results of earlier studies in older patients with more advanced COPD (26). Further randomized controlled trials enrolling large numbers of persons with well-defined COPD are necessary to confirm the effectiveness of this agent.

In conclusion, even if the supportive evidence is still controversial, influenza and pneumococcal vaccinations are recommended by the most recent international guidelines on COPD (1,14,15), particularly in the elderly. In contrast, immunostimulants such as OM-85 are not recommended despite being supported by similarly inconsistent evidence (1,14,15).

## IV. Antioxidant and/or Mucolytic Agents

In the 2006 Cochrane analysis (27) of 26 clinical trials comprising more than 7300 patients with chronic bronchitis and/or COPD, treatment with oral mucolytics was weakly associated with a small reduction in acute exacerbations and a reduction in the total number of days of disability. In contrast, a large placebo-controlled three-year trial showed no significant reduction in the number of exacerbations in COPD patients, even though a post hoc analysis suggested some effect in a subgroup of patients not treated with inhaled glucocorticosteroids (28). However, a properly designed randomized clinical trial showed clearly that carbocisteine reduces the number of exacerbations in properly selected Chinese COPD patients (29). In conclusion, at present, while antioxidants and mucolytics are still largely used, they are not recommended by the major international guidelines on COPD (1,14,15).

## V. Bronchodilators

The pathognomonic pathophysiological abnormality of COPD is poorly reversible airflow limitation caused by increased resistance, mainly of small airways, and decreased elastic recoil due to parenchymal destruction. Considering the irreversible or poorly reversible nature of the airflow limitation, the rationale for using bronchodilators in COPD is shaky at best. The principal symptom reported by COPD patients is dyspnea, an unpleasant sensation in breathing that is essentially due to hyperinflation rather than airflow limitation per se. In fact, in patients with airflow limitation there is air trapping that results in increased work of breathing, and it places respiratory muscles at a mechanical disadvantage that is believed to contribute to the sensation of breathlessness. Interestingly, lung inspiratory capacity correlates reasonably well with exercise endurance time and exertion, whereas $FEV_1$ does not. Changes in inspiratory volumes also contribute to the perceived benefits of bronchodilator therapy.

In a recent study, the perceived benefit of inhaling 400 µg of salbutamol in patients with COPD was based on a significant correlation between symptom score and changes in forced inspiratory volume that was much closer than the correlation with expiratory volume. This result suggested that the symptomatic effect of bronchodilators on dyspnea in COPD patients is mainly related to reduction of inspiratory volumes (30). Having said that, the Global Initiative on Chronic Obstructive Lung Disease (GOLD) guidelines (1) recommends the use of bronchodilators for the symptomatic management of COPD and assigns an evidence level of "A" for this recommendation. These drugs are given both on an as-needed basis and on a regular basis to prevent symptoms and exacerbations. Thus, inhaled bronchodilators remain the mainstay therapy for symptomatic COPD patients.

### A.  Short-Acting Bronchodilators

Short-acting bronchodilators, both $\beta_2$-agonists and anticholinergics, reduce symptoms and improve the quality of life in COPD patients (31–34). A post hoc analysis claimed that regular long-term use of ipratropium, alone or in combination with albuterol, was associated with fewer exacerbations than the use of albuterol alone (35); however, the sample sizes in each population were not matched. No randomized clinical trial on the effects of short-acting bronchodilators on COPD exacerbations has been adequately powered, and thus firm conclusions are not possible. In contrast, the combination of ipratropium and a short-acting $\beta_2$-agonist showed benefits over those of a short-acting $\beta_2$-agonist alone in terms of postbronchodilator lung function and a reduced requirement for oral glucocorticosteroids; however, no significant benefits in subjective improvements in health-related quality of life were seen (36).

   In conclusion, while short-acting bronchodilators are still used, regularly, the major international guidelines recommend them only for symptom relief and not for regular treatment of COPD (1,14,15).

### B.  Long-Acting Bronchodilators

More data on the efficacy of inhaled bronchodilators in preventing COPD exacerbations became available when long-acting bronchodilators were developed. Several studies (37–40) suggest a possible role for long-acting bronchodilators in preventing COPD exacerbations.

   Although salmeterol and ipratropium were equally effective in reducing dyspnea and the use of rescue medications in patients with mild to moderate COPD, salmeterol was superior to ipratropium both in improving lung function and in reducing the time to first COPD exacerbation (37). The positive effect of salmeterol alone on COPD exacerbations was recently confirmed by the TORCH (TOwards a Revolution in COPD Health) study (*vide infra*) (41). In contrast, in two large studies, formoterol failed to reduce time to first exacerbation and the number of severe exacerbations (8,9). However, formoterol may reduce the number of "bad days" (comparable to mild exacerbations), daily symptoms, and use of rescue medications, suggesting that it might be effective in reducing the severity of exacerbations (39).

   Long-acting anticholinergic drugs, such as tiotropium, are also effective in reducing COPD exacerbations. Vincken and colleagues reported a reduction of 24% in COPD exacerbations and 38% in hospitalizations due to COPD exacerbations in patients treated with tiotropium compared with patients treated with ipratropium (42). Furthermore, the time to first hospitalization due to a COPD exacerbation was significantly longer in the tiotropium group than in the placebo group. The role of tiotropium in reducing the frequency and the severity of COPD exacerbations was recently confirmed by Niewoehner and colleagues (43). They evaluated the number of COPD exacerbations and the number of hospitalizations due to COPD exacerbation in more than 1800 patients with moderate to severe COPD; patients were randomly treated with tiotropium once daily or with placebo for six months. Tiotropium significantly reduced the percentage of patients who experienced at least one COPD exacerbation during the six-month treatment period. Furthermore, tiotropium prolonged the time to first exacerbation and the time to first hospitalization due to COPD exacerbation, although this relationship was of borderline statistical significance. Tiotropium also decreased the number of exacerbation days and the duration of antibiotic treatment (43). The combined analysis of 1207 patients included in two studies examining the effects of tiotropium or salmeterol versus placebo on exacerbations, health resource use, dyspnea, health-related quality of life, and lung function showed that, compared with salmeterol, tiotropium was associated with longer time to onset of the first exacerbation, fewer hospital admissions, fewer days during which patients were unable to perform their usual daily activities, and better lung function (44). The differences between tiotropium and salmeterol were small, and the tolerability of the two treatments was similar. Neither tiotropium nor salmeterol markedly reduced exacerbations, suggesting that, in patients with severe COPD, it is not particularly relevant to choose between these two long-acting bronchodilators with different mechanisms of action. The clinically relevant question would be whether the combination of the two is more effective than each single agent alone. Unfortunately, the only long-term study adequately powered to address this question failed to show an additive effect on exacerbations of combining salmeterol and tiotropium (45).

In conclusion, inhaled bronchodilators, particularly the inhaled long-acting $\beta_2$-agonist salmeterol or the anticholinergic tiotropium, are effective in reducing exacerbations of COPD. The evidence for the inhaled long-acting $\beta_2$-agonist formoterol is less documented and more controversial. Most recent international guidelines recommend regular treatment with long-acting bronchodilators for patients with moderate to severe COPD (1,14,15), and the evidence supporting this recommendation is quite strong. In contrast, the recommendation of the same guidelines to combine bronchodilators, particularly long-acting $\beta_2$-agonists and anticholinergics, is not supported by any published evidence.

## VI. Theophylline

In patients with COPD, theophylline has some beneficial functional and clinical effects, such as on lung function, arterial blood gas tensions, and exercise tolerance, but most studies have been conducted in patients receiving a variety of concomitant therapies (46). Therefore, data on the effect of theophylline on COPD exacerbations are lacking.

The efficacy of low-dose theophylline in reducing COPD exacerbations was shown in a randomized, double-blind, parallel-group, placebo-controlled study of low-dose, slow-release theophylline given to COPD patients for one year (47). In a comparison study, Rossi et al. showed that formoterol was more effective than adequate doses of theophylline in reducing COPD exacerbations (48). One study showed that adding salmeterol to adequate doses of theophylline further reduced COPD exacerbations compared with theophylline alone, but the cumulative effect was no different from that of salmeterol alone (49).

Considering the evidence available, the recommendation of recent guidelines (1,14,15) to add theophylline for patients who are still symptomatic while receiving regular long-acting bronchodilator therapy may be useful for symptom control, but this agent has not been proved to be associated with a reduction in COPD exacerbations.

## VII. Phosphodiesterase Inhibitors

New and more specific phosphodiesterase inhibitors, namely cilomilast and roflumilast, may be the only new treatments expected to become available within the next five years (50). The preclinical pharmacology and phase II and phase III studies strongly support the potential of this new class of drugs in the treatment of COPD. Few recent large clinical trials have shown a significant effect of roflumilast or cilomilast on COPD exacerbations. In a large six-month double-blind, randomized, placebo-controlled study powered on lung function, Rabe et al. reported that roflumilast, in addition to improving lung function, significantly reduced the number of mild exacerbations compared with placebo in patients with moderate COPD (51). However, in a large 12-month double-blind, randomized, placebo-controlled study powered on both lung function and exacerbations, Calverley et al. reported that roflumilast had no effect on COPD exacerbations in patients with moderate to severe COPD (52). In that study, however, the subgroup of patients with very severe COPD experienced fewer exacerbations with roflumilast than with placebo. Finally, in a large six-month double-blind, randomized, placebo-controlled study powered on lung function and quality of life, Rennard et al. reported that cilomilast not only had a positive, significant effect on lung function and quality of life but also reduced the total number of exacerbations in patients with to severe COPD (53).

In conclusion, the new and more specific phosphodiesterase inhibitors, cilomilast and roflumilast, have been shown to have inconsistent effects on COPD exacerbations (51–53). More studies are required to understand the role of these new drugs in the management of COPD.

## VIII. Inhaled Corticosteroids

The role of inhaled corticosteroids (ICS) in COPD has been the subject of much controversy (5). The reasons for the widespread use of ICS in COPD include the efficacy and well-established safety of these agents in asthma (54), their anti-inflammatory effects, and the efficacy of systemic corticosteroids for the treatment of acute exacerbations of COPD. Indeed, the fact that COPD is associated with pulmonary and systemic inflammation has provided a major rationale for conducting studies on the effects of ICS in COPD. Unfortunately, the strong anti-inflammatory effect of inhaled glucocorticosteroids observed in asthma (54) has not been confirmed in COPD (55), and that might explain their frequently reported negative effects.

The several excellent, large randomized clinical trials that aimed to investigate the effect of ICS in the natural course of COPD were consistently negative (56–58), proving that inhaled glucocorticosteroids have no effect on the excessive decline in lung function associated with COPD. In contrast, several studies on ICS have shown a consistent though small increase in lung function, some improvements in cough and dyspnea, and a slower decline in the quality of life (59).

The causes of COPD exacerbations are often unclear, and the definition of COPD exacerbations varies. However, several studies have clearly demonstrated that (*i*) in addition to the chronic bronchopulmonary and systemic inflammation associated with the disease, COPD exacerbations are associated with transient acute bronchopulmonary and systemic inflammation, and that (*ii*) systemic and inhaled glucocorticosteroids may suppress this transient acute inflammation, thus providing a strong rationale for examining the effect of inhaled glucocorticosteroids on COPD exacerbations. Additional support for this rationale comes from studies that examined the effect of withdrawal of ICS from COPD patients who were being treated with it; all consistently showed an increased rate of exacerbations after cessation of treatment (60,61).

A recent systematic review that was aimed at determining the efficacy of regular use of ICS in patients with stable COPD included 47 studies with 13,139 participants (59). The review showed that long-term use of ICS does not significantly reduce the rate of decline in $FEV_1$ and has no effect on mortality, but does reduce the mean rate of exacerbations. The authors' conclusion was that patients and clinicians should balance the potential benefits of inhaled glucocorticosteroids in COPD, particularly the reduced rate of exacerbations, against the known increase in local side effects (oropharyngeal candidiasis and hoarseness)—and, we would add, the increased risk of pneumonia (41,62). The firm conclusion of the authors, however, has to be balanced with the strong methodological concerns expressed by Suissa et al. (5–7), who came to the opposite conclusion. By reanalyzing the most recent large studies (57,58,63), they concluded that inhaled glucocorticosteroids have no effect on exacerbations in COPD.

On the basis of all the evidence described above, the most recent guidelines (1,14,15) suggest that treatment with ICS be used only in combination with long-acting bronchodilators and only in patients with severe or very severe COPD who experience repeated exacerbations.

## IX. Combination Therapy

Combination therapy—a long-acting $\beta_2$-agonist and a glucocorticosteroid together in one inhaler—has been available for more than 10 years. Two types of combined inhalers have been studied in COPD: budesonide/formoterol and salmeterol/fluticasone. Several large clinical trials (9,64–66) have consistently shown that combination therapy is more effective than the single components in reducing the frequency and severity of exacerbations in patients with severe to very severe COPD; now this effect has been confirmed in moderate to severe COPD (41).

The first pivotal study was TRISTAN (Trial of Inhaled Steroids and Long-Acting Beta2 Agonists) (64). In that study the combination of inhaled fluticasone and inhaled salmeterol reduced the rate of severe exacerbations by approximately 40% compared with placebo, whereas fluticasone alone reduced the exacerbations rate by 34% and salmeterol alone reduced it by only 29% (Fig. 1). The recent TORCH study, in which the same combination of salmeterol/fluticasone was compared with salmeterol or fluticasone alone, confirmed the superior effect of this combination in a very large population of patients with moderate to very severe COPD (postbronchodilator $FEV_1$ 44% predicted) (41) (Fig. 2).

Two large 12-month double-blind, randomized, placebo-controlled studies, both powered on exacerbations, investigated the effect of the combination of formoterol and

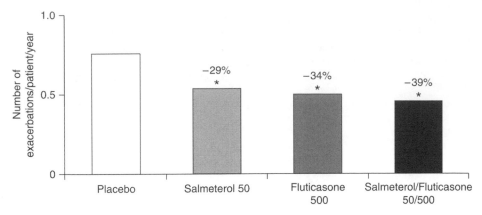

*p ≤ 0.001 vs placebo

**Figure 1** The annual rate of COPD exacerbations in the placebo, salmeterol/fluticasone, and combination-therapy group, respectively. All active treatments were effective in preventing exacerbations compared with placebo, but the effect of combination treatment was no different from the effect of monotherapy (TRISTAN). *Source*: From Ref. 64.

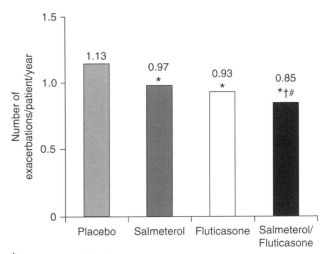

\* $p < 0.001$ vs Placebo,
† $p = 0.002$ vs Salmeterol,
# $p = 0.024$ vs Fluticasone

**Figure 2** Reduction of acute exacerbations requiring oral corticosteroids in the placebo, salmeterol/fluticasone, and combination-therapy groups, respectively. All active treatments were effective in preventing exacerbations compared with placebo, and the combination treatment was significantly more effective and better than individual treatment (TORCH). *Source*: From Ref. 41.

budesonide in a single inhaler in patients with severe to very severe COPD (8,9). The design of the two studies differed in the prerandomization phase: in one (8), patients were pretreated with oral glucocorticosteroids and high-dose combination therapy, whereas in the other (9), all preventative medications were withdrawn. Also, one study was powered on $FEV_1$ and time to first exacerbation (8), whereas the other was powered on $FEV_1$ and rate of severe exacerbations (9). Both studies clearly showed that the budesonide/formoterol combination in a single inhaler was effective in treating severe exacerbations. The time to first severe exacerbation requiring an oral corticosteroid course was prolonged by 28.2%, 30.5%, and 44.7%, with the use of the budesonide/formoterol combination in a single inhaler versus budesonide alone, formoterol alone, and placebo, respectively. The number of severe exacerbations per patient per year in those using the budesonide/formoterol combination in a single inhaler was reduced by 24% versus placebo and 23% versus formoterol alone (9).

Because tiotropium alone was shown to be quite effective in reducing COPD exacerbations (43,67)—to an extent similar to that of the combination of long-acting $\beta_2$-agonists and glucocorticosteroids in a single inhaler—the INSPIRE (Investigating New Standards for Prophylaxis in Reduction of Exacerbations) study was conducted to compare the efficacy of salmeterol/fluticasone and tiotropium in more than 1300 patients with severe COPD (mean age 64 years; postbronchodilator $FEV_1$ 39% predicted). Patients were followed for two years. Unfortunately, the study showed no difference in the primary outcome: the percentage of patients who had at least one exacerbation requiring therapeutic intervention was 62% in the combination therapy group and 59% in the tiotropium group (66).

None of the above-cited studies showed a decrease in exacerbations of more than 30%, suggesting the possibility that an additional effect could be achieved by adding long-acting bronchodilators with different mechanisms of action (e.g., tiotropium and either salmeterol or formoterol) to inhaled glucocorticosteroids. The effect of the triple combination was examined in the Canadian Optimal Therapy of COPD Trial (45), which showed that the addition of the salmeterol/fluticasone combination to tiotropium did not further decrease the rate of exacerbations (Fig. 3) or time to the next exacerbation (Fig. 4).

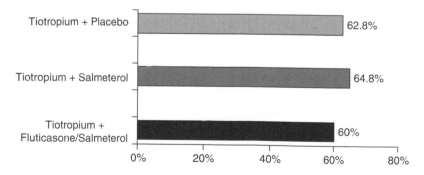

**Figure 3** Proportions of one year COPD exacerbations defined as those that required treatment with oral corticosteroids and/or antibiotics or required hospitalization. No difference was found in the overall rate of exacerbations between treatment groups, suggesting that both treatments reduced exacerbations frequency by similar magnitude (OPTIMAL) *Source*: From Ref. 66.

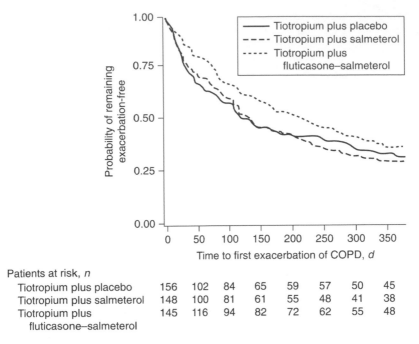

Patients at risk, *n*

| | | | | | | | | |
|---|---|---|---|---|---|---|---|---|
| Tiotropium plus placebo | 156 | 102 | 84 | 65 | 59 | 57 | 50 | 45 |
| Tiotropium plus salmeterol | 148 | 100 | 81 | 61 | 55 | 48 | 41 | 38 |
| Tiotropium plus fluticasone–salmeterol | 145 | 116 | 94 | 82 | 72 | 62 | 55 | 48 |

**Figure 4** Kaplan–Maier estimates of the probability of remaining free of exacerbations according to treatment assigned. The median time to first exacerbation was not statistically significant among the three treatments. *Source*: From Ref. 45.

The 2007 Cochrane analysis on combination therapy in COPD patients (68,69) concluded that the combination of inhaled glucocorticosteroids and long-acting bronchodilators significantly reduces morbidity and mortality when compared with single-component glucocorticosteroids.

On the basis of the evidence cited above, the most recent guidelines (1,14,15) recommend treatment with a combination of inhaled long-acting bronchodilators and glucocorticosteroids in patients with moderate to very severe COPD and a history of repeated exacerbations. While the GOLD guidelines limit this recommendation to patients with severe or very severe COPD (FEV$_1$ <50% predicted) (1), the Canadian guidelines consider the TORCH and Optimal Therapy studies sufficient evidence to recommend the same treatment also for patients with moderate COPD (15).

## X.  Importance of Comorbidities and Their Treatment

Comorbidities markedly affect health outcomes in COPD (70); in fact, patients with COPD mainly die of no respiratory diseases (71–73), such as cardiovascular diseases ($\sim$25%), cancer (mainly lung cancer, 20–33%), and other causes (30%). Considering that the pharmacological treatment of COPD to date is primarily symptomatic, a more comprehensive approach to the frequent comorbidities of COPD may provide an opportunity to modify the natural history of patients with COPD and to identify novel targets for treatment. This is particularly relevant for those conditions that appear more preventable and treatable than COPD, such as cardiovascular and metabolic disorders.

Interestingly, Mancini et al. (74), in a retrospective study, examined the effect of statins, angiotensin-converting enzyme inhibitors, and angiotensin receptor blockers in COPD patients with and without concomitant heart disease. The results showed a reduction in COPD hospitalization and total mortality with the use of these agents, suggesting that they may have dual cardiopulmonary protective properties and have the potential to alter the prognosis of patients with COPD. The reported effects need to be assessed in properly designed and powered randomized clinical trials, but preliminary results suggest that these agents may reduce COPD exacerbations.

## XI. Conclusion

The prevention of exacerbations of respiratory symptoms in COPD patients is an important aim of treatment, as COPD exacerbations are a major cause of morbidity, mortality, and poor quality of life in these patients. Inhaled long-acting bronchodilators and inhaled glucocorticosteroids are the first choice of drugs recommended for the treatment of COPD by the most influential and recent guidelines. In independent studies, both long-acting bronchodilators and inhaled glucocorticosteroids have been shown to prevent COPD exacerbations, although the effects of inhaled glucocorticosteroids are less reproducible in some studies. Several studies have consistently shown that the combination of a long-acting $\beta_2$-agonist and an inhaled glucocorticosteroid in a single inhaler provides a more effective preventative treatment of COPD exacerbations than does a single component. However, recent studies have shown that the combination of a long-acting $\beta_2$-agonist and an inhaled glucocorticosteroid is not more effective than the long-acting anticholinergic tiotropium. Whatever the treatment, the maximum percentage of prevention of COPD exacerbations is in the range of 30%, suggesting that there is still much room for improvement.

## References

1. A collaborative project of the National Heart, Lung and Blood Insitute, National Institutes of Health, and the World Health Organization. Bethesda (MD): National Institutes of Health, National Heart, Lung, and Blood Institute. 2007. Global Initiative for Chronich Obstructive Lung Disease. Available at: www.goldcopd.org.
2. Donaldson GC, Wedzicha JA. COPD exacerbations.1: Epidemiology. Thorax 2006; 61(2): 164–168.
3. Donaldson GC, Seemungal TA, Bhowmik A, et al. Relationship between exacerbation frequency and lung function decline in chronic obstructive pulmonary disease. Thorax 2002; 57(10): 847–852.
4. Fabbri LM, Luppi F, Beghé B, et al. Complex chronic comorbidities of COPD. Eur Respir J 2008; 31(1):204–212.
5. Suissa S. Observational studies of inhaled corticosteroids in chronic obstructive pulmonary disease: misconstrued immortal time bias. Am J Respir Crit Care Med 2006; 173(4):464; author reply 464–465.

6.   Suissa S. Statistical treatment of exacerbations in therapeutic trials of chronic obstructive pulmonary disease. Am J Respir Crit Care Med 2006; 173(8):842–846.
7.   Suissa S, Ernst P, Vandemheen KL, et al. Methodological issues in therapeutic trials of chronic obstructive pulmonary disease. Eur Respir J 2008; 31(5):927–933.
8.   Calverley PM, Boonsawat W, Cseke Z, et al. Maintenance therapy with budesonide and formoterol in chronic obstructive pulmonary disease. Eur Respir J 2003; 22(6):912–919.
9.   Szafranski W, Cukier A, Ramirez A, et al. Efficacy and safety of budesonide/formoterol in the management of chronic obstructive pulmonary disease. Eur Respir J 2003; 21(1):74–81.
10.  Aaron SD, Vandemheen KL, Hebert P, et al. Outpatient oral prednisone after emergency treatment of chronic obstructive pulmonary disease. N Engl J Med 2003; 348(26):2618–2625.
11.  Anthonisen NR, Connett JE, Kiley JP, et al. Effects of smoking intervention and the use of an inhaled anticholinergic bronchodilator on the rate of decline of FEV1. The Lung Health Study. JAMA 1994; 272(19):1497–1505.
12.  Anthonisen NR, Connett JE, Murray RP. Smoking and lung function of Lung Health Study participants after 11 years. Am J Respir Crit Care Med 2002; 166(5):675–679.
13.  Bourbeau J, Julien M, Maltais F, et al. Reduction of hospital utilization in patients with chronic obstructive pulmonary disease: a disease-specific self-management intervention. Arch Intern Med 2003; 163(5):585–591.
14.  Celli BR, MacNee W. Standards for the diagnosis and treatment of patients with COPD: a summary of the ATS/ERS position paper. Eur Respir J 2004; 23(6):932–946.
15.  O'Donnell DE, Aaron S, Bourbeau J, et al. Canadian Thoracic Society recommendations for management of chronic obstructive pulmonary disease - 2007 update. Can Respir J 2007; 14 (suppl B):5B–32B.
16.  Nichol KL, Baken L, Nelson A. Relation between influenza vaccination and outpatient visits, hospitalization, and mortality in elderly persons with chronic lung disease. Ann Intern Med 1999; 130(5):397–403.
17.  Poole PJ, Chacko E, Wood RW-Baker, et al. Influenza vaccine for patients with chronic obstructive pulmonary disease. Cochrane Database Syst Rev 2006; (1):CD002733.
18.  Prevention of pneumococcal disease: recommendations of the Advisory Committee on Immunization Practices (ACIP). MMWR Recomm Rep 1997; 46(RR-3):1–24.
19.  Targonski PV, Poland GA. Pneumococcal vaccination in adults: recommendations, trends, and prospects. Cleve Clin J Med 2007; 74(6):401–406, 408–410, 413–414.
20.  Schenkein JG, Nahm MH, Dransfield MT. Pneumococcal vaccination for patients with COPD: current practice and future directions. Chest 2008; 133(3):767–774.
21.  Alfageme I, Vazquez R, Reyes N, et al. Clinical efficacy of anti-pneumococcal vaccination in patients with COPD. Thorax 2006; 61(3):189–195.
22.  Granger R, Walters J, Poole PJ, et al. Injectable vaccines for preventing pneumococcal infection in patients with chronic obstructive pulmonary disease. Cochrane Database Syst Rev 2006; (4):CD001390.
23.  Steentoft J, Konradsen HB, Hilskov J, et al. Response to pneumococcal vaccine in chronic obstructive lung disease: the effect of ongoing, systemic steroid treatment. Vaccine 2006; 24(9):1408–1412.
24.  Sprenkle MD, Niewoehner DE, MacDonald R, et al. Clinical efficacy of OM-85 BV in COPD and chronic bronchitis: a systematic review. COPD 2005; 2(1):167–175.
25.  Soler M, Mutterlein R, Cozma G. Double-blind study of OM-85 in patients with chronic bronchitis or mild chronic obstructive pulmonary disease. Respiration 2007; 74(1):26–32.
26.  Collet JP, Shapiro P, Ernst P, et al. Effects of an immunostimulating agent on acute exacerbations and hospitalizations in patients with chronic obstructive pulmonary disease. The PARI-IS Study Steering Committee and Research Group. Prevention of Acute Respiratory Infection by an Immunostimulant. Am J Respir Crit Care Med 1997; 156(6):1719–1724.

27. Poole PJ, Black PN. Mucolytic agents for chronic bronchitis or chronic obstructive pulmonary disease. Cochrane Database Syst Rev 2006; 3:CD001287.

28. Decramer M, Rutten-van Molken M, Dekhuijzen PN, et al. Effects of N-acetylcysteine on outcomes in chronic obstructive pulmonary disease (Bronchitis Randomized on NAC Cost-Utility Study, BRONCUS): a randomised placebo-controlled trial. Lancet 2005; 365 (9470):1552–1560.

29. Zheng JP, Kang J, Huang SG, et al. Effect of carbocisteine on acute exacerbation of chronic obstructive pulmonary disease (PEACE Study): a randomised placebo-controlled study. Lancet 2008; 371(9629):2013–2018.

30. Taube C, Lehnigk B, Paasch K, et al. Factor analysis of changes in dyspnea and lung function parameters after bronchodilation in chronic obstructive pulmonary disease. Am J Respir Crit Care Med 2000; 162(1):216–220.

31. Guyatt GH, Townsend M, Pugsley SO, et al. Bronchodilators in chronic air-flow limitation. Effects on airway function, exercise capacity, and quality of life. Am Rev Respir Dis 1987; 135 (5):1069–1074.

32. Higgins BG, Powell RM, Cooper S, et al. Effect of salbutamol and ipratropium bromide on airway calibre and bronchial reactivity in asthma and chronic bronchitis. Eur Respir J 1991; 4 (4):415–420.

33. O'Donnell DE, Lam M, Webb KA. Measurement of symptoms, lung hyperinflation, and endurance during exercise in chronic obstructive pulmonary disease. Am J Respir Crit Care Med 1998; 158(5 pt 1):1557–1565.

34. Ram FS, Sestini P. Regular inhaled short acting beta2 agonists for the management of stable chronic obstructive pulmonary disease: Cochrane systematic review and meta-analysis. Thorax 2003; 58(7):580–584.

35. Friedman M, Serby CW, Menjoge SS, et al. Pharmacoeconomic evaluation of a combination of ipratropium plus albuterol compared with ipratropium alone and albuterol alone in COPD. Chest 1999; 115(3):635–641.

36. Appleton S, Jones T, Poole P, et al. Ipratropium bromide versus long-acting beta-2 agonists for stable chronic obstructive pulmonary disease. Cochrane Database Syst Rev 2006; 3:CD006101.

37. Mahler DA, Donohue JF, Barbee RA, et al. Efficacy of salmeterol xinafoate in the treatment of COPD. Chest 1999; 115(4):957–965.

38. Rennard SI, Anderson W, ZuWallack R, et al. Use of a long-acting inhaled beta2-adrenergic agonist, salmeterol xinafoate, in patients with chronic obstructive pulmonary disease. Am J Respir Crit Care Med 2001; 163(5):1087–1092.

39. Dahl R, Greefhorst LA, Nowak D, et al. Inhaled formoterol dry powder versus ipratropium bromide in chronic obstructive pulmonary disease. Am J Respir Crit Care Med 2001; 164(5): 778–784.

40. Casaburi R, Mahler DA, Jones PW, et al. A long-term evaluation of once-daily inhaled tiotropium in chronic obstructive pulmonary disease. Eur Respir J 2002; 19(2):217–224.

41. Calverley PM, Anderson JA, Celli B, et al. Salmeterol and fluticasone propionate and survival in chronic obstructive pulmonary disease. N Engl J Med 2007; 356(8):775–789.

42. Vincken W, van Noord JA, Greefhorst AP, et al. Improved health outcomes in patients with COPD during 1 yr's treatment with tiotropium. Eur Respir J 2002; 19(2):209–216.

43. Niewoehner DE, Rice K, Cote C, et al. Prevention of exacerbations of chronic obstructive pulmonary disease with tiotropium, a once-daily inhaled anticholinergic bronchodilator: a randomized trial. Ann Intern Med 2005; 143(5):317–326.

44. Brusasco V, Hodder R, Miravitlles M, et al. Health outcomes following treatment for six months with once daily tiotropium compared with twice daily salmeterol in patients with COPD. Thorax 2003; 58(5):399–404.

45. Aaron SD, Vandemheen KL, Fergusson D, et al. Tiotropium in combination with placebo, salmeterol, or fluticasone-salmeterol for treatment of chronic obstructive pulmonary disease: a randomized trial. Ann Intern Med 2007; 146(8):545–555.

46. Ram FS, Jones PW, Castro AA, et al. Oral theophylline for chronic obstructive pulmonary disease. Cochrane Database Syst Rev 2002; (4):CD003902.

47. Zhou Y, Wang X, Zeng X, et al. Positive benefits of theophylline in a randomized, double-blind, parallel-group, placebo-controlled study of low-dose, slow-release theophylline in the treatment of COPD for 1 year. Respirology 2006; 11(5):603–610.

48. Rossi A, Kristufek P, Levine BE, et al. Comparison of the efficacy, tolerability, and safety of formoterol dry powder and oral, slow-release theophylline in the treatment of COPD. Chest 2002; 121(4):1058–1069.

49. ZuWallack RL, Mahler DA, Reilly D, et al. Salmeterol plus theophylline combination therapy in the treatment of COPD. Chest 2001; 119(6):1661–1670.

50. Boswell-Smith V, Cazzola M, Page CP. Are phosphodiesterase 4 inhibitors just more theophylline? J Allergy Clin Immunol 2006; 117(6):1237–1243.

51. Rabe KF, Bateman ED, O'Donnell D, et al. Roflumilast–an oral anti-inflammatory treatment for chronic obstructive pulmonary disease: a randomised controlled trial. Lancet 2005; 366 (9485):563–571.

52. Calverley PM, Sanchez-Toril F, McIvor A, et al. Effect of 1-year treatment with roflumilast in severe chronic obstructive pulmonary disease. Am J Respir Crit Care Med 2007; 176(2): 154–161.

53. Rennard SI, Schachter N, Strek M, et al. Cilomilast for COPD: results of a 6-month, placebo-controlled study of a potent, selective inhibitor of phosphodiesterase 4. Chest 2006; 129(1): 56–66.

54. Djukanovic R, Wilson JW, Britten KM, et al. Effect of an inhaled corticosteroid on airway inflammation and symptoms in asthma. Am Rev Respir Dis 1992; 145(3):669–674.

55. Keatings VM, Jatakanon A, Worsdell YM, et al. Effects of inhaled and oral glucocorticoids on inflammatory indices in asthma and COPD. Am J Respir Crit Care Med 1997; 155(2):542–548.

56. Pauwels RA, Lofdahl CG, Laitinen LA, et al. Long-term treatment with inhaled budesonide in persons with mild chronic obstructive pulmonary disease who continue smoking. European Respiratory Society Study on Chronic Obstructive Pulmonary Disease. N Engl J Med 1999; 340 (25):1948–1953.

57. Vestbo J, Sorensen T, Lange P, et al. Long-term effect of inhaled budesonide in mild and moderate chronic obstructive pulmonary disease: a randomised controlled trial. Lancet 1999; 353 (9167):1819–1823.

58. Burge PS, Calverley PM, Jones PW, et al. Randomised, double blind, placebo controlled study of fluticasone propionate in patients with moderate to severe chronic obstructive pulmonary disease: the ISOLDE trial. BMJ 2000; 320(7245):1297–1303.

59. Yang IA, Fong KM, Sim EH, et al. Inhaled corticosteroids for stable chronic obstructive pulmonary disease. Cochrane Database Syst Rev 2007; (2):CD002991.

60. O'Brien A, Russo-Magno P, Karki A, et al. Effects of withdrawal of inhaled steroids in men with severe irreversible airflow obstruction. Am J Respir Crit Care Med 2001; 164(3):365–371.

61. van der Valk P, Monninkhof E, van der Palen J, et al. Effect of discontinuation of inhaled corticosteroids in patients with chronic obstructive pulmonary disease: the COPE study. Am J Respir Crit Care Med 2002; 166(10):1358–1363.

62. Ernst P, Gonzalez AV, Brassard P, et al. Inhaled corticosteroid use in chronic obstructive pulmonary disease and the risk of hospitalization for pneumonia. Am J Respir Crit Care Med 2007; 176(2):162–166.

63. Paggiaro PL, Dahle R, Bakran I, et al. Multicentre randomised placebo-controlled trial of inhaled fluticasone propionate in patients with chronic obstructive pulmonary disease. International COPD Study Group. Lancet 1998; 351(9105):773–780.

64. Calverley P, Pauwels R, Vestbo J, et al. Combined salmeterol and fluticasone in the treatment of chronic obstructive pulmonary disease: a randomised controlled trial. Lancet 2003; 361 (9356):449–456.
65. Kardos P, Wencker M, Glaab T, et al. Impact of salmeterol/fluticasone propionate versus salmeterol on exacerbations in severe chronic obstructive pulmonary disease. Am J Respir Crit Care Med 2007; 175(2):144–149.
66. Wedzicha JA, Calverley PM, Seemungal TA, et al. The prevention of chronic obstructive pulmonary disease exacerbations by salmeterol/fluticasone propionate or tiotropium bromide. Am J Respir Crit Care Med 2008; 177(1):19–26.
67. Brusasco V, Hodder R, Miravitlles M, et al. Health outcomes following treatment for 6 months with once daily tiotropium compared with twice daily salmeterol in patients with COPD. Thorax 2006; 61(1):91.
68. Nannini LJ, Cates CJ, Lasserson TJ, et al. Combined corticosteroid and long-acting beta-agonist in one inhaler versus long-acting beta-agonists for chronic obstructive pulmonary disease. Cochrane Database Syst Rev 2007; (4):CD006829.
69. Nannini LJ, Cates CJ, Lasserson TJ, et al. Combined corticosteroid and long-acting beta-agonist in one inhaler versus inhaled steroids for chronic obstructive pulmonary disease. Cochrane Database Syst Rev 2007; (4):CD006826.
70. Sin DD, Anthonisen NR, Soriano JB, et al. Mortality in COPD: Role of comorbidities. Eur Respir J 2006; 28(6):1245–1257.
71. Hansell AL, Walk JA, Soriano JB. What do chronic obstructive pulmonary disease patients die from? A multiple cause coding analysis. Eur Respir J 2003; 22(5):809–814.
72. Mannino DM, Doherty DE, Sonia A Buist. Global Initiative on Obstructive Lung Disease (GOLD) classification of lung disease and mortality: findings from the Atherosclerosis Risk in Communities (ARIC) study. Respir Med 2006; 100(1):115–122.
73. Mannino DM, Watt G, Hole D, et al. The natural history of chronic obstructive pulmonary disease. Eur Respir J 2006; 27(3):627–643.
74. Mancini GB, Etminan M, Zhang B, et al. Reduction of morbidity and mortality by statins, angiotensin-converting enzyme inhibitors, and angiotensin receptor blockers in patients with chronic obstructive pulmonary disease. J Am Coll Cardiol 2006; 47(12):2554–2560.

# 32
## Self-Management in Prevention and Early Intervention of Exacerbations

**JEAN BOURBEAU**
Respiratory Epidemiology and Clinical Research Unit, Montreal Chest Institute, McGill University Health Center, Montréal, Québec, Canada

**ERIK W. M. A. BISCHOFF**
Department of Primary Care, Centre of Evidence Based Medicine, Radboud University Nijmegen Medical Centre, Nijmegen, The Netherlands

**MARIA SEDENO**
Respiratory Epidemiology and Clinical Research Unit, Department of Medicine, McGill University, Montréal, Québec, Canada

## I. Introduction

Exacerbation of chronic obstructive pulmonary disease (COPD) is usually defined as an acute episode of sustained deterioration of symptoms, i.e., worsening of dyspnea and change in sputum, beyond normal day-to-day variations (1). Although many exacerbations are successfully managed in primary care, they are yet a common cause of hospital admission, often after failed initial therapy in the community. Exacerbations are severely distressing events that impact greatly on health status, loss of symptom control, and activities of daily live. Frequent exacerbations significantly diminish patients' health status (2), and moderate to severe COPD patients have a mean of two exacerbations a year (3). Patients' symptom recovery time varies between 4 and 14 days (3,4) except that activities of daily living and mental state can take longer to recover, up to 18 and 39 days (4). Decreasing the rate of exacerbations is associated with improved quality of life (5,6) and thus would be expected to reduce hospitalizations and benefit health care costs (7). Furthermore, early report and treatment have been shown to reduce the length of an exacerbation, to improve patients' health status, and to decrease hospital admissions (8).

If we are to progress in the management of COPD exacerbations, treatment goals should not only aim to treat the acute episode but the focus should also be on prevention and early treatment. New strategies that will help patients to recognize their exacerbation and to initiate treatment promptly may have great potential. Self-management education programs with a written action plan that includes rapid access and/or standing prescriptions for antibiotics and/or prednisone in the event of an exacerbation have been proposed as a strategy for early treatment of exacerbations (9–11). Such a strategy may be effective in reducing hospital admissions (12), presumably by decreasing the severity and duration of exacerbations.

In this chapter, the concept and practice of self-management and its potential role in the prevention and early treatment of COPD exacerbation is discussed on the basis of the most recent medical literature. This chapter will give practical advices for implementation of self-management strategies, given rapid access to treatment by the means of a written action plan as an option, and suggestions for future research.

## II.  Self-Management in COPD

### A.  The Self-Management Model

Self-management can be described as a set of skilled behaviors and refers to the various tasks that individuals carry out for the management of their condition (13). A self-management program in COPD targets the integration of effective interventions that are recognized to be effective in disease control, such as healthy life habits (smoking cessation, regular exercise) and self-management skills (adherence to medication, breathing techniques, and positioning early recognition and prompt treatment of exacerbations) (9,14).

Self-management is not only about education (teaching effective interventions), but it is aiming at behavior modification and maintenance. Self-management in chronic disease requires a process that can be illustrated as a causal chain (Fig. 1). Self-management skills are not enough to bring about change in behavior and produce health impacts. Many so called self-management programs rely on merely passing information to the patient, and consider that success is attained if patient's disease knowledge has improved. A meta-analysis of 30 studies of chronic disease (15) showed that efforts to improve health by improving knowledge alone were rarely successful, meaning that people may memorize information well, but are not necessarily able to put the information into use. Behavioral-oriented programs (regimen-oriented) and sustainability in the education process are

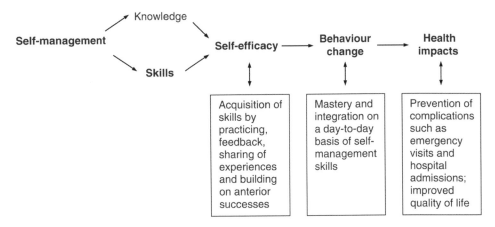

**Figure 1**  Effective chronic illness care model—self-management. *Source*: Adapted from Ref. 13.

consistently more successful at improving the clinical course of chronic disease. These are keys to the success of any self-management education program.

Improving disease knowledge is one important target, but it is only the beginning of the process. In a chronic disease such as COPD, it is important to work at improving patients' confidence in their own ability to modify and maintain a specific behavior. A self-management program should be designed to increase self-efficacy (Fig. 1), which is the individual's belief in his or her ability to execute necessary actions in response to specific situations. Self-efficacy is task related and is considered in the social cognitive theory (16) a predictor of behavioral change; individuals choose and invest the effort to maintain a specific action only if they believe that they are capable of doing it and will benefit from it. The limited numbers of studies evaluating the role of self-efficacy in COPD have consistently reported it as a significant predictor of adherence to exercise programs and pulmonary rehabilitation (17,18). There is also indication that a self-management program can result in lifestyle changes. In a qualitative study by Nault and colleagues (19), the majority of COPD patients educated via the self-management program "Living Well with COPD" reported experiencing lifestyle modifications, such as learning to breathe and maintaining exercise. It is only when the new behaviors have been mastered and integrated to the patient's daily life that we could expect improvements on health status and health care utilization.

## B. Self-Management and High-Quality Chronic Disease Care

The chronic care model has been a proposed solution for effective management of patients with chronic diseases. This model identifies essential elements that encourage high-quality chronic disease care: (*i*) self-management approach, (*ii*) delivery system design, (*iii*) decision support, and (*iv*) clinical information systems (20). *Self-management* interventions include education, behavioral support, and motivation. The *care delivery system* must be designed to provide "advanced" access to chronic care. Patient interactions with an integrated team that includes a skilled health professional who acts as "case manager" are a key component. Therapies given should be based on *evidence-based practice guidelines*, and support from specialists must be assured. The final component of the chronic care model, which is often lacking, involves integrating a computerized *clinical information system* into clinical practice to plan care, implement automated reminders to comply with clinical guidelines, and provide individual feedback to care providers regarding their performance (14). The four components of the chronic care model are not independent. A recent systematic review by Adams (21) suggested that implementing an intervention that includes at least two of these components is an effective preventative strategy to reduce health care use in COPD, while interventions that only apply one of the components (self-management without the delivery system and decision support) will not have a clear benefit on outcomes such as emergency department visits and hospital admissions.

This is why one of the minimum requirements for implementing a successful self-management education program is to have a continuum of care which includes access and continuous communication with a case manager, as already shown in chronic diseases such as arthritis and diabetes (22–24). A case manager within a multidisciplinary care team ensures that some critical elements of care that physicians may not have the training or time to do are competently performed (25). In self-management programs, case managers are used to empower patients with the knowledge and skills necessary to manage their own illness and, more importantly, to gain the confidence to apply these skills on a daily basis (26) by using various strategies such as practice, feedback, reattribution of the perceived causes of failure, and role modeling (13). Case managers evaluate patient comprehension, beliefs and, self-efficacy throughout the self-management program, while making sure those healthy behaviors and self-management skills are integrated. Case managers play as well an important role in facilitating and coordinating care activities, monitoring patient's progress, and modifying the delivery of services as needed.

### C.  Self-Management Effectiveness

When studying the literature on self-management, several trials have described the effects of self-management strategies on COPD exacerbations. With regard to the model of self-management, these studies show major differences in intensity of the programs, educational processes, and role of care providers. In addition, studies often have methodological limitations in statistical power, sustainability of the education program, and outcomes measured, which makes it difficult to compare the trials and may explain their failure to show positive results (27). Usually, no information is provided on patient self-efficacy or on methods used to enhance it as part of the self-management education program. Many of these studies may have simply failed to intervene. Instead of pooling the results of individual trials, it is perhaps of more interest to scrutinize the few successful interventions and explain their success by using the self-management model.

The Canadian Living Well with COPD program was one of the first self-management interventions, which clearly demonstrated a significant reduction in health care use and an improvement in health status (28), even after a two-year follow-up period (29). These results were confirmed by a self-management intervention from New Zealand (30) and an integrated care plan tested in Spain and Belgium (31). The latter has also been demonstrated to improve COPD knowledge, exacerbation identification and early treatment, as well as inhaler adherence and proper use (32). The contents of these programs are similar to those with inconclusive results (33,34); they mainly focus on proven effective topics, such as smoking cessation, accurate use of medication, promotion of exercise, and early recognition and treatment of exacerbations. However, in the successful programs the education plan was customized to each individual patient and aimed at enhancing self-efficacy and behavior modification by setting achievable goals. The self-management strategies were embedded in an integrated health care system coordinated by a case manager who provided a continuum of care throughout the follow-up period. By regular contacts with the patient, the case manager ensures the maintenance of self-management skills, provides empowerment, and is able to respond to changes in the trajectory of the disease.

### III.  Self-Management to Prevent Exacerbation

Preventing acute exacerbations in COPD should be as important as it is to prevent myocardial infarction in patients with cardiovascular disease. Behavioral interventions based on the self-efficacy theory, such as self-management, show enormous potential as part of the continuum of care to improve adherence to preventive strategies for acute exacerbations such as smoking cessation, vaccination, and regular pharmacotherapy.

Poor adherence in patients with COPD entails risk of adverse health outcomes, including suboptimal treatment leading to COPD exacerbations, emergency department visits, and hospitalizations. Making sure patients are adherent to their therapy should be as important as prescribing the right medication. Important lessons have been learned from COPD and other chronic disease self-management programs. For example, providing information in both written and oral forms and allowing an opportunity for discussion can increase knowledge and adherence (35,36). The effectiveness of counseling is maximized when information is presented in a structured manner over a period of at least 15 minutes. Interventions that include prescribed behavioral components (e.g., keeping medications in one place, self-monitoring of symptoms, and medication use, etc.) are more effective.

Self-management groups led by professional staff or trained lay patients can provide a cost-effective (29,35–38) and enjoyable way for patients to learn about managing their disease and rehearse (13,39) new behaviors while receiving support from other families and patients with COPD.

Having opportunities to regularly discuss the use of self-management strategies and problem-solving skills with the physician and the case-manager enhances patient self-efficacy, and it is also of great importance.

## IV. Self-Management and Early Treatment

### A. Importance of Early Treatment

To date, treatment has focused mostly on therapy to decrease admissions, reduce length of hospital stay, and hasten recovery. More attention needs to be paid to the early treatment of exacerbations to prevent complications such as deterioration in quality of life and hospitalizations. However, to be able to intervene early, patients have to recognize and to report promptly their symptoms. Under-reporting of COPD exacerbations seems to be a widespread phenomenon, as 30% of patients have problems in recognizing warning signs when an exacerbation is imminent (40) and less than 50% of patients report to the health care provider (3,4).

Failure to report exacerbations has been shown to be associated with an increased risk of emergency hospitalization (8) due to a delay or a failure in treatment. Unreported exacerbations are very similar with reported exacerbations in terms of severity and duration of symptoms and changes in lung function (3). Although unreported exacerbations may not be serious enough to warrant an emergency visit or hospitalization, they may still have an important impact on health status for a given patient (41). The high incidence of unreported exacerbations may indicate an unmet health care need. Improving patient understanding of the nature of an exacerbation and improving early recognition of its symptoms could benefit reporting and early treatment. Patient recognition of exacerbation symptoms and prompt treatment has been shown to improve exacerbation recovery, reduce risks of hospitalization, and it is associated with better health status (8).

### B. Use of Tailored Action Plans

Early treatment of exacerbations can only be accomplished when patients undertake immediate actions to respond to changes in their baseline symptoms. This requires knowledge of exacerbations, skills for proper management, and self-confidence to start

**Table 1**  Essential Components of a Written Plan of Action and Required Skills for the Prevention and Early Treatment of COPD Exacerbations

| Component | Required self-management skill |
|---|---|
| How to remain stable and prevent exacerbations | Knowledge of baseline symptoms |
| | Adherence to medication |
| | Maintenance of healthy behaviors (e.g., healthy diet, quit smoking, exercise) |
| | Identification and avoidance of factors that make symptoms worse (e.g., indoor and outdoor pollutants, emotions, changes in temperature, respiratory infections) |
| How to manage an acute exacerbation | Recognition of symptoms deterioration |
| | Knowledge of contact resources (case manager) |
| | Knowledge of medication to be increased or added depending on symptom presentation and within recommended delay |
| | Use of breathing, relaxation, and energy conservation techniques |
| How to manage a nonimprovement or worsening of exacerbation | Recognition of nonimprovement or worsening in symptoms within expected delay |
| | Knowledge of contact resources (case manager, treating physician, emergency department) |
| How to manage an emergency situation regarding the exacerbation | Recognition of life-threatening symptoms |
| | Knowledge of contact resources (emergency services) |

prompt action. Action plans, whether embedded or not in a comprehensive self-management intervention, are useful in providing the patient a guideline for proper management of an exacerbation. Although early treatment is mainly focused on appropriate medication changes, an action plan is more than simply prescribing the use of rescue medication, antibiotics, or oral prednisone. An action plan should include key components that will facilitate patients managing the exacerbation, such as recognition of symptom deterioration, medication to be adjusted or added depending on symptoms presentation, proper response timing, resources to contact, and other important self-management strategies to be applied and/or maintained in case of exacerbation (e.g., breathing and relaxation techniques). In addition, action plans should include a section in which the baseline symptoms are identified and the actions to remain stable are addressed (e.g., healthy lifestyle and medication compliance). Table 1 shows the essential components of a written action plan and required skills for the prevention and early treatment of COPD exacerbations.

The use of an action plan also requires a proper delivery structure with support by a case manager to assure that the response to treatment is adequate and to promote long-term adherence case managers should be accessible to patients, and, if possible, provide a close follow-up at the time of an exacerbation (Fig. 2). As with any other skill, patients experience a learning curve, and need to practice on using their action plans. Case managers help patients in this process, building on previous success to improve self-confidence, and reassuring them when bad experiences occur. In this way, the action plan becomes a streamlined intervention that summarizes the full self-management education program.

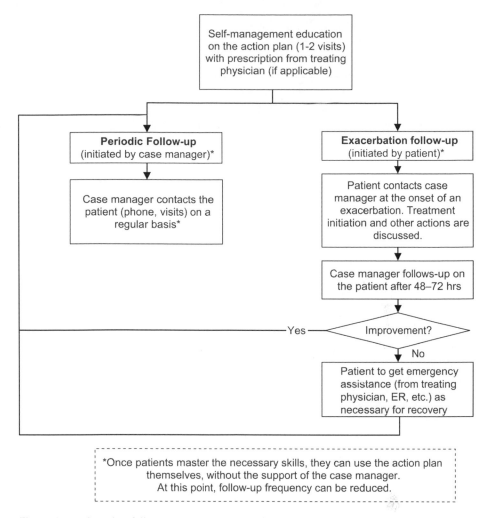

**Figure 2** Action plan follow-up process as part of a self-management education program: shared decision-making and close follow-up during the event of an exacerbation, as well as planned contacts are necessary to assure proper response to treatment and to promote long-term adherence.

Individualized action plans have been shown to help patients recognize and react appropriately to an exacerbation by promptly self-initiating antibiotics and oral steroids (42). Although the studies showed that patients provided with an action plan have a better knowledge of the importance of early intervention and how to implement appropriate treatment for an exacerbation, they could not show benefit in reducing health service use. New study results suggest that a written action plan embedded in a comprehensive self-management intervention can considerably contribute to reduce health care utilization (43). The use of action plans to help patients recognize symptom changes, to implement self-care behaviors, and to promptly self-initiate a customized prescription in the event of an exacerbation is a promising strategy.

## V. Practice Advice in Using an Action Plan

Since its development in 1996, much experience has been gained with the implementation of the self-management program Living Well with COPD. The program has been evaluated (28), adjusted to meet the needs of health care professionals and patients, and approved by the health ministry in Québec, Canada. Nowadays, most of the health professionals in Québec use this evidence-based program to educate their COPD patients. The full educational material as well as reference guides describing its implementation (individual and group education) can be found on the website www.livingwellwithcopd .com (password: copd).

One of the patient learning modules specifically addresses the use of a tailored action plan for acute exacerbations. The matching reference guide describes a step-by-step process in which the health professional (case manager) guides the patient in the learning process (Table 2). At first, the case manager evaluates patient's present knowledge and behaviors (e.g., understanding of exacerbations and actions taken to prevent or manage them). By doing this, the case manager is able to identify patients' learning needs. Subsequently, each

**Table 2** Structure of the Educational Session on the Action Plan (Living Well with COPD): Interventions and Suggested Questions

| Intervention | Suggested questions |
|---|---|
| 1. Explore present patient's knowledge and behaviors | According to you, what is a COPD exacerbation? What do you usually do when your symptoms get worse? |
| 2. i. Present/demonstrate technique/discuss topic | Why should you use an action plan? What is included in an action plan? |
| ii. Evaluate patient's comprehension | Who are your resource persons, how and when should you contact them? Could you describe your daily symptoms? What should you do to keep your health condition stable? Which changes in your COPD symptoms tell you that you may have a respiratory infection? When should you start your additional treatment? How do you know that your symptoms improved? What should you do if you feel you are in danger? |
| 3. Explore possible barriers to integration of skills and behaviors learned | What prevents you from using your action plan? |
| 4. Evaluate patient's level of self-efficacy | Do you believe that you will be able to use your action plan to prevent or manage an exacerbation at home? Do you believe that an action plan can help to prevent or manage a worsening of COPD symptoms? |
| 5. Reference to other health professionals if needed | Did you get your prescription from your physician? Is your action plan prescription on file at the pharmacy? |

*Source*: From Ref. 45.

of the session's topics is discussed; e.g., importance and structure of an action plan, recognition of an exacerbation, and actions to manage it. The reference guide identifies learning objectives for each topic and suggests questions to evaluate patient comprehension and beliefs, identify barriers, and solutions to them. The educational session ends with an evaluation of the patient's self-efficacy (beliefs with respect to the value of an action plan and own capabilities to use it). Additional references are described; in this case, the case manager should communicate with the treating physician to discuss rapid access and/or the use of a self-administered prescription.

The case manager should remain accessible to the patient for support and close follow-up at the time of an exacerbation (Fig. 2). In addition, at periodic scheduled telephone calls, the case manager reviews the patient's general health condition and the use of self-management strategies to reinforce the acquired skills. When the patient demonstrates a complete integration of the appropriate skills to manage an exacerbation, the role of the case manager has been fulfilled.

## VI. Conclusion

Providing COPD patients with the self-management skills they need to properly manage their COPD should be considered as important as writing the correct prescription. Besides enhancing patient self-efficacy as part of self-management education, shared decision-making during the initial and regular follow-up is also important to promote long-term adherence.

The use of action plans to help patients recognize symptom changes, to implement self-care, and to self-initiate a customized prescription (antibiotics and corticosteroids) in the event of an exacerbation has been suggested as a promising strategy. So far, there is growing evidence that self-management influences COPD exacerbation management and decreases health care utilization. Successful programs are based on organization and practice that include accurate self-management strategies, enhance patients' self-efficacy and specific skills, and are supported by a practice team and a case manager to optimize disease control and follow-up. Studies have shown that patients can learn how to recognize symptom changes and to react promptly. The results of effective studies show that implementation of self-management programs and written action plans in primary and secondary care is possible. However, well-designed and adequately powered studies are still needed to strengthen the positive results and to resolve remaining questions.

## VII. Needs for Research

Further research is undoubtedly needed to strengthen the results of the positive studies on which current guidelines are mainly based. Research needs to be carried out to gain insight on health behavior change interventions in COPD in order to design more effective self-management programs. For future studies it is imperative to realize that a self-management strategy must enhance self-efficacy and behavior modification before it can affect exacerbation outcomes. Therefore, self-efficacy and behavior modification should be measured as outcomes. Future clinical trials need to be planned and designed more carefully; studies should be powered properly.

Furthermore, future studies must avoid the methodological pitfalls, which might have caused equivocal and inconclusive results in previous studies. Benefits of a self-management program on health care utilization and health status are more likely to be observed in a study population consisting of patients with moderate to severe COPD, and previous hospitalization due to exacerbations. Only few studies consider comorbidities as possible confounders, whereas depression and anxiety can inhibit self-management (44). A recent review on the effects of action plans demonstrated that exacerbation severity and duration were not used as outcomes in any of the reviewed trials (42). This is conspicuous, as early symptom recognition and prompt treatment of exacerbations affect health care utilization and health status by decreasing the severity and length of an exacerbation. If we are to progress in the management of acute exacerbation, it is evident that the effect of early interventions on symptom recovery and health status should be considered as an essential component of clinical trials.

## References

1.  Global Initiative for Chronic Obstructive Lung Disease. Global strategy for the diagnosis, management and prevention of chronic obstructive pulmonary disease: NHLBI/WHO workshop report, updated 2005. Bethesda, MD: National Heart, Lung and Blood Institute, 2005. GOLD-Wkshp05Clean.pdf. Available at: www.goldcopd.com/download.asp?intID_231. Accessed June 28, 2006.
2.  Miravitlles M, Ferrer M, Pont A, et al. Effect of exacerbations on quality of life in patients with chronic obstructive pulmonary disease: a 2 year follow up study. Thorax 2004; 59(5):387–395.
3.  Seemungal TA, Donaldson GC, Bhowmik A, et al. Time course and recovery of exacerbations in patients with chronic obstructive pulmonary disease. Am J Respir Crit Care Med 2000; 161 (5):1608–1613.
4.  Bourbeau J, Ford G, Zackon H, et al. Impact on patient's health status following early identification of a COPD exacerbation. Eur Respir J 2007; (30):907–913.
5.  Burge P, Calverley P, Jones P, et al. Randomised, double blind, placebo controlled study of fluticasone propionate in patients with moderate to severe chronic obstructive pulmonary disease: the ISOLDE trial. BMJ 2000; 320(7245):1297–1303.
6.  Calverley P, Pauwels R, Vestbo J, et al. Combined salmeterol and fluticasone in the treatment of chronic obstructive pulmonary disease: a randomised controlled trial. Lancet 2003; 361(9356): 449–456.
7.  Wedzicha JA, Seemungal TA. COPD exacerbations: defining their cause and prevention. Lancet 2007; 370(9589):786–796.
8.  Wilkinson TM, Donaldson GC, Hurst JR, et al. Early therapy improves outcomes of exacerbations of chronic obstructive pulmonary disease. Am J Respir Crit Care Med 2004; 169(12): 1298–1303.
9.  Nici L, Donner C, Wouters E, et al. American Thoracic Society/European Respiratory Society statement on pulmonary rehabilitation. Am J Respir Crit Care Med 2006; 173(12):1390–1413.
10. O'Donnell DE, Aaron J, Bourbeau J, et al. Canadian Thoracic Society recommendations for management of chronic obstructive pulmonary disease - 2007 update. Can Respir J 2007; 14(suppl B):5B–32B.
11. Scullion JE. NICE guidelines: the management, treatment and care of COPD. Br J Nurs 2004; 13(18):1100–1103.
12. Effing T, Monninkhof E, van d V, et al. Self-management education for patients with chronic obstructive pulmonary disease. Cochrane Database Syst Rev 2007; (4):CD002990.
13. Bourbeau J, Nault D, Dang-Tan T. Self-management and behaviour modification in COPD. Patient Educ Couns 2004; 52(3):271–277.

14. Bourbeau J, Nault D. Self-management strategies in chronic obstructive pulmonary disease. Clin Chest Med 2007; 28(3):617–628.
15. Mazzuca S. Does patient education in chronic disease have therapeutic value? J Chronic Dis 1982; 35(7):521–529.
16. Bandura A. The assessment and predictive generality of self-percepts of efficacy. J Behav Ther Exp Psychiatry 1982; 13(3):195–199.
17. Atkins C, Kaplan R, Timms R, et al. Behavioral exercise programs in the management of chronic obstructive pulmonary disease. J Consult Clin Psychol 1984; 32:591–603.
18. Kaplan RM, Ries AL, Prewitt LM, et al. Self-efficacy expectations predict survival for patients with chronic obstructive pulmonary disease. Health Psychol 1994; 13(4):366–368.
19. Nault D, Dagenais J, Perreault V, et al. Qualitative evaluation of a disease specific self-management program "Living well with COPD". Eur Resp J 2000; 16:317S.
20. Wagner EH. Chronic disease management: what will it take to improve care for chronic illness? Eff Clin Pract 1998; 1(1):2–4.
21. Adams SG, Smith PK, Allan PF, et al. Systematic review of the chronic care model in chronic obstructive pulmonary disease prevention and management. Arch Intern Med 2007; 167(6):551–561.
22. Piette JD, Weinberger M, Kraemer FB, et al. Impact of automated calls with nurse follow-up on diabetes treatment outcomes in a Department of Veterans Affairs Health Care System: a randomized controlled trial. Diabetes Care 2001; 24(2):202–208.
23. Simon GE, VonKorff M, Rutter C, et al. Randomised trial of monitoring, feedback, and management of care by telephone to improve treatment of depression in primary care. BMJ 2000; 320(7234):550–554.
24. Weingarten SR, Henning JM, Badamgarav E, et al. Interventions used in disease management programmes for patients with chronic illness-which ones work? Meta-analysis of published reports. BMJ 2002; 325(7370):925–928.
25. Wagner EH. The role of patient care teams in chronic disease management. BMJ 2000; 320 (7234):569–572.
26. Zwarenstein M, Stephenson B, Johnson L. Case management: effects on professional practice and health care outcomes. Cochrane Database Syst Rev 2000; 4:CD002797.
27. Taylor SJ, Candy B, Bryar RM, et al. Effectiveness of innovations in nurse led chronic disease management for patients with chronic obstructive pulmonary disease: systematic review of evidence. BMJ 2005; 331(7515):485–488.
28. Bourbeau J, Julien M, Maltais F, et al. Reduction of hospital utilization in patients with chronic obstructive pulmonary disease: a disease-specific self-management intervention. Arch Intern Med 2003; 163(5):585–591.
29. Gadoury MA, Schwartzman K, Rouleau M, et al. Self-management reduces both short- and long-term hospitalisation in COPD. Eur Respir J 2005; 26(5):853–857.
30. Rea H, McAuley S, Stewart A, et al. A chronic disease management programme can reduce days in hospital for patients with chronic obstructive pulmonary disease. Intern Med J 2004; 34(11): 608–614.
31. Casas A, Troosters T, Garcia-Aymerich J, et al. Integrated care prevents hospitalisations for exacerbations in COPD patients. Eur Respir J 2006; 28(1):123–130.
32. Garcia-Aymerich J, Lange P, Benet M, et al. Regular physical activity modifies smoking-related lung function decline and reduces risk of chronic obstructive pulmonary disease: a population-based cohort study. Am J Respir Crit Care Med 2007; 175(5):458–463.
33. Coultas D, Frederick J, Barnett B, et al. A randomized trial of two types of nurse-assisted home care for patients with COPD. Chest 2005; 128(4):2017–2024.
34. Monninkhof E, van der Valk P, van der Palen J, et al. Effects of a comprehensive self-management programme in patients with chronic obstructive pulmonary disease. Eur Respir J 2003; 22(5):815–820.
35. Ley P. Communicating with patients [magazine article]. London: Croom Helm, 1988.

36. Morris LA, Halperin JA. Effects of written drug information on patient knowledge and compliance: a literature review. Am J Public Health 1979; 69(1):47–52.
37. Bourbeau J, Collet JP, Schwartzman K, et al. Economic benefits of self-management education in COPD. Chest 2006; 130:1704–1711.
38. Bourbeau J, Maltais F, Julien M, et al. Predictors of high utilization of health care services in patients with chronic obstructive pulmonary disease. Abstract. Can Respir J 2003; 10(4):207
39. Gallefoss F, Bakke PS, Rsgaard PK. Quality of life assessment after patient education in a randomized controlled study on asthma and chronic obstructive pulmonary disease. Am J Respir Crit Care Med 1999; 159(3):812–817.
40. Kessler R, Stahl E, Vogelmeier C, et al. Patient understanding, detection, and experience of COPD exacerbations: an observational, interview-based study. Chest 2006; 130(1):133–142.
41. Langsetmo L, Platt RW, Ernst P, et al. Underreporting exacerbation of chronic obstructive pulmonary disease in a longitudinal cohort. Am J Respir Crit Care Med 2008; 177(4):396–401.
42. Turnock AC, Walters EH, Walters JA, et al. Action plans for chronic obstructive pulmonary disease. Cochrane Database Syst Rev 2005; 4:CD005074.
43. Sedeno MF, Nault D, Hamd DH, et al. A written action plan for early treatment of COPD exacerbations: an important component to the reduction of hospitalizations. Proc Am Thorac Soc 2006; 3:A603.
44. Dowson CA, Town GI, Frampton C, et al. Psychopathology and illness beliefs influence COPD self-management. J Psychosom Res 2004; 56(3):333–340.
45. Living Well With COPD. Individual Reference Guide: Integrating a Plan of Action for life; October 20, 2006. Available at: www.livingwellwithcopd.com (password: copd).

# 33
# Immunological Interventions

**PHILLIPPA J. POOLE**
Department of Medicine, Faculty of Medical and Health Sciences, University of Auckland, Auckland, New Zealand

## I. Introduction

Reasons for reducing the burden of chronic obstructive pulmonary disease (COPD) exacerbations on patient morbidity and mortality and scarce health care resources have been outlined in earlier chapters. There is considerable appeal in the use of low-risk and low-cost immunological interventions to prevent, or at least minimize, clinical effects resulting from respiratory infection in COPD patients. To date, inactivated influenza vaccination is the most successful and widely used immunization, with other immunological interventions against respiratory bacteria not yet shown to reduce exacerbations in COPD. This chapter will discuss the evidence for effectiveness of immunization on clinical outcomes related to acute exacerbation in COPD and some practical considerations.

## II. Influenza Vaccination

The recommendation for annual influenza vaccination in recent COPD guidelines is supported by evidence from observational studies as well as from randomized controlled trials (RCTs). Many countries provide the vaccine free to those with chronic respiratory diseases such as COPD.

### A. Diagnosing Influenza as a Cause of COPD Exacerbation

Many respiratory viruses cause fever, myalgia, and cough, making it difficult to attribute an infective COPD exacerbation specifically to influenza infection. Confirmation of influenza as the cause of an infection requires laboratory documentation, so-called laboratory-documented influenza (LDI). In the past, this was done using serological techniques, although newer techniques allow direct detection of influenza antigens or cellular material in respiratory cells or secretions. The presentation of symptomatic LDI was assessed as part of two RCTs of influenza vaccine, and both of these concluded that while myalgia and fever were fairly specific, these symptoms had a low positive predictive value for LDI (1,2).

## B. How Influenza Vaccines Work

Most national vaccination programs use a trivalent inactivated split vaccine containing two type A and one type B influenza strains administered in one intramuscular injection. The component strains are selected each year by the World Health Organization according to the estimate of the influenza viruses most likely to circulate in the upcoming winter.

Selected influenza viruses are grown in the allantoic cavity of embryonated eggs, before being inactivated, then disrupted. Protection by influenza vaccines occurs from development of circulating antibodies to the hemagglutinin and neuraminidase glycoproteins found on the surface of influenza viruses. Stimulation of cytotoxic T-cell responses may also be important (3).

As it takes up to three weeks to develop maximal immunity, vaccination needs to occur well in advance of the anticipated arrival of the winter influenza season, around November in the Northern Hemisphere and May in the Southern Hemisphere. Annual vaccination is required as immunity is relatively short lived and specific to the strains in the vaccine.

As most COPD patients are elderly, they will, in general, have lower phagocytic function and mount less of an immune response to vaccination than younger people. In an attempt to improve vaccine efficacy, live attenuated viruses have been trialled, both alone and in combination with inactivated virus vaccines. Live attenuated virus vaccines have the additional advantage of being administered intranasally. At this time nasal spray attenuated influenza vaccine is approved in the United States for use only in healthy people aged between 5 and 49 years (4).

## C. Effectiveness of Influenza Vaccines in COPD

The effectiveness of influenza vaccine in reducing influenza-related COPD exacerbations will depend on

1.  how much influenza-related acute respiratory infection is present. This in turn is affected by whether there is an influenza epidemic and/or vaccination coverage in the population, including those with COPD;
2.  the match of vaccine with circulating strains; and
3.  the immunocompetence of the vaccine recipient cohort.

Influenza vaccine is effective at preventing influenza in the majority of the population, but there is still significant benefit to be had where the match is poor and/or patients are older. A meta-analysis of 20 cohort studies showed that influenza vaccination in the elderly was associated with a 56% reduction in respiratory illness, a 53% reduction in pneumonia, a 50% reduction in hospitalization, and a 68% reduction in deaths from all causes during influenza outbreaks (5). Greater benefit was seen in epidemic years when the vaccine strain was identical or similar to the epidemic strain. In an observational study of more than 20,000 senior citizens enrolled with a health care plan in the United States conducted over six influenza seasons, the vaccination rate was 60% (6). Compared with nonvaccinated subjects, in the season after vaccination, those who had received influenza vaccination had a 39% reduction in hospitalizations for pneumonia or influenza ($p < 0.001$), 32% fewer hospitalizations for respiratory conditions ($p < 0.001$), and a reduction of 50% in all-cause mortality ($p < 0.001$). Benefits were greater in people with more serious underlying disease. In the subgroup of 1898 older people with chronic lung disease, there was a vaccination rate of over 70%. During the ensuing influenza season, vaccinated subjects had a 52% reduction in hospitalizations for pneumonia and influenza ($p = 0.008$) and a 70% reduction in death from all causes ($p < 0.001$) over unvaccinated subjects (7). A recent cohort study conducted over three years in 260,000 Swedes older than 65 years showed that the number needed to treat with influenza vaccination to prevent one death lay between 50 and 300 in an epidemic season (8). Sixty-four studies of efficacy/effectiveness of influenza vaccine in the elderly have been combined in a Cochrane systematic review (9). A key finding is that influenza vaccine is more effective at preventing pneumonia, hospitalization, or death when study subjects live in residential homes for the elderly, rather than independently in the community.

As cohort studies are liable to bias from unmeasured factors, the best method for assessing the effectiveness of vaccines is a randomized placebo-controlled trial with careful matching of the intervention and control groups (10).

A Cochrane systematic review evaluating the RCT evidence for influenza vaccination in COPD patients was first published in 2001 and has been updated regularly since (11). The review focuses on clinical outcomes such as acute exacerbations, hospitalization, and mortality. The reviewers found six RCTs of influenza vaccine, involving a total of 2649 chronic bronchitics or people with COPD (2,12–16). Each of the studies is too small to have detected any effect on mortality.

The two RCTs of inactivated virus vaccine in COPD were conducted in very different settings. The first (13) took place in a general practice in Wolverhampton, United Kingdom, in the winter of 1960. Fifty chronic bronchitics (37 men, mean age 53 years) were followed for four months after vaccination. The other (2) in Thailand in 1997–1998 was felt ethically justified as influenza vaccination had not been available in that country previously. The investigators enrolled 125 university hospital outpatients with COPD (94% male, mean age 68 years) and followed the subjects for one year.

In these two trials, exacerbations were classified as either "early" or "late" (after 3 of 4 weeks). This stratification was to explore the commonly held yet scientifically implausible concern that inactivated virus vaccination causes exacerbations. Meta-analysis of these two studies showed no statistically significant effect of vaccination on early exacerbation rates [weighted mean difference (WMD) 0.01; 95% CI, $-0.11$–$0.13$; $p = 0.87$].

Despite the trials being small, there was a significant reduction in the total number of exacerbations per vaccinated subject compared with those who received placebo; WMD $-0.37$; 95% CI, $-0.64$ to $-0.11$; $p = 0.006$. This was nearly all due to the reduction in late exacerbations; WMD $-0.39$; 95% CI, $-0.61$ to $-0.18$; $p = 0.0004$. In the Howells study, the total number of patients experiencing late exacerbations was significantly fewer; odds ratio (OR) = 0.13; 95% CI, $0.04$–$0.45$; $p = 0.002$. The two studies carefully assessed the clinical presentations for presence of LDI. Howells used serology, and Wongsurakiat used both serology and virology swabs. Overall, inactivated influenza vaccination resulted in a marked decrease in influenza-related respiratory infections; OR = 0.19; 95% CI, $0.07$–$0.48$; $p = 0.0005$. The effect was similar whether the subjects had mild, moderate, or severe COPD or chronic bronchitis. Influenza accounted for 8% (13 of 161) of the acute exacerbations in the Wongsurakiat study. Although this was not an influenza epidemic year, there was a good match between vaccine and virus strains. On the other hand, influenza was responsible for 37% of the acute exacerbations in the Howells study.

The other four RCTs (12,14–16) assessed the effects of live attenuated intranasal virus vaccines. None of these studies showed a clinical benefit of intranasal live attenuated virus in COPD patients compared with placebo, whether given alone or in conjunction with inactivated influenza virus vaccine.

### D.   Contraindications and Adverse Effects of Influenza Vaccination

The only absolute contraindication to vaccination is chicken egg allergy, although as vaccines may include traces of polymixin and neomycin, people with known sensitivities to these agents should also avoid influenza vaccination. Among relative contraindications are acute feverish illness (temperature over 38.5°C), although mild upper respiratory infections should not preclude vaccination. Influenza vaccine may impair metabolism by the hepatic P4-50 system, hence patients on warfarin, theophylline, phenytoin, or carbamazepine should have closer monitoring of the effects of these medicines in the early postvaccination period.

Adverse effects usually become manifest within 24 hours of vaccination and may be local or systemic. Local effects at the site of injection are more common in vaccinated patients than those given placebo, but these are mild and transient (17,18). Systemic reactions include myalgia, fatigue, headache, and low-grade fever, but as discussed above, these should not be attributed to influenza infection arising "from the vaccine." It is of course possible that vaccination occurs during the prodromal phase of influenza infection, especially during epidemic seasons.

The most feared complication of influenza vaccination is Guillain-Barre syndrome (GBS). In the early 1990s, there were reports of an excess of one to two cases of GBS per million persons vaccinated, but the Advisory Committee on Immunization Practices (ACIP) concluded subsequently that the benefits of the vaccine far outweigh the risks for developing vaccine-associated GBS (19).

### E.   Cost-Effectiveness Considerations

Most studies estimate that that influenza vaccination results in net cost savings. In her serial cohort studies, Nichol estimated a saving of about U.S. $170 per year per high-risk person vaccinated (6). In a study from Taiwan, savings for each elderly person vaccinated were at least three times the cost of vaccination (20). A cost-effectiveness analysis based on an RCT suggested that inactivated virus vaccination is highly cost effective in COPD patients, particularly those with severe airways obstruction (21). This analysis took into account direct health care costs, but not indirect costs, or future health care costs that might be incurred by COPD patients living longer. It was conducted in a nonepidemic year and will underestimate the benefits that would be gained in an epidemic year. More than 90% of the costs of an influenza-related COPD exacerbation were costs of hospitalization. In patients with moderate or severe COPD, more than 90% of the hospital costs were due to costs of treating those who required mechanical ventilation. Cost savings were seen in all grades of severity, more so in those with more severe COPD.

### F.   Influenza Vaccine Coverage

Despite evidence of effectiveness and concerted public health initiatives, only about two-thirds of elderly people are vaccinated, with this marginally higher in those with COPD (6). Barriers include difficulties in accessing health care, uncertainty about the degree and longevity of protection, concern about adverse effects (including infection from the vaccine), and, perhaps, palliative treatment intent. Supply chain issues emerged as another major barrier in the developed world in 2006. Arguably, people with COPD and other chronic diseases should be a high priority for receiving the vaccine, along with health care workers and others in essential services.

## III. Pneumococcal Vaccination

People with COPD are at significantly higher risk for hospitalization for pneumococcal pneumonia than non-COPD controls (22). Injectable pneumococcal vaccines are manufactured using several capsular polysaccharide extracts and have been shown to reduce invasive pneumococcal disease in young adults working in close quarters. The recommendation for a pneumococcal vaccine every five years in high-risk elderly (including COPD) (23), while well intentioned, is not well supported by evidence in the COPD population, and coverage rates remain relatively low. A recent Cochrane systematic review identified four RCTs of pneumococcal vaccination in people with COPD (24). The two older trials used a 14-valent vaccine (25,26), with the more recent ones using a 23-valent vaccine (27,28). Information on acute exacerbations of COPD was available from only one small study ($n = 49$), with this showing no effect of vaccination on exacerbations over that seen in the control group; OR $= 1.43$; 95% CI, 0.31–6.69 (28). Vaccination had no effect on the number of COPD subjects developing pneumonia, on hospitalization rates, all-cause mortality, or death from cardiorespiratory causes.

There were no reports of an increased rate of major adverse effects in vaccinated subjects in either the Cochrane review or in a meta-analysis of nine RCTs in adults (29). The main adverse effect was erythema at the injection site.

## IV. Haemophilus Influenzae Vaccination

A Cochrane systematic review has summarized the six RCTs conducted in Australia and Papua New Guinea in the 1980s comparing the effects of an oral, monobacterial whole-cell, killed, nontypeable *H. influenzae* formulation with placebo on acute exacerbations in chronic bronchitis (30). While there was a trend for the vaccine to reduce the incidence and severity of bronchitic episodes at three and six months after vaccination, none of the results reached statistical significance, and results were heterogeneous.

## V. Other Immunostimulants

There have been a number of oral bacterial extracts developed with the aim of stimulating the immune system via the mucosa to prevent infection. A systematic review evaluated 13 RCTs involving approximately 2000 subjects taking agents such as OM-85 BV, LW-50020 or SL-04, or placebo (31). The reviewers found the methodological quality of the included studies was poor and results heterogeneous; signs that any findings should be interpreted with caution. On the basis of three studies, it was seen that there was no difference between the use of active extracts and placebo for the prevention of exacerbation; RR $= 0.66$; 95% CI, 0.41–1.08. There was a significant reduction in exacerbation duration of about three days with active extracts compared with placebo. While skin itching, cutaneous eruptions, or urologic problems were experienced significantly more by those receiving bacterial extracts than those receiving placebo, there was no increase in other major adverse events. Since that review was undertaken, there have been further two RCTs of oral bacterial extracts; one with OM-85 (32) showing a 23% reduction in acute exacerbations with the active treatment ($p = 0.03$), and the other with AM3 showing no difference in exacerbation frequency between treatment and control groups (33).

## VI. Conclusion

The strength of evidence and cost savings for inactivated influenza vaccination mandate a redoubling of efforts to ensure a near-to-universal coverage for people with COPD, especially those with severe disease and/or in long-term care. Instead of further RCTs of effectiveness of this vaccine, research should focus on improving coverage rates and boosting the immunological responses to the vaccine. People in the developing world will carry a disproportionate burden of COPD in the next few decades, and the particular difficulties of distributing a refrigerated vaccine cannot be underestimated.

Other immunological interventions, while safe and relatively cheap, have not yet been shown to prevent exacerbations of COPD. The lack of evidence for injectable and oral vaccines against respiratory bacteria suggests two possibilities either the studies have been underpowered to detect any differences in exacerbations or pneumonia; or the vaccines are not sufficiently immunogenic. Before deciding whether or not they have any place in COPD management, a two-pronged approach seems necessary:

1. To better understand the mechanisms and immunogenicities of vaccines, specifically in COPD patients;
2. To conduct larger clinical trials with clinically relevant endpoints, such as exacerbations.

If new immunological interventions or vaccinations are developed, for example, against agents such as rhinovirus or respiratory syncytial virus, these should be subject to large, well-conducted RCTs, specifically in people with COPD, before they are recommended by public health authorities or in guidelines.

## References

1. Neuzil K, O'Connor T, Gorse G, et al. Recognizing influenza in older patients with chronic obstructive pulmonary disease who have received influenza vaccine. Clin Infect Dis 2003; 36(2): 169–174. (Epub 2003, Jan 8).
2. Wongsurakiat P, Maranetra K, Wasi C, et al. Acute respiratory illness in patients with COPD and the effectiveness of influenza vaccination: a randomized controlled study. Chest 2004; 125:2011–2020.
3. Patriarcha P. A randomized controlled trial of influenza vaccine in the elderly. JAMA 1994; 272 (21):1700–1701.
4. The Nasal-Spray Flu Vaccine (Live Attenuated Influenza Vaccine [LAIV]). Available at: http://www.cdc.gov/flu/about/qa/nasalspray.htm. Accessed June 2008.
5. Gross P, Hermogenes A, Sacks H, et al. The efficacy of influenza vaccine in elderly persons. Ann Intern Med 1995; 123:518–527.

6. Nichol K, Wuorenma J, von Sternberg T. Benefits of influenza vaccination for low-, intermediate-, and high-risk senior citizens. Arch Intern Med 1998; 158:1769–1776.

7. Nichol K, Baken L, Nelson A. Relation between influenza vaccination and outpatient visits, hospitalization, and mortality in elderly persons with chronic lung disease. Ann Intern Med 1999; 130:397–403.

8. Ortqvist A, Granath F, Askling J, et al. Influenza vaccination and mortality in elderly subjects: prospective cohort study of the elderly in a large geographical area. Eur Respir J 2007; 30:414–422.

9. Rivetti D, Jefferson T, Thomas R, et al. Vaccines for preventing influenza in the elderly. Cochrane Database Syst Rev 2006; 3:CD004876.

10. Jefferson T. Influenza vaccination: policy versus evidence. BMJ 2006; 333:912–915.

11. Poole P, Chacko E, Wood-Baker R, et al. Influenza vaccine for patients with chronic obstructive pulmonary disease. Cochrane Database Syst Rev 2006; 1:CD002733.

12. Fell P, O'Donnell H, Watson N, et al. Longer term effects of live influenza vaccine in patients with chronic pulmonary disease. Lancet 1977; 1(8025):1282–1284.

13. Howells C, Tyler L. Prophylactic use of influenza vaccine in patients with chronic bronchitis. A pilot trial. Lancet 1961; 2:1428–1432.

14. Gorse G, Otto E, Daughaday C, et al. Influenza virus vaccination of patients with chronic lung disease. Chest 1997; 112(5):1221–1233.

15. Gorse G, O'Connor T, Young S, et al. Efficacy trial of live, cold-adapted and inactivated influenza virus vaccines in older adults with chronic obstructive pulmonary disease: a VA cooperative study. Vaccine 2003; 21:2133–2144.

16. Advisory Group on Pulmonary Function Tests in Relation to Live Influenza Virus Vaccines. A study of live influenza virus vaccine in patients with chronic bronchitis. Report to Medical Research Council's committee on influenza and other respiratory virus vaccines. Br J Dis Chest 1980; 74(2):121–127.

17. Govaert M, Dinant G, Aretz K, et al. Adverse reactions to influenza vaccine in elderly people: randomised double blind placebo controlled trial. BMJ 1993; 307:988–990.

18. Wongsurakiat P, Maranetra K, Gulprasutdilog P, et al. Adverse effects associated with influenza vaccination in patients with COPD: a randomized controlled study. Respirology 2004; 9:550–556.

19. Advisory Committee on Immunization Practices (ACIP). Prevention and control of influenza: recommendations of the Advisory Committee on Immunization Practices (ACIP). Morbidity & Mortality Weekly Report 1999; 48(RR-4):1–28.

20. Wang C, Wang S, Chou P. Efficacy and cost-effectiveness of influenza vaccination of the elderly in a densely populated and unvaccinated community. Vaccine 2002; 20(19–20):2494–2499.

21. Wongsurakiat P, Lertakyamanee J, Maranetra K, et al. Economic evaluation of influenza vaccination in Thai chronic obstructive pulmonary disease patients. J Med Assoc Thai 2003; 86(6): 497–508.

22. Lee T, Weaver F, Weiss K. Impact of pneumococcal vaccination on pneumonia rates in patients with COPD and asthma. JGIM 2007; 22:62–67.

23. Centers for Disease Control and Prevention. Prevention of pneumococcal disease: recommendations of the Advisory Committee on Immunization Practices (ACIP). MMWR 1995; 44: 561–563.

24. Granger R, Walters J, Poole P, et al. Injectable vaccines for preventing pneumococcal infection in patients with chronic obstructive pulmonary disease. Cochrane Database Syst Rev 2006; 4: CD001390.

25. Davis A, Aranda C, Schiffman G, et al. Pneumococcal infection and immunologic response to pneumococcal vaccine in chronic obstructive pulmonary desease. A pilot study. Chest 1987; 92(2): 204–212.

26. Leech J, Gervais A, Ruben F. Efficacy of pneumococcal vaccine in severe chronic obstructive pulmonary disease. CMAJ 1987; 136(4):361–365.

27. Alfageme I, Vazquez R, Reyes N, et al. Clinical efficacy of anti-pneumococcal vaccination in patients with COPD. Thorax 2006; 61:189–195.
28. Steentoft J, Konradsen H, Hilskov J, et al. Response to pneumococcal vaccine in chronic obstructive lung disease - the effect of ongoing, systemic steroid treatment. Vaccine 2006; 24:1408–1412.
29. Fine M, Smith M, Carson C, et al. Efficacy of pneumococcal vaccination in adults; a meta-analysis of randomized controlled trials. Arch Intern Med 1994; 154:2666–2677.
30. Foxwell A, Cripps A, Dear K. Haemophilus influenzae oral whole cell vaccination for preventing acute exacerbations of chronic bronchitis. Cochrane Database Syst Rev 2006; 4:CD001958.
31. Steurer-Stey C, Bachmann L, Steurer J, et al. Oral purified bacterial extracts in chronic bronchitis and COPD: systematic review. Chest 2004; 126:1645–1655.
32. Solèr M, Mütterlein R, Cozma G, et al. Double-blind study of OM-85 in patients with chronic bronchitis or mild chronic obstructive pulmonary disease. Respiration 2007; 74(1):26–32. (Epub 2006, Jun 12).
33. Alvarez-Mon M, Miravitlles M, Morera J, et al. Treatment with the immunomodulator AM3 improves the health-related quality of life of patients with COPD. Chest 2005; 127:1212–1218.

# 34
## Oxygen Therapy and Home Mechanical Ventilation

**NATHANIEL MARCHETTI and GERARD J. CRINER**
Division of Pulmonary and Critical Care Medicine, Temple University School
of Medicine, Philadelphia, Pennsylvania, U.S.A.

## I. Introduction

Chronic obstructive pulmonary disease (COPD) is a common, chronic, and disabling disease with significant morbidity and mortality. Much of the associated morbidity and mortality of COPD is a direct consequence of exacerbations of the disease. Additionally, COPD is extremely costly to the health care system with direct costs in the United States estimated to be $21.8 billion annually (1). COPD exacerbations are extremely costly and account for 35% to 68% of the total direct cost of COPD in the United States (2,3). In the United Kingdom alone, more than £235 million is spent on COPD exacerbations per year (4). Because of the high cost of COPD exacerbations, both clinical and financial, there is great interest in preventing exacerbations from occurring in the first place. The focus of this chapter is to review the role of oxygen and mechanical ventilation in preventing and treating COPD exacerbations.

## II. Oxygen Therapy

Oxygen therapy is the commonly prescribed therapy for COPD. Approximately, 800,000 patients were prescribed home oxygen therapy in the United States in 1993 at a cost of $1.2 billion annually (5). The use of oxygen in COPD has been shown to prolong life (6,7) and to improve exercise performance, dyspnea, and neurocognitive function (8,9). The indications for oxygen use in COPD, shown in Table 1, are based on the Nocturnal Oxygen Therapy Trial (7) and subsequent consensus conferences on the use of oxygen in COPD (10). The utility of oxygen to prevent COPD exacerbations has not been directly addressed in randomized controlled study because of the potential ethical concerns of withholding oxygen from hypoxemic patients. Despite these potential ethical concerns, there is some indirect evidence that the use of oxygen may prevent exacerbations, or at least severe exacerbations, that require hospital admission. One of the initial studies to report a decrease in hospital admissions was by Stewart et al. (11) who studied the long-term effect of oxygen therapy in 12 men with advanced COPD [mean forced expiratory volume in one second ($FEV_1$) 0.68 L ± 0.15] and hypoxemia ($PaO_2 \leq 55$ mm Hg). In order to be included in the study, subjects had to show improvement in hypoxemia and exercise tolerance while

**Table 1** Indications for Long-Term Oxygen Use

| Length of oxygen use | Indication |
| --- | --- |
| Continuous | $PaO_2 \leq 55$ mm Hg or $O_2$ saturation $< 88\%$ |
| | $PaO_2$ 56–59 mm Hg or $O_2$ saturation 89% with any of following: |
| | Lower extremity edema suggesting cor pulmonale |
| | P pulmonale on ECG |
| | Hematocrit above 56% |
| During exercise | $PaO_2 \leq 55$ mm Hg or $O_2$ saturation $< 88\%$ with minimal exertion |
| During sleep | $PaO_2 \leq 55$ mm Hg or $O_2$ saturation $< 88\%$ with associated symptoms |
| | Pulmonary hypertension |
| | Daytime somnolence |
| | Cardiac arrhythmias |

*Abbreviation*: ECG, electrocardiogram.

using oxygen at 2 liters per minute (LPM) via nasal cannula. Patients were asked to wear oxygen continuously, and they underwent treatment for a mean duration of 25.2 months with a range of 4–40 months. During the first year of receiving continuous oxygen, patients exhibited a 14.8 (SD not provided by the investigators) day reduction in hospitalization days compared with the year preceding oxygen initiation. This effect appeared to be cumulative as there was 16.4 and 28.8 day reduction in hospitalization duration at years 2 and 3, respectively. Garcia-Aymerich et al. performed a case control study designed to determine which factors are most responsible to trigger a hospitalization for COPD exacerbation (12). They included 86 COPD patients (70 ± 8 years; $FEV_1$ 34% ± 16) and 86 control patients (69 ± 9 years; $FEV_1$ 43% ± 19). They found that a lower $FEV_1$, more than three prior admissions for COPD, and underprescription of long-term oxygen therapy (LTOT) were independently associated with an increased risk for hospitalization to treat a COPD exacerbation. Underprescription of LTOT, defined as having a $PaO_2$ less than or equal to 55 mm Hg without a prescription for oxygen, had the highest-adjusted risk associated with admission for a COPD exacerbation [OR 26.92 (1.89–382.9); $p = 0.015$] (12). However, appropriate oxygen use ($PaO_2 < 60$ mm Hg) or, conversely, inappropriate use ($PaO_2 > 60$ mm Hg) was not protective against admission for COPD exacerbation. It is possible that patients underprescribed oxygen, defined as having a $PaO_2$ less than or equal to 55 mm Hg without a prescription for oxygen, were also underprescribed other medications or did not have equal access to health care that may have also contributed to the need for hospitalization to treat an exacerbation. The same authors also followed 340 patients who had been admitted for a COPD exacerbation for 410 ± 181 days to understand the risk factors for readmission to the hospital for COPD management (13). They found that patients with a lower $PaO_2$ had an increased risk for hospital readmission, but using LTOT did not protect against readmission for exacerbation management.

Ringbaek et al. (13) also studied the effect of LTOT on hospital admission rate in 246 COPD patients; 162 that used oxygen for more than or equal to 15 hr/day [continuous oxygen therapy (COT)] and 84 that used oxygen for less than or equal to 15 hr/day [noncontinuous oxygen therapy (NCOT)] were included in the study. They examined hospital admission rates and hospitalization days for a 10-month period prior to and following the initiation of oxygen therapy. Among all 246 patients, LTOT reduced hospital admission rates by 23.8%, hospitalization days by 43.5%, and the number of patients undergoing at least one hospitalization by 31.2% (14). Whether patients were on COT or NCOT did not matter as both groups had a reduction in hospitalization days and the number of patients with one hospitalization. However, only those receiving COT had a significant reduction in the total number of admissions.

Not all studies support the notion that oxygen use decreases either the number of COPD exacerbations or the number of hospital admissions related to COPD. The British Medical Research Council (MRC) domiciliary study not only sought to examine the effect of oxygen use on mortality but also looked at hospital admissions as a secondary endpoint (6). The patients studied all had advanced obstructive lung disease, ($FEV_1$ 0.58–0.76 L), hypoxemia ($PaO_2$ 49.4–51.8 mm Hg), and hypercapnia ($PaCO_2$ 53.2–54.9 mm Hg). The major finding of the study was that the mortality in the control group was significantly higher with 30 of 45 (66%) patients dying as compared with 19 of 42 (45%) dying in the oxygen group. Despite the improvement in mortality, there was no difference in the number of days patients spent in the hospital due to exacerbations of COPD (6). One possible explanation provided by the authors was that patients were followed more closely than normally and likely had earlier admission for treatment of any exacerbation.

Kessler et al. studied a series of 64 COPD patients (age 63.5 ± 9 years, $FEV_1$ 39 ± 20% predicted) prospectively to determine the predictive factors for hospitalization due to a COPD exacerbation (15). All subjects had right heart catheterization, 10 patients were on LTOT for at least 16 hr/day, and 5 were treated with nocturnal oxygen. Patients were followed for an average of 30 months, and 45% of patients required hospitalization for treatment of an exacerbation. Patients admitted were hypoxemic ($PaO_2$ 55 ± 15 mm Hg) and hypercapnic ($PaCO_2$ 61 ± 22 mm Hg). Univariate analysis showed that LTOT was a significant risk for admission with 38.5 ± 13% of patients on LTOT being free from hospitalization at one year; while 77 ± 6% of patients not on LTOT were free from hospitalization at one year ($p = 0.01$) (15). However, a Cox proportional hazards model revealed that only a $PaCO_2$ above 44 mm Hg and a mean pulmonary artery pressure greater than 18 mm Hg were independent predictors of hospitalization, suggesting that the patients treated with LTOT were also more hypercapnic with higher mean pulmonary artery pressures.

## A. Potential Adverse Effects of Oxygen

The most significant adverse effects of oxygen are the potential for worsening hypercapnia and the possibility of increased oxidative stress leading to airway inflammation. Hypercapnia is a significant concern in this patient population, as it has been associated with increased mortality in COPD patients both in the stable and exacerbated state (6,16,17). Furthermore, the level of $PaCO_2$ has been found to be an independent predictor of hospitalization, secondary to an acute exacerbation (15). Initially, the increase in $PaCO_2$ was felt to be due to the loss of hypoxic ventilatory drive, but other mechanisms clearly contribute. Aubier et al. administered 100% oxygen to COPD patients in respiratory failure noninvasively and found that the minute ventilation ($V_E$) did fall 18% below the baseline $V_E$ (18). Although the $V_E$ returned nearly to normal after 15 minutes, the $PaCO_2$ still rose by 23 mm Hg. The authors found that 22% of the increase was secondary to the decrease in $V_E$, and 30% was due to the Haldane effect, which occurs because oxyhemoglobin reduces the affinity of hemoglobin to bind $CO_2$, thus shifting the $CO_2$ hemoglobin dissociation curve to the right. The majority of the hypercapnia (48%) was due to increased dead space ventilation. Hyperoxia results in release of hypoxic vasoconstriction, which ultimately causes slightly worsened ventilation/perfusion matching, thereby increasing dead space.

## B. Increased Oxidative Stress and Inflammation Secondary to Oxygen Use

COPD exacerbations are recognized as inflammatory events, and many investigators have found inflammatory markers to be elevated both locally in the lung and systemically (19–24). There is further evidence from animal studies that hyperoxia results in increased cell apoptosis (25) and the production of reactive oxygen species (26). Both cell apoptosis and the production of reactive oxygen species could theoretically lead to an inflammatory response. Phillips et al. studied the effect of oxygen delivered via nasal cannula at 2 LPM on exhaled markers of oxidative stress in normal subjects and found that they were significantly elevated (27). In both normal subjects and COPD patients breathing 28% oxygen for one hour, evidence of increased oxidative stress and inflammation (IL-6 levels) in exhaled breath condensates have been reported (28). However, short-term oxygen (1 hour at 4 LPM) has been reported in nine muscle-wasted normoxemic COPD patients to actually reduce plasma markers of oxidative stress and inflammation at rest and following exercise (29).

## III. Home Mechanical Ventilation

### A. Noninvasive Positive Pressure Ventilation

Noninvasive positive pressure ventilation (NPPV) is an effective and widely accepted therapy in the treatment of COPD exacerbations that has been well studied in the acute setting. A recent meta-analysis comparing eight randomized controlled trials of NPPV to standard medical care has demonstrated that NPPV decreased pH, $PaCO_2$, and respiratory rate within the first hour of use (30). More importantly, NPPV reduced mortality, intubation rate, treatment failure rate, hospital stay, and associated complications. The natural progression would be to extend the use of NPPV to the outpatient setting, but the evidence supporting its use has been inconsistent. NPPV would be expected to reduce the number of exacerbations because of its ability to reduce hypercapnia, unload respiratory muscles, decrease end-expiratory lung volumes, and reset central respiratory drive (31). Particularly interesting is the reduction in $PaCO_2$, because the $PaCO_2$ has been shown to be a predictor of admission for COPD exacerbation as well as mortality (6,15–17).

Leger et al. retrospectively reviewed their single center experience with 276 patients treated (50 from COPD) with nocturnal NPPV for hypercapnia secondary to a variety of illnesses (32). Patients were referred on the basis of development of acute hypercapnic respiratory failure or if they had repeated exacerbations of chronic respiratory failure despite therapy. Most of the COPD patients (88%) were also being treated with LTOT and had a $PaO_2$ of $47 \pm 7$ mm Hg with a $PaCO_2$ of $53 \pm 9$ mm Hg on room air. In the COPD patients that died or were converted to invasive mechanical ventilation within two years, there was no difference in hospital days during the study period as compared with the time prior to NPPV initiation. However, in the 15 patients that were able to tolerate the NPPV for at least two years, there was a significant decline in the number of hospitalizations during the first year ($49 \pm 51$ vs. $17 \pm 22$ days; $p < 0.002$), but not the second year ($49 \pm 51$ vs.

$25 \pm 51$ days, $p = $ ns). It is possible that the patients that tolerated NPPV for the two years were not as ill as those that died or were switched to invasive mechanical ventilation, thus explaining why there was a decrease in hospital days during the first year. A prospective descriptive study of NPPV use in Geneva included 211 patients treated for chronic respiratory failure with NPPV for a variety of diagnoses, of which 58 had COPD (51 emphysema or chronic bronchitis, 4 bronchiectasis, and 3 cystic fibrosis) (33). The patients with COPD were aged $63 \pm 13$ years with an $FEV_1$ of $29 \pm 14\%$ predicted and used NPPV an average of $6.6 \pm 3.9$ hr/day. Hospital admissions secondary to cardiac or respiratory illness were available for only 24 patients being treated for COPD. Compared with the number of hospital days in the year preceding initiation of NPPV ($42 \pm 9$ days, 24 patients), there was a decrease in hospital days during the first year ($22 \pm 5$ days, $p = 0.02$, 24 patients), the second year ($22 \pm 7$ days, $p = 0.03$, 18 patients), but not the third year ($37 \pm 14$ days, $p = 0.3$, 12 patients), following the initiation of NPPV.

Jones et al. studied 11 patients ($60 \pm 10$ years with an $FEV_1$ $34.5 \pm 11.2\%$ predicted) that developed symptomatic hypercapnia after initiating LTOT to maintain an arterial saturation greater than 90% (34). Patients were electively admitted to the hospital for titration of NPPV and then discharged to home once they were comfortable with the therapy and the desired treatment effect on diurnal measurement of $PaCO_2$. There was a significant improvement in both the $PaO_2$ and $PaCO_2$ after 6, 12, and 24 months of therapy. The investigators also compared the number of admissions and visits with a general practice physician during the one year preceding initiation of NPPV to the year following initiation and found that there were less admissions and visits to the general practitioner. The small number of patients and lack of a control group limit the generalization of these results.

None of the previously mentioned studies were primarily designed to assess the effect of NPPV on hospital admissions specifically due to exacerbations nor did they address COPD exacerbations that were treated as an outpatient. To date, there have been two studies published that attempted to answer this question directly. Casanova et al. prospectively randomized 52 patients to nocturnal NPPV plus standard therapy or standard therapy alone with the primary outcomes being the effect on rate of COPD exacerbations, hospital admissions, intubations, as well as mortality at 3, 6, and 12 months (35). All patients were maximally treated with bronchodilators, oxygen when clinically indicated, and were stable at the time of enrollment (no acute exacerbation in the preceding 3 months). NPPV was initiated as an inpatient and was titrated until there was less accessory muscle use, less dyspnea, and a 20% fall in the respiratory rate. Twenty-six patients were randomized to each treatment arm but six patients from the treatment group and two from the control group dropped out of the study because of an inability to tolerate NPPV (5 patients) or because of new echocardiographic findings (3 patients). There was only one female enrolled, and all patients were Caucasian. The NPPV group was significantly younger ($64 \pm 5$ vs. $68 \pm 4$ years, $p = 0.005$), but there was no difference in $FEV_1$ ($29 \pm 8\%$ predicted in NPPV and $31 \pm 7\%$ in the controls) or the level of hypercapnia ($50.7 \pm 7.9$ mm Hg in NPPV and $53.2 \pm 8.6$ mm Hg) at baseline. After three months of therapy, there were less hospital admissions and endotracheal intubations, but this difference was not statistically significant (Fig. 1). There was no difference at 6 or 12 months in the number of acute exacerbations, hospital admissions, or episodes of tracheal intubation. Additionally, there was no difference in mortality at 3, 6, or 12 months.

Clini et al. published the largest prospective multicenter randomized controlled trial comparing NPPV and usual care to usual care alone (36). All patients had stable COPD,

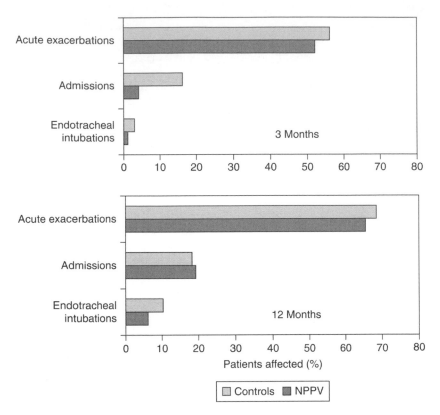

**Figure 1** Long-term outcome of patients treated with NPPV plus standard care versus standard care alone. There was no statistical difference at 3 or 12 months in acute exacerbations, hospital admissions, or endotracheal intubations. *Abbreviation*: NPPV, noninvasive positive pressure ventilation. *Source*: From Ref. 35.

were hypercapnic, and were treated maximally with bronchodilators. Initially, 122 patients were recruited for the study, but after a one-month run, 32 of the patients failed to meet the inclusion criteria. Forty-three patients were randomized to the NPPV + LTOT group, but four dropped out of the study early, leaving 39 subjects. The remaining 47 subjects were randomized to the LTOT group. Patients were followed every three months for two years, and only 23 patients remained in the NPPV + LTOT group, while 24 remained in the LTOT control group. There was no difference in baseline characteristics between the NPPV (64 ± 7 years, $FEV_1$ 27 ± 8% predicted, $PaCO_2$ 54.0 ± 4.5 mm Hg) and the LTOT (66 ± 14 years, $FEV_1$ 31 ± 11% predicted, $PaCO_2$ 55.5 ± 45 mm Hg) treatment groups. The NPPV group was treated for 9 ± 2 hours per night with an average inspiratory positive airway pressure (IPAP) of 14 ± 3 and an EPAP of 2 ± 1 cm $H_2O$, and there was no difference in LTOT use between groups (19 ± 1 hours in NPPV and 20 ± 2 hours in LTOT group). The $PaCO_2$, dyspnea at rest, and quality of life scores were improved in the NPPV group, but there was no difference in lung function, sleep quality, exercise tolerance, or survival. Furthermore, there was no difference in the number of hospital admissions or ICU

**Table 2**   Comparison of Randomized Controlled Trials in NPPV and COPD Exacerbations

| Study | $n$ at start | $n$ at study end | FEV$_1$ (%) predicted | IPAP cm H$_2$O EPAP cm H$_2$O | Duration NPPV | Outcome |
|---|---|---|---|---|---|---|
| Casanova | 52 | 44 | 29 ± 8 NPPV arm | 12 ± 2 | 1 yr | [a]Decreased admissions at 3 mo |
| | | | 31 ± 7 controls | All set at 4 | | No difference at 6 or 12 mo |
| Clini | 90 | 47 | 27 ± 8 NPPV arm | 14 ± 3 | 2 yr | No difference in hospital admissions |
| | | | 31 ± 11 controls | 2 ± 1 | | |

[a]not statistically significant.

*Abbreviations*: FEV$_1$, forced expiratory volume in one second; IPAP, inspiratory positive airway pressure; EPAP, expiratory positive airway pressure, NPPV, noninvasive positive pressure ventilation.

admissions between the two groups. When the average number of hospital days over the three years prior to enrollment was compared with the number of hospital days after enrollment, the NPPV group did have a reduction (from 19.9 ± 0.2 to 13.6 ± 18.3 day/yr), but it was not statistically significant.

Table 2 compares the two randomized controlled trials addressing NPPV and COPD exacerbations. Despite two well-done randomized controlled studies examining the role of NPPV in the prevention of COPD exacerbations, questions still remain. Neither study mentions specific pharmacologic therapies (inhaled corticosteroid or long-acting anticholinergics), which have been shown to reduce COPD exacerbations in their own right that patients in either treatment arm may have taken (37–39). Furthermore, both studies lost a substantial number of patients who had difficulty tolerating NPPV for an extended period of time, which has been previously reported (40). Clini et al. did not record the number of COPD exacerbations that may have been treated as an outpatient, which may have been a significant number of subjects, and finally, neither study accounted for the possibility that the COPD exacerbations that did occur may have been less intense and easier to treat in the patients treated with NPPV. In order to fully answer whether or not NPPV can reduce COPD exacerbations, large multicentered trials will be required to account for the previously discussed confounding variables.

### Complications of NPPV

Complications of NPPV are very frequent and can be divided into problems related to the mask, air pressure, or air leaks (most common) (31). Mask-related problems include facial skin erythema, nasal bridge ulceration, acneiform rash, and claustrophobia. Air pressure issues include nasal congestion, sinus/ear pain, oral dryness, eye irritation, and gastric distension. Fortunately, major complications (aspiration, pneumothorax, and hypotension) are rare and more likely to occur in the acutely hospitalized patient.

### B. Invasive Mechanical Ventilation

Chronic home invasive mechanical ventilation via a tracheostomy has become less commonly used because of the recognition of significant complications and the availability of effective noninvasive ventilation. The French, who have a developed system of caring for mechanically ventilated patients at home, have provided much of the outcome data with this mode of ventilation in COPD and chronic respiratory failure (41). Muir et al. published their experience with 259 severe COPD patients that were mechanically ventilated via a tracheostomy for at least one year (42). These patients (63.3 ± 8.7 years) were severely obstructed ($FEV_1$ 0.73 ± 0.5 L) and hypercapnic ($PaCO_2$ 56.01 ± 8.5 mm Hg). Most of the patients (82%) were able to go home, with the majority unable to return home because of social reasons rather than a medical cause. The investigators also reported the number of hospital days per patient per year and found that the hospital days were highest during the first year following tracheostomy (40.9 day/patient/yr) and decreased during years 2 and 3 (29.8 and 22.8 day/patient/yr). However, by year 5 the number of hospital days had returned to what the rate was during the first year following tracheostomy. These data are limited by the lack of a control group, the fact that information is available for only 74 of the 259 patients, and the reason for admission is not provided.

### Complications of Invasive Mechanical Ventilation

Complications related to invasive mechanical ventilation have been extensively reviewed and can range from mild to severe (43). Muir et al. reported a 6% incidence in pneumothorax and a 4% incidence in ventilator failure occurring at home, but also reported significant complications related to tracheostomy (42). The most common complications were tracheal stenosis, tracheal granulomas, tracheal hemorrhage, and ulceration. Other complications include nosocomial infections (often with resistant organisms, impairment of cardiac function, respiratory muscle dysfunction, immobility, swallowing dysfunction, and speech impediment) (43). Many patients are most disturbed by the loss of basic human tasks such as eating and speaking.

## IV.  Conclusion

Clearly, both oxygen therapy and mechanical ventilation have an important role in reducing COPD mortality, reducing dyspnea, improving gas exchange, and improving the overall quality of life in patients suffering from COPD when clinically indicated. These modalities may even reduce the rate of COPD exacerbations, and there is some indirect evidence to suggest that they do. However, at this point in time neither oxygen nor the initiation of home mechanical ventilation can be recommended to reduce the number of COPD exacerbations. Further, more definitive large multicenter and even international clinical trials are required before using these potentially harmful therapies solely to reduce the frequency or severity of exacerbations.

### References

1.  Miller JD, Foster T, Boulanger L, et al. Direct costs of COPD in the U.S.: an analysis of Medical Expenditure Panel Survey (MEPS) data. COPD 2005; 2(3):311–318.
2.  Andersson F, Borg S, Jansson SA, et al. The costs of exacerbations in chronic obstructive pulmonary disease (COPD). Respir Med 2002; 96(9):700–708.

3. Strassels SA, Smith DH, Sullivan SD, et al. The costs of treating COPD in the United States. Chest 2001; 119(2):344–352.
4. Wedzicha JA, Seemungal TA. COPD exacerbations: defining their cause and prevention. Lancet 2007; 370(9589):786–796.
5. O'Donohue WJ Jr., Plummer AL. Magnitude of usage and cost of home oxygen therapy in the United States. Chest 1995; 107(2):301–302.
6. Long term domiciliary oxygen therapy in chronic hypoxic cor pulmonale complicating chronic bronchitis and emphysema. Report of the Medical Research Council Working Party. Lancet 1981; 1(8222):681–686.
7. Continuous or nocturnal oxygen therapy in hypoxemic chronic obstructive lung disease: a clinical trial. Nocturnal Oxygen Therapy Trial Group. Ann Intern Med 1980; 93(3):391–398.
8. O'Donnell DE, D'Arsigny, Webb KA. Effects of hyperoxia on ventilatory limitation during exercise in advanced chronic obstructive pulmonary disease. Am J Respir Crit Care Med 2001; 163(4):892–898.
9. Lane R, Cockcroft A, Adams L, et al. Arterial oxygen saturation and breathlessness in patients with chronic obstructive airways disease. Clin Sci (Lond) 1987; 72(6):693–698.
10. Petty TL, Casaburi R. Recommendations of the Fifth Oxygen Consensus Conference. Writing and Organizing Committees. Respir Care 2000; 45(8):957–961.
11. Stewart BN, Hood CI, Block AJ. Long-term results of continuous oxygen therapy at sea level. Chest 1975; 68(4):486–492.
12. Garcia-Aymerich J, Monso E, Marrades RM, et al. Risk factors for hospitalization for a chronic obstructive pulmonary disease exacerbation. EFRAM study. Am J Respir Crit Care Med 2001; 164(6):1002–1007.
13. Garcia-Aymerich J, Farrero E, Felez MA, et al. Risk factors of readmission to hospital for a COPD exacerbation: a prospective study. Thorax 2003; 58(2):100–105.
14. Ringbaek TJ, Viskum K, Lange P. Does long-term oxygen therapy reduce hospitalisation in hypoxaemic chronic obstructive pulmonary disease? Eur Respir J 2002; 20(1):38–42.
15. Kessler R, Faller M, Fourgaut G, et al. Predictive factors of hospitalization for acute exacerbation in a series of 64 patients with chronic obstructive pulmonary disease. Am J Respir Crit Care Med 1999; 159(1):158–164.
16. Seneff MG, Wagner DP, Wagner RP, et al. Hospital and 1-year survival of patients admitted to intensive care units with acute exacerbation of chronic obstructive pulmonary disease. JAMA 1995; 274(23):1852–1857.
17. France AJ, Prescott RJ, Biernacki W, et al. Does right ventricular function predict survival in patients with chronic obstructive lung disease? Thorax 1988; 43(8):621–626.
18. Aubier M, Murciano D, Milic-Emili J, et al. Effects of the administration of O2 on ventilation and blood gases in patients with chronic obstructive pulmonary disease during acute respiratory failure. Am Rev Respir Dis 1980; 122(5):747–754.
19. Bhowmik A, Seemungal TA, Sapsford RJ, et al. Relation of sputum inflammatory markers to symptoms and lung function changes in COPD exacerbations. Thorax 2000; 55(2):114–120.
20. Drost EM, Skwarski KM, Sauleda J, et al. Oxidative stress and airway inflammation in severe exacerbations of COPD. Thorax 2005; 60(4):293–300.
21. Hurst JR, Perera WR, Wilkinson TM, et al. Systemic and upper and lower airway inflammation at exacerbation of chronic obstructive pulmonary disease. Am J Respir Crit Care Med 2006; 173(1):71–78.
22. Perera WR, Hurst JR, Wilkinson TM, et al. Inflammatory changes, recovery and recurrence at COPD exacerbation. Eur Respir J 2007; 29(3):527–534.
23. Qiu Y, Zhu J, Bandi V, et al. Biopsy neutrophilia, neutrophil chemokine and receptor gene expression in severe exacerbations of chronic obstructive pulmonary disease. Am J Respir Crit Care Med 2003; 168(8):968–975.
24. Saetta M, Di Stefano A, Maestrelli P, et al. Airway eosinophilia in chronic bronchitis during exacerbations. Am J Respir Crit Care Med 1994; 150(6 pt 1):1646–1652.

25. Mantell LL, Lee PJ. Signal transduction pathways in hyperoxia-induced lung cell death. Mol Genet Metab 2000; 71(1–2):359–370.
26. Hitka P, Vizek M, Wilhelm J. Hypoxia and reoxygenation increase H2O2 production in rats. Exp Lung Res 2003; 29(8):585–592.
27. Phillips M, Cataneo RN, Greenberg J, et al. Effect of oxygen on breath markers of oxidative stress. Eur Respir J 2003; 21(1):48–51.
28. Carpagnano GE, Kharitonov SA, Foschino-Barbaro MP, et al. Supplementary oxygen in healthy subjects and those with COPD increases oxidative stress and airway inflammation. Thorax 2004; 59(12):1016–1019.
29. van Helvoort HA, Heijdra YF, Heunks LM, et al. Supplemental oxygen prevents exercise-induced oxidative stress in muscle-wasted patients with chronic obstructive pulmonary disease. Am J Respir Crit Care Med 2006; 173(10):1122–1129.
30. Lightowler JV, Wedzicha JA, Elliott MW, et al. Non-invasive positive pressure ventilation to treat respiratory failure resulting from exacerbations of chronic obstructive pulmonary disease: Cochrane systematic review and meta-analysis. BMJ 2003; 326(7382):185.
31. Mehta S, Hill NS. Noninvasive ventilation. Am J Respir Crit Care Med 2001; 163(2):540–577.
32. Leger P, Bedicam JM, Cornette A, et al. Nasal intermittent positive pressure ventilation. Long-term follow-up in patients with severe chronic respiratory insufficiency. Chest 1994; 105(1): 100–105.
33. Janssens JP, Derivaz S, Breitenstein E, et al. Changing patterns in long-term noninvasive ventilation: a 7-year prospective study in the Geneva Lake area. Chest 2003; 123(1):67–79.
34. Jones SE, Packham S, Hebden M, et al. Domiciliary nocturnal intermittent positive pressure ventilation in patients with respiratory failure due to severe COPD: long-term follow up and effect on survival. Thorax 1998; 53(6):495–498.
35. Casanova C, Celli BR, Tost L, et al. Long-term controlled trial of nocturnal nasal positive pressure ventilation in patients with severe COPD. Chest 2000; 118(6):1582–1590.
36. Clini E, Sturani C, Rossi A, et al. The Italian multicentre study on noninvasive ventilation in chronic obstructive pulmonary disease patients. Eur Respir J 2002; 20(3):529–538.
37. Lung Health Study Research Group. Effect of inhaled triamcinolone on the decline in pulmonary function in chronic obstructive pulmonary disease. N Engl J Med 2000; 343(26):1902–1909.
38. Burge PS, Calverley PM, Jones PW, et al. Randomised, double blind, placebo controlled study of fluticasone propionate in patients with moderate to severe chronic obstructive pulmonary disease: the ISOLDE trial. BMJ 2000; 320(7245):1297–1303.
39. Niewoehner DE, Rice K, Cote C, et al. Prevention of exacerbations of chronic obstructive pulmonary disease with tiotropium, a once-daily inhaled anticholinergic bronchodilator: a randomized trial. Ann Intern Med 2005; 143(5):317–326.
40. Criner GJ, Brennan K, Travaline JM, et al. Efficacy and compliance with noninvasive positive pressure ventilation in patients with chronic respiratory failure. Chest 1999; 116(3):667–675.
41. Simonds AK Long-term ventilation in obstructive ventilatory disorders. Respir Care Clin N Am 2002; 8(4):533–544.
42. Muir JF, Girault C, Cardinaud JP, et al. Survival and long-term follow-up of tracheostomized patients with COPD treated by home mechanical ventilation. A multicenter French study in 259 patients. French Cooperative Study Group. Chest 1994; 106(1):201–209.
43. Chatila WM, Criner GJ. Complications of long-term mechanical ventilation. Respir Care Clin N Am 2002; 8(4):631–647.

# 35
## Design of Trials for COPD Exacerbations

**FERNANDO J. MARTINEZ and MEILAN HAN**
Division of Pulmonary and Critical Care Medicine, Department of Internal Medicine, University of Michigan Health System, Ann Arbor, Michigan, U.S.A.

**JEFFREY L. CURTIS**
Pulmonary and Critical Care Medicine Section, Medical Service, Department of Veterans Affairs Health System and the Division of Pulmonary and Critical Care Medicine, Department of Internal Medicine and the Graduate Program in Immunology, University of Michigan Health System, Veterans Administration Medical Center, Ann Arbor, Michigan, U.S.A.

## I. Introduction

Given the potential importance of acute exacerbations of chronic obstructive pulmonary disease (AECOPD) on disease biology, expression, and progression, properly designed studies are crucial. In general, trials in this arena have focused on the treatment of acute episodes or prevention of future events. There are similar issues in the design of trials for both of these clinical scenarios, including case definition and the modalities used to assess response to therapy. On the other hand, distinct differences exist in the statistical approaches used to power studies and the patient populations examined.

## II. Therapeutic Trials of AECOPD

The majority of therapeutic trials of AECOPD have tested bronchodilators, corticosteroids, or antimicrobial agents. An examination of selected studies highlights some of the persistent controversies in this arena, particularly with respect to case definition and definition of response to therapy.

### A. Case Definition and Selection of Subjects

Current therapeutic trials have used a variety of case definitions that have been adapted for the intervention being tested. For example, studies examining the role of various bronchodilators and corticosteroids generally have included AECOPD as defined by health care use (Table 1). In contrast, studies that have addressed the therapeutic role of antimicrobial agents have generally used the definition promulgated by Anthonisen et al. in their sentinel placebo-controlled study of antimicrobial therapy in AECOPD (1). Those investigators defined an AECOPD on the basis of a combination of symptoms that included increased sputum volume, a change in

**Table 1** Varying Definitions for Acute Exacerbations for Chronic Bronchitis in Selected Interventional and Observational Studies

| Reference | Definition | Basis of definition |
|---|---|---|
| *Interventional Studies* | | |
| Anthonisen et al. (1) | Major: dyspnea, sputum volume, sputum purulence Minor: URTI within last five days, unexplained fever, increased wheeze or cough, increased respiratory rate or heart rate by >20% from baseline | Symptom based |
| Thompson et al. (60) | Subjective worsening of baseline dyspnea or cough for more than 24 hr and necessitating a hospital visit; >25% increase in inhaled β-agonist use for more than 24 hr or an increase in sputum production (more than one-fourth cup per day over baseline) and/or purulence (more than 25 neutrophils/field) | Both event based and symptom based |
| Paggiaro et al. (61) | Worsening of COPD symptoms, requiring changes to normal treatment, including antimicrobial therapy, short courses of oral steroids, and other bronchodilator therapy | Event based |
| Niewoehner et al. (62) | Readmission because of COPD or intensification of pharmacological therapy | Event based |
| Mahler et al. (63) | Worsening of symptoms | Event based |
| Vestbo et al. (64) | More cough and phlegm than usual | Symptom based |
| Burge et al. (65) | Worsening of respiratory symptoms that require treatment with oral steroids or antibiotics or both | Event based |
| Van Noord et al. (66) | Increase in symptoms, requiring oral steroids or antibiotics or hospitalization | Event based |
| Gomez et al. (67) | Anthonisen criteria | Symptom based |
| Kanner et al. (68) | Patient-reported bronchitis, pneumonia, influenza, chest colds with MD visits | Event based |
| Woolhouse et al. (69) | 1 or more of increased dyspnea, increased sputum volume, change in sputum purulence | Symptom based |
| Cazzola et al. (70) | Sustained worsening of patient's condition from stable state and beyond normal day-to-day variations, necessitating change in regular medication | Event based |
| Allegra et al. (32) | Increase of at least 3 points in clinical score based on multiple components (temperature, sputum quantity, sputum purulence, dyspnea, and pulmonary physical findings) | Symptom based |
| Gompertz et al. (71) | A combination of worsening respiratory symptoms (including breathlessness, sputum volume, color or viscosity, cough, wheeze, or chest pain), with or without systemic symptoms (malaise, fever, rigors), that caused the patient to seek medical advice | Both event based and symptom based |
| Suzuki et al. (72) | Acute and sustained worsening of COPD symptoms, requiring changes to regular treatment, including antimicrobial therapy and/or short courses of systemic steroids | Both event based and symptom based |
| ZuWallack et al. (73) | Worsening of symptoms, requiring an increase in drug therapy | Event based |
| Rennard et al. (74) | Worsening of symptoms, requiring an increase in drug therapy | Event based |

**Table 1** Varying Definitions for Acute Exacerbations for Chronic Bronchitis in Selected Interventional and Observational Studies (*Continued*)

| Reference | Definition | Basis of definition |
|---|---|---|
| Vincken et al. (75); Casaburi et al. (76) | New or worsening cough, sputum, dyspnea, or wheeze ≥3 days from adverse event monitoring | Symptom based |
| Rossi et al. (77) | 2 individual symptom scores >2 and reduction in peak expiratory flow (bad days); corticosteroids, antibiotics, or oxygen (moderate); COPD-related hospitalization (severe) | Both event based and symptom based |
| Maltais et al. (78) | Unscheduled visit triggered by an exacerbation of respiratory symptoms, requiring additional respiratory medications. | Both event based and symptom based |
| Jones et al. (50) | Chest problems, requiring treatment with antibiotics and/or oral corticosteroids | Event based |
| Brusasco et al. (76) | Complex of respiratory symptoms (new onset or an increase in at least 1 of cough, sputum, dyspnea, wheeze, chest discomfort) lasting at least 3 days | Symptom based |
| Celli et al. (45) | Worsening symptoms requiring drug therapy | Event based |
| Szafranski et al. (79) | Severe: requirement for oral steroids and/or antibiotics and/or hospitalization due to respiratory symptoms Mild: ≥4 inhalations per day of reliever medication above mean run-in use. | Event based |
| Calverley et al. (80) | Worsening of COPD symptoms, requiring treatment with antibiotics, oral corticosteroids, or both | Event based |
| Calverley et al. (81) | Requiring oral antibiotics and/or corticosteroids or hospitalization | Event based |
| Del Negro et al. (82) | Increased use of salbutamol PRN by >2 occasions/24 hr period on 2 or more consecutive days (mild); treatment with antibiotics and/or oral steroids (moderate); emergency treatment and/or hospitalization (severe) | Event based |
| De Melo et al. (83) | Moderate exacerbation: prescriptions for a systemic antibiotic and an oral corticosteroid on the same day Severe exacerbation: hospitalization with a primary discharge diagnosis of COPD | Event based |
| Decramer et al. (54) | Increase in dyspnea, cough, or both with a change in quality and quantity of sputum that lasted for at least 3 days and led to medical attention | Both event based and symptom based |
| Rabe et al. (84) | Increase in bronchodilator use on 2 or more consecutive days (mild); Home management with oral steroids or unscheduled health care contact or both (moderate); Hospitalization or emergency room treatment (severe) | Event based |
| Wouters et al. (51) | ≥3 salbutamol inhalations of ≥2 days (mild); Required oral steroids (moderate); Required hospitalization (severe) | Event based |
| Niewoehner et al. (59) | More than 1 of the cardinal symptoms (cough, sputum, wheezing, dyspnea, or chest tightness) of at least 3-day duration, requiring treatment with antibiotics or systemic steroids, hospitalizations, or both | Both event based and symptom based |

*(Continued)*

**Table 1** Varying Definitions for Acute Exacerbations for Chronic Bronchitis in Selected Interventional and Observational Studies (*Continued*)

| Reference | Definition | Basis of definition |
|---|---|---|
| Briggs et al. (85) | Complex of respiratory symptoms (new onset or an increase in at least 1 of cough, sputum, dyspnea, wheeze, chest discomfort), lasting at least 3 days | Symptom based |
| Dusser et al. (86) | At least 1 clinical descriptor (worsening dyspnea, cough, or sputum: appearance of sputum purulence; fever (>38°C); new chest radiograph abnormality), lasting >2 days and requiring a new prescription or an increase in bronchodilators, antibiotics, or corticosteroids | Both event based and symptom based |
| Stockley et al. (87) | Worsening symptoms, requiring increased salbutamol alone (mild) Worsening symptoms requiring antibiotics and/or oral steroids or increase inhaled steroids (moderate) | Event based |
| Kardos et al. (55) | Worsening of COPD symptoms that required a change of respiratory medications and medical assistance (moderate); requiring emergency room treatment or hospitalization (severe) | Both event based and symptom based |
| Calverley et al. (88) | Symptomatic deteriorations treated with systemic corticosteroids and/or antibiotics (moderate) or hospitalization (severe) | Event based |
| Calverley et al. (46) | Symptomatic deterioration, requiring treatment with antibiotics, systemic corticosteroids, and/or hospitalizations | Event based |
| Aaron et al. (44) | Sustained worsening of patient's condition from stable state and beyond normal day-to-day variations, necessitating change in regular medication | Both event based and symptom based |
| Wedzicha et al. (89) | Required treatment with oral steroids and/or antibiotics or required hospitalizations. Daily diary card data collected | Event based |
| *Observational studies* | | |
| Seemungal et al. (49); Patel et al. (90); Wilkinson et al. (91); Donaldson et al. (92) | Major: dyspnea, sputum volume, sputum purulence Minor: nasal discharge, wheeze, sore throat, cough, fever AECOPD: 2 major or 1 major/1 minor on 2 consecutive days | Symptom based |
| Adams et al. (93) | Anthonisen criteria | Symptom based |
| Miravittles et al. (94) | The presence of any combination of the following symptoms: increased dyspnea and increased production and purulence of sputum, leading to a change or increase in treatment. Severity was classified using Anthonisen criteria | Event based |
| Sethi et al. (95,96) | Symptoms: dyspnea, cough, sputum production, viscosity, and purulence AECOPD: minor worsening of >2 symptoms or major worsening of 1 symptom | Symptom based |
| Wilson et al. (30) | Anthonisen criteria | Symptom based |

**Table 1** Varying Definitions for Acute Exacerbations for Chronic Bronchitis in Selected Interventional and Observational Studies (*Continued*)

| Reference | Definition | Basis of definition |
|---|---|---|
| Miravitlles et al. (97) | Sustained worsening of the patient's condition, from stable state characterized by the increase of a combination of any 3 cardinal symptoms, including dyspnea, sputum purulence, and sputum volume, that is acute in onset and necessitates a change in regular medication. | Both event based and symptom based |
| Tsoumakidou et al. (52) | Anthonisen criteria | Symptom based |

*Abbreviations*: URTI, upper respiratory tract infection; COPD, chronic obstructive pulmonary disease; MD, doctor of medicine; PRN, pro re nata; AECOPD, acute exacerbations of COPD.
*Source*: From Ref. 43.

sputum characteristics, and an increase in dyspnea. Patients with at least two of these cardinal symptoms experienced a benefit with antibiotic therapy in their study.

Subsequent studies provide support for the use of Anthonisen criteria to determine the need for antibiotic use. Stockley et al. also found that sputum purulence identified AECOPD that were more likely to benefit from antibiotic treatment (2). A multicenter Italian study reported that increasing sputum purulence, as defined by a semiquantitative colorimetric scale, was associated with bacterial growth (3). In addition, deepening sputum color was associated with increased yield of gram-negative organisms, including *Pseudomonas aeruginosa* and *Enterobacteriaceae*. Importantly, without the aid of an objective color stick, the definition of color by subjects and by investigators was concordant in this study in only 68% of cases. Recent bronchoscopic sampling in hospitalized patients with multisymptom AECOPD who were stratified by the Anthonisen criteria also confirmed a greater likelihood of bacterial infection in patients with sputum purulence (4). Collectively, these data imply that development of purulent sputum may identify a patient more likely to benefit from antibiotic therapy, although additional data are required to define how this concept should be used into daily decision making. Despite these uncertainties, numerous major multispecialty societies have already incorporated sputum purulence into guidelines regarding who should be treated with antimicrobial agents (5).

Biomarkers have been highly sought to compliment or replace symptom-based methods of identifying patients in whom bacteria are pathogenic during an AECOPD. Measurement of plasma procalcitonin (PCT) levels has been proposed as a means of defining AECOPD patients with a high likelihood of bacterial infection (6). PCT is a small protein (116 amino acids, 13 kDa), which is normally undetectable in plasma (7), but which increases in bacterial infections. Data from single-center, cluster-randomized, single-blinded studies indicate that PCT-guided therapy can safely reduce antibiotic use in patients with lower respiratory infection at low likelihood of bacterial infection (6,8). Stolz et al. randomized 208 consecutive patients admitted to the hospital with an AECOPD either to usual care (management based on standard criteria without access to PCT levels) or to a PCT-guided group in which antibiotic use was based on PCT level at the time of admission (9). In the PCT-guided therapy group, a level less than 0.1 µg/L was considered to be nonbacterial, and antimicrobial use was discouraged. In those with a PCT level greater than 0.25 µg/L, bacterial infection was felt to be present, and antimicrobial therapy was encouraged. For patients with levels between 0.1 and 0.25 μg/L, the use of antimicrobial agents was based on the clinical situation at admission and during early follow-up. Total antimicrobial use was decreased during the hospitalization (72% in usual care group vs. 40% in PCT-guided therapy), at short-term follow-up and through six months. No differences were noted in clinical success rate during the index hospitalization, antimicrobial use during the subsequent six months, or in time to the next exacerbation. Additional investigation is required to assess whether patients with low PCT levels require antimicrobial therapy and if similar results can be achieved in an optimally designed multicenter trial, in settings less accustomed to use of PCT measurement (10).

## B.  Assessment of Response to Therapy

Historically, response to treatment in clinical trials has been based on a global assessment by the investigator (Table 1). This approach, common to studies of bronchodilators, steroids, and antimicrobials, is a crude measure of treatment response. Increasingly, studies have emphasized alternative objective endpoints, such as rapidity of symptom resolution. This method has been included as a secondary endpoint in several antimicrobial studies, with intriguing findings. It has been found that symptoms resolved more rapidly with quinolones than with comparator agents (11,12). A composite of symptoms (breathlessness, cough, and sputum characteristics) has been claimed to demonstrate objectively the natural history of an AECOPD in therapeutic trials (13). A Food and Drug Administration (FDA)-sponsored group [the EXAcerbations of Chronic pulmonary disease Tool-Patient Reported Outcome (EXACT-PRO) initiative] is in the process of refining a patient-reported instrument to define the longitudinal behavior of an AECOPD, as is reviewed elsewhere in this volume. Universal acceptance of such an instrument would significantly advance the field by permitting comparison of different categories of therapeutic agents that may modify disparate aspects of the exacerbation.

Given the accepted systemic nature of COPD (14), there is considerable interest in whether biomarkers of inflammation could be used as surrogate endpoints in future therapeutic trials. Plasma fibrinogen, IL-6, C-reactive protein (CRP), and endothelin-1 have all been reported to increase during AECOPD (15–18). One prospective study showed that the degree of systemic inflammation, manifested by rising serum IL-6 and CRP levels, correlated significantly with sputum and nasal inflammation (19). The same group examined a large number of plasma biomarkers during 90 distinct AECOPD episodes and found that only CRP seemed to exhibit diagnostic accuracy, particularly when combined with increased dyspnea, sputum volume, or purulence (18). The ability of such biomarker approaches to serve as surrogate markers of treatment response requires additional investigation.

In antimicrobial therapeutic trials, the ability of varying agents to "eradicate" bacteria in sputum samples has been suggested as an alternate outcome. A recent comprehensive review of the literature suggests different results depending on the agent studied (20). In this analysis, there was a small but significant effect size favoring quinolones over macrolides, amoxicillin/clavulanate, and cephalosporins in "eradication" of *Haemophilus influenzae*. Importantly, however, the majority of these cases reflected presumed eradication, because most patients were not producing sputum at the follow-up visit. Interpretation of the non-detection of nontypeable *H. influenzae* is also challenged conceptually by the findings that the organism can persist intracellularly within epithelial cells (21) and that its detection by culture seriously underestimates its persistence as assessed by genetic methods (22). Finally, the entire concept that changes in bacterial load are associated with AECOPD occurrence has been challenged recently (23).

Another way of evaluating the success of antimicrobial agents is the disease-free interval (DFI), i.e., the time between successive exacerbations (24–26). The rationale for this outcome relies on the accepted notion that antimicrobial therapy does not necessarily eradicate pathogens completely and that persistent bacterial colonization is associated with an ongoing inflammatory response (27). Hence, antimicrobials that decrease the bacterial load in the lower airways more successfully should result in greater symptomatic resolution and improved long-term clinical outcomes (25,26). Some recent AECOPD clinical trials have assessed how different antibiotics affect the DFI (12,26). The data have been inconclusive, with some studies suggesting a differential effect between different agents (28–30), while others did not (31). It is likely that some of the discordant findings reflect differences in patient characteristics, including severity of underlying COPD. Additional data are required to better establish this novel endpoint as a primary basis for future comparative studies.

### Concomitant Therapy and Other Confounding

The severity of underlying airflow obstruction at baseline likely influences the response of AECOPD to therapy. For example, in one of the larger placebo-controlled trials of antimicrobial therapy, the overall clinical response rate clearly varied by the severity of baseline airflow obstruction, as defined by forced expiratory volume in one second ($FEV_1$) (32). The results of this study and another of severe hospitalized AECOPD (33) imply that patients with more severe airflow obstruction at baseline are more likely to respond favorably to antimicrobial therapy than to placebo therapy. Stratification of patients according to the risk of treatment failure has been suggested as a means of guiding antimicrobial choice (34–36). These stratification schemes have generally relied on features for a high likelihood of infection with organisms that are unlikely to respond to standard antibiotic regimens (e.g., *P. aeruginosa*, drug-resistant bacteria) or on host factors that predict treatment failure. The latter include worse lung function, increased frequency of exacerbation/office visits, ischemic heart disease, and other comorbid conditions (37,38). However, prospective data supporting such an approach are quite limited. A recent prospective study confirmed that patients with a complicated AECOPD experienced inferior clinical response rate compared with those with uncomplicated AECOPD (12). Although tailoring the selection of the initial antimicrobial regimen in individuals at increased risk for treatment failure seems promising, it also still requires additional prospective validation.

### C. Trials of AECOPD Prevention

Given the importance of AECOPDs on disease course, including physiology and health status, as reviewed elsewhere in this tome, it is not surprising that prevention of AECOPDs has increasingly become another target of therapeutic intervention. Such studies also raise numerous methodological issues that impact interpretation (39,40). These include varying definitions for individual events, disparate methodologies used to count events, lack of independent adjudication of episodes, and difference in statistical approaches. The implications of these findings on the analytical approach to studies are highlighted elsewhere.

Identification of patients at higher risk of events has been used as an approach to increase the number of events and provide a clearer definition of therapeutic response.

### Case Definition

The available therapeutic trials that have addressed AECOPD prevention have used a variety of case definitions adapted for the intervention being tested (Table 1). As with trials of treatment of acute episodes, both symptom-based and event-based definitions have been employed. Symptom-based definitions have generally used modifications of the criteria defined by Anthonisen et al. (1). Although symptom-based definitions are the most applicable to patient care, some investigators have shown that a significant proportion of patients may not report these symptoms to health care professionals (41). Not surprisingly, perhaps, observational studies that have used this approach to define individual episodes have identified a greater number of events (Table 2).

To circumvent difficulties with quantifying symptom changes, event-based definitions have been used, particularly in therapeutic trials (Table 1). This approach seems to capture a lesser number of events (Table 2). Interestingly, there is variability in the event-based definitions, with some investigators including "bad days" or "mild" AECOPD to reflect events treated with increased bronchodilation. In general, antibiotics and/or corticosteroids in the outpatient setting have been used to define "moderate" events, while emergency room care or COPD-related hospitalizations have been defined as "severe" events. One investigative group recently compared symptom-based definition from daily diary cards to an event-based definition in a large prospective study of an inhaled steroid/long-acting β-agonist study (42). Interestingly, the correlation between the two definitions was quite weak. Accordingly, intensive investigation continues to develop optimal definitions both for clinical use and research studies (43).

If the goal of a prevention trial is to assess change in exacerbation rates, discrete events must be identified (39). However, it may be difficult to identify when one AECOPD has ended and a new one has begun. Recent trials have defined discrete episodes using arbitrary thresholds ranging from 14 to 28 days (44). Importantly, one group has documented that a significant minority of patients have not returned to their baseline health status for up to three months after an AECOPD (defined by symptoms) (41). Several attempts are under way to develop a patient-reported instrument that can track the longitudinal behavior of symptoms during an exacerbation. One such instrument is the Breathlessness, Cough, and Sputum Scale (BCSS) (13). In three multinational trials, the BCSS demonstrated responsiveness during the natural course of individual events (13). More subtle changes were demonstrated over three months of follow-up in these studies (45). The EXACT-PRO initiative (described elsewhere in this book) is developing a similar multidimensional index that can be used to define discrete events in a clinical trial and to demonstrate responsiveness to intervention.

An alternative and potentially complementary methodology uses an adjudication committee to review data and arbitrate events. This approach has been demonstrated recently to add significant independent value to a large multinational trial, with mortality as the primary endpoint (46). The clinical endpoint committee in this sentinel study identified a cause of death that was equivalent to that provided by the local investigator in only 52% of cases (47). Interestingly, a recent multicenter therapeutic trial with prevention of acute exacerbations as the primary endpoint used a similar approach to adjudicate events (44).

(*text continues on page 403*)

**Table 2** Frequency of AECOPD Episodes Per Year in Selected Observational or Therapeutic Studies

| Reference | n | FEV$_1$ | Previous AECOPD history required? | Therapeutic intervention | Duration of follow-up | Patients withdrawn remained in trial? | AECOPD in previous year | Number of AECOPD/ yr | Proportion with ≥1 AECOPD |
|---|---|---|---|---|---|---|---|---|---|
| *Therapeutic studies* | | | | | | | | | |
| Van Noord et al. (66) | 47 | 41% | No | Salmeterol + ipratropium | 12 wk | Yes | NA | NA | 13% |
| | 47 | 42% | | Salmeterol | | | | | 23% |
| | 50 | 38% | | Placebo | | | | | 36% |
| Kanner et al. (68) | 5887 | 75% | No | Usual care or smoking cessation intervention | 5 yr | | NA | 0.24 MD visits/pt/ yr | |
| ZuWallack et al. (73) | 313 | 40.8% | No | Salmeterol and theophylline | 12 wk | Yes | NA | NA | 13% |
| | 310 | 40.1% | | Salmeterol | | | | | 18% |
| | 315 | 40.7% | | Theophylline | | | | | 20% |
| Rennard et al. (74) | 132 | 1.46 L | No | Salmeterol | 12 wk | No | NA | NA | 28.8% |
| | 138 | 1.52 L | | Ipratropium | | | | | 26.8% |
| | 135 | 1.52 L | | Placebo | | | | | 30.4% |
| Rossi et al. (77) | 214 | 47% | No | Formoterol 24 µg | 1 yr | No | NA | NA | 23% |
| | 211 | 47% | | Formoterol 12 µg | | | | | 32% |
| | 209 | 46% | | Theophylline | | | | | 20% |
| | 220 | 49% | | Placebo | | | | | 34% |
| Vincken et al. (75) | 356 | 41.9% | No | Tiotropium | 1 yr | No | NA | 0.73/pt/yr | 35% |
| | 179 | 39.4% | | Ipratropium | | | | 0.96/pt/yr | 46% |
| Casaburi et al. (76) | 550 | 39.1% | No | Tiotropium | 1 yr | No | NA | 0.76/pt/yr | 5.5%[a] |
| | 371 | 38.1% | | Placebo | | | | 0.95/pt/yr | 9.4%[a] |
| Brusasco et al. (98) | 402 | 39.2% | No | Tiotropium | 6 mo | No | NA | 1.07/pt/yr | 32% |
| | 405 | 37.7% | | Salmeterol | | | | 1.23/pt/yr | 35% |
| | 400 | 38.7% | | Placebo | | | | 1.49/pt/yr | 39% |

*(Continued)*

**Table 2** Frequency of AECOPD Episodes Per Year in Selected Observational or Therapeutic Studies (*Continued*)

| Reference | n | FEV$_1$ | Previous AECOPD history required? | Therapeutic intervention | Duration of follow-up | Patients withdrawn remained in trial? | AECOPD in previous year | Number of AECOPD/yr | Proportion with ≥1 AECOPD |
|---|---|---|---|---|---|---|---|---|---|
| Celli et al. (45) | 543<br>554<br>271 | 42.3%<br>42.1%<br>43.6% | No | Sibenadet<br>Salmeterol<br>Placebo | 12 wk | Unclear | NA | NA | 21.4%<br>17.1%<br>21.9% |
| Jones et al. (50) | 196<br>180<br>195<br>179 | 39%<br>62%<br>39%<br>62% | No | Fluticasone propionate<br>Fluticasone propionate<br>Placebo<br>Placebo | 3 yr | No | NA | 1.47/pt/yr<br>0.99/pt/yr<br>1.75/pt/yr<br>1.32/pt/yr | NA |
| Calverley et al. (80) | 358<br>374<br>372<br>361 | 44.8%<br>45.0%<br>44.3%<br>44.2% | ≥1 AECOPD/yr in each of previous 3 yr; 1 AECOPD in previous year requiring oral steroids, antibiotics, or both | Fluticasone/salmeterol<br>Fluticasone<br>Salmeterol<br>Placebo | 1 yr | No | NA | 0.97/pt/yr<br>1.05/pt/yr<br>1.04/pt/yr<br>1.30/pt/yr | NA |
| Calverley et al. (81) | 254<br>257<br>255<br>256 | 36%<br>36%<br>36%<br>36% | ≥1 AECOPD requiring oral corticosteroids and/or antibiotics in previous year | Budesonide/formoterol<br>Budesonide<br>Formoterol<br>Placebo | 1 yr | No | NA | 1.38/pt/yr<br>1.60/pt/yr<br>1.85/pt/yr<br>1.80/pt/yr | NA |
| Szafranski et al. (79) | 208<br>198<br>201<br>205 | 36%<br>37%<br>36%<br>36% | ≥1 severe AECOPD | Budesonide and formoterol<br>Budesonide<br>Formoterol<br>Placebo | 1 yr | No | NA | 1.42/pt/yr<br>1.59/pt/yr<br>1.84/pt/yr<br>1.87/pt/yr | NA |

| Study | n | % | Inclusion criteria | Treatment | Duration | Dropouts | | | |
|---|---|---|---|---|---|---|---|---|---|
| Dal Negro et al. (82) | 6 | 50% | No | Fluticasone/salmeterol and theophylline | 1 yr | No dropouts | 3.5/pt/yr | 1.2/pt/yr | NA |
| | 6 | 48% | | Salmeterol + theophylline | | | 3.0/pt/yr | 0.9/pt/yr | |
| | 6 | 50% | | Placebo + theophylline | | | 3.2/pt/yr | 4.2/pt/yr | |
| Decramer et al. (99) | 256 | 57% | ≥2 AECOPD/yr during previous 2 yr | N-acetylcysteine | 3 yr | No | 2.4/pt/yr | 1.25/pt/yr | NA |
| | 267 | 57% | | Placebo | | | 2.5/pt/yr | 1.31/pt/yr | |
| Rabe et al. (84) | 555 | 54% | No requirement | Roflumilast 500 µg | 6 mo | No | NA | 0.75/pt/yr | 28% |
| | 576 | 50% | | Roflumilast 250 µg | | | | 1.03/pt/yr | 36% |
| | 280 | 51% | | Placebo | | | | 1/13/pt/yr | 35% |
| Wouters et al. (51) | 189 | 48.1% | ≥2 AECOPD requiring oral steroids and/or antibiotics | Fluticasone/salmeterol | 1 yr | No | NA | 1.3/pt/yr | NA |
| | 184 | 49.0% | | Salmeterol | | | | 1.6/pt/yr | |
| Briggs et al. (85) | 328 | 37.7% | No requirement | Tiotropium | 12 wk | No | NA | NA | 9% |
| | 325 | 37.7% | | Salmeterol | | | | | 11% |
| Niewoehner et al. (59) | 914 | 35.6% | No requirement | Tiotropium | 6 mo | Yes | NA | 0.85/pt/yr | 27.9% |
| | 915 | 35.6% | | Placebo | | | | 1.05/pt/yr | 32.3% |
| Dusser et al. (86) | 500 | 48.0% | ≥1 AECOPD in the previous year | Tiotropium | 1 yr | No | 2.16/pt/yr | 1.57/pt/yr | 49.3% |
| | 510 | 47.6% | | Placebo | | | 2.12/pt/yr | 2.41/pt/yr | 60.3% |
| Stockley et al. (87) | 316 | 46.1% | ≥2 AECOPD requiring antibiotics and/or oral steroids | Salmeterol | 1 yr | No | NA | 0.93/pt/yr | 46% |
| | 318 | 45.8% | | Placebo | | | | 1.18/pt/yr | 51% |
| Kardos et al. (55) | 487 | 40.4% | ≥2 moderate to severe AECOPD in previous year | Fluticasone/salmeterol | 44 wk | No | 2.91/pt/yr | 0.92/pt/yr | NA |
| | 507 | 40.3% | | Salmeterol | | | 2.87/pt/yr | 1.4/pt/yr | |
| Aaron et al. (44) | 156 | 38.7% | ≥1 AECOPD requiring systemic steroids or antibiotics in previous year | Tiotropium + placebo | 1 yr | Yes | NA | 1.61/pt/yr | 62.8% |
| | 148 | 38.0% | | Tiotropium + salmeterol | | | | 1.75/pt/yr | 64.8% |
| | 145 | 39.4% | | Tiotropium + fluticasone/salmeterol | | | | 1.37/pt/yr | 66.2% |
| Calverley et al. (46) | 1533 | 44.3% | No | Fluticasone/salmeterol | 3 yr | No | NA | 0.85/pt/yr | NA |
| | 1534 | 44.1% | | Fluticasone | | | | 0.93/pt/yr | |
| | 1521 | 43.6% | | Salmeterol | | | | 0.97/pt/yr | |
| | 1524 | 44.1% | | Placebo | | | | 1.13/pt/yr | |

*(Continued)*

**Table 2** Frequency of AECOPD Episodes Per Year in Selected Observational or Therapeutic Studies (*Continued*)

| Reference | n | FEV$_1$ | Previous AECOPD history required? | Therapeutic intervention | Duration of follow-up | Patients withdrawn remained in trial? | AECOPD in previous year | Number of AECOPD/yr | Proportion with $\geq$1 AECOPD |
|---|---|---|---|---|---|---|---|---|---|
| Calverley et al. (88) | 761 753 | 41% 41% | No | Roflumilast Placebo | 1 yr | No | NA | 0.857/pt/yr (1.014[b]) 0/918/pt/yr (1.588[b]) | NA |
| Wedzicha et al. (89) | 665 658 | 39.4% 39.1% | History of previous AECOPD required | Fluticasone/salmeterol Tiotropium | 2 yr | No | NA | 1.28/pt/yr 1.32/pt/yr | 62% 59% |
| *Observational studies* | | | | | | | | | |
| Seemungal et al. (49) | 70 | 40% | No | Various | 1 yr | NA | NA | 2.7/pt/yr | NA |
| Donaldson et al. (53) | 132 | 38.4% | No | Various | 918 days | NA | NA | 2.52/pt/yr | NA |
| Tsoumakidou et al. (52) | 67 | GOLD I GOLD II GOLD III | Patients identified at time of hospitalization | Various | 18 mo follow-up | NA | NA | 0/pt/yr[a] 2.07/pt/yr[a] 2.53/pt/yr | NA |

[a] hospitalization
[b] data in patients with GOLD Stage IV disease.
*Abbreviations*: FEV$_1$, forced expiratory volume in 1 second; AECOPD, acute exacerbations of COPD; MD, doctor of medicine; GOLD, global initiative for COPD.

### Factors That Impact AECOPD Frequency

The frequency and severity of exacerbations are quite variable among COPD patients (48). This variability, in part, reflects the nature of data collection (prospective vs. retrospective), disparities in disease severity, medications administered, vaccinations, and smoking status (43,48). Additionally, as noted above, reports that define AECOPD by use of daily diary cards tend to identify more episodes per year (41,49). The most consistent predictor of an increased AECOPD frequency is more severely impaired pulmonary function. Several studies have clearly documented that a greater number of yearly episodes is noted in patients with more impaired $FEV_1$ (50,51), although the various international disease severity classification schemes are associated with a differing relationship with the frequency of hospitalizations (52). One group examined 132 patients during three years of follow-up, carefully documenting exacerbations through the use of diary cards (53). They found that patients with severe COPD ($FEV_1$ <30% predicted) experienced a higher exacerbation frequency (3.43/yr) than those with moderate COPD ($FEV_1$ >30% but <80% predicted) (2.68/yr). Troublesomely, the annual exacerbation frequency remained constant throughout the period of study, while the time to physiological and clinical recovery from exacerbations grew significantly longer each year.

A previous history of frequent AECOPD has been loosely associated with a subsequent increase in AECOPD rate during a clinical trial. Table 2 demonstrates this relationship. This association is likely confounded by the level of pulmonary dysfunction, the duration of the trial, the modality used to ascertain the AECOPD history (patient self-report vs. prospective documentation), and the severity of AECOPD (mild, moderate, or severe). For example, the proportion of individuals with an AECOPD during a clinical trial appears higher in studies with longer duration. This finding is also supported by studies that use a time-to-event format. Importantly, the relationship between a previous AECOPD history and subsequent documentation of exacerbation in a rigorous clinical trial is quite weak (54,55).

Additional factors may identify individuals at a higher risk of subsequent AECOPD. In a large, predominantly male cohort followed in a U.S.-based Veterans Administration Health System study, multivariate modeling for AECOPD during six months of follow-up identified the following independent predictors: older age, lower $FEV_1$ percent predicted, longer COPD duration, productive cough, antibiotic or systemic use for COPD in the previous year, hospitalization for COPD in the prior year, and baseline theophylline use (56). In the same cohort, hospitalization for AECOPD was predicted by older age, lower $FEV_1$ % predicted, unscheduled clinic/emergency visit in the previous year, any cardiovascular comorbidity, and prednisone use at baseline. In a separate cohort of both male and female patients with severe emphysema, worse baseline spirometry, lower $PaO_2$, greater dyspnea, prior hospitalization/emergency room visit, and comorbidity all predicted an emergency room visit or hospitalization during one year of follow-up (57). In COPD patients who are identified at the time of an exacerbation, subsequent readmission is predicted by worse dyspnea, higher $PaCO_2$ at discharge, depression, cor pulmonale, chronic oxygen use, and worse quality of life (58). These results argue for the use of multiple factors for enrichment or stratification in future studies of AECOPD.

Conversely, it is likely that a series of therapeutic interventions can decrease the risk of subsequent AECOPD. Elsewhere in this volume, discussions are presented highlighting the potential AECOPD-ameliorating effects of long-acting bronchodilators, inhaled corticosteroids, theophylline, and vaccination. As such, studies that target therapeutic interventions to decrease AECOPD rate or severity must consider baseline medications in the cohort. In secondary analyses, one such large therapeutic trial suggested that baseline use of inhaled steroids decreased the therapeutic effect of a long-acting anticholinergic in minimizing subsequent AECOPD (59).

## III. Conclusions

Appropriate therapy and prevention of AECOPD are becoming important primary endpoints in therapeutic trials. Rigorous attention to the details of study design and standardized analytical approaches are essential. A trial of adequate duration (at least 1 year), with a predefined patient population (worse spirometric severity and previous history of AECOPD), an explicitly predefined standardized definition of an AECOPD (event based or, ideally, using a validated patient-reported instrument), and careful inclusion criteria (standardization of baseline medications) are required to maximize the likelihood of identifying a therapeutic effect. Similarly, careful attention to statistical design should be considered.

## References

1. Anthonisen N, Manfreda J, Warren C, et al. Antibiotic therapy in exacerbations of chronic obstructive pulmonary disease. Ann Intern Med 1987; 106:196–204.
2. Stockley RA, O'Brien C, Pye A, et al. Relationship of sputum color to nature and outpatient management of acute exacerbations of COPD. Chest 2000; 117(6):1638–1645.
3. Allegra L, Blasi F, Diano P, et al. Sputum color as a marker of acute bacterial exacerbations of chronic obstructive pulmonary disease. Respir Med 2005; 99:742–747.
4. Soler N, Agusti A, Angrill J, et al. Bronchoscopic validation of the significance of sputum purulence in severe exacerbations of chronic obstructive pulmonary disease (COPD). Thorax 2007; 62:29–35.
5. Blasi F, Ewig S, Torres A, et al. A review of guidelines for antibacterial use in acute exacerbations of chronic bronchitis. Pulm Pharmacol Ther 2006; 19(5):361–369. (Epub 2005, Nov 10.)
6. Christ-Crain M, Jaccard-Stolz D, Bingisser R, et al. Effect of procalcitonin-guided treatment on antibiotic use and outcome in lower respiratory tract infections: cluster-randomised, single-blinded interventional trial. Lancet 2004; 363:600–607.
7. Maruna P, Nedelnikova K, Gurlich R.Physiology and genetics of procalcitonin. Physiol Rev 2000; 49(suppl 1):S57–S61.
8. Christ-Crain M, Stolz D, Bingisser R, et al. Procalcitonin guidance of antibiotic therapy in community-acquired pneumonia: a randomized trial. Am J Respir Crit Care Med 2006; 174:84–93.
9. Stolz D, Christ-Crain M, Leuppi J, et al. Antibiotic treatment of exacerbations of COPD: a randomized, controlled trial comparing procalcitonin-guidance with standard therapy. Chest 2007; 131:9–19.
10. Martinez F, Curtis J.Procalcitonin-guided antibiotic therapy in COPD exacerbations: closer but not quite there. Chest 2007; 131:1–2.
11. Miravitlles M, Llor C, Naberan K, et al. Effect of various antimicrobial regimens on the clinical course of exacerbations of chronic bronchitis and chronic obstructive pulmonary disease in primary care. Clin Drug Investig 2004; 24(2):63–72.
12. Martinez F, Grossman R, Zadeikis N, et al. Patient stratification in the management of acute bacterial exacerbation of chronic bronchitis: the role of levofloxacin 750 mg. Eur Respir J 2005; 25: 1001–1010.
13. Leidy N, Rennard S, Schmier J, et al. The breathlessness, cough, and sputum scale: the development of empirically based guidelines for interpretation. Chest 2003; 124:2182–2191.

14. Agusti A. COPD, a multicomponent disease: implications for management. Respir Med 2005; 99:670–682.
15. Dev D, Wallace E, Sankaran R, et al. Value of C-reactive protein measurements in exacerbations of chronic obstructive pulmonary disease. Respir Med 1998; 92(4):664–667.
16. Wedzicha J. The heterogeneity of chronic obstructive pulmonary disease. Thorax 2000; 5:631–632.
17. Roland M, Bhowmik A, Sapsford R, et al. Sputum and plasma endothelin-a levels in exacerbations of chronic obstructive pulmonary disease. Thorax 2001; 56:30–35.
18. Hurst J, Donaldson G, Perera W, et al. Utility of plasma biomarkers at exacerbations of chronic obstructive pulmonary disease. Am J Respir Crit Care Med 2006; 174:867–874.
19. Hurst J, Perera W, Wilkinson T, et al. Systemic and upper and lower airway inflammation at exacerbation of chronic obstructive pulmonary disease. Am J Respir Crit Care Med 2005; 173:71–78.
20. Martinez F, Han M, Flaherty K, et al. Role of infection and antimicrobial therapy in acute exacerbations of chronic obstructive pulmonary disease. Expert Rev Anti Infect Ther 2006; 4(1): 101–124.
21. van Schilfgaarde M, Eijk P, Regelink A, et al. Haemophilus influenzae localized in epithelial cell layers is shielded from antibiotics and antibody-mediated bactericidal activity. Microb Pathog 1999; 26(5):249–262.
22. Murphy T, Brauer A, Schiffmacher A, et al. Persistent colonization by Haemophilus influenzae in chronic obstructive pulmonary disease. Am J Respir Crit Care Med 2004; 170:266–272.
23. Anzueto A, Sethi S, Martinez F. Exacerbations of chronic obstructive pulmonary disease. Proc Am Thorac Soc 2007; 4(7):554–564.
24. Saint S, Flaherty K, Abrahamse P, et al. Acute exacerbations of chronic bronchitis: disease-specific issues that influence the cost-effectiveness of antimicrobial therapy. Clin Ther 2001; 23(3):499–512.
25. Anzueto A, Rizzo J, Grossman R. The infection-free interval: its use in evaluating antimicrobial treatment of acute exacerbations of chronic bronchitis. Clin Infect Dis 1999; 28:1344–1345.
26. Chodosh S. Clinical significance of the infection-free interval in the management of acute bacterial exacerbations of chronic bronchitis. Chest 2005; 127:2231–2236.
27. White AJ, Gompertz S, Bayley DL, et al. Resolution of bronchial inflammation is related to bacterial eradication following treatment of exacerbations of chronic bronchitis. Thorax 2003; 58(8):680–685.
28. Chodosh S, McCarty J, Farkas S, et al. Randomized, double-blind study of ciprofloxacin and cefuroxime axetil for treatment of acute bacterial exacerbations of chronic bronchitis. The Bronchitis Study Group. Clin Infect Dis 1998; 27(4):722–729.
29. Wilson R, Schentag J, Ball P, et al. A comparison of gemifloxacin and clarithromycin in acute exacerbations of chronic bronchitis and long-term clinical outcomes. Clin Ther 2002; 24(2): 639–652.
30. Wilson R, Allegra L, Huchon G, et al., and MOSAIC Study Group. Short-term and Long-term outcomes of moxifloxacin compared to standard antibiotic treatment in acute exacerbations of chronic bronchitis. Chest 2004125:953–964.
31. Lode H, Eller J, Linnhoff A, et al. and the Evaluation of Therapy-Free Interval in COPD Patients Study Group. Levofloxacin versus clarithromycin in COPD exacerbation: focus on exacerbation-free interval. Eur Respir J 2004; 24:947–953.
32. Allegra L, Blasi F, de Bernardi B, et al. Antibiotic treatment and baseline severity or disease in acute exacerbations of chronic bronchitis: a re-evaluation of previously published data of a placebo-controlled randomized study. Pulm Pharmacol Ther 2001; 14:149–155.
33. Nouira S, Marghli S, Belghith M, et al. Once daily oral ofloxacin in chronic obstructive pulmonary disease exacerbation requiring mechanical ventilation: a randomised placebo-controlled trial. Lancet 2001; 358:2020–2025.
34. Martinez F. Acute bronchitis: state of the art diagnosis and therapy. Compr Ther 2004; 30:55–69.

35. Balter M, La Forge J, Low D, et al. Canadian guidelines for the management of acute exacerbations of acute exacerbations of chronic bronchitis. Can Respir J 2003; 10 (suppl B):3B–32B.
36. Global Initiative for Chronic Obstructive Lung Disease. Executive Summary: Global Initiative for Chronic Obstructive Lung Disease.
37. Ball P. Epidemiology and treatment of chronic bronchitis and its exacerbations. Chest 1995; (108): 43S–52S.
38. Wilson R, Kubin R, Ballin I, et al. Five day moxifloxacin therapy compared with 7 day clarithromycin therapy for the treatment of acute exacerbations of chronic bronchitis. J Antimicrob Chemother 1999; 44:501–513.
39. Aaron S, Fergusson D, Marks G, et al. Counting, analyzing and reporting exacerbations of COPD in randomized, controlled trials. Thorax 2008; 63:122–128.
40. Suissa S. Statistical treatment of exacerbations in therapeutic trials of chronic obstructive pulmonary disease. Am J Respir Crit Care Med 2006; 173(8):842–846.
41. Seemungal T, Donaldson G, Bhowmik A, et al. Time course and recovery of exacerbations in patients with chronic obstructive pulmonary disease. Am J Respir Crit Care Med 2000; 161: 1608–1613.
42. Calverley P, Pauwels R, Lofdahl C, et al. Relationship between respiratory symptoms and medical treatment in exacerbations of COPD. Eur Respir J 2005; 26:406–413.
43. Pauwels R, Calverley P, Buist A, et al. COPD exacerbations: the importance of a standard definition. Respir Med 2004; 98(2):99–107.
44. Aaron S, Vanderheen K, Fergusson D, et al. and the Canadian Thoracic Society/Canadian Respiratory Clinical Research Consortium. Tiotropium in combination with placebo, salmeterol, or fluticasone-salmeterol for the treatment of chronic obstructive pulmonary disease. A randomized trial. Ann Int Med 2007; 146:546–555.
45. Celli B, Halpin D, Hepburn R, et al. Symptoms are an important outcome in chronic obstructive pulmonary disease clinical trials: results of a 3-month comparative study using the Breathlessness, Cough and Sputum Scale (BCSS). Respir Med 2003; 97(suppl A):S35–S43.
46. Calverley P, Anderson J, Celli B, et al. and for the TORCH investigators. Salmeterol and fluticasone propionate and survival in chronic obstructive pulmonary disease. N Eng J Med 2007; 356:775–789.
47. McGarvey, L, John M, Anderson J, et al. and TORCH Clinical Endpoint Committee. Ascertainment of cause-specific mortality in COPD: operations of the TORCH Clinical Endpoint Committee. Thorax 2007; 62:411–415.
48. Burge S, Wedzicha J. COPD exacerbations: definitions and classifications. Eur Respir J 2003; 21(suppl 41):46s–53s.
49. Seemungal T, Donaldson G, Paul E, et al. Effect of exacerbation on quality of life in patients with chronic obstructive pulmonary disease. Am J Respir Crit Care Med 1998; 157: 1418–1422.
50. Jones P, Willits L, Burge P, et al. and on behalf of the Inhaled Steroids in Obstructive Lung Disease in Europe study investigators. Disease severity and the effect of fluticasone propionate on chronic obstructive pulmonary disease exacerbations. Eur Respir J 2003; 21:68–73.
51. Wouters E, Postma D, Fokkens B, et al. and for the COSMIC (COPD and Seretide: a Multi-Center Intervention and Characterization) Study Group. Withdrawal of fluticasone propionate from combined salmeterol/fluticasone treatment in patients with COPD causes immediate and sustained disease deterioration: a randomised controlled trial. Thorax 2005; 60:480–487.
52. Tsoumakidou M, Tzanakis N, Voulgaraki O, et al. Is there any correlation between the ATS, BTS, ERS and GOLD COPD's severity scales and the frequency of hospital admissions? Respir Med 2004; 98(2):178–183.
53. Donaldson G, Seemungal T, Patel I, et al. Longitudinal changes in the nature, severity and frequency of COPD exacerbations. Eur Respir J 2003; 22:931–936.

54. DeCramer M,Rutten-van Molken M, Dekhuijzen P, et al. Effect of N-acetylcysteine on outcomes in chronic obstructive pulmonary disease (Bronchitis Randomized on NAC Cost-Utility Study, BRONCUS): a randomised placebo-controlled trial. Lancet 2005; 365:1552–1560.

55. Kardos P, Wencker M, Glaab T, et al. Impact of salmeterol/fluticasone propionate versus salmeterol on exacerbations in severe COPD. Am J Respir Crit Care Med 2007; 175:144–149.

56. Niewoehner D, Loknygina Y, Rice K, et al. Risk indexes for exacerbations and hospitalizations due to COPD. Chest 2007; 131:20–28.

57. Fan V, Ramsey S, Make B, et al. Physiologic variables and functional status independently predict COPD hospitalizations and emergency department visits in patients with severe COPD. COPD 2007; 4:29–39.

58. Almagro P, Barreiro B, Ochoa de Echaguen A, et al. Risk factors for hospital readmission in patients with chronic obstructive pulmonary disease. Respiration 2006; 73:311–317.

59. Niewoehner D, Rice K, Cote C, et al. Prevention of exacerbations of chronic obstructive pulmonary disease with tiotropium, a once-daily anticholinergic bronchodilator. A randomized trial. Ann Intern Med 2005; 143:317–326.

60. Thompson W, Nielson C, Carvalho P, et al. Controlled trial of oral prednisone in outpatients with acute COPD exacerbation. Am J Respir Crit Care Med 1996; 154:407–412.

61. Paggiaro P, Dahle R, Bakran I, et al. and I. C. S. Group. Multicenter randomised placebo-controlled trial of inhaled fluticasone propionate in patients with chronic obstructive pulmonary disease. Lancet 1998; 351:773–780.

62. Niewoehner D, Erbland M, Deupree R, et al. Effect of systemic glucocorticoids on exacerbations of chronic obstructive pulmonary disease. N Engl J Med 1999; 340:1941–1947.

63. Mahler D, Donohue J, Barbee R, et al. Efficacy of salmeterol xinafoate in the treatment of COPD. Chest 1999; 115:957–965.

64. Vestbo J, Sorensen T, Lange P, et al. Long-term effect of inhaled budesonide in mild and moderate chronic obstructive pulmonary disease: a randomized controlled trial. Lancet 1999; 353:1819–1823.

65. Burge P, Calverley P, Jones P, et al. Randomised, double blind, placebo controlled study of fluticasone propionate in patients with moderate to severe chronic obstructive pulmonary disease: the ISOLDE trial. BMJ 2000; 320:1297–1303.

66. Van Noord J, Bantje T, Eland M, et al., and D. T. S. Group. 2000. A randomised controlled comparison of tiotropium and ipratropium in the treatment of chronic obstructive pulmonary disease. Thorax 2000; 55:289–294.

67. Gomez J, Banos V, Simarro E, et al. Estudio prospectivo y comparativo (1994–1998) sobre la influencia del tratamiento corto profilactico con azitromicina en pacientes con EPOC evolucionada. Rev Esp Quimioter 2000; 13(4):379–383.

68. Kanner R, Anthonisen N, Connett J. Lower respiratory illnesses promote $FEV_1$ decline in current smokers but not ex-smokers with mild chronic obstructive pulmonary disease. Am J Respir Crit Care Med 2001; 164:358–364.

69. Woolhouse I, Hill S, Stockley R. Symptom resolution assessed using a patient directed diary card during treatment of acute exacerbations of chronic bronchitis. Thorax 2001; 56:947–953.

70. Cazzola M, Di Perna F, D'Amato M, et al. Formoterol turbuhaler for as-needed therapy in patients with mild acute exacerbations of COPD. Respir Med 2001; 95:917–921.

71. Gompertz S, O'Brien C, Bayley D, et al. Changes in bronchial inflammation during acute exacerbations of chronic bronchitis. Eur Respir J 2001; 17:1112–1119.

72. Suzuki T, Yanai M, Yamaya M, et al. Erythromycin and common cold in COPD. Chest 2001; 120: 730–733.

73. ZuWallack R, Mahler D, Reilly D, et al. Salmeterol plus theophylline combination therapy in the treatment of COPD. Chest 2001; 119(6):1661–1670.

74. Rennard S, Anderson W, ZuWallack R, et al. Use of a long-acting inhaled $\beta_2$-adrenergic agonist, salmeterol xinafoate, in patients with chronic obstructive pulmonary disease. Am J Respir Crit Care 2001; 163:1087–1092.

75.  Vincken W, Van Noord J, Greefhorst A, et al., and on behalf of the Dutch/Belgian Tiotropium Study Group.Improved health outcomes in patients with COPD during 1 yr's treatment with tiotropium. Eur Respir J 2002; 19:209–216.
76.  Casaburi R, Mahler D, Jones P, et al. A long-term evaluation of once-daily tiotropium in chronic obstructive pulmonary disease. Eur Respir J 2002; 19:217–224.
77.  Rossi A, Kristufek P, Levine B, et al. Comparison of the efficacy, tolerability, and safety of formoterol dry powder and oral, slow-release theophylline in the treatment of COPD. Chest 2002; 121:1058–1069.
78.  Maltais F, Ostinelli J, Bourbeau J, et al. Comparison of nebulized budesonide and oral prednisolone with placebo in the treatment of acute exacerbations of chronic obstructive pulmonary disease. A randomized controlled trial. Am J Respir Crit Care Med 2002; 165:698–703.
79.  Szafranski W, Cukier A, Ramirez A, et al. Efficacy and safety of budesonide/formoterol in the management of chronic obstructive pulmonary disease. Eur Respir J 2003; 21:74–81.
80.  Calverley P, Pauwels R, Vestbo J, et al., and for the TRISTAN (Trial of inhaled steroids and long-acting β2 agonists) Study Group. Combined salmeterol and fluticasone in the treatment of chronic obstructive pulmonary disease: a randomised controlled trial. Lancet 2003; 361:449–456.
81.  Calverley P, Boonsawat W, Cseke Z, et al. Maintenance therapy with budesonide and formoterol in chronic obstructive pulmonary disease. Eur Respir J 2003; 22:912–919.
82.  Dal Negro R, Pomari C, Tognella S, et al. Salmeterol & fluticasone 50 µg/250 µg bid combination provides a better long-term control than salmeterol 50 µg bid alone and placebo in COPD patients already treated with theophylline. Pulm Pharmacol Ther 2003; 16:241–246.
83.  de Melo M, Ernst P, Suissa S. Inhaled corticosteroids and the risk of a first exacerbation in COPD patients. Eur Respir J 2004; 23:692–697.
84.  Rabe K, Bateman E, O'Donnell D, et al. Roflumilast-an oral anti-inflammatory treatment for chronic obstructive pulmonary disease: a randomised controlled trial. Lancet 2005; 366:563–571.
85.  Briggs DD Jr., Covelli H, Lapidus R, et al. Improved daytime spirometric efficacy of tiotropium compared with salmeterol in patients with COPD. Pulm Pharmacol Ther 2005; 18:397–404.
86.  Dusser D, Bravo M, Iacono P, and on behalf of the MISTRAL study group. The effect of tiotropium on exacerbations and airflow in patients with COPD. Eur Respir J 2006; 27:547–555.
87.  Stockley R, Chopra N, Rice L, and on behalf of the SMS40026 Investigator Group. Addition of salmeterol to existing treatment in patients with COPD: a 12 month study. Thorax 2006; 61: 122–128.
88.  Calverley P, Sanchez-Toril F, McIvor A, et al. Effect of 1-year treatment with roflumilast in severe chronic obstructive pulmonary disease. Am J Respir Crit Care Med 2007; 176:154–161.
89.  Wedzicha J, Calverley P, Seemungal T, et al. The prevention of COPD exacerbations by salmeterol/fluticasone propionate or tiotropium bromide. Am J Respir Crit Care Med 2008; 177:19–26.
90.  Patel I, Seemungal T, Wilks M, et al. Relationship between bacterial colonisation and the frequency, character, and severity of COPD exacerbations. Thorax 2002; 57:759–764.
91.  Wilkinson T, Donaldson G, Hurst J, et al. Early therapy improves outcomes of exacerbations of chronic obstructive pulmonary disease. Am J Respir Crit Care Med 2004; 169:1298–1303.
92.  Donaldson G, Seemungal T, Bhowmik A, et al. Relationship between exacerbation frequency and lung function decline in chronic obstructive pulmonary disease. Thorax 2002; 57:847–852.
93.  Adams S, Melo J, Luther M, et al. Antibiotics are associated with lower relapse rates in outpatients with acute exacerbations of COPD. Chest 2000; 117:1345–1352.
94.  Miravitlles M, Murio C, Guerrero T. Factors associated with relapse after ambulatory treatment of acute exacerbations of chronic bronchitis. DAFNE Study Group. Eur Respir J 2001; 17(5): 928–933.
95.  Sethi S, Evans N, Grant B, et al. New strains of bacteria and exacerbations of chronic obstructive pulmonary disease. N Engl J Med 2002; 347:465–471.

96. Sethi S, Muscarella K, Evans N, et al. Airway inflammation and etiology of acute exacerbations of chronic bronchitis. Chest 2000; 118(6):1557–1565.
97. Miravitlles M, Ferrer M, Pont A, et al., and for the IMPAC Study Group. Effect of exacerbations on quality of life in patients with chronic obstructive pulmonary disease: a 2 year follow up study. Thorax 2004; 59:387–395.
98. Brusasco V, Hodder R, Miravitlles M, et al. Health outcomes following treatment for six months with once daily tiotropium compared with twice daily salmeterol in patients with COPD. Thorax 2003; 58:399–404.
99. DeCramer M, Dekhuijzen P, Troosters T, et al., and the BRONCUS-trial Committee. The Bronchitis Randomized on NAC Cost-Utility Study (BRONCUS): hypothesis and design. Eur Respir J 2001; 17:329–336.

# 36
## Statistical Considerations for COPD Exacerbation Trials

**SHAWN D. AARON**
The Ottawa Health Research Institute, University of Ottawa, Ottawa, Ontario, Canada

## I. Introduction

Many earlier trials of chronic obstructive pulmonary disease (COPD) therapy assessed lung function as a primary outcome to demonstrate evidence of efficacy of therapy (1,2). However, given the global health, social, and economic importance of COPD exacerbations, the prevention of exacerbations is now recognized as a primary goal of COPD therapy (3). Accordingly, recent clinical trials of maintenance medications for COPD have evaluated their effects on the incidence of COPD exacerbations as a primary study outcome. Because prevention of exacerbations is now being relied upon to demonstrate efficacy of new treatments for COPD, it becomes extremely important for investigators to ensure that correct statistical methods are being used to assess this outcome. If clinical trials are not been consistent in how they count, record, or analyze COPD exacerbation rates, then methodological errors in the assessment of COPD exacerbations can potentially lead to biased or spurious results.

The objectives of this chapter will be to describe preferred statistical approaches for the analysis of COPD exacerbations. In addition, this chapter will discuss methodological issues related to how COPD exacerbations are counted and recorded and also issues related to correct reporting of exacerbation results.

## II. Distribution of the Data

COPD exacerbations occur as recurrent events in individual patients. The data is organized as a "counting outcome," i.e., patients can have zero exacerbations or alternatively one or several exacerbations over a given time period. Counting outcomes are often characterized by a large proportion of values at zero, with the remaining values skewed toward the right (4). Typical recent COPD trials, such as the TRISTAN trial or the Optimal trial, follow this distribution; among patients randomized into these studies, 40% to 45% experienced no exacerbations within the first year (5,6). However a small minority of patients in these trials experienced multiple exacerbations, often more than five over a single year. Clearly, these data do not follow a normal distribution, and therefore many standard statistical tests, which rely on the usual normality assumption, cannot be applied to COPD exacerbation data.

When faced with this problem, statisticians have three options: (*i*) They can rely on a transformation of the data to induce normality, however this approach often does not work; (*ii*) They can categorize the outcome and use nonparametric methods to analyze ranks, however this results in considerable loss of information, and this method often does not provide an appropriate method to estimate treatment effects since the exacerbation rates are bounded by zero; or (*iii*) Statisticians can assume a Poisson or negative binomial distribution that is better suited to the distribution of the data.

## III. Approaches to Determining Rates

### A. Time-Weighting

A typical COPD clinical trial will assess each patient's duration of participation in the trial, along with a count of the number of COPD exacerbations that occurred for that patient within the trial time period. This will generate a subject-event rate; i.e., the number of events per unit time.

Mean COPD exacerbation rates can be analyzed using an unweighted or weighted approach. The unweighted approach estimates the rate for each patient individually by dividing each patient's number of exacerbations during follow-up by the length of time each patient remained in the trial. The mean rate for the group is then estimated by taking the average of the individual patient rates. For example, assume three patients are randomized to a treatment in a one-year trial. Patient 1 experiences two exacerbations in the first month of the study and is then withdrawn from the study; he has been followed for only one month, which equals 0.083 years. Patient 1's exacerbation rate would be calculated as two exacerbations per 0.083 years, which equals 24 exacerbations per patient-year. Patients 2 and 3 experience one exacerbation each over the entire 12-month trial period (i.e., 1 exacerbation/patient-year). The mean unweighted exacerbation rate for these three patients would be (24+1+1)/3, which equals 8.67 exacerbations per patient-year.

In contrast, a weighted statistical approach adjusts for asymmetry in follow-up times by accounting for each patient's time spent in the trial. Using this approach, the mean rate would be calculated by pooling all events in the group and dividing the total number of exacerbations in the pooled group by the total follow-up time of the pooled group. For the example above, the weighted mean rate would be calculated as (2+1+1) exacerbations/ 2.083 years = 1.92 exacerbations per patient-year.

Clearly a comparison of the results obtained using an unweighted mean rate (8.67 exacerbations/patient-year) and the weighted mean rate (1.92 exacerbations/patient-year) reveals that the unweighted mean rate is heavily biased because it overestimates exacerbations that occur in patients who drop out early. The unweighted statistical approach does not adjust for time spent in the trial, and therefore only weighted statistical approaches should be used since this approach produces the correct estimate (7). Studies using actual clinical trial results from the Optimal trial confirm that using an unweighted analysis leads to a biased rate ratio and falsely exaggerates the benefits of treatment (8).

### B. Overdispersion of the Data

The Poisson distribution is most suitable to analyze counting data such as COPD exacerbation data. The Poisson distribution assumes that exacerbations can occur repeatedly but that they occur randomly and independently of each other. However the usual Poisson regression technique also assumes that the variance of the rate of exacerbations is less than and is proportional to the mean (4), but in COPD this is unusual. Clinicians who treat COPD are aware that there is considerable between-subject variability in COPD exacerbations; two patients taking similar treatments with the same degree of lung dysfunction may have markedly different rates of exacerbation.

To account for this heterogeneity in exacerbation rates between patients, statisticians can employ an overdispersion parameter. The overdispersion parameter accounts for intersubject variability, which cannot be explained by covariates. The overdispersion correction is estimated by the square root of either the deviance or Pearons' chi-square, divided by the degrees of freedom. It should be noted that the overdispersion parameter is applied only to the standard error of the treatment estimates. Thus use of the overdispersion parameter does not affect the estimate of treatment effect (i.e., the rate ratio); however, its use does typically widen the confidence intervals, and hence increases the *p* value, around the rate ratio by accounting for this extra source of variability in the data.

An alternative to using the Poisson model with overdispersion is to use a negative binomial model (9). The negative binomial model uses a more flexible regression model that assumes that for each patient, exacerbations follow an underlying Poisson rate, and that the set of rates is distributed across subjects in a gamma distribution. As such, the negative binomial regression model incorporates a parameter that represents the degree of overdispersion. Either model, the Poisson with overdispersion, or the negative binomial, is therefore acceptable for determining the confidence interval (and hence the *p* value) for rates of COPD exacerbations in clinical trials.

## IV. Counting Individual COPD Exacerbations

### A. Independence of Events

Both the Poisson and negative binomial distributions assume that exacerbations happen randomly and independently of each other over the follow-up time. However, patients may present to health care providers recurrently with symptoms of an acute exacerbation over short periods of time. For instance, a patient may present with symptoms of cough, dyspnea, and sputum to a physician on March 1 and be given an antibiotic, then present again on March 7 for identical symptoms and be given a second antibiotic, then present again on March 14 with the same symptoms and be treated with oral steroids. The question is: are these truly independent events or are these latter two events simply relapses or continuations of the original exacerbation? The negative binomial and Poisson distributions assume that individual events will be independent of prior events. This assumption can only be satisfied if it is clear that the patient had reverted to his or her baseline between events.

A recently published study using an actual clinical trial dataset has shown that failure to determine independence of events may artificially inflate the rate of exacerbations in each treatment group (8). Theoretically, failure to determine independence of event could produce biased estimates, if more relapses occur systematically in one treatment group compared with another.

How to avoid this problem? The Canadian Optimal study considered patients to have experienced a new COPD exacerbation if they had been off of oral steroids and antibiotics for at least 14 days following their previous exacerbation (6). Other options to determine independence of events could include an assessment of patient symptoms using symptom diaries with a reversion of symptoms to baseline before a new event can be said to occur (10,11). To ensure the best quality data analysis, future clinical trials should incorporate methods to ensure that individual events are independent.

## B.  Adjudication of Events

In any trial, investigators need to be sure that they are actually measuring what they think they are measuring. Hence, quality control measures should be incorporated to ensure that events counted as exacerbations are consistent with the study definition of exacerbation. Problems can arise with diagnostic exchange; e.g., should a respiratory event be classified as a COPD exacerbation, or an upper respiratory tract infection, or pneumonia? One approach to help avoid mistakes, inconsistencies, and diagnostic exchange is for studies to use blinded Adjudication Committees, which review clinical and radiographic data surrounding each suspected respiratory event to determine if a COPD exacerbation, or conversely an adverse event, such as pneumonia, had occurred (6).

## C.  Counting Events That Occur After Patients Prematurely Discontinue Study Treatment

Most clinical trials of drug therapies for COPD have excluded patients from the study analysis after they prematurely stopped study medications. Premature exclusion of patients may be inappropriate since it precludes an effectiveness analysis of the medication in question—how the drug will act in real world circumstances when some patients are noncompliant. In addition, early exclusion of patients can introduce bias because the factors that determined whether a patient might be excluded may often also be related to the outcome. For instance, some patients may prematurely discontinue a study medication because they are doing poorly and about to have an exacerbation in the near future. Premature exclusion of these patients after they stop study drugs introduces bias since the subsequent exacerbation is not counted and is not attributed to the study drug in question. To be consistent with CONSORT guidelines (12), patients who prematurely stop a study medication should not be considered "dropouts" unless they absolutely refuse permission for the study to continue to follow them. Ideally, these patients should be retained in the study for its duration, and any subsequent COPD exacerbations should be counted and attributed to their randomized group.

In the Optimal COPD trial, the rate ratio for exacerbations per patient-year was 0.85 when all patients who consented were followed until the end of the trial. In other words, the study showed that patients who were randomized to tiotropium + fluticasone/salmeterol had a 15% relative risk reduction in exacerbation rates compared with those patients who were randomized to tiotropium + placebo. Alternatively, if patients had instead been excluded when they prematurely stopped study medications, the relative risk reduction would have been overestimated as 21% (8).

A similar paper by Kesten et al. analyzed clinical trial data and showed that the bias can also work in the opposite direction (13). In the Kesten study, higher incidence rates of fatal events occurred following premature discontinuation of study medication. The authors concluded that failure to consider outcomes of patients who discontinue early from clinical trials might bias results against effective therapies.

It should be acknowledged that an intention-to-treat approach that follows all patients to the end of the study, regardless of whether they prematurely discontinue study medications is correct, but it is also conservative. In some COPD clinical trials proportionately more patients randomized to the placebo limb have exited the study early. Many of these patients subsequently used active open-label therapies for the duration of the study. If such therapies are effective at reducing exacerbations then an intention-to-treat analysis might reduce the possibility of a difference being found between the placebo group and the active arms in these instances. Since it is impossible to know a priori the direction and magnitude of the effect of patient noncompliance, and because of the potential biases involved in premature exclusion of patients, it is preferable for investigators to report two separate analyses, a true intention-to-treat effectiveness analysis as well as a secondary efficacy analysis that excludes patients when they stop study medications. If results of both analyses are reported, then the reader can make up his or her mind to decide on the effectiveness of the intervention in question.

## V.  Reporting Exacerbations

COPD exacerbation data can be reported in various formats: (*i*) as rates per person-year; (*ii*) as proportions who experience an exacerbation; (*iii*) as time to first exacerbation and; (*iv*) as number needed to treat to prevent exacerbations.

Most commonly exacerbations are reported as rates, typically expressed as rates of exacerbations per patient-year of follow-up. Rates for two different treatments are then compared and expressed as rate ratios. An example of how to calculate weighted mean exacerbation rates and a rate ratio is presented in Table 1.

**Table 1**  Calculation of Exacerbation Rates and Rate Ratios from the Optimal Study Clinical Trial Data

| Number of exacerbations during the 1-yr study | Tiotropium + placebo group ($N = 156$ patients) | Tiotropium + fluticasone/salmeterol group ($N = 145$ patients) |
|---|---|---|
| 0 | 37.2% | 40.0% |
| 1 | 28.8% | 23.4% |
| 2 | 13.5% | 17.9% |
| 3 | 9.6% | 10.3% |
| 4 | 2.6% | 3.4% |
| 5 | 4.5% | 3.4% |
| 6 | 2.6% | 1.4% |
| 7 | 0.6% | 0.0% |
| 8 | 0.6% | 0.0% |
| Total no. of adjudicated exacerbations | 222 | 188 |
| Total person-yr of follow-up | 138.0 | 137.0 |
| Weighted mean adjudicated exacerbation rate/patient-yr | 222/138 = 1.61 | 188/137 = 1.37 |

*Note:* Rate ratio = 1.37/1.61 = 0.85.
95% CI around the rate ratio (using Poisson regression analysis with overdispersion) = 0.65 to 1.11.

An alternative method to present exacerbations is to determine the proportion of patients who experienced one or more exacerbations over the trial treatment period. The results can then be compared between treatment groups using a chi-square analysis or alternatively using a Mantel-Haenszel test to compare odd ratios for the treatments. An example would be clinical trial data generated by Niewoehner et al. The investigators randomized patients with COPD to six months of treatment with tiotropium or placebo. After six months, 27.9% of patients in the tiotropium group, and 32.3% of patients in the placebo group had experienced one or more COPD exacerbations. The odds ratio for exacerbation was 0.81 (0.66–0.99), indicating that treatment with tiotropium significantly decreased the percentage of patients having one or more exacerbations over the six-month trial period (14).

A third method of reporting exacerbations is to examine the time to first exacerbation. This method uses survival analysis, and data is then analyzed using Kaplan–Meier curves with a log-rank test of hazard ratios. In addition multivariate survival models of time to first exacerbation can be constructed and analyzed using Cox proportional regression methods.

A final method of reporting exacerbations results is to calculate a number needed to treat (NNT). The NNT represents the estimated number of patients who need to be treated with a new treatment, rather than a standard treatment, for one additional patient to benefit (15). The NNT is defined as the reciprocal of the absolute risk reduction. It can be obtained for trials that report a binary patient outcome, such as death. In the case of COPD exacerbations the NNT can be calculated from data that report the proportion of patients in each treatment group who experience one or more COPD exacerbations.

Each method of reporting COPD exacerbations has its merits and disadvantages. The rate of exacerbations per patient-year captures patients with multiple exacerbations, which may be clinically and economically important. However measurement of the mean number of exacerbations per patient-year can be heavily influenced by a small minority of patients who experience multiple exacerbation events, and it cannot yield an NNT since this can only be derived from the absolute difference in the proportions of patients who experience at least one exacerbation (16,17). Conversely, the proportion of patients who experience at least one exacerbation is not always an ideal measurement since it is heavily influenced by the duration of the trial; for instance, if the study continues for an extended time period, then most or all patients will eventually experience an exacerbation. Both the survival time to first exacerbation and the proportion of patients who experience at least one exacerbation exclude information, since exacerbation events that occur after the first COPD exacerbation are not considered.

It might be preferable if trials be designed, and sample sizes calculated, using the mean number of exacerbations per patient-year as the primary outcome. However it is also important for studies to report the proportion of patients who experienced at least one exacerbation over the trial period as a secondary outcome, along with a properly calculated NNT. Presenting the data in these multiple formats will allow the reader to determine whether treatment may prevent some patients from having multiple exacerbations and also how many patients need to be treated to prevent an individual patient from having an exacerbation.

## A.  Misapplication of the NNT in COPD Clinical Trials

Recently, several articles have been published in the pulmonary literature advocating an alternative method for calculating the NNT that does not involve differences in proportions (18,19). Instead, these articles provide directions for how to calculate the NNT to reduce

COPD exacerbations in patients who may experience recurrent exacerbations over a single time period. The articles define "event-based NNTs" as "the reciprocal of the difference between the treatment and control groups in the rate of a particular outcome per patient within a given time frame." Using this definition the rate of COPD exacerbations per patient-year is calculated for the treatment and control groups and the reciprocal of the difference in rates is used to calculate an event-based NNT (18,19).

The above definition for an event-based NNT has been used by several authors in prominent publications. For example, the TORCH trial (TOwards a Revolution in COPD Health) observed an annual rate of exacerbations of 0.85 in the fluticasone/salmeterol group and 1.13 in the placebo group, respectively. The authors calculated an NNT of $1/(1.13-0.85) = 4$, implying that the clinician needs to treat four additional patients with fluticasone/salmeterol rather than placebo to prevent an exacerbation event over one year (20).

The problem is that the above calculation is incorrect. The NNT statistic cannot be correctly applied to repeated events in the same patient. Consider the example outlined in Table 2, where 10 patients are randomized to placebo for one year and 10 patients are randomized to treatment for one year. The treatment is designed to prevent COPD exacerbations. One patient in the placebo group experiences a single exacerbation over one year, two patients experience eight exacerbations over one year, and the rest have none. In contrast, two patients in the treatment group each experience two exacerbations over the year, and the rest have none. Calculation of the traditional NNT yields an NNT of 10; however, the alternative event-based NNT is 0.77. This suggests that 0.77 patients have to be treated to prevent a single exacerbation. Clearly, it is impossible to treat 0.77 of a patient, and the statistic therefore has no meaning. If the NNT of 0.77 is rounded up to 1, this would falsely imply that treatment is indicated in every patient, since treatment will prevent

**Table 2**  Biased Results from the "Event-Based NNT" statistic

| Placebo treatment patient no. | Number of COPD exacerbations in 1 yr | Treatment patient no. | Number of COPD exacerbations in 1 yr |
|---|---|---|---|
| P1 | 0 | T1 | 0 |
| P2 | 0 | T2 | 0 |
| P3 | 0 | T3 | 0 |
| P4 | 0 | T4 | 0 |
| P5 | 0 | T5 | 0 |
| P6 | 0 | T6 | 0 |
| P7 | 0 | T7 | 0 |
| P8 | 1 | T8 | 0 |
| P9 | 8 | T9 | 2 |
| P10 | 8 | T10 | 2 |
| Annual rate of COPD exacerbations/ patient-yr | 17 exacerbations/10 patient-yr = 1.7 | | 4 exacerbations/10 patient-yr = 0.4 |
| Traditional NNT | $1/(0.3-0.2) = 10$ | | |
| Event-based NNT | $1/(1.7-0.4) = 0.77$ | | |

*Abbreviation*: NNT, number needed to treat.

exacerbations in all. The event-based NNT is heavily influenced by a minority of patients who may experience multiple exacerbations, and the statistic therefore provides biased information since it does not correctly describe the effect of extending treatment out to the population at large.

The NNT should only be calculated on the basis of the difference in proportions of patients who experience one or more COPD exacerbations during the trial period. An example of the correct use of the NNT statistic to describe COPD exacerbations can be taken directly from previous clinical trials. As described in the Kardos' trial, 241 of 487 patients treated with salmeterol (49.5%) and 210 of 507 patients treated with salmeterol/fluticasone (41.4%) had at least one exacerbation over the 44-week trial (21). Therefore the absolute risk reduction is equal to 8.1%, and the number of patients needed to treat with salmeterol/fluticasone (rather than salmeterol) to prevent one additional patient from experiencing an exacerbation in 44 weeks is equal to 12.3.

## VI.  Summary

Improper methods for counting, analyzing, and reporting COPD exacerbation rates can lead to biased estimates of treatment effects and/or spurious results. In addition, differences in ascertainment of events and differences in statistical methodology make comparisons of exacerbation rates between trials difficult. Without use of consistent methodologies it is impossible to compare one trial with another, or even one medication against another, to determine the relative efficacy of different therapies in reducing the rate of COPD exacerbations.

Future clinical trials should strive to incorporate parameters in their definition that assure independence of events and use blinded adjudication committees to ensure that suspected COPD exacerbations meet study definitions. These measures will help avoid counting a single COPD exacerbation multiple times, and will help avoid misclassification of events and diagnostic exchange.

In addition, trials should use intention-to-treat approaches to discourage premature exclusion of patients from a study analysis after they stop study medications. Correct statistical analysis, using weighted mean rates and employing statistical corrections for between-patient variability, using the Poisson distribution with an overdispersion correction, or using the negative binomial distribution, should be encouraged. This will help avoid inappropriate narrowing of confidence intervals around the estimate, with false assumptions of statistical significance. Numbers needed to treat should be reported on the basis of differences in proportions, not differences in rates. Use of these standardized measures for defining, counting, and analyzing COPD exacerbations should help ensure unbiased estimates and would ensure comparability of clinical trial results.

## References

1.  Anthonisen NR, Connet JE, Murray RP. Smoking and lung function of lung health study participants after 11 years. Am J Respir Crit Care Med 2002; 166:675–679.
2.  Mahler DA, Barbee RA, Gross NJ, et al. Efficacy of salmeterol xinafoate in the treatment of COPD. Chest 1999; 115:957–965.

3. Pauwels R, Calverley P, Buist AS, et al. COPD exacerbations: the importance of a standard definition. Respir Med 2004; 98(2):99–107 (review).

4. Slymen D, Ayala G, Arredondo EM, et al. Analytic perspective: a demonstration of modeling count data with an application to physical activity. Epidemiol Perspect Innnov 2006; 3(3):1–9.

5. Calverley P, Pauwels R, Vestbo J, et al. Combined salmeterol and fluticasone in the treatment of chronic obstructive pulmonary disease: a randomised controlled trial. Lancet 2003; 361:449–456.

6. Aaron SD, Vandemheen K, Fergusson D, et al. Tiotropium in combination with placebo, salmeterol, or fluticasone/salmeterol for treatment of chronic obstructive pulmonary disease: a randomized trial. Ann Intern Med 2007; 146:545–555. (epub 2007, Feb 19).

7. Suisa S. Statistical treatment of exacerbations in therapeutic trials of chronic obstructive pulmonary disease. Am J Respir Crit Care Med 2006; 173:842–846.

8. Aaron SD, Fergusson D, Marks GB, et al. Counting, analyzing and reporting exacerbations of COPD in randomized, controlled trials. Thorax 2008; 63:122–128.

9. Keene ON, Jones MRK, Lane PW, et al. Analysis of exacerbation rates in asthma and chronic obstructive pulmonary disease: example from the TRISTAN study. Pharm Stat 2007; 6:89–97.

10. Spencer S, Jones PW. Globe Study Group. Time course of recovery of health status following an infective exacerbation of chronic bronchitis. Thorax 2003; 58(7):589–593.

11. Seemungal TAR, Donaldson GC, Bhowmik A, et al. Time course and recovery of exacerbations in patients with chronic obstructive pulmonary disease. Am J Respir Crit Care Med 2000; 161: 1608–1613.

12. Moher D, Schulz KF, Altman DG. The CONSORT statement: revised recommendations for improving the quality of reports of parallel-group randomized trials. Ann Intern Med 2001; 134(8): 657–662.

13. Kesten S, Plautz M, Piquette CA, et al. Premature discontinuation of patients: a potential bias in COPD clinical trials. Eur Respir J 2007; 30(5):898–906.

14. Niewoehner DE, Rice KL, Cote CG, et al. Prevention of exacerbations of chronic obstructive pulmonary disease with tiotropium, a once-daily inhaled anticholinergic bronchodilator. A randomized trial. Ann Intern Med 2005; 143:317–326.

15. Laupacis A, Sackett DL, Roberts RS. An assessment of clinically useful measures of the consequences of treatment. N Engl J Med 1988; 318:1728–1733.

16. Altman DG. Confidence intervals for the number needed to treat. Br Med J 1998; 317:1309–1312.

17. Cook RJ, Sackett DL. The number needed to treat: a clinically useful measure of treatment effect. Br Med J 1995; 310:452–454.

18. Halpin DMG. Evaluating the effectiveness of combination therapy to prevent COPD exacerbations: the value of NNT analysis. Int J Clin Pract 2005; 59(10):1187–1194.

19. Cazzola M. Application of Number Needed to Treat (NNT) as a measure of treatment effect in respiratory medicine. Treat Respir Med 2006; 5(2):79–84.

20. Calverley PM, Anderson JA, Celli B, et al. Salmeterol and fluticasone propionate and survival in chronic obstructive pulmonary disease. NEJM 2007; 356(8):775–789.

21. Kardos P, Wencker M, Glaab T, et al. Impact of salmeterol/fluticasone propionate versus salmeterol on exacerbations in severe chronic obstructive pulmonary disease. Am J Respir Crit Care Med 2007; 175:144–149.

# 37
## Future Developments in Acute Exacerbations of COPD

**PETER J. BARNES**

National Heart and Lung Institute, Imperial College, London, U.K.

## I. Introduction

Current therapies are poorly effective in both preventing and treating acute exacerbations of COPD (AECOPD) (1). This indicates the need to find more effective drug therapies, and this will depend on a better understanding of the cellular and molecular mechanisms involved in acute exacerbations and improved diagnosis of the causal mechanisms involved. An exacerbation may be an amplification of existing pathology and may include additional pathological mechanisms that are added to existing pathology.

In this chapter, some of the research approaches that may be useful in better understanding exacerbations and some of the novel therapies that may be introduced in the future are discussed.

## II. Inflammatory Mechanisms

### A. Inflammatory Cells and Mediators

In chronic stable COPD, there is chronic inflammation in the airways and lung parenchyma, which involves multiple cells and inflammatory mediators, including cytokines and chemokines (2,3). There appears to be an amplification of this underlying inflammatory process during an exacerbation, with increased numbers of neutrophils, T cells, and macrophages. Indeed, the increase in neutrophils, with release of green myeloperoxidase, accounts for the purulence (yellow color) of sputum during an exacerbation. This reflects an increase in several neutrophil chemotactic factors during an exacerbation. In acute exacerbations there are increases in the concentrations of all of the mediators detected in stable disease in sputum and bronchoalveolar lavage (BAL), including CXCL8 (interleukin-8), tumor necrosis factor alpha (TNF-$\alpha$), interleukin (IL)-6, and granulocyte-macrophage colony–simulating factor (GM-CSF) (4–8). There is also an increase in the concentrations of LTB$_4$ during an exacerbation (9,10). This suggests that an acute exacerbation of COPD represents a further amplification of the inflammatory response to inhaled irritants (usually cigarette smoke) (Fig. 1).

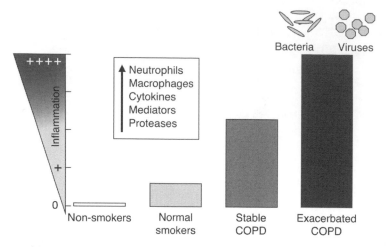

**Figure 1** Further amplification of the inflammatory response during exacerbations of COPD.

During AECOPD, the pattern of inflammation may also change. An increase in eosinophils has been reported in bronchial biopsies and BAL fluid (8,11). Increased eosinophils have also been found in sputum during exacerbations secondary to viral rather than bacterial infections (12). This may reflect increased expression of the eosinophil chemotactic factor CCL5 [RANTES (regulated upon activation, normal T cell expressed and secreted)] (13). However, whether the pattern of inflammation can discriminate between different causal mechanisms is not yet certain.

## B.  Transcription Factors

Transcription factors play a critical role in the activation of inflammatory genes that orchestrate the chronic inflammatory process. Many of the inflammatory cytokines involved in COPD are regulated by the transcription factor nuclear factor-kappa B (NF-κB) and there is evidence that it is activated to a greater extent in macrophages and airway epithelial cells during acute exacerbations (14). NF-κB may be activated by bacterial and viral infections and by oxidative stress, thus providing a molecular basis for exacerbations (Fig. 2) (15–17). Mitogen-activated protein (MAP) kinase pathways, particularly p38 MAP kinase, are also activated by these agents, providing further molecular targets for new therapies (15).

## C.  Oxidative Stress

Oxidative stress is increased in stable COPD but increased to a greater extent during acute exacerbations, as measured by increased concentrations of hydrogen peroxide ($H_2O_2$) (18) and 8-isoprostane (8-epi prostaglandin $F_{2\alpha}$) in exhaled breath condensate (10). The increase in oxidative stress during an exacerbation may play an important role in its pathophysiology since $H_2O_2$ is able to activate NF-κB and thus further increase the expression of inflammatory

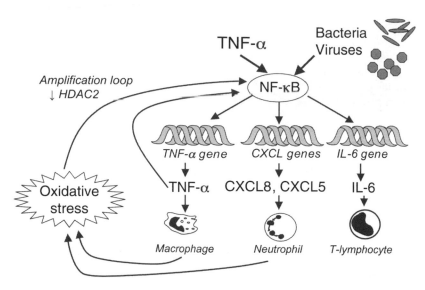

**Figure 2** Critical role of NF-κB in the inflammatory response in acute exacerbations of COPD. NF-κB is activated by bacteria and viruses and switches on several inflammatory genes, including TNF-α, CXC chemokines and IL-6. Oxidative stress produced from recruited inflammatory cells amplifies the inflammatory response by reducing HDAC2. *Abbreviations*: NF-κB, nuclear factor-kappa B; TNF-α, tumor necrosis factor-alpha; IL, interleukin; HDAC2, histone deactylase-2.

mediators, such as TNF-α and CXCL8 (Fig. 2). Oxidative stress reduces the activity and expression of histone deacetylase (HDAC)-2, a critical nuclear enzyme involved in switching off activated inflammatory genes and in this way leads to amplification of the inflammatory response as well as resistance to the anti-inflammatory effects of cortico-steroids (19). HDAC2 activity and expression are markedly reduced in peripheral lungs and macrophages of patients with severe COPD (20). Bacterial infections also decrease HDAC2 activity in airway epithelial cells (16).

## D. Causal Mechanisms

Although both upper respiratory tract viruses and bacteria may induce exacerbations, it is often difficult to distinguish these causal agents on clinical grounds, so treatment with antibiotics is often inappropriate. Future research may identify noninvasive markers that might differentiate between bacterial and viral infections, so antibiotics may be used more selectively. Noninvasive markers may include the profile of inflammatory mediators in exhaled breath, or protein products of specific bacteria detected by proteomic analysis of sputum samples. The pathogen may influence the nature of the inflammatory response. For example, acute exacerbations associated with *Haemophilus influenzae* were associated with higher concentrations of IL-8, TNF-α, and neutrophil elastase in sputum compared with infection with *H. parainfluenzae* (21).

## III.  Novel Therapeutic Approaches

A better understanding of the cellular and molecular mechanism involved in COPD may identify novel therapeutic targets (Fig. 3). Although several new drugs are currently in development for the treatment of stable COPD and the prevention of AECOPD (22), little attention has been paid to the more effective treatment of exacerbations.

### A.  New Bronchodilators

Bronchodilators are the current mainstay of management of exacerbations. It has proved very difficult to find more effective drugs than $\beta_2$-agonists. There may be advantages to using the rapid-onset long-acting $\beta_2$-agonist (LABA) formoterol as a treatment for acute exacerbations compared with short-acting $\beta_2$-agonists, such as albuterol, as has already been shown for asthma (23). The active [R,R]-enantiomer of formoterol (arformoterol) is now available for treatment of COPD but has not yet been studied in treating acute exacerbations (24). Longer-acting $\beta_2$-agonists (ultra-LABAs), with a duration of over 24 hours, such as indacaterol which are now under development for the treatment of COPD have not yet been tested in acute exacerbations (25). In patients with asthma, the combination of a corticosteroid and rapid-acting $\beta_2$-agonost is much more effective than conventional $\beta_2$-agonist therapy alone in preventing exacerbations (26,27). Whether this strategy would be effective in COPD is not yet known, however. The long-acting muscarinic antagonist tiotropium is an effective bronchodilator for stable COPD and reduces exacerbations, but is not suited as a reliever for acute exacerbations because of its slow onset of action. Aclidinium bromide is a new anticholinergic with a long duration of action like tiotropium, but with a more rapid onset of action, so may be suited for relief of acute symptoms (28).

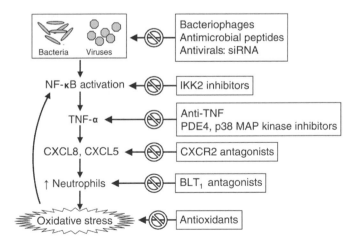

**Figure 3**  There are several targets for the development of novel treatments of acute exacerbations of COPD based on the cellular and molecular pathways involved. *Abbreviations*: IKK2, inhibitor of NF-κB kinase-2; TNF, tumor necrosis factor; PDE, phosphodiesterase; MAP, mitogen-activated protein; BLT, leukotriene $B_4$ receptor.

Novel classes of bronchodilator have been difficult to develop as they often have greater effects on vascular smooth muscle and so produce postural hypotension and headaches. Inhibition of smooth muscle myosin by inhibitors of the signal transduction pathways involved, such as Rho-kinase, myosin light chain kinase or smooth muscle myosin inhibitors, are currently being investigated for inhaled delivery (29).

## B.  New Anti-infective Therapies

Antibiotic resistance is a major and increasing barrier to the effective treatment of bacterial infections, so there is a need for more effective antibacterial agents, particularly those that are not likely to induce resistance. It has become increasingly difficult to develop new antibiotics, so that there is a need for novel types of therapy.

### Bacteriophages

Bacteriophages are bacterial viruses that are approximately 10 times more numerous than bacteria in nature. Although they have been used in Russia for many decades as antibacterial agents, they have been largely ignored in Western medicine (30). Lytic phages are highly specific to particular bacteria and are well tolerated, with no risk of overgrowth of intestinal flora. They can be administered by inhalation, so may be effective in the treatment of respiratory bacterial infections. It is possible to give cocktails of phages to cover several likely organisms. It is also possible to genetically engineer phages to increase their efficacy. More research is now needed to explore the potential of bacteriophages in the treatment of respiratory infections.

### Antimicrobial Peptides

Antimicrobial peptides, including $\alpha$- and $\beta$-defensins and cathelicidins, are produced from epithelial and other cells in the respiratory tract and play a key role in innate immunity and stimulating adaptive immune responses (31). These peptides may also be considered as therapies since they are small peptides and there is a low probability of resistance. They are effective against bacteria and viruses through various molecular mechanisms. Several antimicrobial peptides, including those derived from amphibians, are now in clinical trials for infection, but none have been studied in COPD so far. The role of antimicrobial peptides in COPD is uncertain, however (32). It is possible that they could have a detrimental effect through increased recruitment of inflammatory and immune cells into the airways.

### Antiviral siRNA

There have been few developments in antiviral therapies, particularly against rhinovirus, which is the commonest single cause of COPD exacerbations. Interference RNA is an endogenous defense mechanism against viral infection and small interfering virus RNA (siRNA) sequences may therefore block viral infections, but the problem is efficient delivery to cells infected by virus. siRNA directed against respiratory syncytial virus is now in phase I clinical trials and a similar strategy may be directed to other respiratory viruses (33,34). siRNA appears to be successful in knocking down specific proteins in airway epithelial cells of intrapulmonary airways when delivered to the nasal mucosa of mice (35).

### TLR Antagonists

Another approach is to block Toll-like receptors (TLRs) that recognize and are activated by infectious agents, including bacteria and viruses. It is very likely that TLRs are activated during exacerbations of COPD, with activation of several signal transduction pathways, including NF-κB and MAP kinase pathways, as well as type I interferon pathways in the case of viruses (36). The predominant targets are TLR2 for gram-positive bacteria, TLR4 for gram-negative bacteria, and TLR3 for viruses. It has proved to be extremely difficult to discover specific TLR antagonists, although the role if specific TLRs is currently under investigation using a siRNA approach. A specific antagonist of TLR4, *Bartonella quintalis* lipopolysaccharide, has been shown to inhibit inflammation in rheumatoid arthritis (37).

### Nonantibiotic Macrolides

Fourteen- and fifteen-membered ring macrolide antibiotics have several anti-inflammatory effects in addition to their antibacterial actions, although the molecular mechanisms for these effects are not yet clear (38). For example, macrolides inhibit neutrophil chemotaxis, mucus hypersecretion, and the release of proinflammatory cytokines such as CXCL8, TNF-$\alpha$, and IL-6, all of which are increased in COPD exacerbations. However, resistance to the antibiotic effect of macrolides develops rapidly. This has led to the identification of nonantibiotic macrolides, such as EM704 derived from the structure of erythromycin, that retains anti-inflammatory effects. This derivative has been shown to inhibit neutrophilic inflammation, the release of TGF-$\beta$ and fibrosis in a bleomycin model of pulmonary fibrosis (39). Such non-antibiotic macrolides may be delivered by inhalation during an exacerbation. Further research in this area is warranted as several nonantibiotic macrolides have now been synthesized.

## C. Mediator Antagonists

Because many inflammatory mediators are involved in exacerbations, it is unlikely that blocking a single mediator will have a major clinical impact (3).

### BLT Antagonists

LTB$_4$ activates BLT$_1$-receptors, which are expressed on neutrophils and T lymphocytes, and as LTB$_4$ is elevated during exacerbations, specific BLT antagonists may be beneficial in the treatment of exacerbations (7). Although BLT$_1$-antagonists have a relatively small effect on neutrophil chemotaxis in response to COPD sputum (40) and have not proved to be effective in treating stable COPD, it is possible that they would have greater efficacy if used acutely in exacerbations.

### Anti-TNF

Although blocking TNF-$\alpha$ was not effective in COPD patients (41), it is possible that administration during an acute exacerbation might be effective in view of the increased TNF-$\alpha$ concentrations during exacerbations.

### Anti-CXC Chemokines

The concentrations of CXC chemokines, including CXCL5 and CXCL8, are increased during exacerbations and, since they all signal through a common CXCR2, specific antagonists of this receptor may be useful in treating exacerbations. A small molecule CXCR1/2 antagonist (AZD8309) shows promise in inhibiting sputum neutrophils after inhaled endotoxin by approximately 80% (42), suggesting that this could be useful in exacerbations and has the advantage of oral administration.

### Anti-IL-6

IL-6 concentrations are increased in sputum during exacerbations and the increase in pulmonary IL-6 may also account for the increase in systemic CRP concentrations. A humanized antibody against the IL-6 receptors (tocilizumab) is effective in several other inflammatory diseases (43), but there are no studies in COPD.

### D. Antioxidants

Increased oxidative stress may play a critical role in COPD exacerbations in amplifying the inflammatory response and may also inhibit the anti-inflammatory effects of corticosteroids even in high doses. This suggests that antioxidants may be a useful therapeutic approach, but it has been difficult to develop more effective antioxidants. *N*-acetylcysteine has antioxidant properties and, although systematic reviews and meta-analyses have suggested that it may prevent AECOPD, this was not confirmed in a three-year controlled study (44). However, *N*-acetylcysteine and other thiol-based antioxidants are inactivated by oxidative stress and so have limited utility when oxidative stress is markedly increased. More effective antioxidants, including more stable glutathione compounds, superoxide dismutase analogs, and radical scavengers are in development (45). Spin-trap antioxidants, such as α-phenyl-*N*-tert-butyl nitrone, are more potent and inhibit the formation of intracellular reactive oxygen species by forming stable compounds but have toxicity that may preclude clinical development.

### E. Novel Anti-inflammatory Therapies

Since corticosteroids are only poorly effective in treating stable COPD and exacerbations, there has been a search for alternative anti-inflammatory treatments. These may be effective in treating the increased inflammation that occurs during an exacerbation and may be effective via inhaled delivery. However, a concern that applies to all anti-inflammatory approaches is whether this may potentially increase the extent of infection by blunting host defense mechanisms.

### Phosphodiesterase-4 Inhibitors

PDE4 inhibitors have a broad spectrum of anti-inflammatory effects and are effective in animal models of COPD, but in human studies, their effectiveness has been limited by side effects, such as nausea, diarrhea, and headaches (46). PDE4 inhibitors are effective in inhibiting neutrophil recruitment and activation (47). Their use as an acute anti-inflammatory therapy has not yet been investigated, but side effects of current drugs when given systemically make it unlikely that they will be useful in the acute situation. In the future inhaled PDE4 inquisitors may be developed as a way of reducing side effects. A PDE4 inhibitor markedly increased the lethality of *Klebsiella pneumoniae* pulmonary infection, as a result of TNF-α inhibition and reduced neutrophil phagocytosis (48), so these drugs may need to be used cautiously in the treatment of bacterial exacerbations.

### NF-κB Inhibitors

As discussed above, NF-κB appears to play a key role in regulating the expression of many inflammatory genes that are upregulated in AECOPD and is activated during exacerbations (49). It is likely that bacteria, viruses, and oxidatives activate NF-κB, so that it is a logical target for inhibition. Selective inhibitors of I kappa B kinase-2 (IKK2) have now been developed and may be predicted to have anti-inflammatory effects n COPD inflammation (50,51). IKK2 inhibitors have not yet been tested clinically, but there are concerns about their long-term safety in view of impaired innate immunity. However, they could be useful in acute treatment of exacerbations, especially if given by inhaled delivery.

### p38 MAP Kinase Inhibitors

p38 MAP kinase is also activated by bacteria and viruses and hence is another target for inhibition. Indeed, the activation of NF-κB by bacteria is completely inhibited by selective p38 inhibitors (15). A selective p38 inhibitor is effective in inhibiting TNF-α release from pulmonary macrophages (52). Several p38 MAP kinase inhibitors are now in clinical development, but the problem is likely to be toxicity so that inhaled administration may be necessary (50,51). Like IKK2 inhibitors, these drugs could be effective in AECOPD as an acute inhaled treatment.

### Theophylline

High doses of theophylline were previously given as a bronchodilator, but there is no evidence that this has any clinical benefit when added to standard treatment with nebulized albuterol in AECOPD (53). In lower doses, theophylline has been shown to reverse corticosteroid resistance in COPD cells by restoring HDAC2 activity to normal (54). Theophylline may therefore reverse corticosteroid resistance in COPD, thus making acute treatment with corticosteroids more effective in the treatment of acute exacerbations. The mechanism of action of theophylline to increase HDAC activity is still not understood but appears to be related to an inhibitory effect of theophylline on the δ-isoform of phosphoinositide-3-kinase

## IV.  Conclusions and Future Directions

Although acute exacerbations have a major impact on patients with COPD and account for a large proportion of associated health care costs, still there is relatively little research into underlying mechanisms, as it is difficult to study patients who are acutely ill and exacerbations are unpredictable.

It is likely that there will be developments in noninvasive biomarkers to detect causative agents and to monitor the inflammatory response (55). It is possible that exhaled hydrocarbon patterns may reflect infection with different organisms, and there are important advances in metabolomics to detect multiple metabolites in the breath using NMR spectroscopy (56). This may lead to more selective use of therapy such as antibiotics, and in the future, antiviral agents. A detailed proteomic analysis of plasma was unable to identify any increase of any individual protein that was specific for an exacerbation, apart from CRP in conjunction with an increase in symptoms (57), so it is likely that measurements need to be made in lung samples.

There is a pressing need for more effective therapies for AECOPD. Several new treatments are now in development for stable COPD, but few are under consideration as acute treatment for an exacerbation. There are no useful animal models of acute exacerbations, but this should be possible with viral or bacterial infection in chronic cigarette smoke exposure models. Most emphasis has been placed on prevention of exacerbations, which is a worthy aim as this may reduce disease progression, mortality, and costs. However, current therapies for acute exacerbation are not very effective and most exacerbations follow a protracted course with an adverse effect on the quality of life over several weeks. An effective anti-inflammatory therapy is likely to reduce symptoms to a greater extent, perhaps avoiding hospital admission and to shorten their duration. It is also possible that more effective suppression of the inflammation in an exacerbation will reduce disease progression. Understanding the inflammatory components of COPD is likely to lead to the development of more effective anti-inflammatory approaches. More effective treatments against causal mechanism, particularly viruses such as rhinovirus, are also needed.

Against the potential benefits of treating exacerbations with anti-inflammatory treatment, consideration needs to be given to any detrimental effect on the causative infection. Suppression of neutrophils and macrophages might increase the spread or multiplication of bacteria and viruses since these cells play an important role in the phagocytosis and clearing of these organisms. Any new therapy for COPD exacerbations will therefore need to be evaluated very carefully.

## References

1. Celli BR, Barnes PJ. Exacerbations of chronic obstructive pulmonary disease. Eur Respir J 2007; 29:1224–1238.
2. Barnes PJ, Shapiro SD, Pauwels RA. Chronic obstructive pulmonary disease: molecular and cellular mechanisms. Eur Respir J 2003; 22:672–688.
3. Barnes PJ. Mediators of chronic obstructive pulmonary disease. Pharm Rev 2004; 56:515–548.
4. Bhowmik A, Seemungal TA, Sapsford RJ, et al. Relation of sputum inflammatory markers to symptoms and lung function changes in COPD exacerbations. Thorax 2000; 55(2):114–120.
5. Aaron SD, Angel JB, Lunau M, et al. Granulocyte inflammatory markers and airway infection during acute exacerbation of chronic obstructive pulmonary disease. Am J Respir Crit Care Med 2001; 163:349–355.
6. Hill AT, Bayley D, Stockley RA. The interrelationship of sputum inflammatory markers in patients with chronic bronchitis. Am J Respir Crit Care Med 1999; 160:893–898.
7. Crooks SW, Bayley DL, Hill SL, et al. Bronchial inflammation in acute bacterial exacerbations of chronic bronchitis: the role of leukotriene B4. Eur Respir J 2000; 15:274–280.
8. Balbi B, Bason C, Balleari E, et al. Increased bronchoalveolar granulocytes and granulocyte/macrophage colony-stimulating factor during exacerbations of chronic bronchitis. Eur Respir J 1997; 10:846–850.
9. Gompertz S, O'Brien C, Bayley DL, et al. Changes in bronchial inflammation during acute exacerbations of chronic bronchitis. Eur Respir J 2001; 17:1112–1119.
10. Biernacki WA, Kharitonov SA, Barnes PJ. Increased leukotriene B4 and 8-isoprostane in exhaled breath condensate of patients with exacerbations of COPD. Thorax 2003; 58:294–298.

11. Saetta M, Di Stefano A, Maestrelli P, et al. Airway eosinophilia and expression of interleukin-5 protein in asthma and in exacerbations of chronic bronchitis. Clin Exp Allergy 1996; 26:766–774.
12. Papi A, Bellettato CM, Braccioni F, et al. Infections and airway inflammation in chronic obstructive pulmonary disease severe exacerbations. Am J Respir Crit Care Med 2006; 173:1114–1121.
13. Zhu J, Qiu YS, Majumdar S, et al. Exacerbations of bronchitis: bronchial eosinophilia and gene expression for interleukin-4, interleukin-5, and eosinophil chemoattractants. Am J Respir Crit Care Med 2001; 164:109–116.
14. Caramori G, Romagnoli M, Casolari P, et al. Nuclear localisation of p65 in sputum macrophages but not in sputum neutrophils during COPD exacerbations. Thorax 2003; 58:348–351.
15. Watanabe T, Jono H, Han J, et al. Synergistic activation of NF-κB by nontypeable Haemophilus influenzae and tumor necrosis factor a. Proc Natl Acad Sci U S A 2004; 101:3563–3568.
16. Slevogt H, Schmeck B, Jonatat C, et al. Moraxella catarrhalis induces inflammatory response of bronchial epithelial cells via MAPK and NF-kappaB activation and histone deacetylase activity reduction. Am J Physiol Lung Cell Mol Physiol 2006; 290:L818–L826.
17. Edwards MR, Hewson CA, Laza-Stanca V, et al. Protein kinase R, IκB kinase-β and NF-κB are required for human rhinovirus induced pro-inflammatory cytokine production in bronchial epithelial cells. Mol Immunol 2007; 44:1587–1597.
18. Dekhuijzen PNR, Aben KHH, Dekker I, et al. Increased exhalation of hydrogen peroxide in patients with stable and unstable chronic obstructive pulmonary disease. Am J Respir Crit Care Med 1996; 154:813–816.
19. Barnes PJ. Reduced histone deacetylase in COPD: clinical implications. Chest 2006; 129:151–155.
20. Ito K, Ito M, Elliott WM, et al. Decreased histone deacetylase activity in chronic obstructive pulmonary disease. New Engl J Med 2005; 352:1967–1976.
21. Sethi S, Muscarella K, Evans N, et al. Airway inflammation and etiology of acute exacerbations of chronic bronchitis. Chest 2000; 118:1557–1565.
22. Barnes PJ, Hansel TT. Prospects for new drugs for chronic obstructive pulmonary disease. Lancet 2004; 364:985–996.
23. Pauwels RA, Sears MR, Campbell M, et al. Formoterol as relief medication in asthma: a worldwide safety and effectiveness trial. Eur Respir J 2003; 22:787–794.
24. Baumgartner RA, Hanania NA, Calhoun WJ, et al. Nebulized arformoterol in patients with COPD: a 12-week, multicenter, randomized, double-blind, double-dummy, placebo- and active-controlled trial. Clin Ther 2007; 29:261–278.
25. Matera MG, Cazzola M. Ultra-long-acting beta2-adrenoceptor agonists: an emerging therapeutic option for asthma and COPD? Drugs 2007; 67:503–515.
26. Barnes PJ. Scientific rationale for using a single inhaler for asthma control. Eur Resp Dis 2007; 29:587–595.
27. Papi A, Canonica GW, Maestrelli P, et al. Rescue use of beclomethasone and albuterol in a single inhaler for mild asthma. N Engl J Med 2007; 356:2040–2052.
28. Joos GF, Schelfhout VJ, Kanniess F. Bronchodilator effects of aclidinium bromide, a novel long-acting anticholinergic, in COPD patients: a phase II study. Eur Resp J 2007; 30 (suppl 51):1299.
29. Gosens R, Schaafsma D, Meurs H, et al. Role of Rho-kinase in maintaining airway smooth muscle contractile phenotype. Eur J Pharmacol 2004; 483:71–78.
30. Hanlon GW. Bacteriophages: an appraisal of their role in the treatment of bacterial infections. Int J Antimicrob Agents 2007; 30:118–128.
31. Jenssen H, Hamill P, Hancock RE. Peptide antimicrobial agents. Clin Microbiol Rev 2006; 19:491–511.
32. Bals R, Hiemstra PS. Antimicrobial peptides in COPD: basic biology and therapeutic applications. Curr Drug Targets 2006; 7:743–750.
33. Barik S, Bitko V. Prospects of RNA interference therapy in respiratory viral diseases: update 2006. Expert Opin Biol Ther 2006; 6:1151–1160.

34. de Fougerolles A, Vornlocher HP, Maraganore J, et al. Interfering with disease: a progress report on siRNA-based therapeutics. Nat Rev Drug Discov 2007; 6:443–453.
35. Moschos SA, Jones SW, Perry MM, et al. Lung delivery studies using siRNA conjugated to TAT (48–60) and penetratin reveal peptide induced reduction in gene expression and induction of innate immunity. Bioconj Chem 2007; 18:1450–1459.
36. Chaudhuri N, Whyte MK, Sabroe I. Reducing the toll of inflammatory lung disease. Chest 2007; 131:1550–1556.
37. Abdollahi-Roodsaz S, Joosten LA, Roelofs MF, et al. Inhibition of Toll-like receptor 4 breaks the inflammatory loop in autoimmune destructive arthritis. Arthritis Rheum 2007; 56:2957–2967.
38. Tamaoki J, Kadota J, Takizawa H. Clinical implications of the immunomodulatory effects of macrolides. Am J Med 2004; 117(suppl 9A):5S–11S.
39. Li YJ, Azuma A, Usuki J, et al. EM703 improves bleomycin-induced pulmonary fibrosis in mice by the inhibition of TGF-β signaling in lung fibroblasts. Respir Res 2006; 7:16.
40. Beeh KM, Kornmann O, Buhl R, et al. Neutrophil chemotactic activity of sputum from patients with COPD: role of interleukin 8 and leukotriene B4. Chest 2003; 123:1240–1247.
41. Rennard SI, Fogarty C, Kelsen S, et al. The safety and efficacy of infliximab in moderate-to-severe chronic obstructive pulmonary disease. Am J Respir Crit Care Med 2007; 175:926–934.
42. O'Connor BJ, Leaker BR, Barnes PJ, et al. Inhibition of LPS-induced neutrophilic inflammation in healthy volunteers. Eur Resp J 2007; 30 (suppl 51):1294.
43. Paul-Pletzer K. Tocilizumab: blockade of interleukin-6 signaling pathway as a therapeutic strategy for inflammatory disorders. Drugs Today (Barc) 2006; 42:559–576.
44. Decramer M, Rutten-van Molken M, et al. Effects of N-acetylcysteine on outcomes in chronic obstructive pulmonary disease (Bronchitis Randomized on NAC Cost-Utility Study, BRON-CUS): a randomised placebo-controlled trial. Lancet 2005; 365:1552–1560.
45. Cuzzocrea S, Riley DP, Caputi AP, et al. Antioxidant therapy: a new pharmacological approach in shock, inflammation, and ischemia/reperfusion injury. Pharmacol Rev 2001; 53:135–159.
46. Fan CK. Phosphodiesterase inhibitors in airways disease. Eur J Pharmacol 2006; 533:110–117.
47. Hatzelmann A, Schudt C. Anti-inflammatory and immunomodulatory potential of the novel PDE4 inhibitor roflumilast in vitro. J Pharmacol Exp Ther 2001; 297:267–279.
48. Soares AC, Souza DG, Pinho V, et al. Impaired host defense to Klebsiella pneumoniae infection in mice treated with the PDE4 inhibitor rolipram. Br J Pharmacol 2003; 140:855–862.
49. Caramori G, Romagnoli M, Casolari P, et al. Nuclear localisation of p65 in sputum macrophages but not in sputum neutrophils during COPD exacerbations. Thorax 2003; 58:348–351.
50. Barnes PJ. Novel signal transduction modulators for the treatment of airway diseases. Pharmacol Ther 2006; 109:238–245.
51. Adcock IM, Chung KF, Caramori G, et al. Kinase inhibitors and airway inflammation. Eur J Pharmacol 2006; 533:118–132.
52. Smith SJ, Fenwick PS, Nicholson AG, et al. Inhibitory effect of p38 mitogen-activated protein kinase inhibitors on cytokine release from human macrophages. Br J Pharmacol 2006; 149:393–404.
53. Duffy N, Walker P, Diamantea F, et al. Intravenous aminophylline in patients admitted to hospital with non-acidotic exacerbations of chronic obstructive pulmonary disease: a prospective randomised controlled trial. Thorax 2005; 60:713–717.
54. Barnes PJ. Theophylline for COPD. Thorax 2006; 61:742–743.
55. Kharitonov SA, Barnes PJ. Exhaled biomarkers. Chest 2006; 130:1541–1546.
56. Carraro S, Rezzi S, Reniero F, et al. Metabolomics applied to exhaled breath condensate in childhood asthma. Am J Respir Crit Care Med 2007; 175:986–990.
57. Hurst JR, Donaldson GC, Perea WR, et al. Utility of plasma biomarkers at exacerbation of chronic obstructive pulmonary disease. Am J Respir.Crit Care Med 2006; 174:867–874.

# Index

Printed and bound by CPI Group (UK) Ltd, Croydon, CR0 4YY

21/10/2024

01777089-0002